Fundamentals
of URINE &
BODY FLUID
Analysis

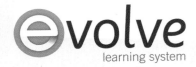
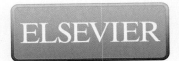
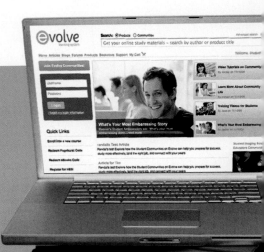

Third Edition

Fundamentals

of # URINE & BODY FLUID *Analysis*

Nancy A. Brunzel, MS, MLS(ASCP)CM

Assistant Professor
University of Minnesota
Minneapolis, Minnesota

ELSEVIER
SAUNDERS

3251 Riverport Lane
St. Louis, Missouri 63043

FUNDAMENTALS OF URINE AND BODY FLUID ANALYSIS, THIRD EDITION

ISBN: 978-1-4377-0989-6

Library of Congress Cataloging-in-Publication Data

Brunzel, Nancy A.
 Fundamentals of urine & body fluid analysis / Nancy A. Brunzel.—3rd ed.
     p. ; cm.
 Fundamentals of urine and body fluid analysis
 Urine & body fluid analysis
 Urine and body fluid analysis
 Includes bibliographical references and index.
 ISBN 978-1-4377-0989-6 (pbk. : alk. paper)
 I. Title. II. Title: Fundamentals of urine and body fluid analysis. III. Title: Urine & body fluid analysis. IV. Title: Urine and body fluid analysis.
 [DNLM: 1. Urinalysis. 2. Body Fluids—chemistry. QY 185]
 616.07′566—dc23

2012005517

Content Manager: Ellen Wurm-Cutter
Developmental Editor: Beth LoGuidice, Spring Hollow Press, LLC
Publishing Services Manager: Catherine Jackson
Senior Project Manager: Karen M. Rehwinkel
Design Direction: Ashley Eberts

Printed in the United States of America

Last digit is the print number: 9 8 7 6 5 4 3 2

SDG—for your inspiration, guidance, and never-ending support.

CONTRIBUTORS AND REVIEWERS

CONTRIBUTOR

Charlotte Janita, MT(ASCP)
Clinical Pathology Operations Manager
Regions Hospital
St. Paul, Minnesota

REVIEWERS

Donna Marie Duberg, MA, MS, MT(ASCP)SM, CLS(NCA)
Assistant Professor
Saint Louis University
St. Louis, Missouri

Debbie Heinritz, MS, MLS(ASCP)^{CM}
CLT Instructor
Northeast Wisconsin Technical College
Green Bay, Wisconsin

Joel D. Hubbard, MT(ASCP), PhD
Associate Professor
Texas Tech University Health Sciences Center
Lubbock, Texas

Michele B. Zitzmann, MHS, MT(ASCP)
Associate Professor
LSUHSC Department of Clinical Laboratory Sciences
New Orleans, Louisiana

This book is designed as a teaching and reference text for the analysis of urine and body fluids. The intended audience is students in clinical/medical laboratory science programs and practicing laboratory professionals. However, other health care professionals—physicians, physician assistants, nurse practitioners, and nurses—can also benefit from the information provided.

As with previous editions, the task of achieving a balance in depth and breadth of content to meet all needs is challenging. I believe that to gain a true understanding of a subject requires more than the mere memorization of facts. Therefore, a guiding principle in the format and writing of this book was to present comprehensive information in a manner that arouses interest, enhances learning, and facilitates understanding and mastery of the content. Although the content is comprehensive and detailed, educators can easily adapt it to the level of content desired.

ORGANIZATION

The organization is similar to previous editions, with a couple of minor changes: the *Urine Sediment Image Gallery* has been centralized for easy access and two new chapters are present. As in previous editions, the first two chapters cover general topics that are important in laboratories that perform urine and body fluid analyses, namely microscopy, quality assurance, and safety. Chapter 1 describes various types of microscopy, proper microscope handling and care, including important do's and don'ts, as well as step-by-step instructions for properly adjusting a binocular microscope for optimal viewing (i.e., Kohler illumination). Chapter 2 reviews quality assurance and safety concerns that apply to laboratories that perform urine and body fluid analyses.

Chapters 3 through 9 focus on the study of urine—preanalytical considerations, analysis, and the role urinalysis plays in the diagnosis and monitoring of disorders. Chapter 3 provides a thorough discussion of urine specimen collection, handling, and preservation; chapters 4 and 5 review the anatomy and physiology of the urinary system. Together, these chapters set the stage for an in-depth discussion of the three components of a complete urinalysis, namely the physical examination (Chapter 6), chemical examination (Chapter 7), and microscopic examination (Chapter 8). Located between Chapters 8 and 9 is a *Urine Sediment Image Gallery* containing *more than 100* urine sediment photomicrographs to be used as a teaching tool and reference for the

identification of urine sediment elements. Chapter 9 completes the study of urine with a discussion of the clinical features of renal and metabolic disorders and their associated urinalysis results.

Chapters 10 through 16 are dedicated to the study of body fluids (other than urine) frequently encountered in the clinical laboratory. Each chapter describes the physiology, normal composition, and clinical value associated with laboratory analysis of the fluid. Preanalytical factors in specimen collection and handling are discussed along with the significance of specific tests that provide clinically useful information. Note that laboratory tests routinely performed on one body fluid may not have clinical value when analyzing another body fluid.

Chapter 17 provides a snapshot of automation currently available for the analysis of urine and body fluids. Because of the robust and dynamic nature of laboratory instrumentation, the content of this chapter will quickly outdate. However, the intent is to provide an understanding of the analytical principles used in semi- and fully automated instruments. In this regard, the basic analytical principles for chemical (reflectance photometry) and microscopic (digital microscopy, flow cytometry) analyses have stood the test of time and will endure. Future improvements in the application of these analytical techniques for the analysis of urine and body fluids will undoubtedly bring to the marketplace new analyzers and manufacturers.

For a variety of reasons, manual cell counts of body fluids using a hemacytometer persist today. Chapter 18 and Appendix C are resources for the preparation of dilutions and the performance of manual body fluid cell counts. Pretreatment solutions and a variety of diluents for body fluids are discussed, as are step-by-step instructions and calculations for performing manual cell counts. This chapter ends with a discussion of cytocentrifugation and the preparation of slides for a leukocyte differential.

Three appendices are provided to complement the chapters. As previously stated, Appendix C *Body Fluid Diluent and Pretreatment Solutions* supplements Chapter 18 by providing detailed instructions for the preparation and use of diluents and pretreatment solutions. Appendix A, *Reagent Strip Color Charts*, supplements the chemical examination of urine (see Chapter 7) by providing figures of manufacturer color charts used to manually determine reagent strip results. These figures are a useful reference and assist in highlighting differences in reagent strip brands such as physical orientation of strip to chart and variations in result reporting. Appendix B serves as a handy resource for the Reference Intervals that are provided in the various chapters.

The book ends with two additional sections, a Glossary and Answer Key. The glossary includes the key terms that are bolded in each chapter and additional important clinical and scientific terms that may be new to readers. The Answer Key provides the answers and explanations (when necessary) to the end-of-chapter study questions and cases in a convenient, readily accessible location.

NEW TO THIS EDITION

- Throughout the text, content has been updated and numerous tables have been revised or added to supplement and enhance mastery of the material.
- In Chapter 8, *Microscopic Examination of Urine Sediment,* some content was reorganized and figures added.
- The alphabetized *Urine Sediment Image Gallery* was relocated to follow Chapter 8, which will greatly assist users in quickly and easily locating additional photomicrographs for reference when performing microscopic examinations.
- *Quick Reference Tables* added to the inside front cover assist in finding figures (i.e., photomicrographs of interest).
- Returning to the third edition is a chapter discussing automation in the analysis of urine and other body fluids and the principles involved in automated systems (see Chapter 17, *Automation of Urine and Body Fluid Analysis*).
- A new Chapter 18 covers manual hemacytometer counts (previously an appendix) of body fluids and

differential slide preparation using cytocentrifugation. This chapter is complemented by a new Appendix C, *Body Fluid Diluent and Pretreatment Solutions,* which provides detailed instructions for the preparation and use of diluents and pretreatment solutions.

LEARNING AIDS

Each chapter includes the following aids to enhance mastery of the content:

- *Learning Objectives* at three cognitive levels (Recall, Application, Analysis)
- *Key Terms* that are bold in the chapter and defined at the front of the chapter and in the Glossary
- Many *Tables* that capture and summarize content
- Numerous high-quality *Figures* in full color
- *Study Questions* at three cognitive levels (Recall, Application, Analysis)
- *Case Studies,* when applicable to content

EVOLVE INSTRUCTOR RESOURCES

New for this edition, downloadable instructor content specific to this text is available on the companion Evolve site (http://evolve.elsevier.com/Brunzel). This includes the following ancillary material for teaching and learning:

- *PowerPoint presentations* for all chapters to aid in lecture development
- *Test Banks* that tie exam questions directly to book content, making exam development easier and faster
- *Image Collection* that includes all illustrations in the book in various formats, offering a closer look at hundreds of microscopic slides.

ACKNOWLEDGMENTS

I have fond memories of performing my first urinalyses in a small hospital laboratory in Kansas City, Missouri. When I reflect on the beginnings of this love for the study of urine, one individual comes to mind—Mary Abts, MT(ASCP). She was my urinalysis instructor at the bench and she made it so exciting! So, I thank her for her guidance, professionalism, and infectious enthusiasm, which ignited the spark that eventually developed into this book.

Throughout the years, numerous colleagues have also blessed me personally and professionally. A special acknowledgement to Karen Karni—my mentor—who nurtured the writer and educator within me, a process that continues to impact what I do today. I am grateful to Charlotte Janita for sharing her expertise in body fluid analysis and contributing photomicrographs. To the many laboratory scientists and students that ask questions, provide feedback, and make suggestions, I take my hat off to you.

To Ellen Wurm-Cutter, a special thank you for her steadfast and patient guidance in directing this new edition, and to Beth LoGiudice, for her encouragement and capable assistance. Finally, I express my appreciation to Karen Rehwinkel and the entire production team at Elsevier for their expertise and creativity.

Nancy A. Brunzel

CONTENTS

CONTENTS

Fundamentals
of URINE &
BODY FLUID
Analysis

Microscopy

LEARNING OBJECTIVES

After studying this chapter, the student should be able to:

1. Identify and explain the functions of the following components of a microscope:
   - Aperture diaphragm
   - Condenser
   - Eyepiece (ocular)
   - Field diaphragm
   - Mechanical stage
   - Objective
2. Describe Köhler illumination and the microscope adjustment procedure used to ensure optimal specimen imaging.
3. Describe the daily care and preventive maintenance routines for microscopes.
4. Compare and contrast the principles of the following types of microscopy:
   - Brightfield
   - Phase-contrast
   - Polarizing
   - Interference contrast
   - Darkfield
   - Fluorescence
5. List an advantage of and an application for each type of microscopy discussed.

CHAPTER OUTLINE

Brightfield Microscope
  Eyepiece
  Mechanical Stage
  Condenser
  Illumination System
  Objectives

Ocular Field Number
Microscope Adjustment Procedure
Care and Preventive Maintenance
Types of Microscopy
  Brightfield Microscopy
  Phase-Contrast Microscopy

Polarizing Microscopy
Interference Contrast Microscopy
Darkfield Microscopy
Fluorescence Microscopy

KEY TERMS

aperture diaphragm Microscope component that regulates the angle of light presented to the specimen. The diaphragm is located at the base of the condenser and changes the diameter of the opening through which source light rays must pass to enter the condenser.

birefringent (also called *doubly refractile*) The ability of a substance to refract light in two directions.

brightfield microscopy Type of microscopy that produces a magnified image that appears dark against a bright or white background.

chromatic aberration Unequal refraction of light rays by a lens that occurs because the different wavelengths of light refract or bend at different angles. As a result, the image produced has undesired color fringes.

condenser Microscope component that gathers and focuses the illumination light onto the specimen for viewing. The condenser is a lens system (a single lens or a combination of lenses) that is located beneath the microscope stage.

darkfield microscopy Type of microscopy that produces a magnified image that appears brightly illuminated against a dark background. A special condenser presents only oblique light rays to the specimen. The specimen interacts with these rays (e.g., refraction, reflection), causing visualization of the specimen. Darkfield microscopy is used on unstained specimen preparations and is the preferred technique for identification of spirochetes.

eyepiece (also called ocular) The microscope lens or system of lenses located closest to the viewer's eye. The eyepiece produces the secondary image magnification of the specimen.

field diaphragm Microscope component that controls the diameter of light beams that strike the specimen and hence reduces stray light. The diaphragm is located at the light exit of the illumination source. With Köhler illumination, the field diaphragm is used to adjust and center the condenser appropriately.

field number A number assigned to an eyepiece that indicates the diameter of the field of view, in millimeters, that is observed when using a 1× objective. This diameter is determined by a baffle or a raised ring inside the eyepiece and sometimes is engraved on the eyepiece.

field of view The circular field observed through a microscope. The diameter of the field of view varies with the eyepiece field number and the magnifications of the objective in use, plus any additional optics before the eyepiece. The field of view (FOV) is calculated using the following formula: FOV (in millimeters) = Field number/M, where M is the sum of all optics magnifications, except that of the eyepiece.

fluorescence microscopy Type of microscopy modified for visualization of fluorescent substances. Fluorescence microscopy uses two filters: one to select a specific wavelength of illumination light (excitation filter) that is absorbed by the specimen, and another (barrier filter) to transmit the different, longer-wavelength light emitted from the specimen to the eyepiece for viewing. The fluorophore (natural or added) present in the specimen determines the selection of these filters.

interference contrast microscopy Type of microscopy in which the difference in optical light paths through the specimen is converted into intensity differences in the specimen image. Three-dimensional images of high contrast and resolution are obtained, without haloing. Two types available are modulation contrast (Hoffman) and differential interference contrast (Nomarski).

Köhler illumination Type of microscopic illumination in which a lamp condenser (located above the light source) focuses the image of the light source (lamp filament) onto the front focal plane of the substage condenser (where the aperture diaphragm is located). The substage condenser sharply focuses the image of the field diaphragm (located at or slightly in front of the lamp condenser) at the same plane as the focused specimen. As a result, the filament image does not appear in the field of view, and bright, even illumination is obtained. Köhler illumination requires appropriate adjustments of the condenser and of the field and aperture diaphragms.

mechanical stage Microscope component that holds the microscope slide with the specimen for viewing. The stage is adjustable, front to back and side to side, to enable viewing of the entire specimen.

numerical aperture Number that indicates the resolving power of a lens system. The numerical aperture (NA) is derived mathematically from the refractive index (n) of the optical medium (for air, n = 1) and the angle of light (μ) made by the lens: NA = n × sin μ.

objective The lens or system of lenses located closest to the specimen. The objective produces the primary image magnification of the specimen.

parcentered Term describing objective lenses that retain the same field of view when the user switches from one objective to another of a differing magnification.

parfocal Term describing objective lenses that remain in focus when the user switches from one objective to another of a differing magnification.

phase-contrast microscopy Type of microscopy in which variations in the specimen's refractive index are converted into variations in light intensity or contrast. Areas of the specimen appear light to dark with haloes of varying intensity related to the thickness of the component. Thin, flat components produce less haloing and the best-detailed images. Phase-contrast microscopy is ideal for viewing low-refractile elements and living cells.

polarizing microscopy Type of microscopy that illuminates the specimen with polarized light. Polarizing microscopy is used to identify and classify birefringent substances (i.e., substances that refract light in two directions) that shine brilliantly against a dark background.

resolution Ability of a lens to distinguish two points or objects as separate. The resolving power (R) of a microscope depends on the wavelength of light used (λ) and the numerical aperture of the objective lens. The greater the resolving power, the smaller the distance distinguished between two separate points.

spherical aberration Unequal refraction of light rays when they pass through different portions of a lens such that the light rays are not brought to the same focus. As a result, the image produced is blurred or fuzzy and cannot be brought into sharp focus.

A high-quality brightfield microscope is required for the microscopic examination of urine and other body fluids. One must give considerable care to its selection because its use is an integral part of laboratory work, and microscopes with quality objective lenses are costly. Because some brightfield microscopes can be modified to allow several types of microscopy from a single instrument—brightfield, phase-contrast, polarization—good planning ensures selection of the most appropriate instrument. Whereas acquiring a suitable microscope is of utmost importance, appropriate training on its use and proper maintenance and cleaning of the microscope are crucial to ensure maximization of its potential. The user must be familiar with each microscope component and its function, as well as with proper microscope adjustment and alignment procedures.

BRIGHTFIELD MICROSCOPE

A brightfield microscope (Figure 1-1) produces a magnified specimen image that appears dark against a brighter background. A simple brightfield microscope consisting of only one lens is known as a *magnifying glass*. In the clinical laboratory, however, compound brightfield microscopes predominate and consist of two lens systems. The first lens system, located closest to the specimen, is the objective mounted in the nosepiece. The objective produces the primary image magnification and directs this image to the second lens system, the eyepiece, or ocular.

The eyepiece further magnifies the image received from the objective lens. Total magnification of a specimen is the product of these lens systems, that is, multiplication of the objective lens magnification by the eyepiece lens magnification. For example, a 10× objective with a 10× eyepiece produces a 100× magnification. In other words, the viewed image is 100 times larger than its actual size.

The eyepiece also determines the diameter of the field of view (FOV) observed. This diameter is established by a round baffle or ridge inside the eyepiece and is indicated by the field number assigned to the eyepiece. Field numbers that predominate in clinical laboratory microscopes typically range from 18 to 26. This number indicates the diameter of the FOV, in millimeters (mm), when a 1× objective is used. To determine the diameter of any FOV the following equation is used

Equation 1-1

$$FOV = \frac{Field\ number}{M}$$

where M is the magnification of the objective and any additional optics. (*Note:* This sum does not include the eyepiece magnification.)

For example, an eyepiece with a field number of 18 has a diameter of 18 mm when a 1× objective is used, a diameter of 1.8 mm when a 10× objective is used, and a diameter of 0.18 mm when a 100× objective is used. Some manufacturers engrave the field number on the eyepiece along with the eyepiece magnification. For those that do not, a small ruler can be placed on the stage to measure the diameter, or the manufacturer can be contacted. As the field number increases, so does the cost of the eyepiece. Before about 1990, microscopes used in the clinical laboratory had eyepieces with a field

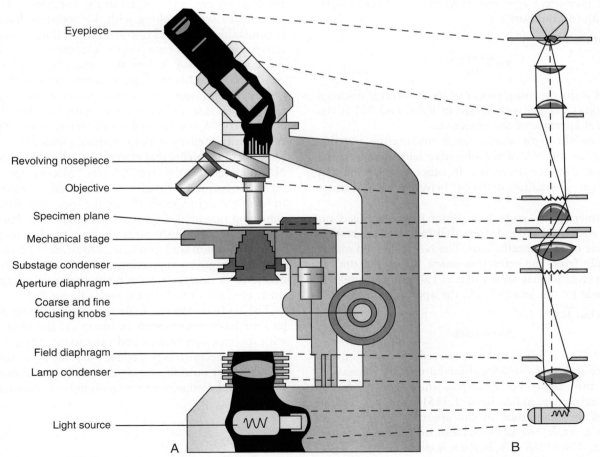

Eyepiece

Revolving nosepiece

Objective

Specimen plane

Mechanical stage

Substage condenser

Aperture diaphragm

Coarse and fine focusing knobs

Field diaphragm

Lamp condenser

Light source

A

B

FIGURE 1-1 A, A schematic representation of a brightfield microscope and its components. **B,** Path of illumination using Köhler illumination.

number of 18. Most microscopes purchased after that time have field numbers of 20 or 22.

In areas of the laboratory where results are reported as the number of elements observed per FOV (e.g., urinalysis, number per high-power or low-power field), performing a microscopic examination on the same or equivalent microscopes is crucial. If this is not done, results depend on the microscope used and can be significantly different even with evaluation of the same specimen. In other words, two microscopes with the same objective magnification and the same eyepiece magnification (e.g., 10×) but with different field numbers will have different diameters for their FOVs. Therefore standardizing microscopic examinations reported as the number of elements observed per FOV requires that microscopes with the same eyepiece field number are used.

The purpose of the microscope lens system (i.e., eyepiece and objective) is to magnify an object sufficiently for viewing with maximum resolution. Resolution, or resolving power, describes the ability of the lens system to reveal fine detail. Stated another way, resolution is the smallest distance between two points or lines at which they are distinguished as two separate entities. Resolving power (R) depends on the wavelength (λ) of light used and the numerical aperture (NA) of the objective lens, according to Equation 1-2.

Equation 1-2

$$R = \frac{0.612 \times \lambda}{NA}$$

where R is the resolving power or the resolvable distance in microns, λ is the wavelength of light, and NA is the numerical aperture of the objective.

Because the light source on a microscope remains constant, as the NA of the objective lens increases, the resolution distance decreases. In other words, one can distinguish a smaller distance between two distinct points.

A numerical aperture is a designation engraved on objective lenses and condensers that indicates the resolving power of each specific lens. The NA is derived mathematically from the refractive index (n) of the optical medium (e.g., air has an n value of 1.0) and the angle of light made by the lens (μ) (i.e., the aperture angle).

Equation 1-3

$$NA = n \times \sin\mu$$

The NA of a lens can be increased by changing the refractive index of the optical medium or by increasing the aperture angle. For example, immersion oil has a greater refractive index (n = 1.515) than air, and it increases the magnitude of the aperture angle (Figure 1-2). As a result, use of immersion oil effects a greater NA (e.g., 100×, NA = 1.2) than is possible with high-power dry lenses. An increase in NA equates with greater magnification and resolution.

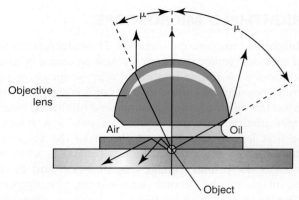

FIGURE 1-2 Drawing depicting changes in numerical aperture. Note the increase in light angle (μ) attained and therefore in the numerical aperture when immersion oil is used.

As previously discussed, the ability of a lens to resolve two points increases with the NA increases. However, to achieve the maximal resolution of a microscope the NA of the microscope condenser must be equal to or slightly greater than the NA of the objective lens used. This requirement is necessary to ensure adequate illumination to the objective lens and can be understood better by reviewing the dynamics involved. Illumination light from the light source is presented to the condenser. The condenser lens system, along with the aperture diaphragm, is adjustable and serves to converge the illumination light into a cone-shaped focus on the specimen for viewing. If the condenser NA is less than the objective NA, the condenser presents inadequate illumination light to the objective lens, and one cannot attain maximal resolution. In contrast, objective lenses with NAs less than the condenser NA are optimal on the microscope. This can be accomplished by making routine condenser and diaphragm adjustments that effectively reduce the condenser NA to match the objective NA (see "Microscope Adjustment Procedure"). Condenser height adjustments serve to focus the light specifically on the specimen plane, thus achieving maximal resolution. Optimal field diaphragm adjustments diminish stray light, thereby increasing image definition and contrast. Adjustment of the aperture diaphragm to approximately 75% of the NA of the objective is necessary to achieve increased image contrast, increased focal depth, and a flatter FOV.

The body or frame of the microscope serves to hold its four basic components in place: (1) the optical tube with its lenses (eyepieces and objectives); (2) a stage on which the specimen is placed for viewing; (3) a condenser to focus light onto the specimen; and (4) an illumination source. Each component and its unique features are discussed next.

Eyepiece

Whereas some microscopes have only one eyepiece (monocular), those used in most clinical laboratories have two eyepieces (binocular). However when using a monocular microscope, always view with both eyes open to reduce eyestrain. Initially this may be difficult, but with practice the image seen by the unused eye will be suppressed. With a binocular microscope, adjustments to the oculars are necessary to ensure optimal viewing. The interpupillary distance of the eyepiece tubes is adjusted by simply sliding them together or apart. Because vision in both eyes usually not the same, each individual eyepiece is adjustable to compensate using the diopter adjustment. To adjust the eyepieces, first view the image using only the right eye and eyepiece. Look at a specific spot on the specimen, and bring it into sharp focus using the fine adjustment knob. Next, close the right eye, and while looking with the left eye through the left eyepiece, rotate the diopter adjustment ring on this eyepiece until the same spot on the specimen is also in sharp focus (Figure 1-3). Each technologist must make the interpupillary and diopter adjustments to suit his or her eyes. To eliminate eyestrain or tired eyes when performing microscopic work, always look through the microscope with eyes relaxed, and continually focus and re-focus the microscope as needed using the fine adjustment control.

Eyeglass wearers should consider keeping their glasses on when performing microscopic work. Rubber guards are available that fit over the eyepieces and prevent scratching of the eyeglasses. People with only spherical corrections (nearsighted or farsighted) can work at the microscope without their glasses. Focus adjustments of the microscope compensate for these visual defects. However, those with an astigmatism that requires a toric lens for correction should do microscopic work while wearing their eyeglasses, because the microscope cannot compensate for this. To determine whether eyeglasses have any toric correction in them, hold the glasses in front of some lettering at arm's length. The eyeglass will magnify or reduce the lettering. Now, rotate the glasses 45 degrees. If the lettering changes in length and width, the glasses contain toric correction and should be worn when one uses the microscope; if the lettering does not change, the eyeglasses have only spherical correction and do not need to be worn for microscopic work.

Mechanical Stage

The microscope mechanical stage is designed to hold firmly in place the slide to be examined. The stage has conveniently located adjustment knobs to move the slide front to back and side to side. When viewing the slide, the user views the image upside down. Moving the slide in one direction causes the image to move in the opposite direction. Some stages have a vernier scale on a horizontal and a vertical edge to facilitate relocation of a particular FOV. By recording the horizontal and vertical vernier scale values, the slide can be removed and at a later time be placed back onto the stage and the identical FOV can be found and reexamined.

Condenser

The condenser, located beneath the mechanical stage, consists of two lenses (Figure 1-4). The purpose of the condenser is to evenly distribute and optimally focus light from the illumination source onto the specimen. This is achieved by adjusting the condenser up or down using the condenser adjustment knob. The correct position of the condenser is always at its uppermost stop; it is slightly lowered only with Köhler illumination. The aperture diaphragm, located at the base of the condenser, regulates the beam of light presented to the specimen. The aperture diaphragm is usually an iris diaphragm made up of thin metal leaves that can be adjusted to form an opening of various diameters. Some microscopes use a disk diaphragm, consisting of a movable disk with openings of various sizes, for placement in front of the condenser (Figure 1-5). The purpose of the aperture diaphragm is to control the angle of the illumination light presented to the specimen and the objective lens. When the user properly adjusts the aperture diaphragm, he or she achieves maximal resolution, contrast, and definition of the specimen. One of the most common mistakes is to use the aperture diaphragm to reduce the brightness of the image field; in so doing, resolution is decreased. Instead, the user should decrease the light source intensity or place a neutral density filter over the source.

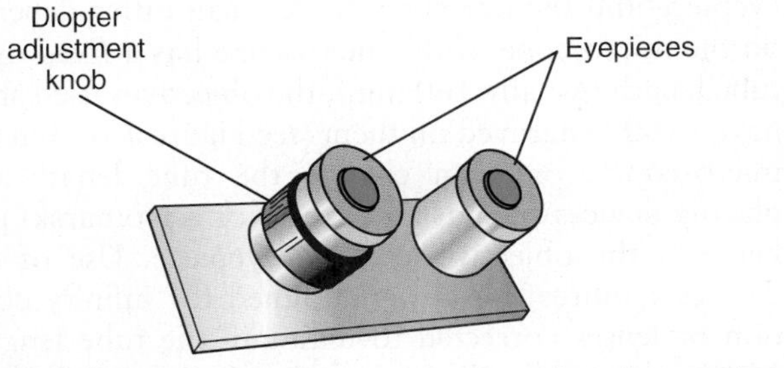

FIGURE 1-3 Schematic representation of a binocular eyepiece shows the location of the diopter adjustment ring.

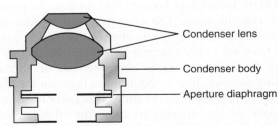

FIGURE 1-4 Schematic diagram of a condenser and an aperture diaphragm located beneath the mechanical stage of the microscope.

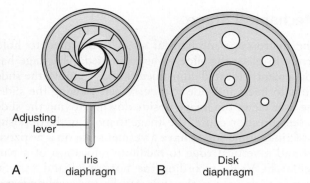

FIGURE 1-5 Two types of aperture diaphragms. **A,** An iris diaphragm. **B,** A disk diaphragm.

Illumination System

Microscopes today usually have a built-in illumination system. The light source is a tungsten or tungsten-halogen lamp located in the microscope base. These lamps often are manufactured specifically to ensure alignment of the lamp filament when a bulb requires changing. Dual controls are usually available: one to turn the microscope on, and another to adjust the intensity of the light. One should adjust the illumination intensity at the light source by turning down the lamp intensity, or by placing neutral density filters over the source. Neutral density filters do not change the color of the light but reduce its intensity. The filters are marked to indicate the reduction made, for example, a neutral density of 25 allows 75% of the light to pass. Some microscopes come with a daylight blue filter that makes the light slightly bluish. This color has been found to be restful to the eyes and is desirable for prolonged microscopic viewing.

Most clinical microscopes have a field diaphragm located at the light exit of the illumination source. The purpose of this diaphragm is to control the diameter of the light beam that strikes the specimen. The diaphragm is an iris type that when properly adjusted is just slightly larger than the FOV and serves to reduce stray light. See Box 1-1 for a procedure used to properly adjust a microscope for optimal viewing.

Objectives

The objectives are the most important optical components of the microscope because they produce the primary image magnification. The objectives are located on a rotatable nosepiece; only one objective is used at a time. Objectives are easily changed by simple rotation of the nosepiece; however, each objective has a different *working distance,* that is, the distance between the objective and the coverslip on the slide. This working distance decreases as the magnification of the objective used increases, for example, a 10× objective has a working distance of 7.2 mm, whereas a 40× objective has only 0.6 mm clearance. Therefore to prevent damage to the

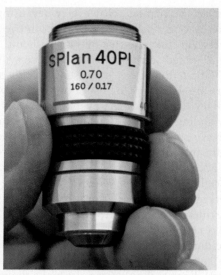

FIGURE 1-6 Engravings on this objective indicate that it is a planachromat lens (SPlan); the initial magnification is 40×; the numerical aperture is 0.70; the objective is designed for a microscope with an optical tube length of 160 mm; and the coverslip thickness should be 0.17 ± 0.01 mm.

objective or to the slide that is being observed, care must be taken when changing or focusing objectives.

A microscope has coarse and fine focus adjustment knobs. The user can focus the microscope by moving the mechanical stage holding the specimen up and down. Coarse focusing adjustments are made first, followed by any necessary fine adjustments.

Various engravings found on the objective indicate its magnification power, the NA, the optical tube length required, the coverglass thickness to be used, and the lens type (if not an achromat). Most often, the uppermost or largest number inscribed on the objective is the magnification power. Following this number is the NA, inscribed on the same line or just beneath it (Figure 1-6). As already discussed, the objective produces the primary magnification of the specimen, and the NA mathematically expresses the resolving power of the objective. Most objectives, designed for use with air between the lens and the specimen, are called *dry objectives.* In contrast, some objectives require immersion oil to achieve their designated NA. These objectives are inscribed with the term *oil* or *oel.*

The optical tube length—the distance between the eyepiece and the objective in use—can differ depending on the microscope. If the microscope has a fixed optical tube length (usually 160 mm), the objectives used should have "160" engraved on them (see Figure 1-6). On some microscopes, one can change the tube length when placing devices such as a polarizer or a Nomarski prism between the objective and the eyepiece. Use of these devices requires objectives designed for infinity correction or lenses corrected to maintain the tube length of 160 mm optically. Objectives designed for infinity correction have an infinity symbol (∞) engraved on them.

BOX 1-1 | Binocular Microscope Adjustment Procedure With Köhler Illumination

Preparing the Microscope

1. Turn on the light source. Adjust the intensity to a comfortable level.
2. Position the low-power (10×) objective in place by rotating the nosepiece.
3. Place a specimen slide on the mechanical stage. Be sure the slide is seated firmly in the slide holder. Position the specimen on the slide directly beneath the objective using the mechanical stage adjustment knobs.

Interpupillary Adjustment

4. Looking through the eyepieces with both eyes, adjust the interpupillary distance until perfect binocular vision is obtained (i.e., left and right images are fused together). Using coarse and fine adjustment knobs, bring the specimen into focus.

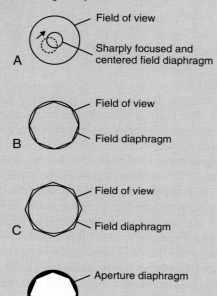

Diopter Adjustment

5. While closing the left eye, look through the right eyepiece with the right eye and bring the specimen into sharp focus using the fine adjustment knob.
6. Now, using only the left eye, bring the image into sharp focus by rotating the diopter adjustment ring located on the left eyepiece. (Do not use the adjustment knobs.)

Condenser Adjustment

(Note: If at any point during adjustment, the light intensity is very bright and uncomfortable, decrease the lamp voltage or insert a neutral density filter.)

Condenser Height and Centration

1. Close the field diaphragm.
2. Using the condenser height adjustment knob, bring the edges of the diaphragm into sharp focus.
3. Center the condenser, if necessary, using the condenser centration knobs (see Figure A).

Field Diaphragm Adjustment

4. Open the field diaphragm to just inside the edges of the field of view to confirm adequate centration (see Figure B). Re-center if necessary.
5. Now, open the field diaphragm until it is slightly larger than the field of view (see Figure C).

Condenser Aperture Diaphragm Adjustment

6. Depending on the microscope, perform one of the following:
   a. On microscopes with a numerical scale on the condenser, open the diaphragm to 70% or 80% of the objective NA (e.g., for 80% of 40× NA 0.65, adjust condenser aperture to 0.52).
   b. Alternatively, remove one eyepiece from the observation tube. While looking down the tube at the back of the objective, adjust the diaphragm until 70% to 80% of the field is visible (approximately 25% less than fully opened). See Figure D.
7. Note that each time an objective is changed, both field and aperture diaphragms should be readjusted.

Some objectives are designed to be used with a coverglass. If a coverglass is required, its thickness is engraved on the lens after the optical tube length (e.g., 160/0.17). Objectives that do not use a coverglass are designated with a dash (e.g., ∞/– or 160/–). A third type of objective is designed to be used with or without a coverglass. These objectives have no inscription for coverglass thickness; rather, they have a correction collar on them with which to adjust and fine-focus the lens appropriately for either application.

Objectives are corrected for two types of aberrations: chromatic and spherical. Chromatic aberration occurs because different wavelengths of light bend at different angles after passing through a lens (Figure 1-7). This results in a specimen image with undesired color fringes. Objectives corrected to bring the red and blue components of white light to the same focus are called *achromats* and may not have a designation engraved on them. Objectives that bring red, blue, and green light to a common focus are termed *apochromats* and are identified by the inscription "apo." Spherical aberration occurs when light rays pass through different parts of the lens and therefore are not brought to the same focus (Figure 1-8). As a result, the specimen image appears blurred and cannot be focused sharply. Objectives are corrected to bring all light entering the lens, regardless of whether the light is at the center or the periphery, to the same central focus. Achromat objectives are corrected spherically for green light, whereas apochromats are corrected spherically for green and blue light.

Other abbreviations may be engraved on the objective to indicate specific lens types. For example, "Plan" indicates that the lens is a planachromat, achromatically corrected and designed for a flat FOV over the entire

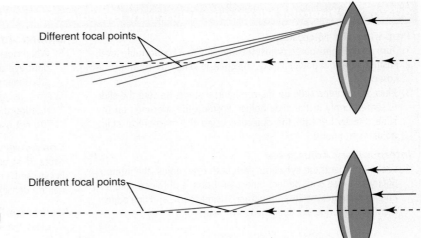

FIGURE 1-7 An illustration of chromatic aberration. Each wavelength of light is bent to a different focal point after passing through an uncorrected lens.

FIGURE 1-8 An illustration of spherical aberration. Each light ray is bent toward a different focal point, depending on where the ray enters an uncorrected lens.

area viewed. "Ph" indicates that the objective lens is for phase-contrast microscopy. Regardless of the manufacturer, the same basic information is engraved on all objective lenses, with only the format varying slightly. To ensure a compatible system, use of objectives and eyepieces designed by the same manufacturer that designed the microscope is advisable.

Two final features of objective lenses need to be discussed. The first characteristic is termed *parcentered* and relates to the ability of objective lenses to retain the same central FOV when the user switches from one objective to another. In other words, when an objective is changed to one of higher magnification for a closer look, the object does not move from the center of the FOV. The second feature, termed *parfocal,* refers to the ability of objectives to remain in focus regardless of the objective used. This allows initial focusing at low power; changing to other magnifications requires only minimal fine focus adjustment. Whereas both of these features are taken for granted today, in the recent past, each objective required individual centering and focusing.

When using a microscope, adjustments must be made with each objective to produce optimal viewing. These adjustments strive to equate the NA of the objective lens in use (e.g., 10×, NA 0.25) with the condenser NA (NA 0.9), thereby achieving maximal magnification and resolution. On current microscopes that use Köhler illumination, once the condenser height adjustment is made, it remains unchanged regardless of the objective used. The user lowers the effective NA of the condenser by decreasing the light the condenser receives (i.e., closing the field diaphragm) and by adjusting the aperture diaphragm for the objective. On microscopes with which Köhler illumination is not possible, use of low-power objectives may require (1) reducing the illumination source light, if possible; (2) slightly lowering (by approximately 1.0 mm) the condenser from its uppermost position; or (3)

minimally closing the aperture diaphragm. An adjustment error that users frequently make is lowering the condenser too much, resulting in loss of resolution as contrast is increased.

When high-power dry objectives are used (e.g., 40×, NA 0.65), the NA is closer to that of the condenser (NA 0.9). Therefore the condenser NA needs less reduction to achieve maximal viewing. Because going from a low-power to a high-power objective means changing from a low NA to a higher NA, more illumination is required. Microscopes using Köhler illumination require only field and aperture diaphragm adjustments with each objective change. When high-power objectives are used on a microscope without Köhler illumination, the user should put the condenser all the way up and close the aperture diaphragm just enough to attain effective contrast. Never use the condenser or the aperture diaphragm to reduce image brightness; rather, decrease the illumination intensity or use neutral density filters.

OCULAR FIELD NUMBER

The eyepieces or oculars together with the objective lenses perform two important functions. They determine (1) the diameter of the **field of view** (FOV) and (2) the total magnification of a specimen. The diameter of the FOV is determined by the round baffle or ridge inside each ocular, and its numerical value is known as the ocular **field number.** Before 1990, most laboratory microscopes had an ocular field number of 18, which means that the diameter of the FOV when a 1× objective is used is 18 mm (or 1.8 mm with a 10× objective). In other words, if a metric ruler were placed on the stage and a 1× objective used, the diameter of the circle of view observed when looking through the eyepieces would measure 18 mm. Typically, the higher the field number, the more expensive the microscope. Areas of high microscope use, such as hematology and pathology laboratories, may be able to justify the expense of microscopes with even higher ocular field numbers of 22 to 26 or larger.

When multiple microscopes are used in the laboratory for urine sediment examination, it is of paramount importance that their FOVs are the same, because clinically significant sediment components are reported as the number present per low-power field or per high-power field. The larger the ocular field number, the larger the FOV, and the greater the number of components that may be observed. Note that two microscopes with equivalent magnifying power (e.g., 100× and 400×) can have FOVs that differ! In other words, the magnification of the oculars on both microscopes is the same, but their field numbers are not. Unfortunately, most microscope manufacturers do not engrave the field number on the oculars, and if needed, it must be obtained from the original purchase information, by measuring the diameter using a ruler and a 1× objective, or by contacting the manufacturer.

MICROSCOPE ADJUSTMENT PROCEDURE

Clinical microscopes today primarily use Köhler illumination. With this type of illumination, the light source image (light filament) is focused onto the front focal plane of the substage condenser at the aperture diaphragm by a lamp condenser, located just in front of the light source. The substage condenser then focuses this image onto the back of the objective in use (see Figure 1-1). As a result, this illumination system produces bright, uniform illumination at the specimen plane even when a coil filament light source is used. Proper use of this illuminating system is just as important as selection of a microscope and its objectives. To use a microscope with Köhler illumination, the microscopist must know how to set up and optimally adjust the condenser and the field and aperture diaphragms. Manufacturers supply instructions with the microscope that are clear and easy to follow. In addition, online interactive tutorials are available that demonstrate the improved optical performance of a microscope when adjusted to achieve Köhler illumination.[1] Box 1-1 gives a basic procedure for adjustment of a typical binocular microscope with a Köhler illumination system. Whereas initially these steps may feel cumbersome, with use they become routine. When using other types of microscopy, additional adjustment procedures may be necessary to ensure optimal viewing. For example, phase-contrast microscopy requires that the phase rings are checked and aligned, if necessary.

Each day, before setting up and adjusting the microscope, the user should check it to ensure that it is clean. The microscopist should look for dust or dirt on the illumination source port, the filters, and the upper condenser lens. The user should check the eyepiece and the objectives, especially any oil immersion objective, to be sure that they are clean and free of oil and fingerprints. By routinely inspecting the microscope and optical surfaces before adjustment, valuable time can be saved in microscope setup and in troubleshooting problems. In laboratories in which the entire staff uses the same microscope, inspection before use helps identify people who need to be reminded of proper microscope care and maintenance.

CARE AND PREVENTIVE MAINTENANCE

The microscope is a precision instrument. Therefore, ensuring long-term mechanical and optical performance requires care, including routine cleaning and maintenance. Dust is probably the greatest cause of harm to the mechanical and optical components of a microscope. Dust settles in mechanical tracks and on lenses. Although dust can be removed from lenses by cleaning, the less cleaning of lenses performed, the better. To remove dust, dirt, or other particulate matter, the microscopist should use a grease-free brush (camel hair) or an air syringe (e.g., an infant's ear syringe). If compressed air is used, the air should be filtered (e.g., with cotton wool) to remove any contaminating residues or moisture. Using a microscope dust cover when the instrument is not in use or placing it in a storage cabinet eliminates dust buildup.

On microscopes, all mechanical parts are lubricated with special long-lasting lubricants. Therefore the user should never use grease or oils to lubricate the microscope. When mechanical parts are dirty, cleaning and regreasing should be performed by the manufacturer or by a professional service representative.

In climates in which the relative humidity is consistently greater than 60%, precautions must be taken to prevent fungal growth on optical surfaces. In these areas, a dust cover or a storage cabinet may reduce ventilation and enhance fungal growth. Therefore microscopes may require storage with a desiccant, or in an area with controlled temperature and air circulation. In addition to high humidity, microscopes should be protected from direct sunlight and high temperatures.

When handling the microscope, for example, when removing it from a storage cupboard or when changing work areas, the user must always carry it firmly using both hands and must avoid abrupt movements. The counter on which the microscope is placed should be vibration free. This eliminates undesired movement in the FOV when viewing wet preparations as well as the detrimental effects that long-term vibration can have on precision equipment.

All optical surfaces must be clean to provide crisp brilliant images. Because the nosepiece is rotated by hand, the objectives are constantly in danger of becoming smeared with skin oils. The user should avoid all handling of optical surfaces with the fingers. Should a lens need cleaning, the user should follow the manufacturer's suggested cleaning protocol. Optical lenses are easily scratched; therefore one must remove all particulate matter from the lens before cleaning. Some residues may be removed simply by breathing on the lens surface and polishing with lens paper. Others may require a commercial lens cleaner. The microscopist should never use gauze, facial tissue, or lint-free tissue to clean optical surfaces. After using oil immersion objective lenses, the microscopist should remove the oil carefully using a dry lens paper and should repeat this procedure using a lens paper moistened with lens cleaner. The microscopist must store oil immersion objectives dry, because oil left on the lens surface can impair its optical performance. Whereas some manufacturers suggest the use of xylene to clean oil immersion lenses, this practice is not recommended for several reasons. If residual xylene is left on the objective, it destroys the adhesive that holds the lens in place. In addition, xylene fumes are toxic and should be avoided.

The eyepiece is particularly susceptible to becoming dirty, especially when the user wears mascara. Therefore when performing microscopy, people should avoid wearing mascara. If an eyepiece is removed for cleaning, care must be taken to prevent dust from entering the microscope tube and settling on the back lens of the objective.

When the specimen image shows a visual aberration, and a dirty lens is suspected, the following procedure can help identify which lens needs attention. Specks appearing in the FOV are most often noted on the eyepiece or the coverglass. The user should rotate the eyepiece; if the speck moves, the eyepiece lens requires cleaning. If the speck moves when the slide position is changed, the coverglass is dirty. If the objective lens is dirty, the speck will not be present when a different objective is used. Often the image is blurred or hazy (i.e., decreased sharpness or contrast) when an objective lens is dirty, as with a fingerprint.

Replacement of the light source is easy to perform when the manufacturer's directions are followed. Use only replacement lamps designated by the manufacturer to ensure compatibility and proper light source alignment. Any other repair that requires microscope disassembly should be performed only by a professional service representative. As with other instrumentation, microscope cleaning, maintenance, and problems should be documented. In addition, service to clean, lubricate, and align components should be performed annually by the manufacturer or a professional service representative.

Box 1-2 lists the dos and don'ts of good microscope care. As with any precision instrument, the microscope will give long-lasting and optimal performance if it is maintained and cared for properly.

BOX 1-2 | Microscope Dos and Don'ts

Dos
- Always use lens paper on optical surfaces.
- Always use a commercial lens cleaner to clean optical surfaces.
- Protect the microscope from dust when not in use. Avoid temperature extremes and direct sunlight.
- Document all cleaning and maintenance; have microscope professionally serviced annually.

Don'ts
- Never use gauze, facial tissue, or lint-free tissue on lens surfaces.
- Never touch optical surfaces with fingers or hands.
- Never wipe off dust or particulate matter; remove using suitable brush or air syringe.
- Never wear mascara while performing microscopy.
- Never clean the back lens of the objectives.
- Never use grease or oil on mechanical parts.
- Never disassemble the microscope for repair; call a service representative.
- Never leave microscope tubes without eyepieces; insert dust plugs as necessary.

TYPES OF MICROSCOPY

All types of microscopy (with the exception of electron microscopy) use the same basic magnification principles used in the compound brightfield microscope. Different types of microscopy—phase-contrast, polarizing, interference contrast, darkfield, and fluorescence—are achieved by changing the illumination system or the character of the light presented to the specimen. In research and in the clinical laboratory, some of these techniques are being used for new applications. As their usage grows, the different types of microscopy become increasingly commonplace.

Brightfield Microscopy

Brightfield microscopy is the oldest and most common type of illumination system used on microscopes. The name refers to the dark appearance of the specimen image against a brighter background. This remains the principal type of microscopy used in the clinical laboratory. Historically, room light was used as the illumination source. A major disadvantage of this procedure was uneven and variable illumination of the FOV. Now with Köhler illumination, the light is focused not at the specimen plane, but at the condenser aperture diaphragm. This allows bright, even illumination of the specimen field despite the use of a coil filament lamp.

Phase-Contrast Microscopy

Often in the clinical laboratory, a microscopist encounters components with a low refractive index (e.g., hyaline casts in urine) that are difficult to view without staining.

With phase-contrast microscopy, variations in refractive index are converted into variations in light intensity or contrast. This permits detailed viewing of low-refractile components and of living cells (e.g., trichomonads). In equivalently detailed imaging performed with other techniques, cells are no longer living because normal fixation and staining has killed them.

Briefly, phase microscopy is based on the wave theory of light. If light waves are in "phase," the intensity of the light observed is the sum of all the individual waves (Figure 1-9, *A*). If some of the light waves are slowed, as from passing through an object, the light intensity observed will be less (Figure 1-9, *B*). If some waves are retarded exactly one-half of a wavelength, they will cancel out completely an unaffected light wave, thereby further reducing the light intensity (Figure 1-9, *C*).

Components retard light to different degrees depending on their unique shape, refractive index, and absorbance properties. The best contrast is achieved when light retardation is one-quarter of a wavelength; however, this retardation is not possible without modification to the brightfield microscope.

Converting a brightfield microscope for phase-contrast microscopy requires changes in the condenser and in the objective. The condenser must be fitted with an annular diaphragm in the condenser itself or below it. As depicted in Figure 1-10, the annular diaphragm resembles a target and produces a light annulus or ring. Illumination light can pass through only this central clear ring of the diaphragm before penetrating the specimen. The objective used must be fitted with a phase-shifting element, also depicted in Figure 1-10. Note that the phase-shifting element also resembles a target. However, its central ring retards light by one-quarter of a wavelength, producing a dark annulus or ring. The light and dark annuli produced on the back of the objective can be seen by removing an eyepiece. This enables proper alignment of the condenser and objective, that is, the light annulus of the condenser is adjusted until light and dark annuli are concentric and superimposed (Figure 1-11).

Normally in brightfield microscopy, undiffracted and diffracted light rays are superimposed to produce the magnified image. In phase-contrast microscopy, light is presented to the specimen only from the central light annulus of the annular diaphragm of the condenser. After passing through the specimen, diffracted light enters the clear rings of the phase-shifting element, and all undiffracted light is shifted one-quarter of a wavelength out of phase. These light rays are recombined,

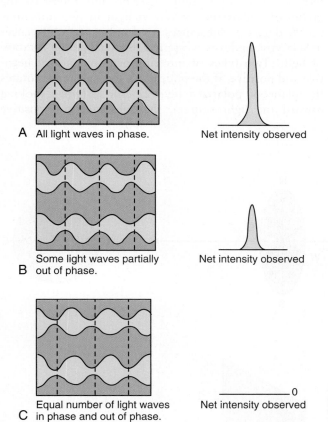

A All light waves in phase.   Net intensity observed

B Some light waves partially out of phase.   Net intensity observed

C Equal number of light waves in phase and out of phase.   Net intensity observed

FIGURE 1-9 The effect of the phase of light waves on the light intensity observed. **A,** All light waves are in phase, and light intensity is maximal. **B,** Some light waves are slower or are partially out of phase, resulting in a decrease in the light intensity observed. **C,** Equal numbers of light waves are in phase and out of phase. As a result, the net intensity observed is zero (i.e., the light waves cancel each other out).

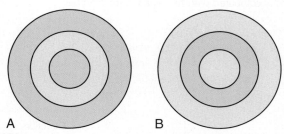

A   **B**

FIGURE 1-10 Schematic representation of **(A)** an annular diaphragm (placed below the condenser) and **(B)** the phase-shifting element (placed in back of the objective).

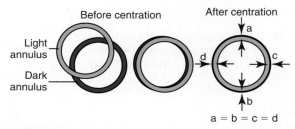

Before centration   After centration

Light annulus

Dark annulus

a = b = c = d

FIGURE 1-11 Phase ring alignment. A schematic representation of the view at the back of the objective when one is looking down the eyepiece tube with the eyepiece removed. The dark annulus is formed by the phase-shifting element in the objective; the light annulus is formed by the annular diaphragm. Phase ring alignment is obtained by adjusting the light annulus until it is centered and superimposed on the dark annulus.

producing varying degrees of contrast in the specimen image (Figure 1-12). Areas of the specimen appear light and dark with haloes of various intensities. Thin, flat specimens that produce less haloing are viewed best by this technique. Bright haloes produced by the optical gradient of some components can reduce visualization of the detail and dimension of the object. When unstained specimens are evaluated, entities with a low refractive index (e.g., hyaline casts, mucus threads) are more visually apparent than when brightfield microscopy is used.

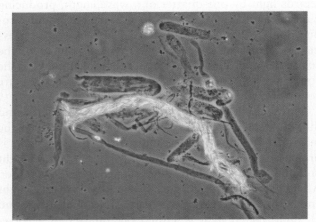

FIGURE 1-12 An example of phase-contrast microscopy. This low-power (100×) view of urine sediment includes a highly refractile fiber revealed by its brightly haloed image. The hyaline casts and mucus threads are less refractile and have haloes of decreased intensity compared with the highly refractile fiber.

Polarizing Microscopy

Understanding the principle of polarizing microscopy requires a fundamental knowledge of polarized light, and this principle can be explained best by comparison. Regular or unpolarized light vibrates in every direction perpendicular to its direction of travel; in contrast, polarized light vibrates in only one direction or plane (Figure 1-13). When polarized light passes through an optically active substance, it is split into two beams. One beam follows the original light path, and the other is rotated 90 degrees. Substances that are not optically active simply permit the light to pass through unchanged.

Polarizing microscopy has widespread application in the clinical laboratory and in pharmaceuticals, forensics, pathology, geology, and other fields. Anisotropic or birefringent substances such as crystals, fibers, bones, or minerals can be identified based on their effects on polarized light. *Anisotropic* is a general term that refers to the ability of a substance to exhibit properties (e.g., refractive index, heat conduction) with different values when measured along axes in different directions. The term *birefringent* is more specific and refers to the ability of a substance to refract light in two directions (at 90 degrees). Substances need only small differences in refractive indexes to appreciably change the rotation of light. Two types of birefringence are known: negative and positive. If the optically active substance rotates the plane of polarized light clockwise (when looking toward the light source), the substance has positive

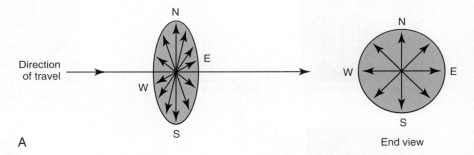

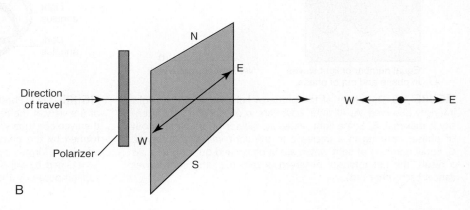

FIGURE 1-13 Comparison of light ray orientation in **(A)** regular light (vibrating in all directions) and **(B)** polarized light (vibrating in only one plane).

birefringence; if rotation is to the left or counterclockwise, the substance has negative birefringence. This optical rotation characteristic provides a means of identifying and distinguishing birefringent substances. For example, monosodium urate crystals exhibit negative birefringence, whereas calcium pyrophosphate crystals are positively birefringent.

To convert a brightfield microscope to a polarizing one requires two filters. One filter, called the *polarizing filter*, is placed below the condenser. Whether placed in a holder below the condenser or directly on the built-in illumination port, the filter is easily added and removed. This filter is adjusted to allow only light vibrating in an East-West direction perpendicular to the light path to pass to the specimen (Figure 1-14). The second filter, called the *analyzer*, is placed between the objective and the eyepiece. Its orientation is such that only light vibrating in the North-South direction can pass. When both filters are in place—and in opposite orientation—they are said to be in a "crossed" position or "crossed pols."

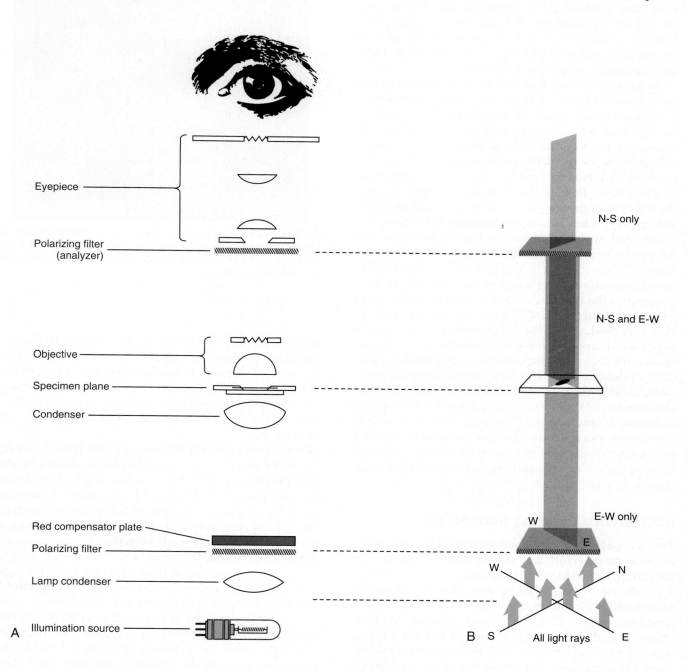

FIGURE 1-14 A, Schematic diagram of a polarizing microscope and its components. **B,** The change in the polarized light rays caused by a birefringent specimen. The polarizer and the analyzer are in a crossed position.

With no optically active specimen in place, the FOV appears black because no light is passing through the analyzer. However, if an optically active specimen is in place, the incident polarized light will be refracted by the specimen into two rays vibrating at 90 degrees to each other. These rays pass through the analyzer and appear as white light.

Many substances found in clinical laboratory specimens are birefringent. Some chemical analyte crystals (e.g., amino acid crystals) have clinical importance in urine, and others (e.g., monosodium urate) have clinical importance in synovial fluid. Because other birefringent substances (e.g., drugs, dyes, starch) may be encountered, technical expertise and training are necessary to ensure proper identification.

To identify a crystal on the basis of its negative or positive birefringence, a first-order red compensator or a full wave plate is used. This compensator is placed in the light path between the crossed pools. When the compensator is in place, the FOV is no longer black but is red-violet, hence the name *red compensator*. This color results from removal of the blue-green color component of white light. Besides changing the background color, the red compensator splits the polarized light into slow and fast rays. The direction of vibration of the slow rays is indicated by an inscription on the compensator. This inscription enables the microscopist to orient the birefringent substance parallel and perpendicular to the slow ray component for observation of the characteristic birefringence of the substance. The refracted rays originating from a birefringent substance can be additive with the slow rays produced by the red compensator, causing the substance to appear blue-green (positive birefringence) against the red-violet background; or the refracted rays can be subtractive with the slow rays of the red compensator, causing the substance to appear yellow (negative birefringence). In the clinical laboratory, this microscopic technique is used primarily for urine and synovial fluid microscopic examinations. For gout studies, the use of a red compensator predominates in the differentiation of monosodium urate crystals from calcium pyrophosphate crystals in synovial fluid.

Interference Contrast Microscopy

Two types of interference contrast microscopy are modulation contrast (Hoffman) and differential interference contrast (Nomarski). In interference contrast microscopy, the microscope converts differences in the optical path through the specimen to intensity differences in the specimen image. Both techniques achieve specimen images of high contrast and resolution without haloing, superior to those obtained with phase-contrast microscopy. These methods also enable optical sectioning of a specimen because the image at each depth of field level is unaffected by material above or below the plane of focus (Figure 1-15). Images have a three-dimensional

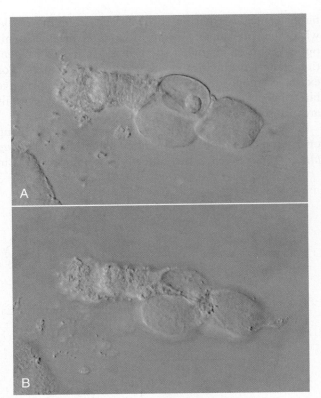

FIGURE 1-15 An example of differential interference contrast (Nomarski) microscopy and its optical sectioning ability. The different plane of focus captured in each photomicrograph allows for greatly detailed imaging.

appearance that readily reveals the contour details of a specimen. Interference contrast microscopy is excellent for detailed viewing of unstained specimens. Its superior visualization of all components, including living cells and substances of low refractive indexes, makes it particularly useful for microscopic examinations of wet preparations.

Modulation Contrast Microscopy (Hoffman). Modulation contrast microscopy can be performed on a brightfield microscope with three modifications: (1) a special slit aperture is placed below the condenser; (2) a polarizer, to control contrast, is placed below this slit aperture; and (3) a special amplitude filter, called a *modulator*, is placed in the back of each objective. Once the microscope has been adapted for modulation contrast microscopy, simply removing the slit aperture from the light path allows the instrument to be used for brightfield, darkfield, polarizing, or fluorescence techniques.

The basic principle of modulation contrast microscopy is presented schematically in Figure 1-16. Illumination light enters the polarizer, becomes polarized, and passes to the special slit aperture at the front focal plane of the condenser. This polarizer is rotatable, and because the slit aperture is covered partially with a second polarizer, rotating it achieves variations in contrast and spatial

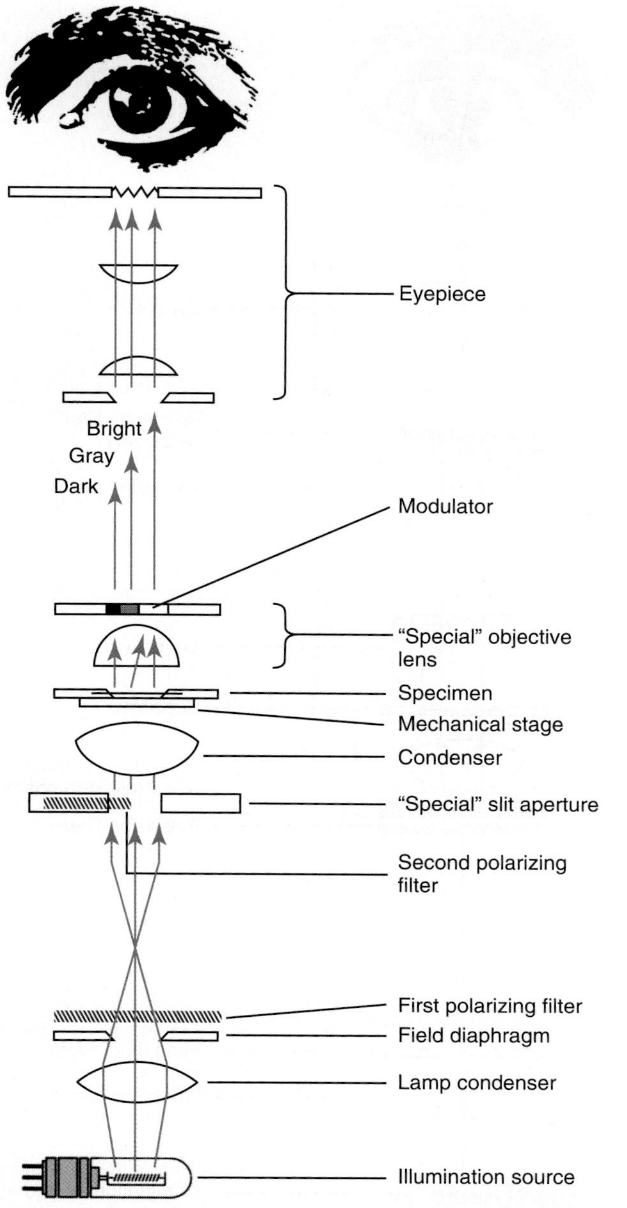
Eyepiece
Bright
Gray
Dark
Modulator
"Special" objective lens
Specimen
Mechanical stage
Condenser
"Special" slit aperture
Second polarizing filter
First polarizing filter
Field diaphragm
Lamp condenser
Illumination source

FIGURE 1-16 Schematic representation of a modulation contrast microscope and its components.

coherence (i.e., reduction of scattering effects such as flare and fringes at specimen edges). The light rays proceed through and interact with the specimen. Where they enter the objective lens depends on their interaction (i.e., diffraction) with the specimen. As a result, light rays pass through different parts of the modulator located at the back of the objective. The modulator is divided into three regions of different size and light transmission (i.e., dark region, approximately 1% transmission; gray region, approximately 15% transmission; and bright region, 100% transmission). The modulator determines the intensity gradients of light to dark observed in the three-dimensional image but does not effect a change in light phase. The modulator is also the component from which this technique derives its name. "When light intensity varies above and below an average value, the light is said to be modulated—thus the name *modulation contrast*."[2]

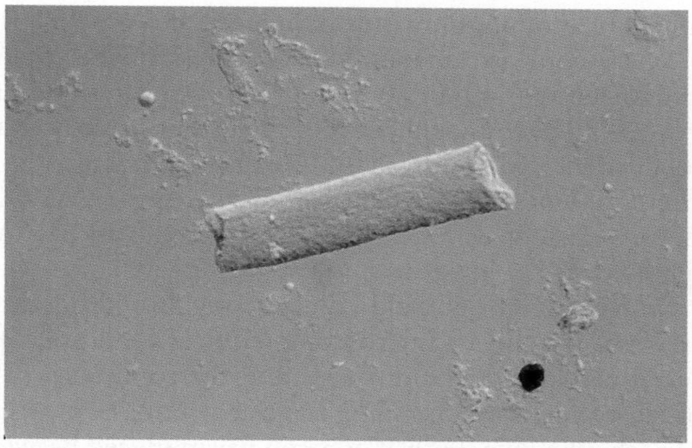

FIGURE 1-17 Example of the three-dimensional image produced by differential interference. This view shows a waxy cast at a magnification of 200×.

Microscope modifications made for modulation contrast are located at the same optical planes as in phase-contrast microscopy. The modulator and the phase-shifting element are located at the back of their respective objectives, whereas the special slit aperture and the annular diaphragm (light annulus) are located in the condenser focal plane. Each system also requires alignment of these conjugate planes for optimal specimen imaging. Modulation contrast produces three-dimensional images that reveal contours and details not possible with phase-contrast microscopy. However, for viewing essentially flat, thin specimens, images using phase-contrast microscopy—with which the halo effect is minimal—can be equivalent to those seen with modulation contrast. Differential interference contrast microscopy can produce specimen images comparable with those seen with modulation contrast. However, because differential interference contrast uses polarization to achieve its three-dimensional image, any birefringent substance present in the specimen plane compromises the image. In these latter situations, modulation contrast microscopy produces an image of superior detail and contrast.

Differential Interference Contrast Microscopy (Nomarski). In differential interference contrast microscopy, intensity differences in the specimen image are attained through the use of birefringent crystal prisms (i.e., modified Wollaston prisms) as beam splitters. One prism placed before the specimen plane splits the illumination light into two beams, whereas the second prism placed after the objective recombines them. The split beams follow different light paths through the specimen plane. They are rejoined before the eyepiece to produce a three-dimensional image (Figure 1-17). Images obtained with differential interference contrast microscopy are similar to modulation contrast images and are superior to phase-contrast images because no halo formation occurs. As with modulation contrast, optical sectioning or layer-by-layer imaging of specimens is possible because the depth of focus is small. Another characteristic of differential interference contrast microscopy is that specimens with low or high refractive indexes can produce equally detailed images.

Converting brightfield microscopy to differential interference contrast microscopy requires (1) a polarizer placed between the light source and the condenser, (2) a special condenser containing modified Wollaston prisms for each objective, (3) a Wollaston prism placed between the objective and the eyepiece, and (4) an analyzer (polarizing filter) placed behind this Wollaston prism and before the eyepiece (Figure 1-18). Illumination light becomes polarized and enters the special condenser, where it is split into two beams. The two beams traverse slightly different parts of the specimen and are recombined at the prism located after the objective. From the prism, the recombined rays (with directions of vibration that are perpendicular and do not interfere with each other) enter the analyzer. The analyzer produces the interference image observed by changing the direction of vibration of the recombined rays, so that they interfere with each other. In reality, two images are formed, but human eyes are unable to resolve them to produce a double image. As a result, the specimen image observed appears to be in relief, or three-dimensional.

When differential interference contrast microscopy is used, the background FOV can be changed from black or dark gray to various colors (e.g., yellow, blue, magenta) by simply rotating the prism located after the objective; this alters the path differences of the split light waves. In this way, specimen images similar to those obtained using darkfield microscopy can be attained, as can brilliantly colored ones. Gray backgrounds result in the most detailed three-dimensional images.

Darkfield Microscopy

As the name implies, **darkfield microscopy** produces a bright specimen image against a dark or black background. In the clinical laboratory, this method is used only on unstained specimens and is the preferred technique for identifying spirochetes. To obtain the specimen image, a special condenser directs the illumination source light through the specimen plane only from oblique angles (Figure 1-19). When light passes through a specimen, the light interacts with the specimen. This interaction, whether refraction, reflection, or diffraction, results in light entering the objective. The resultant image, a shining specimen on a black background, is enhanced visually by the increased contrast. If no specimen is present, the FOV appears black because no light is entering the objective lens.

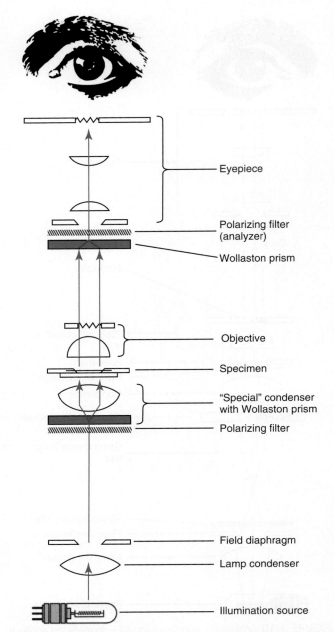

FIGURE 1-18 Schematic representation of a differential interference contrast (Nomarksi) microscope and its components.

Darkfield microscopy is an inexpensive means of obtaining increased contrast to facilitate visualization of specimen details. The technique is beneficial in clarifying edges and boundaries but is not as good as phase-contrast microscopy or interference contrast microscopy in revealing internal structural detail. To convert a brightfield microscope for darkfield microscopy, the condenser must be replaced with a special darkfield condenser. Two types of darkfield condensers are available: one type uses air between it and the specimen slide, as in brightfield microscopy, whereas the second, an immersion darkfield condenser, requires placement of oil

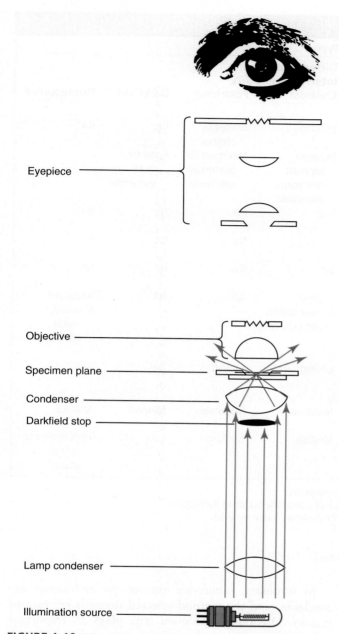

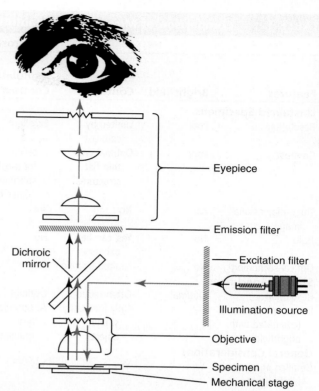

FIGURE 1-19 Schematic representation of a darkfield microscope and its components.

FIGURE 1-20 Schematic representation of a reflected illumination fluorescence microscope and its components.

Fluorescence Microscopy

Fluorescence microscopy allows the visualization of fluorescent substances. Light of a selected wavelength is presented to the specimen. If a specific fluorescent substance is present in the specimen, then light is absorbed and emitted at a different, longer wavelength. Any emitted light is transmitted to the eyepiece for viewing. To accomplish this task, two filters are used (Figure 1-20). The first filter, called the *excitation filter,* selects the wavelength of the excitation light presented to the specimen. The second filter, called the *barrier* or *emission filter,* selects a specific wavelength of emitted light from the specimen. Whereas some biological substances are naturally fluorescent (e.g., vitamin A), most applications of this technique require staining of the specimen with fluorescent dyes called *fluorophores* (e.g., quinacrine).

Each fluorophore has a unique excitation and emission wavelength. Consequently, the filters selected vary with the fluorophore used in the procedure. Historically, excitation and emission filters were made of glass and were not wavelength selective enough for some applications. Today, selective interference filters made from metallic salts are available and greatly increase wavelength specificity.

Two types of illumination systems that differ in the path of the excitation light are available for fluorescence microscopy. A transmitted illumination system is similar

between the condenser and the specimen slide. The advantage of the immersion condenser is the ability to use objectives of high NAs (NA values >0.65) and therefore to achieve greater magnification and resolution of the specimen.

By design, darkfield microscopy requires bright illumination sources because only small amounts of light ever reach the objective lens. In addition, the glass slides used must be meticulously clean, because any particles of dust or dirt present in the specimen plane will shine brightly against the dark background.

TABLE 1-1 | Comparison of Microscopic Capabilities

				Microscopy Types			
Features	**Brightfield**	**Phase Contrast**	**Modulation Contrast**	**Differential Interference Contrast**	**Polarizing**	**Darkfield**	**Fluorescence**
Unstained Specimens							
Resolution	Poor	Limited by contrast	Excellent	Excellent	Limited by contrast	Fair	NA*
Contrast	Poor	Optimal with thin flat structures†	Excellent for most specimens; adjustable	Excellent for most specimens; adjustable	Maximum for birefringent specimens	Good for most specimens	—
Three-dimensional image	No	No	Yes	Yes	No	No	No
Halo	No	Yes, can be excessive	No	No	No	No	No
Optical sectioning	No	Limited by halo	Yes	Yes	No	No	No
Stained Specimens							
Resolution	Optimal	Often reduced	Optimal	Optimal	NA‡	NA‡	Adequate§
Image enhancement (compared with brightfield)	—	Only for faintly stained objects	At boundaries and gradients	At boundaries and gradients	—	—	Maximal, not visible otherwise
General Considerations							
Detailed imaging of birefringent specimens	Yes	Yes	Yes	Limited	Limited	Yes	No
Technical training required¶	Minimal	Moderate	Moderate	Moderate	Moderate	Minimal	Minimal
Comparative cost	Low	Medium	Medium	Medium	Medium	Low	High (owing to cost of source)

Modified from Hoffman Modulation Contrast System, Modulation Optics, Inc., Greenvale, NY.
*Not applicable; technique requires staining with a fluorescent dye or the presence of a naturally occurring fluorophore.
†Contrast is optimal in thin sections, where structures are flat and differences in the refractive index are small.
‡Not applicable; technique used only to observe unstained specimens.
§Stained with a fluorescent dye.
¶Training includes microscope setup, alignment, and adjustment for optimized image.

to other microscopy systems in which the excitation light is presented to the condenser, focused, and passed through the specimen. In contrast, the excitation light in a reflected illumination system is presented to the specimen from above the specimen via the objective lens. In this case, a dichroic mirror reflects excitation light from the illumination source, and the objective focuses light onto the specimen (see Figure 1-20). The dichroic mirror has a dual role: first, to reflect excitation light to the specimen, and second, to allow passage of emitted light to the selective barrier filter.

Reflected fluorescence microscopy is currently the method of choice. Its illumination sources vary from halogen-quartz lamps to mercury or xenon arc lamps. Fluorescence microscopy is sensitive to minute quantities of fluorophores present on antibodies, antigens, viruses, or any other entity with which they become associated. As a result, fluorescence microscopy frequently is used in microbiological and immunologic procedures in the clinical laboratory.

In summary, numerous microscopic techniques are available, and the method selected depends on various factors. Obviously, specimen type plays an important role in determining the microscopic technique used. Some techniques cannot produce detailed images of unstained living materials or of components with a low refractive index. Other methods require the presence of specific substances, such as a fluorescent dye or a birefringent entity, to produce an image. The ability to produce a three-dimensional image or to section a specimen optically may not be necessary in some applications. Each feature plays an important part in the selection of a microscope to suit the needs of each laboratory: instrumentation cost, amount of technical training required, ability of the instrument to convert to other types of microscopy, and the need for adequate or more enhanced imaging. Table 1-1 lists each of the techniques discussed, compares their capabilities with different specimen types, and provides several general considerations.

STUDY QUESTIONS

1. In a brightfield microscope, which lens produces the primary image magnification?
   A. Condenser
   B. Eyepiece (ocular)
   C. Numerical aperture
   D. Objective

2. A microscope has a 10× magnification eyepiece and a 100× objective lens. What is the total magnification of the specimen when viewed using this microscope?
   A. 0.1×
   B. 10×
   C. 100×
   D. 1000×

3. Select the numerical aperture that has the ability to distinguish the smallest distance between two distinct points, that is, the greatest resolving power (R).
   A. 0.25
   B. 0.65
   C. 0.85
   D. 1.25

4. The numerical aperture of a lens can be increased by
   A. decreasing the angle of light made by the lens.
   B. increasing the refractive index of the optical medium.
   C. increasing the illumination intensity.
   D. decreasing the interpupillary distance.

5. Which parameter(s) will increase with an increase in the numerical aperture of an objective lens?
   A. Magnification and resolution
   B. Field of view and resolution
   C. Magnification and field of view
   D. Magnification

6. Match the microscope component with its primary function.

Function	Microscope Component
__ A. Produces primary image magnification	1. Aperture diaphragm
__ B. Produces secondary image magnification	2. Condenser
__ C. Moves the specimen for viewing	3. Eyepiece
__ D. Optimally focuses light onto the specimen	4. Field diaphragm
__ E. Controls the angle of light presented to the specimen	5. Mechanical stage
__ F. Controls the diameter of light rays that strike the specimen	6. Light source
	7. Objective

7. Which of the following components should be adjusted to decrease the illumination light or field brightness?
   A. Aperture diaphragm
   B. Condenser
   C. Field diaphragm
   D. Light source

8. Which lens characteristic is described as the ability to keep a specimen image in focus regardless of which objective lens is used?
   A. Parcentered
   B. Parfocal
   C. Chromatic aberration
   D. Spherical aberration

9. To achieve maximal image magnification and resolution, the
   A. condenser should be in its lowest position.
   B. condenser numerical aperture must be equal to or greater than the objective numerical aperture.
   C. aperture diaphragm should be used to decrease field brightness.
   D. field diaphragm should be opened fully.

10. Various inscriptions may be found on an objective lens. Select the objective lens inscription that indicates a numerical aperture of 0.25.
    A. SPlan40PL
       0.65
       160/025
    B. 25
       0.10
       160/0.17
    C. E10
       0.25
       160/0.20
    D. DPlan25
       0.10
       25/160

11. When a microscope with Köhler illumination is adjusted, the
    A. condenser is adjusted up or down until the field diaphragm is focused sharply.
    B. field diaphragm is opened until it is slightly smaller than the field of view.
    C. illumination intensity is adjusted using the field and aperture diaphragms.
    D. aperture diaphragm is opened until 25% of the field is in view.

12. Microscope lenses should be cleaned or polished using
    1. gauze.
    2. facial tissue.
    3. lint-free tissues.
    4. lens paper.
    A. 1, 2, and 3 are correct.
    B. 1 and 3 are correct.
    C. 4 is correct.
    D. All are correct.

13. When viewing a focused specimen in the microscope, the user sees a speck in the field of view. The speck remains in view when the objective is changed and when the specimen is moved. The speck is most likely located on the
    A. condenser.
    B. eyepiece.
    C. objective.
    D. specimen coverslip.

14. Which type of microscopy converts differences in refractive index into variations in light intensity to obtain the specimen image?
    A. Brightfield
    B. Interference contrast
    C. Phase-contrast
    D. Polarizing

15. A birefringent substance is one that
    A. vibrates light in all directions.
    B. vibrates light at two different wavelengths.
    C. refracts light in two different directions.
    D. shifts light one-half wavelength out of phase.

16. Which type of microscopy is able to produce three-dimensional images and perform optical sectioning?
    A. Brightfield
    B. Interference contrast
    C. Phase-contrast
    D. Polarizing

17. The principle of fluorescence microscopy is based on
    A. a substance that causes the rotation of polarized light.
    B. differences in the optical light path being converted to intensity differences.
    C. differences in refractive index being converted into variations in light intensity.
    D. the absorption of light and its subsequent emission at a longer wavelength.

18. Converting a brightfield microscope for polarizing microscopy requires
    A. two polarizing filters—one placed below the condenser and one placed between the objective and the eyepiece.
    B. a special condenser, two polarizing filters, and a Wollaston prism between the objective and the eyepiece.
    C. an annular diaphragm in the condenser and a phase-shifting element in the objective.
    D. a slit aperture below the condenser, a polarizing filter, and a modulator.

19. Which type of microscopy uses a special condenser to direct light onto the specimen from oblique angles only?
    A. Darkfield
    B. Interference contrast
    C. Phase-contrast
    D. Polarizing

20. Match the type of microscopy with the characteristic.

    Characteristic
    ___ A. Is the preferred technique for identifying spirochetes.
    ___ B. Is used often to visualize antigens, antibodies, and viruses.
    ___ C. Enables three-dimensional viewing of unstained, low-refractile specimens.
    ___ D. Is used to identify negative and positive birefringence.
    ___ E. Produces less haloing with thin, flat specimens.

    Microscopy Type
    1. Brightfield
    2. Darkfield
    3. Fluorescence
    4. Phase-contrast
    5. Polarizing
    6. Interference contrast

REFERENCES

1. Nikon Microscopy U: Microscope Alignment for Köhler Illumination (website): http://www.microscopyu.com/tutorials/java/kohler/index.html. Accessed July 7, 2011.
2. Hoffman R: The modulation contrast microscope: principles and performance. J Microsc 110:205-222, 1977.

BIBLIOGRAPHY

Abramowitz MJ: Koehler illumination. Am Lab 21:106, 1989.
Abramowitz MJ: Microscope objectives. Am Lab 21:81, 1989.
Abramowitz MJ: The first order red compensator. Am Lab 21:110, 1989.
Abramowitz MJ: Fluorescence filters. Am Lab 22:168, 1990.
Abramowitz MJ: The polarizing microscope. Am Lab 22:72, 1990.
Abramowitz MJ: Darkfield illumination. Am Lab 23:60, 1991.
Brown B: Basic laboratory techniques. In Hematology: principles and procedures, ed 5, Philadelphia, 1988, Lea & Febiger.
Foster B, ASCLS: Optimizing light microscopy for biological and clinical laboratories, Dubuque, IA, 1997, Kendall/Hunt Publishing.
Mollring FK: Microscopy from the very beginning, Oberkochen, West Germany, 1981, Carl Zeiss.
Olympus instruction manual: differential interference contrast attachment for transmitted light model BH2-NIC, AX5349, Tokyo, 1988, Olympus Optical Company.
Olympus Microscopy Resource Center: Interactive Java tutorials (website): http://www.olympusmicro.com/primer/java/index.html. Accessed July 7, 2011.
Physician's office laboratory guidelines, tentative guideline, POL 1-T, Villanova, PA, 1989, National Committee for Clinical Laboratory Standards.
Smith RF: Microscopy and photomicroscopy: a working manual, ed 2, Boca Raton, FL, 1994, CRC Press.

Quality Assurance and Safety

LEARNING OBJECTIVES

After studying this chapter, the student should be able to:

1. Define and explain the importance of quality assurance in the laboratory.
2. Identify and explain preanalytical, analytical, and postanalytical components of quality assurance.
3. Differentiate between internal and external quality assurance and discuss how each contributes to an overall quality assurance program.
4. Define and discuss the importance of the following:
   - Critical values
   - Documentation
   - Ethical behavior
   - Preventive maintenance
   - Technical competence
   - Test utilization
   - Turnaround time
5. Discuss the relationship of the Occupational Safety and Health Administration to safety and health in the workplace.
6. Define and give an example of the following terms:
   - Biological hazard
   - Chemical hazard
   - Decontamination
   - Personal protective equipment (PPE)
7. Describe a Standard Precautions policy and state its purpose.
8. Discuss the three primary routes of transmission of infectious agents and a means of controlling each route in the clinical laboratory.
9. Describe appropriate procedures for the handling, disposal, decontamination, and spill control of biological hazards.
10. Discuss the source of potential chemical and fire hazards encountered in the laboratory and the procedures used to limit employee exposure to them.
11. State the purpose of and the information contained in a material safety data sheet.

CHAPTER OUTLINE

Quality Assurance
  Quality Assurance: What Is It?
  Preanalytical Components of Quality Assurance
  Analytical Components of Quality Assurance

Monitoring Analytical Components of Quality Assurance
Postanalytical Components of Quality Assurance

Safety in the Urinalysis Laboratory
  Biological Hazards
  Chemical Hazards
  Other Hazards

KEY TERMS

biological hazard A biological material or an entity contaminated with biological material that is potentially capable of transmitting disease.

Chemical Hygiene Plan An established protocol developed by each facility for the identification, handling, storage, and disposal of all hazardous chemicals. The Occupational Safety and Health Administration established the plan in January 1990 as a mandatory requirement for all facilities that deal with chemical hazards.

critical value A patient test result representing a life-threatening condition that requires immediate attention and intervention.

decontamination A process to remove a potential chemical or biological hazard from an area or entity (e.g., countertop, instrument, materials) and render the area or entity "safe." One may use various processes in decontamination, such as autoclaving, incineration, chemical neutralization, and disinfecting agents.

documentation A written record. In the laboratory, documentation includes written policies and procedures, quality control, and maintenance records. Documentation may encompass the recording of any action performed or observed, including verbal correspondence, observations, and corrective actions taken.

external quality assurance The use of materials (e.g., specimens, Kodachrome slides) from an external unbiased source to monitor and determine whether quality goals (i.e., test results) are being achieved. Results are compared with results from other facilities performing the same function. Proficiency surveys are one form of external quality assurance.

infectious waste disposal policy A procedure outlining the equipment, materials, and steps used in the collection, storage, removal, and decontamination of infectious materials and substances.

material safety data sheet (MSDS) A written document provided by the manufacturer or distributor of a chemical substance listing information about the characteristics of that chemical. An MSDS includes the identity and hazardous ingredients of the chemical, its physical and chemical properties including reactivity, any physical or health hazards, and precautions for safe handling, storage, and disposal of the chemical.

Occupational Safety and Health Administration (OSHA) Established by Congress in 1970, OSHA is a division of the U.S. Department of Labor that is responsible for defining potential safety and health hazards in the workplace, establishing guidelines to safeguard all workers from these hazards, and monitoring compliance with these guidelines. The intent is to alert, educate, and protect all employees in every environment from potential safety and health hazards.

personal protective equipment Items used to eliminate exposure of the body to potentially infectious agents. These barriers include protective gowns, gloves, eye and face protectors, biosafety cabinets (fume hoods), and splash shields.

preventive maintenance The performance of specific tasks in a timely fashion to eliminate equipment failure. These tasks vary with the instrument and include cleaning procedures, inspection of components, and component replacement when necessary.

procedure manual A written document describing in detail all aspects of each policy and procedure performed in the laboratory. For example, the manual includes supplies needed, reagent preparation procedures, specimen requirements, mislabeled and unlabeled specimen protocols, procedures for the storage and disposal of wastes, technical procedures, quality control criteria, reporting formats, and references.

quality assurance An established protocol of policies and procedures for all laboratory actions performed to ensure the quality of services (i.e., test results) rendered.

quality control materials Materials used to assess and monitor the accuracy and precision (i.e., analytical error) of a method.

Standard Precautions One tier of the *Guidelines for Isolation*

Precautions from the Healthcare Infection Control Practices Advisory Committee (HICPAC) and the Centers for Disease Control and Prevention (CDC) that describes procedures to prevent transmission of infectious agents when obtaining, handling, storing, or disposing of all blood, body fluid, or body substances, regardless of patient identity or patient health status. All body fluids including secretion and excretions should be treated as potentially infectious.

technical competence The ability of an individual to perform a skilled task correctly. Technical competence also includes the ability to evaluate results, such as recognizing discrepancies and absurdities.

test utilization The frequency with which a test is performed on a single individual and how it is used to evaluate a disease process. Repeat testing of an individual is costly and may not provide additional or useful information. Sometimes a different test may provide more diagnostically useful information.

turnaround time To the laboratorian, the time that elapses from receipt of the specimen in the laboratory to reporting of test results on that specimen. Physicians and nursing personnel assign a broader time frame.

QUALITY ASSURANCE

Quality Assurance: What Is It?

Quality assurance (QA) is a program of checks and balances designed to ensure the quality of a laboratory's services. All laboratorians must be aware of the effects that their services have on the diagnosis and treatment of patients. These services must be monitored to ensure that they are appropriate and effective, and that they meet established standards for laboratory practice. The QA program must involve a mechanism for the detection of problems and must provide an opportunity to improve services. In essence, "quality assurance is a broad spectrum of plans, policies, and procedures that

together provide an administrative structure for a laboratory's efforts to achieve quality goals."[1] On a larger scale, all components of health care, including physicians, nurses, clinics, hospitals, and their services, are involved in QA. The laboratory is only part of a larger program to ensure quality health care.

Quality assurance has been an important part of the clinical laboratory since the first laboratory surveys of the 1940s. These early surveys revealed that not all laboratories reported the same results on identical blood specimens submitted for hematologic and chemical analyses. Since the time of those first surveys, all sections of the clinical laboratory have become involved in ensuring the quality, accuracy, and precision of the laboratory results they generate. The urinalysis laboratory is no exception.

A QA program encompasses all aspects of the urinalysis laboratory. Specimen collection, storage, and handling; instrumentation use and maintenance; reagent quality and preparation; and the laboratorian's knowledge and technical skills must meet specific minimum criteria to ensure the quality of the results generated. To achieve the goals set forth in a QA program, a commitment by all laboratory personnel, including those in administration and management, is necessary. This dedication must be evident in management decisions, including the allocation of laboratory space, the purchase of equipment and supplies, and the budget. Without adequate resources, the quality of laboratory services is compromised. Properly educated and experienced laboratory personnel with a high level of evaluative skills are essential to ensure the quality of laboratory results. "Many studies have shown that the standards of specimen collection technique and analytical performance are generally inferior to those obtained by skilled laboratorians."[2] Because of the dynamic environment of clinical laboratory science, it is imperative that laboratorians have access to reference books and opportunities for continuing education to assist them in skill maintenance and development. Not only do continuing education opportunities provide intellectual stimulation and challenges for laboratorians, they also facilitate the development of quality employees and ensure that maintenance of the urinalysis laboratory is kept abreast of technological advances.

A QA program for the urinalysis laboratory consists of three principal aspects: (1) preanalytical components—procedures that occur before testing; (2) analytical components—aspects that directly affect testing; and (3) postanalytical components—procedures and policies that affect reporting and interpretation of results. Because an error in any component will directly affect the quality of results, each component must be monitored, evaluated, and maintained.

Preanalytical Components of Quality Assurance

The preanalytical components involve numerous laboratory and ancillary staff and, in many instances, multiple departments. Because of the importance of cost-effective practices in test ordering, the laboratory plays a role in monitoring test utilization, that is, avoiding duplicate testing and ensuring test appropriateness whenever possible. Each laboratory is unique, and procedures to intercept and eliminate unnecessary testing must be designed to fit the workflow of each laboratory.

The importance of timely result reporting cannot be overemphasized. A delay in specimen transport and processing directly affects specimen **turnaround time**. The definition of turnaround time differs for the laboratorian as opposed to physicians or nursing personnel. For example, a laboratorian defines turnaround time as the time from receipt of the specimen in the laboratory to reporting of results to a patient care area or into a data information system. In contrast, physicians view turnaround time as the time from when they write the order for the test until the result is communicated to them for action. To nursing personnel, turnaround time is the time that elapses from actual specimen collection until the results are communicated to them. To monitor and address potential delays that directly involve the laboratory, a policy for the documentation of specimen collection, receipt, and result report times is necessary.

Specimen collection techniques differ, are often controlled by medical personnel outside of the laboratory, and can have a direct effect on laboratory results. In addition, numerous factors can affect the urine specimen obtained (e.g., diet, exercise, hydration, medications), and appropriate patient preparation may be needed. To ensure an appropriate specimen, collection instructions (including special precautions and appropriate labeling) must be well written and must be distributed to and used by all personnel involved in specimen collection.

Laboratory staff who receive specimens must be educated to identify and handle inappropriate or unacceptable specimens. In addition, they must document any problems encountered, so that these problems can be addressed and corrected. The procedure the staff should follow involves (1) correlation of the patient's name on the request slip with the patient's name on the specimen container; (2) evaluation of elapsed time between collection and receipt of the specimen in the laboratory; (3) the suitability of specimen preservation, if necessary; and (4) the acceptability of the specimen (e.g., the volume collected, the container used, its cleanliness, any evidence of fecal contamination). If the specimen is not acceptable, a procedure must be in place to ensure that the physician or nursing staff is informed of the problem, the problem or discrepancy is documented, and appropriate action is taken. Written guidelines that give the criteria for specimen rejection, as well as the procedure for handling of mislabeled specimens, are required to ensure consistent treatment by all personnel (Box 2-1 and Table 2-1).

Processing of urine specimens within the laboratory is another potential source of preanalytical problems.

BOX 2-1 | Criteria for Urine Specimen Rejection

- Insufficient volume of urine for requested test(s)
- Inappropriate specimen type or collection
- Visibly contaminated (e.g., by fecal material, debris) specimen
- Incorrect urine preservative
- Specimen not properly preserved for transportation delay
- Unlabeled or mislabeled specimen or request form
- Request form incomplete or lacking

TABLE 2-1	Definitions and an Example of Policy for Handling Unlabeled or Mislabeled Specimens
Definitions	
Unlabeled	No patient identification is placed directly on the container or tube containing the specimen. To place the label on the plastic bag that holds the specimen is inadequate.
Mislabeled	The name or identification number on the specimen label does not agree with that on the test request form.
Policy Features	
Notification	Contact the originating nursing station or clinic and indicate that the specimen must be recollected. Document the name of the individual contacted.
Document	Order the requested test and write CANCEL on the document with the appropriate reason for the cancellation, that is, specimen unlabeled or specimen mislabeled, identification questionable. Initiate an incident report and include names, dates, times, and all circumstances.
Specimen	Do not discard the specimen. Process and perform analyses on those specimens that cannot be saved, but do not report the results. Properly store all other specimens. On specimens that cannot be recollected (e.g., cerebrospinal fluid): 1. The patient's physician must: • contact the appropriate laboratory supervisor and request approval for tests on the "questionable" specimen • sign documentation of the incident 2. The individual who obtained the specimen must come to the laboratory to: • identify the specimen • properly label the specimen or correctly label the test request form • sign documentation of the incident
Reporting Results	All labeling and signing of documentation must take place before results are released (except in cases of life-threatening emergencies, for example, cardiac arrest, when verbal specimen identification is acceptable and the documentation is completed later). All reported results must include comments describing the incident. For example, "Specimen was improperly labeled, but was approved for testing. The reported value may not be from this patient."
Quality Assurance Report	Forward a copy of the incident to the Quality Assurance committee and to the patient care unit involved (e.g., nursing station, clinic, physician's office).

One should process routine urinalysis specimens immediately to prevent changes in specimen integrity; if delay at the reception area is unavoidable, one must protect the specimens from light and refrigerate them. Timed urine collections require a written protocol to ensure adequate mixing, volume measurement, recording, aliquoting, and preservation if specimen testing is to be delayed. With a written procedure for specimen processing in place, all personnel will perform these tasks consistently, thereby eliminating unnecessary variables.

Because of the multitude of variables and personnel involved in urine specimen collection and processing, adequate training and supervision are imperative. Written procedures must be available; personnel must adhere to equipment manuals and maintenance schedules; personnel must have had appropriate education regarding universal blood and body fluid precautions; and communication to personnel regarding all procedure changes or introduction of new procedures must be consistent. Preanalytical components are a dynamic part of the clinical laboratory and require adherence to protocol to ensure meaningful test results.

Analytical Components of Quality Assurance

Analytical components are those variables that are involved directly in laboratory testing. They include reagents and supplies, instrumentation, analytical methods, monitoring of analytical methods, and the laboratory personnel's technical skills. Because each component is capable of affecting test results, procedures must be developed and followed to ensure acceptable quality.

Equipment. All equipment—such as glassware, pipettes, analytical balances, centrifuges, refrigerators, freezers, microscopes, and refractometers—requires routine monitoring to ensure appropriate function, calibration, and adherence to prescribed minimal standards. **Preventive maintenance** schedules to eliminate equipment failure and downtime are also important aspects of a QA program and should be included in the laboratory procedure manual. Use of instrument maintenance sheets for documentation provides a visual format to remind the staff of maintenance requirements and to record the performance of periodic maintenance. Because the bench technologist is the first individual to be aware of an instrument failure, troubleshooting and "out-of-control" protocols including service and repair documentation should be readily available in the urinalysis laboratory.

The required frequency of maintenance differs depending on the equipment used; the protocol should meet the minimal standards set forth in guidelines provided by The Joint Commission (TJC) (formerly the Joint Commission on Accreditation of Health Care Organizations

TABLE 2-2	Urinalysis Equipment Performance Checks	
Equipment	Frequency	Checks Performed
Automatic pipettes	Initially and periodically thereafter; varies with usage (e.g., monthly)	Check for accuracy and reproducibility.
Balances, analytical	Periodically (e.g., quarterly)	Check with standard weights (National Bureau of Standards Class S).
	Annually	Service and clean.
Centrifuges	Daily	Clean rotor, trunnions, and interior with suitable disinfectant.
	Periodically (e.g., annually)	Check revolutions per minute and timer.
	Periodically	Change brushes whenever needed; frequency varies with centrifuge type and usage.
Fume hoods (i.e., biosafety cabinets)	Periodically (e.g., annually)	Airflow
Microscopes	Daily	Clean and adjust if necessary (e.g., Köhler illumination, phase ring adjustment).
	Annually	Service and clean.
Osmometers	Daily	Determine and record osmolality of control materials.
Reagent strip readers	Daily	Calibrate reflectance meter with standard reagent strip.
	Daily (or periodically)	Clean mechanical parts and optics.
Refractometers	Daily	Read and record deionized water (SG 1.000) and at least one standard of known SG. For example, NaCl 3% (SG 1.015), 5% (SG 1.022), 7% (SG 1.035); or sucrose 9% (1.034). Acceptable tolerance: target $\pm$ 0.001.
Temperature-dependent devices, (e.g., refrigerators, freezers, water baths, incubators)	Daily (or when used)	Read and record temperature.
Thermometers	Initially and annually thereafter	Check against NIST-certified thermometer.

NIST, National Institute of Standards and Technology; *SG,* Specific gravity.

[JCAHO]) or the College of American Pathologists (CAP). Table 2-2 lists equipment often present in the urinalysis laboratory along with the frequency and types of performance checks that should be performed. For example, temperature-dependent devices are monitored and recorded daily, as are refractometers and osmometers. Whereas centrifuges should be cleaned daily, the accuracy of their timers and speed (revolutions per minute) can be checked periodically. Automatic pipettes, analytical balances, and fume hoods also require periodic checks, which are determined by the individual laboratory and often vary according to usage. Microscopes require daily cleaning and sometimes adjustments (e.g., illumination, phase ring alignment) to ensure optimal viewing. Microscopes and balances should undergo annual preventive maintenance and cleaning by professional service engineers to avoid potential problems and costly repairs. A current CAP inspection checklist is an excellent resource for developing an individualized procedure for performing periodic checks and routine maintenance on equipment, and for providing guidelines on the documentation necessary in the urinalysis laboratory.

Reagents. Reliable analytical results obtained in the urinalysis laboratory require the use of quality reagents. The laboratory must have an adequate supply of distilled water, deionized water, or clinical laboratory reagent water (CLRW). Each urinalysis procedure should specify the type and quality of water required for tasks such as reagent preparation or reconstitution of lyophilized materials. The quality of CLRW requires periodic monitoring for ionic and organic impurities as well as for microbial contamination[3] In addition, because CLRW absorbs carbon dioxide, thereby losing its resistivity on storage, it should be obtained fresh daily. CLRW quality tolerance limits and the actions to be taken when these quality limits are exceeded must also be available in a written policy.

Reagent-grade or analytical reagent–grade reagents should be used when reagent solutions are prepared for qualitative or quantitative procedures. Primary standards for quantitative methods, must be made from chemicals of the highest grade available. These can be purchased from manufacturers or agencies such as the National Institute of Standards and Technology (NIST) (formerly the National Bureau of Standards [NBS]) or CAP and can be accurately weighed to produce a standard of a known concentration. From these primary standards, secondary standards or calibration solutions can be made. Any solvents used should be of sufficient purity to ensure appropriate reactivity and to prevent interfering side reactions.

Standard laboratory practice is to check all newly prepared standards and reagents before using them. This is done by analyzing a control material using new and old standards or reagents. If performance of the new standard or reagent is equivalent to performance of the old, it is acceptable and dated as approved for use; if it performs inadequately, it should be discarded and the reagent or standard remade. New lot numbers of commercially prepared reagents and standards, as well as different bottles of a current lot number, must be checked against older, proven reagents before they are placed into use. Documentation of standard and reagent checks must be maintained in the urinalysis laboratory. All standards, reagents, reagent strips, and tablets, whether made in the laboratory or commercially obtained, must be dated when prepared or received, and when their performance is checked and determined to be acceptable. Ensuring the quality of commercial reagent strips and tablet tests used in the urinalysis laboratory is discussed in Chapter 7.

Procedure Manuals. **Procedure manuals** must be available in the urinalysis laboratory and should comply with the Clinical and Laboratory Standards Institute (CLSI) (formerly the National Committee for Clinical Laboratory Standards [NCCLS]) approved guideline GP02-A5 Laboratory Documents: Development and Control.[4] Each manual should be comprehensive and should include details of all procedures performed, proper specimen collection and handling procedures, test principles, reagent preparation, control materials and acceptance criteria, step-by-step performance procedures, calculations, reporting of results, and references. Because the procedure manual is vital to the laboratory, it must be reviewed continually, updated, and adhered to in the performance of all tests. The manual must show documentation of any procedural changes and must be reviewed annually. A well-written procedure manual provides a ready and reliable reference for the veteran technologist, as well as an informational training tool for the novice. The importance of procedure manuals cannot be overemphasized, because uniform performance of testing methods ensures accurate and reproducible results, regardless of changes in personnel.

A routine urinalysis incorporates methods to ensure consistent quality in each of its components. The laboratory procedure manual details all examinations—physical, chemical, and microscopic—and includes quality control checks, acceptable terminology, and tolerances for each. The manual also provides steps to follow when tolerances are exceeded or results are questionable. In addition, procedures include criteria for the correlation of physical, chemical, and microscopic examinations, as well as follow-up actions if discrepancies are discovered. (For instance, if the blood reagent strip test is negative and the microscopic examination reveals red blood cells, the specimen should be checked for ascorbic acid.) Reference materials such as textbooks, atlases, and charts must be available for convenient consultation.

BOX 2-2	Guidelines for Standardizing Microscopic Urinalysis

Procedural Factors
1. Volume of urine examined (10, 12, 15 mL)
2. Speed of centrifugation (400× g, 600× g)
3. Length of centrifugation (3, 5, 10 minutes)
4. Concentration of sediment (10:1, 12:1, 15:1)
5. Volume of sediment examined (0.4, 0.5, 1.0 mL)

Reporting Factors
1. Each laboratory should publish its own normal values (based on system used and patient population).
2. All personnel must use same terminology.
3. All personnel must report results in standard format.
4. All abnormal results should be flagged for easy reference.

From Schweitzer SC, Schumann JL, Schumann GB: Quality assurance guidelines for the urinalysis laboratory. J Med Technol 3:570, 1986.

Monitoring. The microscopic examination requires standardization of technique and adherence to the established procedure by all technologists to ensure consistency in results obtained and in their reporting. Preparing urine for manual microscopy requires written step-by-step instructions that detail the volume of urine to use, the centrifuge speed, the time of centrifugation, the sediment concentration, and the volume of sediment examined, as well as the reporting format, terminology, and grading criteria (Box 2-2). Several standardized manual microscopic slides (e.g., KOVA [Hycor Biomedical Inc, Garden Grove, CA], Urisystem [Fisher Scientific, Waltham, MA]) are commercially available, and all are superior to the traditional glass slide and coverslip technique.[5] In contrast, automated microscopy instruments such as the iQ200 (Iris Diagnostics, Chatsworth, CA) and the UF1000i (bioMérieux, Marcy l'Etoile, France) require minimal specimen preparation and have good accuracy and precision; their performance is easily monitored and documented using quality control materials.

Because many of the procedures performed in the urinalysis laboratory are done manually, it is very important to monitor **technical competence.** Uniformity of technique by all personnel is necessary and can be achieved through (1) proper training, (2) adherence to established protocols, and (3) performance of quality control checks. New technologists should have their technical performance evaluated before they perform routine clinical tests. Similarly, new procedures introduced into the laboratory should be properly researched, written, and proven before they are placed into use.

Before reporting results, technologists must be able to evaluate the results obtained, recognize discrepancies or absurdities, and seek answers or make corrections for those encountered. Performing and recording the results obtained, even when they differ from those expected or desired, is paramount. Because test results have a direct effect on patient diagnosis and treatment, the highest level of ethical behavior is required. Documentation of errors or problems and the actions taken to correct them is necessary to (1) ensure communication with staff and supervisory personnel, (2) prevent the problem from recurring, and (3) provide a paper trail of actual circumstances and corrective actions taken as a result. These policies should be viewed as a means of guaranteeing the quality of laboratory results.

Accurate results depend not only on the knowledge and technical competence of the technologist, but also on the technologist's integrity in reporting what actually is obtained. Circumstances can arise in laboratory testing that appear to contradict expected test results. When these circumstances are appropriately investigated, legitimate explanations that expand the technologist's scope of experience can be obtained. For example, a patient's test results can differ greatly from those obtained previously. Investigation may reveal that a specimen mix-up occurred, or that a drug the patient recently received is now interfering with testing. This highlights the need for good communication among all staff and supervisory personnel, as well as the need for staff meetings or "quality circles" (i.e., a small team of individuals that meet to identify problems and discuss possible solutions) to ensure the dissemination of new information.

Monitoring Analytical Components of Quality Assurance

For internal QA of testing methods, **quality control (QC) materials** are used to assess and monitor analytical error, that is, the accuracy and precision of a method. QC materials serve to alert the laboratorian of method changes that directly affect the quality of results obtained. These materials can be prepared by laboratory personnel or purchased from commercial suppliers. They mimic patient samples in their physical and chemical characteristics, that is, they have the same matrix. For some QC materials, the manufacturer determines and assigns expected values. These values should be confirmed and adjusted if necessary to reflect the method and conditions of each laboratory.

Numerous urinalysis control materials are commercially available. Some control materials monitor only the status of the qualitative chemical examination of urine using reagent strips, whereas other control materials include microscopic entities that can monitor the microscopic examination and the steps involved in processing urine specimens (e.g., centrifugation). The microscopic elements present vary with the manufacturer. Quantimetrix Corporation (Redondo Beach, CA) (DipandSpin, QuanTscopics) uses stabilized human red blood cells, white blood cells, and crystals. In contrast, Hycor Biomedical Inc. (Garden Grove, CA) (KOVA-Trol) includes stabilized red blood cells, organic particles (mulberry spores) to simulate white blood cells, and crystals.

Another means of monitoring the entire urinalysis procedure is to select a well-mixed urine specimen and have each technologist or one from each shift of workers perform the procedure. This provides an intra-laboratory or in-house quality assessment. Results should be recorded and evaluated independently. When multiple laboratory sites within a facility perform urinalysis testing, personnel at each site can test an aliquot of the same urine specimen and compare results. If commercial control materials with sediment constituents are not used to evaluate the microscopic examination, in-house duplicate testing can be instrumental in detecting subtle changes in the processing procedure, such as alterations in centrifugation speed or time. The time and effort involved in intralaboratory testing are worthwhile because it ensures that each laboratory and all staff are consistently obtaining equivalent results.

Results obtained on control materials, as well as from duplicate specimen testing, are recorded daily in a tabular or graphic format. The tolerance limits for these results must be defined, documented, and readily available in the laboratory. When these tolerances are exceeded, corrective action must be taken and documented.

Whether the urinalysis laboratory performs quantitative urine procedures (e.g., total protein, creatinine) depends on the facility. In some settings, the urinalysis laboratory performs only the manual quantitative procedures, whereas the chemistry section performs those procedures that are automated. Regardless, a brief discussion of the QC materials used for quantitative urine methods is necessary. The value assigned to commercial or homemade QC materials is determined in the laboratory by performing repeated analyses over different days. This enables variables such as personnel, reagents, and supplies to be represented in the data generated. After analyses are complete, QC data are tabulated and control limits determined by using the mean and standard deviation (SD). Initial control (or tolerance) limits can be established using a minimum of 20 determinations; as more data are accumulated, the limits can be revised. Because the error distribution is gaussian, control limits are chosen such that 95% to 99% of control values will be within tolerance. This corresponds to the mean value ± 2 SD or ± 3 SD, respectively. Graphs of the QC values obtained over time are plotted and are known as QC or Levey-Jennings control charts. They provide an easy, visual means of identifying changes in accuracy and precision. Changes in accuracy are evidenced by a shift in the mean, whereas changes in precision (random error) are manifested by an increase in scatter or a widening of the distribution of values about the mean (standard deviation).

External quality assurance measures (e.g., proficiency surveys) monitor and evaluate a laboratory's performance as compared with other facilities. These QA measures may take the form of proficiency testing or participation in programs in which each laboratory uses the same lot of QC materials. The latter is used primarily with quantitative urine methods. Monthly, the results obtained by each laboratory are reported to the manufacturer of the QC material. Within weeks, reports summarizing the analytical methods used and the results obtained by each laboratory are distributed. These reports are useful in detecting small continuous changes in systematic error in quantitative methods that may not be evident with internal quality assurance procedures.

For a laboratory to be accredited, periodic interlaboratory comparison testing in the form of proficiency surveys is required by the Clinical Laboratory Improvement Act of 1988 (CLIA 88). This comparison testing involves the performance of routine tests on survey samples provided for a fee to participating laboratories. Each laboratory independently performs and submits results to the survey agency (e.g., CAP, Centers for Disease Control and Prevention [CDC]) for assessment and tabulation. Before distribution of the survey samples, the target value of each sample is determined by testing at selected or reference laboratories. Using the reference laboratory target values and results submitted by the participant laboratories, the survey agency prepares extensive reports and charts for each analyte assessed, the method used, and the values obtained. These surveys provide valuable information on laboratory performance and testing methods—individually, by specific method, and as a whole.

Some urinalysis proficiency surveys include digital images or photographic slides for the identification of urine sediment components, such as casts, epithelial cells, blood cells, and artifacts. One approach used to evaluate these urine sediment images is for each technologist in the laboratory to independently identify the sediment component. Results are reviewed and shared, and a single answer is ultimately submitted to the survey agency. Although limited, this approach enables evaluation of competence in microscopic identification. In addition, if the process of arriving at an answer by consensus is used, it provides an opportunity to maintain and improve the competence of personnel.

Although QC materials and proficiency testing samples help to detect decreased quality in laboratory testing, they do not pinpoint the source of the problem, nor do they solve it. Only with good communication and **documentation** can analytical problems be pursued and continuing education programs developed. Some problems encountered in the laboratory may be approached best by the development of a quality circle team. The involvement of laboratorians in a problem-solving team reaffirms the technologists' self-worth and enhances their commitment to quality goals.

Postanalytical Components of Quality Assurance

Urinalysis results can be communicated efficiently and effectively using a standardized reporting format and terminology. The report should include reference ranges and the ability to add informative statements if warranted, for example, "glucose oxidase/reducing substances questionable owing to the presence of ascorbic acid" or "clumps of white blood cells present." Results should be quantitative (e.g., 100 mg/dL or 10 to 25 RBCs/HPF [red blood cells per high-power field]) wherever possible. All personnel should use the same (i.e., standardized) terminology for test parameters (e.g., color or clarity terms).

Laboratory procedures should describe in detail the appropriate reporting format and should provide criteria for the reporting of any critical values. **Critical values** are significantly abnormal results that exceed the upper or lower critical limit and are life threatening. These results need to be relayed immediately to the health care provider for appropriate action. The laboratorian is responsible for recognizing critical values and communicating them in a timely fashion. Each institution must establish its own list of critical values. For example, the list might include as critical the presence of pathologic urine crystals (e.g., cystine, leucine, tyrosine); a strongly positive test for glucose and ketones; and the presence of a reducing substance, other than glucose or ascorbic acid, in an infant.

Quality assurance measures, whether internal (QC materials) or external (proficiency surveys), require documentation and evidence of active review. When acceptable tolerances are exceeded, they must be recorded and corrective action taken. In the clinical laboratory, documentation is crucial because an action that was not documented essentially has not been performed. The goal of an effective QA program is to obtain consistently accurate and reproducible results. In achieving this goal, test results will reflect the patient's condition, rather than results modified due to procedural or personnel variations.

SAFETY IN THE URINALYSIS LABORATORY

For years the health care industry has been at the forefront in developing policies and procedures to prevent and control the spread of infection in all areas of the hospital to ensure patient and employee safety. Because clinical laboratory employees are exposed to numerous workplace hazards in various forms—biological, chemical, electrical, radioactive, compressed gases, fires, and so on—safety policies are an integral part of the laboratory. With passage of the Occupational Health and Safety Act in 1970, formal regulation of safety and health for all employees, regardless of employer, officially began. This law is administered through the U.S. Department of Labor by the **Occupational Safety and Health Administration (OSHA)**. As a result of the law, written manuals that define specific safety policies and procedures for all potential hazards are required in laboratories. Guidelines for developing these written policies and procedures are provided in several Clinical and Laboratory Standards Institute (CLSI) documents.[6,7,8] An additional requirement of the law is that all employees must document annual review of the safety manual. The next section discusses hazards frequently encountered in the clinical laboratory when working with urine and other body fluids (e.g., feces, amniotic fluid, cerebrospinal fluid), as well as the policies and procedures necessary to ensure a safe and healthy working environment.

Biological Hazards

Biological hazards abound in the clinical laboratory. Today, any patient specimen or body substance (e.g., body fluid, fresh tissue, excretions, secretions, sputum, drainage) is considered infectious, regardless of patient diagnosis. Table 2-3 provides a brief history and key points of safety guidelines and regulations implemented to prevent the transmission of infectious agents in hospitals. In the 1980s, the transmission of disease such as human immunodeficiency virus (HIV), hepatitis B virus (HBV), and hepatitis C virus (HCV) became a major concern for health care workers. To address the issue, in 1987, the Centers for Disease Control and Prevention (CDC) issued practice guidelines known as **Universal Precautions (UP).** UP was intended to protect health care workers, primarily from patients with these bloodborne diseases. Under UP, body fluids and secretions that did not contain visible blood were exempt. At this same time, another system of isolation was proposed and refined; this was called Body Substance Isolation (BSI).[9,10] BSI and UP had similar features to prevent the transmission of bloodborne pathogens but differed with regard to handwashing after glove use. UP recommended handwashing after the removal of gloves, whereas BSI indicated that handwashing was not required unless the hands were visibly soiled. Then in 1991, OSHA enacted the Bloodborne Pathogens Standard (BPS) to address occupational exposure of health care workers to infectious agents, primarily HIV, hepatitis viruses, and retroviruses. BPS requires laboratories to have an exposure control plan that regulates work practices such as handling of needles and sharps and requires hepatitis B vaccinations, training, and other measures.[11,14,15]

This became a time of confusion with hospitals differing in their isolation protocols, as well as in the handling of body fluids and other substances. It was recognized that UP guidelines alone were inadequate because infectious body fluids do not always have or show visible blood. To resolve this conundrum, the Healthcare Infection Control Practices Advisory Committee (HICPAC) and the CDC issued in 1996 a new two-tier practice guideline known as Standard Precautions and Transmission-Based Precautions.[12,13] **Standard Precautions** are infection prevention practices that are applied to all patients in all health care settings and that address not only the protection of health care personnel, but the prevention of patient-to-patient and healthcare worker-to-patient transmission (i.e., nosocomial transmission) of infectious agents. It combines the major features of UP and BSI into a single guideline with feasible recommendations to prevent disease transmission. Standard Precautions also dictate that standards or calibrators, quality control materials, and proficiency testing materials be handled like all other laboratory specimens.[6] The Transmission-Based Precautions of the guideline apply to specific patients with known or suspected infections or colonization with infectious agents (e.g., vancomycin-resistant enterococcus [VRE]). Three categories of transmission-based precautions in the hospital are described and include contact precautions, droplet precautions, and airborne precautions. These additional precautions are used when the potential for disease transmission from these patients or their body fluids is not completely interrupted by using Standard Precautions alone.

It is important to note that Standard Precautions do not affect other necessary types of infection control strategies, such as identification and handling of infectious laboratory specimens or waste during shipment; protocols for disinfection, sterilization, or decontamination; or laundry procedures.[6]

Traditionally, the three routes of infection or disease transmission are (1) inhalation, (2) ingestion, and (3) direct inoculation or skin contact. In the laboratory, aerosols can be created and inhaled when liquids (e.g., body fluids) are poured, pipetted, or spilled. Similarly, centrifugation of samples and removal of tight-fitting caps from specimen containers are potential sources of airborne transmission. Ingestion occurs when infectious agents are taken into the mouth and swallowed, as from eating, drinking, or smoking in the laboratory; mouth pipetting; or hand-to-mouth contact following failure to appropriately wash one's hands. Direct inoculation involves parenteral exposure to the infectious agent as a result of a break in the technologist's skin barrier or contact with the mucous membranes. This includes skin punctures with needles, cuts or scratches from contaminated glassware, and splashes of specimens into the eyes, nose, and mouth. Although it is impossible to eliminate all sources of infectious transmission in the laboratory, the use of protective barriers and adherence to Standard Precautions minimize transmission.

Under Standard Precautions, *all body fluids, secretions, and excretions* (except sweat) are considered potentially infectious and capable of disease transmission. Key components of Standard Precautions are good hand hygiene and the use of barriers (physical, mechanical, or chemical) between potential sources of an infectious agent and individuals. All personnel must adhere to Standard Precautions including ancillary health care staff such as custodial and food service employees, as well as health care volunteers. It is a responsibility of

TABLE 2-3	Selected Evolution History of Isolation Precautions in Hospitals[7,8]	
Year	**Guideline or Regulation**	**Key Points**
1985–1988	Universal Precautions (UP)	• Established in response to HIV/AIDS epidemic • Initiated the application of blood and body fluid precautions to *all* patients • Exempted some specimens from precautions, namely, urine, feces, nasal secretions, sputum, sweat, tears, and vomitus *unless visible blood present* • Included the use of personal protective equipment (PPE) by health care workers to prevent mucous membrane exposures • Recommended handwashing after glove removal • Included recommendations for the handling and disposal of needles and other sharps

1987	Body Substance Isolation (BSI)[9,10]	• Emphasized avoiding contact with potentially infectious, moist body fluids (except sweat), *regardless* of the presence or absence of blood
		• Similar to UP recommendations for the prevention of bloodborne pathogen transmission
		• Handwashing after glove removal *not required* unless hands visibly soiled
		• Inadequate provisions to prevent:
		  • Some droplet transmissions
		  • Direct or indirect contact transmission from dry skin or environmental sources
		  • Airborne droplet nuclei transmission of infection (e.g., tuberculosis) over long distances

1991,[11] (1999,[14] 2001[15])	Bloodborne Pathogens Standard[11,14,15]; OSHA	• Aimed at reducing health care worker exposure to bloodborne pathogens—HIV, hepatitis viruses, and retroviruses—when caring for patients with known infection
		• Requires *employer* to have an Exposure Control Plan to:
		  • Educate workers
		  • Provide necessary supplies and other measures (e.g., PPE, hepatitis B vaccination, signs and labels, medical surveillance)

1996,[12] 2007[13]	Standard Precautions and Transmission-Based Precautions; HICPAC/CDC	• Two-tier approach to prevent disease transmission that emphasizes prevention of nosocomial infection and worker safety
		• Tier 1: Standard Precautions
		  • A synthesis of UP, BSI, and 1983 CDC guidelines
		  • Applies to all body fluids, secretions, excretions (except sweat), and tissue specimens
		  • Applies to human-based standards or calibrators, quality control materials, and proficiency testing materials
		  • Applies to nonintact skin and mucous membranes of patient and health care worker
		• Tier 2: Transmission-Based Precautions
		  • Three categories: airborne, droplet, and contact
		  • Used when Standard Precautions alone are insufficient
		  • Used for patients with known or suspected infection
		• Lists specific syndromes that require temporary isolation precautions until a definitive diagnosis is made

CDC, Centers for Disease Control and Prevention; *HICPAC,* Healthcare Infection Control Practices Advisory Committee; *OSHA,* Occupational Safety and Health Administration.

each health care department to educate, implement, document, and monitor compliance with Standard Precautions. In addition, written safety and infection control policies and procedures must be readily available for reference in the laboratory.

Personal Protective Equipment. When contact with body fluids or other liquids is anticipated, appropriate **personal protective equipment** (PPE) or barriers must be used. Gloves should be worn when assisting patients in collecting specimens, when receiving and processing specimens, when performing any testing procedure, and when cleaning equipment or work areas. In addition, they should be worn at all times in the laboratory, where countertops, chairs, and other surfaces are exposed to these specimens. If the technologist is involved directly with patients, he or she should change gloves and wash or sanitize the hands after each patient. In the laboratory, gloves are changed when they are visibly soiled or physically damaged. Gloves used in the laboratory should not be worn outside of the area. Whenever gloves are removed, or when contact with urine or other body fluids has occurred, hands should be washed with an appropriate antiseptic soap.

Protective laboratory coats must be worn in the laboratory and when necessary must be impermeable to blood and other liquid samples that could be potentially infectious. Lab coats should be changed daily or more often if soiled. These coats should not be worn outside of or be removed from the laboratory area. If splashing of liquids such as urine, body fluids, or chemicals is anticipated, a moisture-resistant (plastic) apron should be worn over the lab coat.

Because processing and performing laboratory procedures on urine and body fluids can often result in sprays, splatters, or aerosols, laboratory employees should wear eyewear, headgear, or masks to protect the eyes, nose, and mouth. Eyeglasses may be sufficient for some situations in the laboratory; however, Plexiglas barriers, safety glasses or goggles, face shields, hood sashes, or particulate respirators may be necessary for protection, depending on the procedure being performed and the substance being handled.

Specimen Processing. All specimens should be transported to the laboratory in sealed plastic bags, with the request slip placed on the outside of the bag. If the outside of the specimen container is obviously contaminated because of leakage or improper collection technique, the exterior of the container can be cleaned using an appropriate disinfectant before processing, or it should be rejected and a new specimen requested. When removing lids or caps from specimens, the technologist should work behind a protective shield or should cover the specimens with gauze or disposable tissues to prevent sprays and splatters. During centrifugation, specimens should be capped or placed in covered trunnions to prevent aerosols. Centrifuges should not be operated with their tops open nor stopped by hand. If a specimen needs to be aliquoted, the technologist should use transfer pipettes or protective barriers when pouring from the specimen container.

Disposal of Waste. To protect all laboratory personnel, including custodial staff, adherence to an **infectious waste disposal policy** is necessary. Because all biological specimens and materials exposed to them (e.g., contaminated needles and glassware) are considered infectious, they must be disposed of properly. Disposal requires leakproof, well-constructed receptacles clearly marked with the universal biohazard symbol and available in all laboratory areas (Figure 2-1). These biohazard containers should not be overfilled. In addition, they should be sealed adequately and enclosed within a clean biohazard

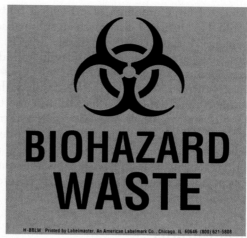

FIGURE 2-1 The universal biohazard symbol. *(Rodak BF: Hematology: clinical principles and applications, ed 2, Philadelphia, 2002, Saunders.)*

bag before removal from the laboratory area by custodial staff.

All biological specimens, except urine, must be sterilized or decontaminated before disposal. Incineration and autoclaving are acceptable, with the latter usually being the most cost-effective. Urine, on the other hand, may be discarded directly down a sink or toilet, with caution taken to avoid splashing. When discarding urine down a sink, the technologist should rinse the sink well with water after discarding specimens and at least daily with 0.5% bleach (sodium hypochlorite).

Contaminated sharps such as needles, broken glass, or transfer pipettes must be placed into puncture-resistant containers for disposal. These containers should not be overfilled. They should be sealed securely and enclosed in a clean infectious waste disposal bag to protect custodial personnel before removal from the laboratory area. Because contaminated sharps are considered infectious, they must be incinerated or autoclaved before disposal.

Noninfectious glass such as empty reagent bottles and nonhazardous waste such as emptied urine containers are considered normal waste and require no special precautions for disposal.

Decontamination. Several agents are available for the daily **decontamination** of laboratory surfaces and equipment. Bleach or a phenolic disinfectant is used most often in the clinical laboratory. A 0.5% bleach solution, prepared by adding 1 part household bleach to 9 parts water (1/10 dilution), is stable for 1 week. Phenolic disinfectants, a combination of phenolic compounds and detergents, are purchased commercially; one makes appropriate dilutions according to the manufacturers' recommendations.

When spills occur, decontaminants are used to neutralize the biological hazard and to facilitate its removal. Because decontaminants are less effective in the presence of large amounts of protein, a body fluid spill should be absorbed first with a solid absorbent powder (e.g., Zorbitrol) or disposable towels. If an absorbent powder is used, the liquid will solidify and can be scooped up and placed into an infectious waste receptacle. If disposable towels are used, allow the spill to be absorbed and pour 0.5% bleach over the towels. Carefully pick up the bleach-soaked towels and transfer them into an infectious waste container. Decontaminate the spill area again using 0.5% bleach and clean it with a phenolic detergent if desired. All disposable materials used to clean the spill area must be placed in infectious waste receptacles.

Chemical Hazards

Chemicals are ubiquitous in the clinical laboratory. Many are caustic, toxic, or flammable and must be specially handled to ensure the safety and well-being of laboratory employees. The OSHA rule of January 1990 requires each facility to have a **Chemical Hygiene Plan** that defines the safety policies and procedures for all hazardous chemicals used in the laboratory. This plan includes the identification of a chemical hygiene officer; policies for handling, storage, and use of chemicals; the use of protective barriers; criteria for monitoring over-exposure to chemicals; and provisions for medical consultations or examinations. Educating personnel about chemical safety policies and procedures is mandatory and requires a documented annual review. By developing and using a comprehensive Chemical Hygiene Plan, chemical hazards are minimized and the laboratory becomes a safe environment in which to work.

The labeling of chemicals is fundamental to a laboratory safety program. Because hazardous chemicals can be classified into several categories—including caustic or corrosive materials, poisons, carcinogens, flammables, explosives, mutagens, and teratogens—each must be appropriately labeled to ensure proper handling. All chemicals are required to have descriptive warning labels on their shipping containers. These labels are color-coded and include a pictorial representation of the hazard (Figure 2-2). However, when a chemical is removed from its original shipping container, its hazard identity is lost unless the laboratory appropriately relabels it. Although OSHA requires the labeling of hazardous chemicals, it does not mandate the type of labeling system to be used. By using a consistent identification system, hazards can be readily identified and appropriate precautions taken. The National Fire Protection Association developed the 704-M Hazard Identification System, using bright, color-coded labels divided into quadrants. These labels are highly visible and identify the health (blue), flammability (red), and reactivity (yellow) hazard for each chemical, as well as any special considerations (white). The system also uses numbers from 0 to 4 to classify hazard severity, with 4 representing extremely hazardous.

A

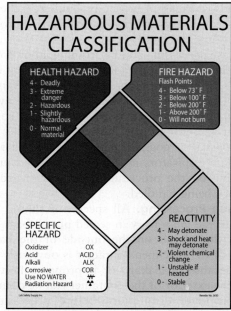

B

FIGURE 2-2 A, Label used by the Department of Transportation to indicate hazardous chemicals. **B,** The label identification system developed by the National Fire Protection Association. *(Courtesy Lab Safety Supply Inc., Janesville, WI.)*

To limit employee exposure, appropriate usage and handling guidelines for each chemical type must be described in the laboratory safety manual. General rules such as prohibiting pipetting by mouth or sniffing of chemicals are mandatory. Because the greatest hazard encountered in the clinical laboratory is that caused by the splattering of acids, alkalis, and strong oxidizers, appropriate use of personal protective equipment is required. Use of gloves, gowns, goggles, and a fume hood or safety cabinet will reduce the potential for injury. Chemical safety tips include (1) never grasp a reagent bottle by the neck or top, and (2) always add acid to water; *never add water to concentrated acid.* Safety equipment such as an eyewash and shower must be readily available and accessible in case of accidental exposure.

The goal of the OSHA hazardous communication rule is to ensure that all employees are aware of potential chemical hazards in their workplace. This employee "right to know" requires chemical manufacturers and suppliers to provide **material safety data sheets (MSDSs)**. These sheets, available for each chemical, include identity information, hazardous ingredients, physical and chemical characteristics, physical hazards, reactivity, health hazards, precautions for safe handling and use, and regulatory information of the chemical. Whereas an MSDS for each hazardous chemical used in all laboratory areas must be available on site, each laboratory section should retain copies of the MSDS for chemicals frequently used in their area for quick reference.

Handling Chemical Spills. In the event of a spill, the MSDS for the chemical should be consulted to determine the appropriate action to take. Each laboratory should have available a chemical spill kit that includes absorbent, appropriate protective barriers (e.g., gloves, goggles), cleanup pans, absorbent towels or pillows, and disposal bags. Frequently, liquids are contained by absorption using a spill compound (absorbent) such as ground clay or a sodium bicarbonate and sand mixture. The latter is generally appropriate for acid, alkali, or solvent spills. Following absorption, the absorbent is swept up and placed into a bag or a sealed container for appropriate chemical disposal, and the spill area is thoroughly washed.

For emergency treatment of personnel affected by chemical splashes or injuries, clear instructions should be posted in the laboratory. Chemical spills of hazardous substances must be reported to supervisory personnel and appropriately documented. This permits a review of the circumstances and facilitates changes to prevent recurrence of the incident. Any injury or illness resulting from the spill or exposure also requires documentation and follow-up.

Disposal of Chemical Waste. All chemicals must be disposed of properly to ensure safety in the workplace and in the environment in general. Because chemical disposal differs according to the chemical type, the amount to be discarded, and local laws, each laboratory must maintain its own policies for disposal. Following performance of laboratory procedures, chemicals often are diluted adequately or neutralized such that disposal in the sewer system is satisfactory. Flushing sinks and drains with copious amounts of water following the disposal of aqueous reagents is a good laboratory practice. Appropriate steps to be followed must be available in a general laboratory policy or in the laboratory procedure that uses the chemical.

Other Hazards

Organic solvents used in the clinical laboratory represent health and fire hazards. As a result, these flammable substances require special considerations regarding storage, use, and disposal. Appropriately vented storage cabinets are necessary to store solvents; the availability of these cabinets dictates the volume of flammables allowed to be stored on the premises. Because of potentially toxic vapors, adequate ventilation during solvent use, such as in a fume hood, is mandatory. Although small quantities of water-miscible solvents may be disposed of in the sewer system with copious amounts of water, disposal of flammable solvents in this fashion is dangerous. All solvent waste should be recovered following procedures in glass or other appropriate containers. Because not all solvents can be mixed together, a written laboratory protocol listing acceptable solvent combinations is necessary. After collection, each solvent waste container must be marked clearly with the solvent type and the relative amount present and must be properly stored until disposal.

Other potential fire hazards in the laboratory include electrical hazards and hazards from flammable compressed gases. Laboratory personnel should report any discovered deterioration in equipment (e.g., electrical shorts) or its connections (e.g., a frayed cord). If a liquid spill occurs on electrical equipment or its connections, appropriate action must be taken to dry the equipment thoroughly before placing it back into use. Compressed gases must be secured at all times, regardless of their contents or the amount of gas in the tank. Their valve caps should be in place except when in use. A procedure for appropriate transport, handling, and storage of compressed gases is necessary to ensure proper usage. All laboratory personnel must be aware of the location of all fire extinguishers, alarms, and safety equipment; must be instructed in the use of a fire extinguisher; and must be involved in laboratory fire drills, at least annually.

STUDY QUESTIONS

1. The ultimate goal of a quality assurance program is to
   A. maximize the productivity of the laboratory.
   B. ensure that patient test results are precise.
   C. ensure appropriate diagnosis and treatment of patients.
   D. ensure the validity of laboratory results obtained.
2. Which of the following is a preanalytical component of a quality assurance program?
   A. Quality control
   B. Turnaround time
   C. Technical competence
   D. Preventive maintenance

3. Which of the following is a postanalytical component of a quality assurance program?
   A. Critical values
   B. Procedure manuals
   C. Preventive maintenance
   D. Test utilization

4. Analytical components of a quality assurance program are procedures and policies that affect the
   A. technical testing of the specimen.
   B. collection and processing of the specimen.
   C. reporting and interpretation of results.
   D. diagnosis and treatment of the patient.

5. The purpose of quality control materials is to
   A. monitor instrumentation to eliminate downtime.
   B. ensure the quality of test results obtained.
   C. assess the accuracy and precision of a method.
   D. monitor the technical competence of laboratory staff.

6. Why are written procedure manuals necessary?
   A. To assist in the ordering of reagents and supplies for a procedure
   B. To appropriately monitor the accuracy and precision of a procedure
   C. To ensure that all individuals perform the same task consistently
   D. To ensure that the appropriate test has been ordered

7. Which of the following is *not* considered to be an analytical component of quality assurance?
   A. Reagents (e.g., water)
   B. Glassware (e.g., pipettes)
   C. Instrumentation (e.g., microscope)
   D. Specimen preservation (e.g., refrigeration)

8. Which of the following sources should include a protocol for the way to proceed when quality control results exceed acceptable tolerance limits?
   A. A reference book
   B. A procedure manual
   C. A preventive maintenance manual
   D. A specimen-processing protocol

9. Technical competence is displayed when a laboratory practitioner
   A. documents reports in a legible manner.
   B. recognizes discrepant test results.
   C. independently reduces the time needed to perform a procedure (e.g., by decreasing incubation times).
   D. is punctual and timely.

10. Quality control materials should have
    A. a short expiration date.
    B. a matrix similar to patient samples.
    C. their values assigned by an external and unbiased commercial manufacturer.
    D. the ability to test preanalytical variables.

11. Within one facility, what is the purpose of performing duplicate testing of a specimen by two different laboratories (i.e., in-house duplicates)?
    A. It provides little information because the results are already known.
    B. It saves money by avoiding the need for internal quality control materials.
    C. It provides a means of evaluating the precision of a method.
    D. It can detect procedural and technical differences between laboratories.

12. Interlaboratory comparison testing as with proficiency surveys provides a means to
    A. identify critical values for timely reporting to clinicians.
    B. ensure that appropriate documentation is being performed.
    C. evaluate the technical performance of individual laboratory practitioners.
    D. evaluate the performance of a laboratory compared with that of other laboratories.

13. The primary purpose of a Standard Precautions policy in the laboratory is to
    A. ensure a safe and healthy working environment.
    B. identify processes (e.g., autoclaving) to be used to neutralize infectious agents.
    C. prevent the exposure and transmission of potentially infectious agents to others.
    D. identify patients with hepatitis B virus, human immunodeficiency virus, and other infectious diseases.

14. Which agency is responsible for defining, establishing, and monitoring safety and health hazards in the workplace?
    A. Occupational Safety and Health Administration
    B. Centers for Disease Control and Prevention
    C. Chemical Hygiene Agency
    D. National Fire Protection Association

15. Match the mode of transmission with the laboratory activity.

Laboratory Activity	Mode of Transmission
___ A. Not wearing gloves when handling specimens	1. Inhalation
___ B. Centrifuging uncovered specimens	2. Ingestion
___ C. Smoking in the laboratory	3. Direct contact
___ D. Being scratched by a broken beaker	
___ E. Having a specimen splashed into the eyes	
___ F. Pipetting by mouth	

CASE 2-1

Both a large hospital and its outpatient clinic have a laboratory area for performance of routine urinalyses. Each laboratory performs daily quality assurance checks on reagents, equipment, and procedures. Because the control material used does not have sediment components, each laboratory sends a completed urinalysis specimen to the other laboratory for testing. After the urinalysis has been performed, results are recorded, compared, and evaluated. The criterion for acceptability is that all parameters must agree within one grade.

Results

One day, all results were acceptable except those of the microscopic examination, which follow:

Hospital Laboratory	Clinic Laboratory
RBCs/hpf: 5–10	RBCs/hpf: 25–50
WBCs/hpf: 0–2	WBCs/hpf: 0–2
Casts/lpf: 0–2 hyaline	Casts/lpf: 5–10 hyaline

On investigation, the results from the clinic were found to be correct; the hospital had a problem, which was addressed and remedied immediately.

1. Which of the following conditions present in the hospital laboratory could cause the observed findings in this case?
   1. The urinalysis centrifuge had its brake left on.
   2. The urinalysis centrifuge was set for the wrong speed or time setting.
   3. Microscopic examination was performed on an unmixed or inadequately mixed specimen.
   4. Microscopic examination was performed using nonoptimized microscope settings for urine sediment viewing (e.g., contrast was not sufficient to view low-refractile components).
   A. 1, 2, and 3 are correct.
   B. 1 and 3 are correct.
   C. 2 and 4 are correct.
   D. 4 is correct.
   E. All are correct.
2. Which of the following actions could prevent this from happening again?
   A. The microscope and centrifuge should be repaired.
   B. The laboratory should participate in a proficiency survey.
   C. A control material with sediment components should be used daily.
   D. All results should be reviewed by the urinalysis supervisor before they are reported.

hpf, High-power field; *lpf,* low-power field; *RBC,* red blood cell; *WBC,* white blood cell.

16. Which of the following is *not* considered personal protective equipment?
    A. Gloves
    B. Lab coat
    C. Disinfectants
    D. Eyeglasses
17. Which of the following actions represents a good laboratory practice?
    A. Washing or sanitizing hands frequently
    B. Wearing lab coats outside of the laboratory
    C. Removing lab coats from the laboratory for laundering at home in 2% bleach
    D. Wearing the same gloves to perform venipuncture on two different patients because the patients are in the same room
18. Which of the following is *not* an acceptable disposal practice?
    A. Discarding urine into a sink
    B. Disposing of used, empty urine containers with nonhazardous waste
    C. Discarding a used, broken specimen transfer pipette with noninfectious glass waste
    D. Discarding blood specimens into a biohazard container

19. Which of the following is *not* part of a Chemical Hygiene Plan?
    A. To identify and label hazardous chemicals
    B. To educate employees about the chemicals they use (e.g., providing material safety data sheets)
    C. To provide guidelines for the handling and use of each chemical type
    D. To monitor the handling of biological hazards
20. Which of the following information is *not* found on a material safety data sheet?
    A. Exposure limits
    B. Catalog number
    C. Hazardous ingredients
    D. Flammability of the chemical

REFERENCES

1. Westgard JO, Klee GG: Quality assurance. In Tietz NW, editor: Fundamentals of clinical chemistry, ed 3, Philadelphia, 1987, WB Saunders.
2. Fraser CG, Petersen PH: The importance of imprecision. Ann Clin Biochem 28:207, 1991.
3. Clinical and Laboratory Standards Institute: Preparation and testing of reagent water in the clinical laboratory: approved

guideline, ed 4, CLSI Document C3-A4, Clinical and Laboratory Standards Institute, Wayne, PA, 2006, CLSI.

4. Clinical and Laboratory Standards Institute: Laboratory documents: development and control: approved guideline, ed 5, CLSI Document GP02-A5, Clinical and Laboratory Standards Institute, Wayne, PA, 2006, CLSI.

5. Schumann GB, Tebbs RD: Comparison of slides used for standardized routine microscopic urinalysis. J Med Technol 3:54–58, 1986.

6. Clinical and Laboratory Standards Institute: Protection of laboratory workers from occupationally acquired infections: approved guideline, ed 3, CLSI Document M29-A3, Clinical and Laboratory Standards Institute, Wayne, PA, 2005, CLSI.

7. Clinical and Laboratory Standards Institute: Clinical Laboratory Safety: approved guideline, ed 2, CLSI Document GP17-A2, Clinical and Laboratory Standards Institute, Wayne, PA, 2004, CLSI.

8. Clinical and Laboratory Standards Institute: Clinical laboratory waste management: approved guideline, ed 2, CLSI Document GP05-A2, Clinical and Laboratory Standards Institute, Wayne, PA, 2002, CLSI.

9. Lynch P, Jackson M, Cummings M, Stamm W: Rethinking the role of isolation precautions in the prevention of nosocomial infections. Ann Intern Med 107:243–246, 1987.

10. Lynch P, Cummings M, Roberts P, et al: Implementing and evaluating a system of generic infection precautions: body substance isolation. Am J Infect Control 18:1–12, 1987.

11. Occupational Safety and Health Administration: Occupational exposure to bloodborne pathogens; final rule. Federal Register 56:64003–640182 (codified at 29 CFR 1910.1030), December 6, 1991.

12. Garner JS: Guideline for isolation precautions in hospitals. Infect Control Hosp Epidemiol 17:53–80, 1996.

13. Center for Disease Control and Prevention: 2007 guideline for isolation precautions: preventing transmission of infectious agents in healthcare settings (website): www.cdc.gov/hicpac/2007IP/2007isolationPrecautions.html. Accessed July 7, 2011.

14. Occupational Safety and Health Administration: Directives: enforcement procedures for the occupational exposure to bloodborne pathogens, CPL 2-2.44D, U.S. Department of Labor, November 5, 1999.

15. Occupational Safety and Health Administration: Directives: enforcement procedures for the occupational exposure to bloodborne pathogens, CPL 2-2.69D, U.S. Department of Labor, November 27, 2001.

BIBLIOGRAPHY

Clinical and Laboratory Standards Institute: Urinalysis: approved guideline, ed 3, CLSI Document GP16-A3, Clinical and Laboratory Standards Institute, Wayne, PA, 2009, CLSI.

Hazardous materials, storage, and handling pocketbook, Alexandria, Va, 1984, Defense Logistics Agency.

National Fire Protection Association: Hazardous chemical data, Boston, 1975, National Fire Protection Association, No. 49.

Occupational exposure to hazardous chemicals in laboratories, final rule. Federal Register 55:3327–3335, 1990.

Schweitzer SC, Schumann JL, Schumann GB: Quality assurance guidelines for the urinalysis laboratory. J Med Technol 3:570, 1986.

Urine Specimen Types, Collection, and Preservation

LEARNING OBJECTIVES

After studying this chapter, the student should be able to:

1. State at least three clinical reasons for performing a routine urinalysis.
2. Describe three types of urine specimens and state at least one diagnostic use for each type.
3. Explain the importance of accurate timing and complete collection of timed urine specimens.
4. Describe the collection technique used to obtain the following specimens:
   - Random void
   - Midstream "clean catch"
   - Catheterized
   - Suprapubic aspiration
   - Pediatric collection
5. Describe materials and procedures used for proper collection and identification of urine specimens.
6. Identify six reasons for rejecting a urine specimen.
7. State the changes possible in unpreserved urine and explain the mechanism for each.
8. Discuss urine preservatives, including their advantages, disadvantages, and uses.
9. List and justify at least three tests that assist in determining whether a fluid is urine.

CHAPTER OUTLINE

Why Study Urine?
Specimen Types
  First Morning Specimen
  Random Urine Specimen
  Timed Collection
Collection Techniques
  Routine Void

Midstream "Clean Catch"
Catheterized Specimen
Suprapubic Aspiration
Pediatric Collections
Reasons for Urine Specimen
  Rejection
Urine Volume Needed for Testing

Urine Specimen Storage and
  Handling
  Containers
  Labeling
  Handling and Preservation
Is This Fluid Urine?

KEY TERMS

catheterized specimen A urine specimen obtained using a sterile catheter (a flexible tube) inserted through the urethra and into the bladder. Urine flows directly from the bladder by gravity and collects in a plastic reservoir bag.

first morning specimen The first urine specimen voided after rising from sleep. The night before the collection, the patient voids before going to bed. Usually the first morning specimen has been retained in the bladder for 6 to 8 hours and is ideal to test for substances that may require concentration (e.g., protein) or

incubation for detection (e.g., nitrites).

midstream "clean catch" specimen A urine specimen obtained after thorough cleansing of the glans penis in the male or the urethral meatus in the female. Following the cleansing procedure, the patient passes the first portion of the urine into the toilet, stops and collects the midportion in the specimen container, then passes any remaining urine into the toilet. Used for routine urinalysis and urine culture, the specimen is essentially free of contaminants from the genitalia and distal urethra.

random urine specimen A urine specimen collected at any time, day or night, without prior patient preparation.

suprapubic aspiration A technique used to collect urine directly from the bladder by puncturing the abdominal wall and distended bladder using a sterile needle and syringe. Aspiration is used primarily to obtain sterile specimens for bacterial cultures from infants and occasionally from adults.

timed collection A urine specimen collected throughout a specific timed interval. The patient voids at the beginning of the collection and discards this urine and then collects all subsequent urine. At the end of the time interval, the patient voids and includes this urine in the collection. This technique is used primarily for quantitative urine assays because it allows comparison of excretion patterns from day to day; the most common are 12-hour and 24-hour collections.

urine preservative A chemical substance or process used to prevent composition changes in a urine specimen (e.g., loss or gain of chemical substances, deterioration of formed elements). The most common form of urine preservation is refrigeration.

The purposes of performing a routine urinalysis are (1) to aid in the diagnosis of disease; (2) to screen for asymptomatic, congenital, or hereditary disease; (3) to monitor disease progression; and (4) to monitor therapy effectiveness or complications.[1] To obtain accurate urinalysis results, urine specimen integrity must be maintained. If the urine specimen submitted for testing is inappropriate (e.g., if a random specimen is submitted instead of a timed collection) or if the specimen has changed because of improper collection or storage conditions, testing will produce results that do not reflect the patient's condition. In such situations, the highest quality reagents, equipment, expertise, and personnel cannot compensate for the unacceptable specimen. Therefore written criteria for urine specimen types, instructions for proper collection and preservation, appropriate specimen labeling, and a handling timeline must be available to all personnel involved in urine specimen procurement.

WHY STUDY URINE?

Urine is actually a fluid biopsy of the kidney and provides a "fountain" of information (Figure 3-1). The kidney is the only organ with such a noninvasive means by which to directly evaluate its status. In addition, because urine is an ultrafiltrate of the plasma, it can be used to evaluate and monitor body homeostasis and many metabolic disease processes.

Usually, urine specimens are readily obtainable, and their collection inconveniences the patient only briefly. Some individuals feel uncomfortable discussing body fluids and body function. Good verbal and written communication with each patient in a sensitive and professional manner ensures collection of the urine specimen desired. The ease with which urine specimens are obtained can lead to laxity or neglect in educating the patient and stressing the importance of a proper collection. Note that if the quality of the urine specimen is compromised, so is the resultant urinalysis.

SPECIMEN TYPES

The type of specimen selected and the collection procedure used are determined by the health care provider and depend on the tests to be performed. The three basic types of urine specimens are first morning, random, and timed (Table 3-1). The ideal urine specimen is adequately concentrated to ensure, upon screening, the detection of analytes and formed elements of interest. These factors, in turn, depend on the patient's state of hydration and the length of time the urine is held in the bladder.

First Morning Specimen

To collect a **first morning specimen,** the patient voids before going to bed, and immediately on rising from sleep collects a urine specimen. Because this urine specimen has been retained in the bladder for approximately 8 hours, the specimen is ideal to test for substances that require concentration or incubation for detection (e.g., nitrites, protein) and to confirm postural or orthostatic proteinuria. Formed elements such as white blood cells, red blood cells, and casts are more stable in these concentrated acidic urine specimens. In addition, these specimens are often preferred for cytology studies because the number of epithelial cells present can be significant. The morphology of cellular components and casts actually is enhanced by the high osmolality of first morning specimens.[2] However, the high concentration of salts in these specimens can crystallize on cooling to room temperature (e.g., amorphous urates) and interfere with routine processing for cytologic studies. If the cellular morphology in this specimen type is determined to be suboptimal (i.e., signs of degeneration present), a random urine specimen can be collected.

Although the first morning urine is usually the most concentrated and is frequently the specimen of choice, it is not the most convenient to obtain. It requires that the patient pick up a container and instructions at least 1 day before his or her appointment; in addition, the specimen must be preserved if it is not going to be analyzed within 2 hours of collection.

Random Urine Specimen

For ease and convenience, routine screening most often is performed on **random urine specimens.** Random specimens can be collected at any time, usually during daytime hours, and without prior patient preparation. Because excessive fluid intake and exercise can affect urine composition directly, these specimens may not accurately reflect the patient's condition. Despite this, random specimens are usually satisfactory for routine screening and

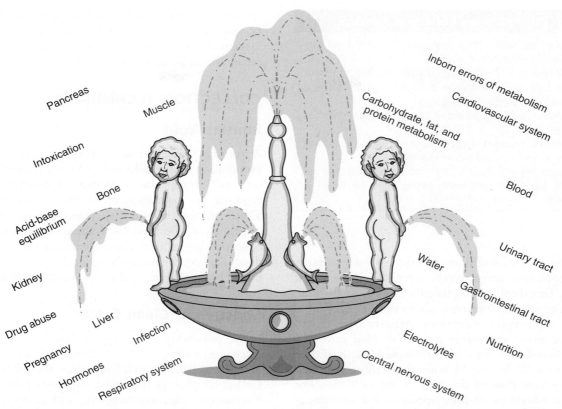

FIGURE 3-1 Urine as a fountain of information. *(Modified from Free AH, Free HM: Urinalysis in clinical laboratory practice, West Palm Beach, FL, 1975, CRC Press. Copyright CRC Press, Boca Raton, FL.)*

TABLE 3-1	Urine Specimen Types	
Specimen Type	**Description**	**Uses**
Random	• Urine collected at any time	• Routine screening • Cytology studies (with prior hydration) • Fluid deprivation tests
First morning	• First urine voided after sleep (≈6 to 8 hours) • Most concentrated urine	• Routine screening; good recovery of cells and casts • To confirm postural or orthostatic proteinuria • Cytology studies
Timed	• Collect all urine during a specific timed interval (e.g., 24-hour, 12-hour, 2-hour) • Preservatives and/or refrigeration during collection may be required	• Quantitative chemical analysis • Clearance tests • Cytology studies • Evaluation of fistula

are capable of detecting abnormalities that indicate a disease process.

With prior hydration of the patient, a random "clean catch" urine specimen is ideal for cytology studies. Hydration consists of instructing the patient to drink 24 to 32 oz of water each hour for 2 hours before urine collection. Most cytologic protocols require collection of these specimens daily for 3 to 5 consecutive days. This increases the number of cells studied, thereby enhancing the detection of abnormality or disease. One method that

can be used to increase the cellularity of the urine specimen is to have the patient exercise for 5 minutes by skipping or jumping up and down before specimen collection.

Timed Collection

Because of circadian or diurnal variation in excretion of many substances and functions (e.g., hormones, proteins, glomerular filtration rate) and the effects of

---

BOX 3-1 | Timed Urine Collection Protocol

- Provide patient with written instructions and collection container (with preservative, if required).
- At start time (e.g., 7 AM), patient empties bladder *into toilet*; afterward, all subsequent urine throughout timed interval is collected in the container provided.
- At end time (e.g., 7 AM), patient empties bladder *into collection container*.
- Specimen is transported to laboratory, where urine is mixed well and the volume is measured and recorded.
- A sufficient aliquot (≈50 mL) is removed for routine testing and possible repeat or additional testing; the remainder is discarded.

---

exercise, hydration, and body metabolism on excretion rates, quantitative urine assays often require a **timed collection.** Timed collections, usually 12-hour or 24-hour, eliminate the need to determine when excretion is optimal and allow comparison of excretion patterns from day to day. Timed urine specimens can be divided into two types: those collected for a predetermined length of time (e.g., 2 hours, 12 hours, 24 hours) and those collected during a specific time of day (e.g., 2 PM to 4 PM). For example, a 4-hour or 12-hour specimen for determination of urine albumin, creatinine, and the albumin-to-creatinine ratio can be collected anytime and is an ideal specimen to screen for microalbuminuria. In contrast, a 2-hour collection for determination of urinary urobilinogen is preferably collected from 2 PM to 4 PM—the time when maximal excretion of urobilinogen is known to occur.

Accurate timing and strict adherence to specimen collection directions are essential to ensure valid results from timed collections. For example, if two first morning specimens are included in a single 24-hour collection, the results will be erroneous because of the additional volume and analyte added. Box 3-1 summarizes a protocol for the timed collection of a 24-hour specimen. This same protocol is applicable to any timed collection. A rule of thumb is to empty the bladder and discard the urine at the beginning of a timed collection and to collect all urine subsequently passed during the collection period. At the end time of the collection, the patient must empty his or her bladder and include that urine in the timed collection.

Depending on the analyte being measured, a urine preservative may be necessary to ensure its stability throughout the collection. In addition, certain foods and drugs can affect the urinary excretion of some analytes. When this influence is known to be significant, the patient needs to be properly instructed to avoid these substances. Written instructions should include the test name, the preservative required, and any special instructions or precautions. The most common errors encountered in quantitative urine tests are related directly to

specimen collection or to handling problems, such as loss of specimen, inclusion of two first morning samples, inaccurate total volume measurement, transcription error, and inadequate preservation.

COLLECTION TECHNIQUES

Routine Void

A routine voided urine specimen requires no patient preparation and is collected by having the patient urinate into an appropriate container. Normally the patient requires no assistance other than clear instructions. These routine specimens, whether random or first morning, can be used for routine urinalysis. For other collection procedures, the patient may require assistance depending on the patient's age and physical condition or the technique to be used for collection (Table 3-2).

Midstream "Clean Catch"

If the possibility of contamination (e.g., from vaginal discharge) exists, or if a bacterial culture is desired, a **midstream "clean catch" specimen** should be obtained. Collection of these specimens requires additional patient instructions, cleaning supplies, and perhaps assistance for elderly patients or young children. Before collection of a midstream clean catch specimen, the glans penis of the male or the urethral meatus of the female is thoroughly cleansed and rinsed. Following the cleansing procedure, a midstream specimen is obtained when the patient first passes some urine into the toilet and then stops and urinates the midportion into the specimen container. Any remaining urine is passed into the toilet. To prevent contamination of the container and specimen, the interior of the container must not come in contact with the patient's hands or perineal area. This midstream technique allows passage of the initial urine that contains any urethral washings (e.g., normal bacterial flora of the distal urethra) into the toilet and allows collection of a specimen that represents elements and analytes from the bladder, ureters, and kidneys. Because an informed patient can obtain these useful specimens with minimal effort, the midstream clean catch specimen is frequently collected. When done properly, the technique eliminates sources of contamination and provides an excellent specimen for routine urinalysis and urine culture.

Catheterized Specimen

A routine voided or midstream clean catch specimen is readily obtained by a well-instructed and physically able patient. In contrast, two collection techniques require medical personnel. A **catheterized specimen** is obtained following catheterization of the patient, that is, insertion of a sterile catheter through the urethra into the bladder.

TABLE 3-2 Urine Collection Techniques

Collection Technique	Description	Use
Routine void	• No preparation before collection	• Routine screening
Midstream clean catch	• Genital area cleansed before collection • Patient passes initial urine into toilet, stops and collects urine in container, then empties any additional urine into toilet	• Bacterial and fungal cultures (sterile container required) • Routine screening • Cytology
Catheterized, urethral	• A catheter is inserted into the bladder via the urethra • Urine flows directly from bladder through catheter into plastic bag	• Bacterial and fungal cultures • Routine screening
Catheterized, ureteral	• A catheter is inserted through the urethra and bladder to collect urine directly from the left and/or right ureters	• To differentiate kidney infections
Suprapubic aspiration	• Using sterile needle and syringe, the abdominal wall is punctured, and urine is directly aspirated from the bladder	• Bacterial and fungal cultures
Pediatric collection bag	• Used with patients unable to urinate voluntarily • Plastic collection bag is adhered to the skin surrounding the genital area • Urine accumulates in plastic bag	• Routine screening • Quantitative assays

Urine flows directly from the bladder through the indwelling catheter and accumulates in a plastic reservoir bag. A urine specimen can be collected at any time from this reservoir. Because urinary tract infections are common in catheterized patients, most often these urine specimens are sent for bacterial culture. However, if additional tests are ordered, the culture should be performed first to prevent possible contamination of the specimen. Any of the specimen types discussed (e.g., random, timed) can be obtained from catheterized patients by following the appropriate collection procedure.

Studies to determine whether one or both kidneys are involved in a disease process can involve collection of urine directly from the ureters. A catheter is threaded up the urethra, through the bladder, and into each ureter, where urine is collected. Urine collected from the left ureter and the right ureter is analyzed, and the results are compared.

Suprapubic Aspiration

Another collection technique, **suprapubic aspiration**, involves collecting urine directly from the bladder by puncturing the abdominal wall and the distended bladder using a needle and syringe. The normally sterile bladder urine is aspirated into the syringe and sent for analysis. This procedure is used principally for bacterial cultures, especially for anaerobic microbes, and in infants, in whom specimen contamination is often unavoidable.

Pediatric Collections

Pediatric and newborn infants pose a challenge in collecting an appropriate urine specimen. Because these patients are unable to urinate voluntarily, commercially available plastic urine collection bags with a hypoallergenic skin adhesive are used. The patient's perineal area is cleansed and dried before the specimen bag is placed onto the skin. The bag is placed over the penis in the male and around the vagina (excluding the anus) in the female, and the adhesive is firmly attached to the perineum. Once the bag is in place, the patient is checked every 15 minutes to see if an adequate specimen has been collected. The specimen should be removed as soon as possible after collection, labeled, and transported to the laboratory. Because of the many possible sources of contamination despite the use of sterile bags and technique, urine for bacterial culture may need to be obtained by catheterization or suprapubic aspiration. However, when the patient is prepared appropriately, these bag specimens are usually satisfactory for routine screening and quantitative assays. The use of disposable diapers to collect urine for quantitative assay also has been reported.[3]

BOX 3-2	Reasons for Urine Specimen Rejection

- Unlabeled urine specimen container
- Mislabeled urine specimen
  - Names on container label and order slip do not match
  - Identification numbers on container label and slip do not match
- Inappropriate urine collection technique or specimen type for test requested
- Specimen not properly preserved during a time delay or inappropriate urine preservative used
- Visibly contaminated urine (e.g., fecal material, toilet tissue)
- Insufficient volume of urine for test(s) requested

Reasons for Urine Specimen Rejection

A urine specimen may be rejected for testing for a variety of reasons (Box 3-2). Each laboratory should have a written protocol that lists each situation and details the steps to follow and the forms to complete to document such specimens when they are encountered. In each instance, the laboratory should keep the urine specimen, notify appropriate personnel, and request collection of a new specimen. Unlabeled and improperly labeled urine specimens (e.g., name or ID number on container label and order slip does not match) are probably the two most common reasons for specimen rejection. Another reason for specimen rejection is a request for a urine culture when the urine specimen was collected in a nonsterile container, or when midstream clean catch instructions were not provided to the patient for collection. Other causes include specimens that have not been properly stored and those visibly contaminated with fecal material or debris (e.g., toilet tissue).

Urine Volume Needed for Testing

Routine urinalysis protocols typically require 10 to 15 mL of urine, but collection of a larger volume is encouraged to ensure sufficient urine for additional or repeat testing. Smaller volumes of urine (<12 mL) hinder performance of the microscopic examination when the urinalysis is performed manually and can limit the chemical tests performed. However, if a fully automated urinalysis system such as the iQ200 system (Iris Diagnostics, Chatsworth, CA) is used, a complete urinalysis can be performed with 4 mL of urine.

With 24-hour urine collection, despite the large volume of urine submitted to the laboratory, only a small amount ($\approx$1 mL) of well-mixed urine is actually required for quantitative urine tests (e.g., creatinine, hormones, electrolytes). A portion of the urine collection (20 to 50 mL) is usually retained to ensure sufficient specimen should repeat or additional testing be required later.

URINE SPECIMEN STORAGE AND HANDLING

Containers

Containers for urine specimen collections must be clean, dry, and made of a clear or translucent disposable material such as plastic or glass. They should stand upright, have an opening of at least 4 to 5 cm, and have a capacity of 50 to 100 mL. A lid or cover that is easily placed onto and removed from the container is needed to prevent spillage. Specimens that are transported require a lid with a leakproof seal. Commercially available, disposable nonsterile containers are available and economical.

Sterile, individually packaged urine containers are available from commercial sources for the collection of specimens for microbial culture. However, if any urine specimen must be stored for a period of time before testing (i.e., longer than 2 hours), the use of a sterile container is recommended, regardless of the tests ordered, because of changes that can occur in unpreserved urine.

Various large containers are available for the collection of 12-hour and 24-hour urine specimens for quantitative analyses. These containers have a capacity of approximately 3000 mL and have a wide mouth and a leakproof screw cap. Usually made of a brown, opaque plastic, they protect the specimen from ultraviolet and white light, and acid preservatives can be added to them.

Clear, pliable, polyethylene urine collection bags are available for collecting specimens from the pediatric patient. These collection bags can be purchased as nonsterile or sterile. After collection, they are self-sealing for transport to the laboratory. For collection of a 24-hour specimen, some brands provide an exit port or tubing attached to the bag base. This port enables transfer of the urine that has accumulated to another collection container, thereby eliminating the need for multiple collection bags. More important, this exit port avoids repeated patient preparation and reapplication of adhesive to the child's sensitive skin.

Labeling

All specimen containers must be labeled before or immediately after collection. Because lids are removed, the patient identification label is always placed directly on the container holding the specimen. Under no circumstances should the label appear only on the removable specimen lid. This practice invites specimen mix-ups; once the lid is removed, such a specimen is technically unlabeled.

Labels must have an adhesive that resists moisture and adheres under refrigeration. The patient identification information required on the label may differ among laboratories. However, the following minimal information should be provided on all labels: the patient's full name, a unique identification number, the date and time of collection, the patient's room number (if applicable), and the preservative used, if any.

Handling and Preservation

Changes in Unpreserved Urine. Urine specimens should be delivered to the laboratory immediately after collection. However, this is not always possible; if a delay in specimen transportation is to be 2 hours or longer, precautions must be taken to preserve the integrity of the specimen, protecting it from the effects of light and room temperature changes. A variety of changes can occur in unpreserved urine (Table 3-3). These changes potentially can affect any aspect—physical, chemical, or microscopic examinations—of a urinalysis. Changes in the physical examination result from (1) alteration of the urine solutes to a different form, resulting in a color change; (2) bacterial growth causing an increased odor because of metabolism or proliferation of bacteria; and (3) solute precipitation in the form of amorphous

material, which decreases urine clarity. Individual components of the chemical examination (e.g., glucose, pH) can also be affected. Most often these changes result in removal of the chemical entity by various mechanisms, leading to false-negative results.

In contrast, urine nitrite and pH increase in unpreserved urine as bacteria proliferate, converting nitrate to nitrite and metabolizing urea to ammonia. The microscopic changes result from disintegration of formed elements, particularly in hypotonic and alkaline urine, or from unchecked bacterial growth. In the latter case, it can be difficult to determine whether the large number of bacteria observed in these specimens results from improper storage or from a urinary tract infection.

In summary, changes will occur in unpreserved urine; which changes occur and their magnitude vary and are impossible to predict. Therefore appropriate specimen collection, handling, and storage are necessary to ensure that these potential changes do not occur, and that accurate results are obtained.

Preservatives. Unfortunately, no single **urine preservative** is available to suit all testing needs (Table 3-4). Hence the preservative used depends on the type of collection, the tests to be performed, and the time delay before testing. The easiest and most common form of preservation, refrigeration at 4° C to 6° C, is suitable for the majority of specimens.[4,5] Any urine specimen for microbiological studies should be refrigerated promptly if it cannot be transported directly to the laboratory. Refrigeration prevents bacterial proliferation, and the specimen remains suitable for culture for up to 24 hours.

Although refrigeration is the easiest means of preserving most urine specimens, refrigeration of routine urinalysis specimens is not recommended if they will be analyzed within 2 hours.[1] Refrigeration can induce precipitation of amorphous urate and phosphate crystals that can interfere substantially with the microscopic examination. For routine urinalysis specimens that must be transported long distances, commercial transport tubes with a preservative are available (Table 3-5).[6-9]

Timed Collections. Timed specimens, particularly 12-hour and 24-hour collections, may require the addition of a chemical preservative to maintain the integrity of the analyte of interest. Regardless of the preservative necessary, urine collections should be kept on ice or refrigerated throughout the duration of the collection.

The collection preservative needed for a particular analyte can differ among laboratories. These variations stem from (1) different test methods, (2) how often the test is performed, and (3) time delays and transportation conditions (e.g., the sample is sent to a reference laboratory). Some laboratories may perform an assay daily in-house and require only refrigeration of the sample during the timed collection. In contrast, a small laboratory may send the assay to a reference facility that requires that a chemical preservative be used during the collection to ensure analyte stability. Each urinalysis

TABLE 3-3	Potential Changes in Unpreserved Urine	
Component	**Observation**	**Mechanism**
Physical Changes		
Color	Darkens or changes	Oxidation or reduction of solutes (e.g., urobilinogen, bilirubin)
Clarity	Decreases	Crystal precipitation; bacterial proliferation
Odor	Ammoniacal, foul smelling	Bacterial conversion of urea to ammonia (and bacterial proliferation)
Chemical Changes		
pH	Increase	Bacterial conversion of urea to ammonia; loss of CO_2
Glucose	Decrease	Consumed by cells and/or bacteria
Ketones	Decrease	Volatilization and bacterial conversion
Bilirubin	Decrease	Photo-oxidation to biliverdin by light exposure
Urobilinogen	Decrease	Oxidation to urobilin
Nitrite	Increase	Bacterial conversion of dietary nitrates
Microscopic Changes		
Blood cells	Decrease	Lysis and/or disintegration, especially in dilute and alkaline urine
Casts	Decrease	Disintegration, especially in dilute and alkaline urine
Bacteria	Increase	Exponential proliferation of bacteria
Trichomonads	Decrease	Loss of characteristic motility and death

TABLE 3-4	Urine Preservatives*			
Type	**Advantages**	**Disadvantages**	**Use**	
Refrigeration	• Acceptable for routine urinalysis for 24 hours[4,9] • Acceptable for urine culture; inhibits bacterial growth for ≈24 hours[5,9] • Inexpensive	• Precipitates amorphous and/or crystalline solutes	• Storage before and after testing	
Commercial transport tubes (see Table 3-5)	• Acceptable for routine urinalysis; preserves chemical and formed elements in urine at room temperature • Boric acid preservative is also acceptable for urine culture[6,7]	• pH and SG may be altered; varies with tube used • Can interfere with chemistry tests (e.g., sodium, potassium, hormone, drug assays)	• Urine transport from off-site to laboratory • Preserve specimen at room temperature for longer time period; varies with tube used	
Thymol	• Preserves sediment elements (e.g., casts, cells) • Inhibits bacterial and yeast growth	• Interferes with protein precipitation tests • In high concentration, can precipitate crystals	• Sediment preservation	
Formalin	• Excellent cellular preservative	• False-negative reagent strip tests for blood and urobilinogen	• Cytology	
Saccomanno's fixative	• Excellent cellular preservative • Commercially available and inexpensive	• Potential chemical hazard	• Cytology	
Acids (HCl, glacial acetic acid)	• Inexpensive • Stabilizes calcium, phosphorus, steroids, hormones, etc.	• Unacceptable for urinalysis testing • Potential chemical hazard	• For quantitative analysis of urine solutes, such as steroids, hormones, etc.	
Sodium carbonate	• Inexpensive • Stabilizes porphyrins, porphobilinogen, etc.	• Unacceptable for urinalysis testing	• For quantitative analysis of porphyrins, porphobilinogen, etc.	

*Time frame of acceptability for urine specimens and the use of preservatives are determined by each laboratory.

TABLE 3-5	Commercial Urine Transport Tubes With Preservative			
Product	**Tube**	**Preservative and Additives**	**Use**	**Comments**
BD VACUTAINER; Plus Plastic Conical UA Preservative Tube (product no. 364946)	Plastic conical tube; yellow and cherry red marble stopper	Chlorhexidine Ethyl paraben Sodium propionate	• Urinalysis • Bactericidal; not acceptable for urine culture	• Stabilizes urine for up to 72 hours at room temperature • Conical bottom designed to fit Kova-pettors
InTac UA System, Therapak Corporation (product no. 94500)	Plastic conical tube; yellow plastic cap	Dowicil 200 (a formaldehyde releasing agent) Mannitol Polyethylene glycol	• Urinalysis • Bactericidal; not acceptable for urine culture	• Stabilizes urine for up to 96 hours at room temperature • No change in pH or SG
BD Vacutainer; C & S Preservative Tube (product no. 364948, 364976)	Glass tube; gray stopper	Boric acid Sodium formate D-Sorbitol Sodium acetate	• Urinalysis • Urine culture and sensitivity • Can be used for urinalysis[7] • Bacteriostatic	• Stabilizes urine for up to 48 hours at room temperature[9] • pH adjusted to 6 to 7 • SG increased by ≈0.006 to 0.007[8]

laboratory must have in its procedure manual a protocol for the collection of all timed urine specimens. The protocol should include the name of the analyte, a description of the appropriate specimen collection technique, the appropriate preservative required, labeling requirements including precautions for certain chemical preservatives, the location at which the test is performed, reference ranges, and the expected turnaround time.

Timed urine collections should be transported to the laboratory as soon as possible after completion of the collection. The total volume is determined, the specimen is well mixed to ensure homogeneity, and aliquots are removed for the appropriate tests. At no point during a timed collection can urine be removed or discarded, even if the volume is recorded. This would invalidate the collection because the concentration of the analyte in any removed aliquot cannot be determined and corrected for.

IS THIS FLUID URINE?

At times it is necessary to verify that the fluid present in a urine container is in fact urine. This may occur in laboratories that perform urine testing for illicit drugs (e.g., amphetamine, cocaine, tetrahydrocannabinol [THC], steroids). In these situations, particularly when the urine collection is not witnessed, the individual may have the opportunity to add a substance to the urine collection (e.g., an adulterated specimen). Another possibility is that the liquid in the container is not urine.

Specific gravity, pH, and temperature can be helpful in identifying urine specimens to which additional liquid has been added. The physiologically possible range for urine pH in a fresh urine specimen is 4.0 to 8.0 and for specific gravity is 1.002 to 1.035. In a normal healthy individual, the temperature of a urine specimen immediately following collection is usually between 32.5° C and 37.5° C. If this range is exceeded and the temperature is lower or higher, the urine has been altered in some way, or the fluid is not urine. Note that urine specific gravity can exceed 1.035 if the patient has had a recent injection of radiographic contrast media (x-ray dye).

Occasionally, when an amniocentesis is performed, concern may be raised regarding whether the fluid collected is amniotic fluid or urine aspirated from the bladder. Another circumstance that may be encountered is receipt in the laboratory of two specimens from the same patient in identical sterile containers for testing, but the fluid source is not clearly evident on either container. In these varied situations, a few simple and easily performed tests can aid in determining whether the fluid is actually urine.

The single most useful substance that identifies a fluid as urine is its uniquely high creatinine concentration (approximately 50 times that of plasma). In addition, concentrations of urea, sodium, and chloride are significantly higher in urine than in other body fluids. Also, in urine from healthy individuals, no protein or glucose is usually present. In contrast, other body fluids such as amniotic fluid or plasma exudates contain glucose and are high in protein.

STUDY QUESTIONS

1. Which of the following is the urine specimen of choice for cytology studies?
   A. First morning specimen
   B. Random specimen
   C. Midstream "clean catch" collection
   D. Timed collection

2. Which of the following specimens usually eliminates contamination of the urine with entities from the external genitalia and the distal urethra?
   A. First morning specimen
   B. Midstream "clean catch" specimen
   C. Random specimen
   D. 4-hour timed collection

3. Substances that show diurnal variation in their urinary excretion pattern are best evaluated using a
   A. first morning specimen.
   B. midstream "clean catch" specimen.
   C. random specimen.
   D. timed collection.

4. Which of the following will not cause erroneous results in a 24-hour timed urine collection?
   A. The collection starts and ends in the evening
   B. Two first morning specimens are included in the collection
   C. Multiple collection containers are not mixed together before specimen testing
   D. A portion of the collection is removed before total volume measurement

5. A 25-year-old woman complains of painful urination and is suspected of having a urinary tract infection. Which of the following specimens should be collected for a routine urinalysis and urine culture?
   A. First morning specimen
   B. Timed collection
   C. Midstream "clean catch" specimen
   D. Random specimen

6. A 35-year-old diabetic woman is suspected of developing renal insufficiency. Which of the following specimens should be obtained to determine the amount of creatinine being excreted in the urine?
   A. 2-hour postprandial
   B. 12-hour timed collection
   C. 24-hour timed collection
   D. Midstream "clean catch"

7. An unpreserved urine specimen collected at midnight is kept at room temperature until the morning hospital shift. Which of the following changes will most likely occur?
   A. Decrease in urine color and clarity
   B. Decrease in pH and specific gravity
   C. Decrease in glucose and ketones
   D. Decrease in bacteria and nitrite

8. A urine specimen containing the substance indicated is kept unpreserved at room temperature for 4 hours. Identify the probable change to that substance.

Substance	Change
__ Bacteria	A. Decrease
__ Bilirubin	B. No change
__ Glucose	C. Increase
__ Ketones	
__ pH	
__ Protein	
__ Urobilinogen	

9. Which of the following is the most common method used to preserve urine specimens?
A. Acid addition
B. Thymol addition
C. Freezing
D. Refrigeration

10. If refrigeration is used to preserve a urine specimen, which of the following may occur?
A. Cellular or bacterial glycolysis will be enhanced.
B. Formed elements will be destroyed.
C. Amorphous crystals may precipitate.
D. Bacteria will proliferate.

11. Which of the following urine preservatives is acceptable for both urinalysis and urine culture?
A. Boric acid
B. Chlorhexidine
C. Dowicil 200
D. Formalin

12. How much urine is usually required for a manually performed routine urinalysis?
A. 5 to 10 mL
B. 10 to 15 mL
C. 20 to 30 mL
D. 50 to 100 mL

13. Which of the following substances is higher in urine than in any other body fluid?
A. Chloride
B. Creatinine
C. Glucose
D. Protein

REFERENCES

1. Clinical and Laboratory Standards Institute: Urinalysis: approved guideline, ed 3, CLSI Document GP16-A3, Clinical and Laboratory Standards Institute, Wayne, PA, 2009, CLSI.
2. Schumann GB, Schumann JL: A manual of cytodiagnostic urinalysis, Salt Lake City, 1984, Cytodiagnostics Company.
3. Roberts SB, Lucas A: Measurement of urinary constituents and output using disposable napkins. Arch Dis Child 60:1021–1024, 1985.
4. Schumann GB, Friedman SK: Specimen collection, preservation and transportation. In Wet urinalysis, Chicago, 2003, ASCP Press.
5. Culhane JK: Delayed analysis of urine. J Fam Pract 30:473–474, 1990.
6. Meers PD, Chow CK: Bacteriostatic and bactericidal actions of boric acid against bacteria and fungi commonly found in urine. J Clin Pathol 43:484–487, 1990.
7. Lum KT, Meers PD: Boric acid converts urine into an effective bacteriostatic transport medium. J Infect 18:51–58, 1989.
8. Kouri T, Vuotari L, Pohjavaara S, Laippala P: Preservation of urine for flow cytometric and visual microscopic testing. Clin Chem 48:900–905, 2002.
9. Becton Dickinson VACUTAINER Systems: Understanding additives: urine preservatives. In Lab notes—a newsletter from Becton Dickinson VACUTAINER Systems, Vol 4 No 2, Franklin Lakes, NJ, 1993, Becton Dickinson VACUTAINER Systems.

BIBLIOGRAPHY

Finnegan K: Routine urinalysis. In Saunders manual of clinical laboratory science, Philadelphia, 1998, WB Saunders.
Kaplan LA, Pesce AJ: Examination of urine. In Kaplan LA, Pesce AJ, Kazmierczak SC, editors: Clinical chemistry: theory, analysis, correlation, ed 4, St Louis, 2003, Mosby.
McPherson RA, Ben-Ezra J, Zhao S: Basic examination of urine. In McPherson RA, Pincus MR, editors: Clinical diagnosis and management by laboratory methods, ed 21, Philadelphia, 2007, Saunders Elsevier.
Ringsrud KM, Linne JJ: Urinalysis and body fluids: a color text and atlas, St Louis, 1995, Mosby-Year Book.

The Kidney

LEARNING OBJECTIVES

After studying this chapter, the student should be able to:

1. Identify and state the primary functions of the macroscopic structures of the kidney and urinary tract.
2. Diagram the structure and state the function of each portion of the nephron.
3. Describe renal blood circulation and its role in renal function.
4. Discuss the components and the process of glomerular filtration and urine formation, including the anatomic structures, the filtration forces, and the substances involved.
5. Describe the transport mechanisms of tubular reabsorption and tubular secretion, including the substances involved.
6. Describe the three secretory mechanisms that the kidney uses to regulate the acid-base equilibrium of the body.
7. Explain tubular transport capacity (Tm) and discuss its relationship to renal threshold.
8. Compare and contrast the countercurrent multiplier mechanism, the countercurrent exchange mechanism, and the urea cycle, and their roles in urine formation and concentration.
9. Briefly summarize the relationship of water reabsorption to antidiuretic hormone and the relationship of sodium reabsorption to renin and aldosterone.

CHAPTER OUTLINE

Renal Anatomy
Renal Circulation
Renal Physiology

Urine Formation
Glomerulus

Tubules
Tubular Function

KEY TERMS

active transport The movement of a substance (e.g., ion, solute) across a cell membrane and against a gradient, requiring the expenditure of energy.

afferent arteriole A small branch of an interlobular renal artery that becomes the capillary tuft within a glomerulus.

antidiuretic hormone Also known as *arginine vasopressin*, a hormone produced in the hypothalamus and released from the posterior pituitary that regulates the reabsorption of water by the collecting tubules. Without adequate arginine vasopressin present, water is not reabsorbed.

basement membrane A trilayer structure located within the glomerulus along the base of the epithelium (podocytes) of the urinary (Bowman's) space. With the overlying slit diaphragm, the basement membrane is the size-discriminating component of the glomerular filtration barrier, limiting the passage of substances to those with an effective molecular radius less than 4 nm. Electron microscopy reveals three distinct layers in the basement membrane: the lamina rara interna (next to the capillary endothelium), the lamina densa (centrally located), and the lamina rara externa (next to the podocytes).

collecting duct The portion of a renal nephron that follows the distal convoluted tubule. Many distal tubules empty into a single collecting duct. The collecting duct traverses the renal cortex and the medulla and is the site of final urine concentration. The collecting ducts terminate at the renal papilla, conveying the urine formed into the renal calyces of the kidney.

countercurrent exchange mechanism A passive exchange by diffusion of reabsorbed solutes and water from the medullary interstitium of the nephron into the blood of its vascular blood supply (i.e., the vasa recta). A requirement of this process is that the flow of blood within the ascending and descending vessels of the U-shaped vasa recta must be in opposite directions, hence the term *countercurrent*. The countercurrent exchange mechanism simultaneously supplies nutrients to the medulla and removes solutes and water reabsorbed into the blood. As a result, the mechanism assists in maintaining medullary hypertonicity.

countercurrent multiplier mechanism A process occurring in the loop of Henle of each nephron that establishes and maintains the osmotic gradient within the medullary interstitium. The medullary osmolality gradient ranges from being isosmotic ($\approx$300 mOsm/kg) at its border with the cortex to approximately 1400 mOsm/kg at the inner medulla or papilla. A requirement of this process is that the flow of the ultrafiltrate in the descending and ascending limbs must be in opposite directions, hence the name *countercurrent*. In addition, active sodium and chloride reabsorption in the ascending limb combined with passive water reabsorption in the descending limb is an essential component of this process. The countercurrent multiplier mechanism accounts for approximately 50% of the solutes concentrated in the renal medulla.

distal convoluted tubule The portion of a renal nephron immediately following the loop of Henle. The tubule begins at the juxtaglomerular apparatus with the macula densa, a specialized group of cells located at the vascular pole. The distal tubule is convoluted and after two to three loops becomes the collecting tubule (or duct).

efferent arteriole The arteriole exiting a glomerulus; the efferent arteriole is formed by rejoining of the anastomosing capillary network within the glomerulus.

glomerular filtration barrier The structure within the glomerulus that determines the composition of the plasma ultrafiltrate formed in the urinary space by regulating the passage of solutes. The glomerular filtration barrier consists of the capillary endothelium, the basement membrane, and the epithelial podocytes, each coated with a "shield of negativity." Solute selectivity by the barrier is based on the molecular size and the electrical charge of the solute.

glomerulus (also called *renal corpuscle*) A tuft or network of capillaries encircled by and intimately related with the proximal end of a renal tubule (i.e., Bowman's capsule). The glomerulus is composed of four distinct structural components: the capillary endothelial cells, the epithelial cells (podocytes), the mesangium, and the basement membrane.

isosmotic Term describing a solution or fluid that has the same concentration of osmotically active solutes as the blood plasma.

juxtaglomerular apparatus A specialized area located at the vascular pole of a nephron. The apparatus is composed of cells from the afferent and efferent arterioles, the macula densa of the distal tubule, and the extraglomerular mesangium. The juxtaglomerular apparatus is actually an endocrine organ and the primary producer of renin.

kidneys The organs of the urinary system that produce urine. Normally, each individual has two kidneys. The primary function of the kidneys is to filter the blood, removing waste products and regulating electrolytes, water, acid-base balance, and blood pressure.

loop of Henle The tubular portion of a nephron immediately following and continuous with the proximal tubule. Located in the renal medulla, the loop of Henle is composed of a thin descending limb, a U-shaped segment (also called a *hairpin turn*), and thin and thick ascending limbs. The thick ascending limb of the loop of Henle (sometimes called *the straight portion of the distal tubule*) ends as the tubule enters the vascular pole of the glomerulus.

maximal tubular reabsorptive capacity Denoted T_m, the maximal rate of reabsorption of a solute by the tubular epithelium per minute (milligrams per minute). Reabsorptive capacity varies with each solute and depends on the glomerular filtration rate.

maximal tubular secretory capacity Also denoted T_m; the maximal rate of secretion of a solute by the tubular epithelium per minute (milligrams per minute). This rate differs for each solute.

mesangium The cells that form the structural core tissue of a glomerulus. The mesangium lies between the glomerular capillaries (endothelium) and the podocytes (tubular epithelium). The mesangial cells derive from smooth muscle and have contractility characteristics and the ability to phagocytize and pinocytize.

nephron The functional unit of the kidney. Each kidney contains approximately 1.3 million nephrons. A nephron is composed of five distinct areas: the glomerulus, the proximal tubule, the loop of Henle, the distal tubule, and the collecting tubule or duct. Each region of the nephron is specialized and plays a role in the formation and final composition of urine.

osmosis The movement of water across a semipermeable membrane in an attempt to achieve an osmotic equilibrium between two compartments or solutions of differing osmolality (i.e., an osmotic gradient). This mechanism is passive, that is, it requires no energy.

passive transport The movement of a substance (e.g., ion, solute) across a cell membrane along a gradient (e.g., concentration, charge). Passive transport does not require energy.

peritubular capillaries The network of capillaries (or plexus) that forms from the efferent arteriole and surrounds the tubules of the nephron in the renal cortex.

podocytes The epithelial cells that line the urinary (Bowman's) space of the glomerulus. These cells completely cover the glomerular capillaries with large finger-like processes that interdigitate to form a filtration slit. The term *podo,* which is Greek for "foot," relates to the footlike appearance of the podocyte when viewed in cross-section. Collectively, the podocytes constitute the glomerular epithelium that forms Bowman's capsule.

proximal tubule The tubular part of a nephron immediately following the glomerulus. The proximal tubule has a convoluted portion and a straight portion, the latter becoming the loop of Henle after entering the renal medulla.

renal threshold level The plasma concentration of a solute above which the amount of solute present in the ultrafiltrate exceeds the maximal tubular reabsorptive capacity. Once the renal threshold level has been reached, increased amounts of solute are excreted (i.e., lost) in the urine.

renin A proteolytic enzyme produced and stored by the cells of the juxtaglomerular apparatus of the renal nephrons. Secretion of renin results in the formation of angiotensin and the secretion of aldosterone; thus renin plays an important role in controlling blood pressure and fluid balance.

shield of negativity A term that describes the impediment produced by negatively charged components (e.g., proteoglycans) of the glomerular filtration barrier. Present on both sides of and throughout the filtration barrier, these negatively charged components effectively limit the filtration of negatively charged substances from the blood (e.g., albumin) into the urinary space.

titratable acids A term that represents H$^+$ ions (acid) excreted in the urine as monobasic phosphate (e.g., NaH$_2$PO$_4$). Urinary excretion of these acids results in the elimination of H$^+$ ions and the reabsorption of sodium and bicarbonate. Titration of urine to a pH of 7.4 (normal plasma pH) using a standard base (e.g., NaOH) will quantitate the number of H$^+$ ions excreted in this form, hence the name *titratable acids*.

tubular reabsorption The movement of substances (by active or passive transport) from the tubular ultrafiltrate into the peritubular blood or the interstitium by the renal tubular cells.

tubular secretion The movement of substances (by active or passive transport) from the peritubular blood or the interstitium into the tubular ultrafiltrate by the renal tubular cells.

urea cycle A passive process occurring throughout the nephron that establishes and maintains a high concentration of urea in the renal medulla. This process accounts for approximately 50% of the solutes concentrated in the medulla. With the countercurrent exchange mechanism, the urea cycle helps establish and maintain the high medullary osmotic gradient. Because urea can passively diffuse into the interstitium and back into the lumen fluid, the selectivity of the tubular epithelium in each portion of the nephron plays an integral part in the urea cycling process.

vasa recta The vascular network of long, U-shaped capillaries that forms from the peritubular capillaries and surrounds the loops of Henle in the renal medulla.

RENAL ANATOMY

The **kidneys** are bean shaped and are located on the posterior abdominal wall in the area known as the *retroperitoneum* (Figure 4-1). An adult human kidney has a mass of approximately 150 g and measures roughly 12.5 cm in length, 6 cm in width, and 2.5 cm in depth. When observed in cross-section, two distinct areas of the kidney are apparent: the cortex and the medulla. The outer cortex layer is approximately 1.4 cm thick and is granular in macroscopic appearance. Because all of the glomeruli are located in the outer cortex, the cortex is the exclusive site of the plasma filtration process. The inner layer, the medulla, consists of renal tissue shaped into pyramids. The apex of each of these pyramids is called a *papilla;* each contains a papillary duct that opens into a cavity called a *calyx*. The normal human kidney consists of about 12 minor calyces, which join together to form two to three major calyces. Each calyx acts as a funnel to receive urine from the collecting tubules and pass it into the renal pelvis.

The funnel-shaped renal pelvis emerges from the indented region of each kidney and narrows to join with the ureter, a fibromuscular tube that is approximately 25 cm long. One ureter extends down from each kidney and connects to the base of the bladder, a muscular sac that is shaped like a three-sided pyramid. The apex of this "bladder pyramid" is oriented downward and is where the urethra originates and extends to the exterior of the body. To review briefly, urine forms as the plasma ultrafiltrate passes through the renal tubules (nephrons) that reside in the renal cortex and the medulla. Thereafter, the urine is transferred via minor and major calyces to the renal pelvis, where peristaltic activity of smooth muscles moves the urine down the ureters into the bladder. The bladder serves as a holding tank for temporary urine storage until it is voided by urination. When approximately 150 mL of urine accumulates, a nerve reflex is initiated. Unless a person overrides the urge to urinate (i.e., the micturition reflex), simultaneous contraction of the bladder muscles and relaxation of the urinary sphincter will result in the passage of urine through the urethra. The urethra, a canal connecting the bladder to the body exterior, is approximately 4 cm long in women and approximately 24 cm long in men.

Note that when an individual is healthy, the composition of urine is not altered appreciably at any point following its introduction into the minor and major calyces. The calyces and subsequent anatomic structures serve only as a conveyance for urine, which is the primary excretory product of the kidneys.

Each kidney contains approximately 1.3 million nephrons, which are the functional units or tubules of the kidney. A **nephron** is composed of five distinct areas,

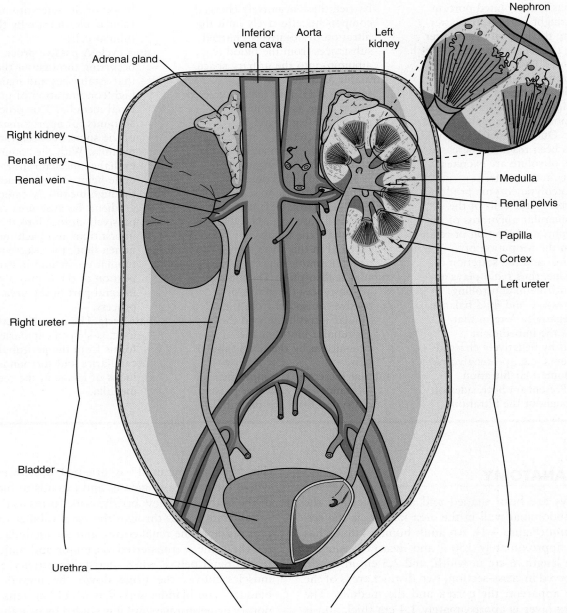

FIGURE 4-1 A schematic representation of the urinary tract. The relationship of the kidneys to the nephrons and the vascular system is shown.

each playing an important part in the formation and final composition of the urine. Figure 4-2 shows a nephron, its component parts, and their physical interrelationships. The glomerulus consists of a capillary tuft surrounded by a thin epithelial layer of cells known as *Bowman's capsule.* Bowman's capsule is actually the originating end of a renal tubule, and its lumen is referred to as *Bowman's space.* The plasma ultrafiltrate of low-molecular-weight solutes initially collects in Bowman's space because of the hydrostatic pressure difference between the capillary lumen and Bowman's space.

The proximal convoluted tubule begins at the glomerulus and extends from it in a circuitous route through the cortex. Eventually the tubule straightens and turns downward, entering the medulla to become the **loop of Henle.** The loop of Henle has anatomically distinct areas: thin descending and ascending limbs that include a sharp hairpin turn, and thick descending and ascending limbs that are actually straight portions of the proximal and distal tubules (Box 4-1). Upon reentry into the cortex at the macula densa—adjacent to the glomerulus—the straight distal tubule becomes the distal convoluted tubule. Anatomically up to this point, each nephron is structurally and functionally distinct. After this point, the distal convoluted tubules join to a "shared" collecting tubule or duct that conveys the urine produced in several nephrons through the medulla for a second time. These collecting tubules fuse to become the larger

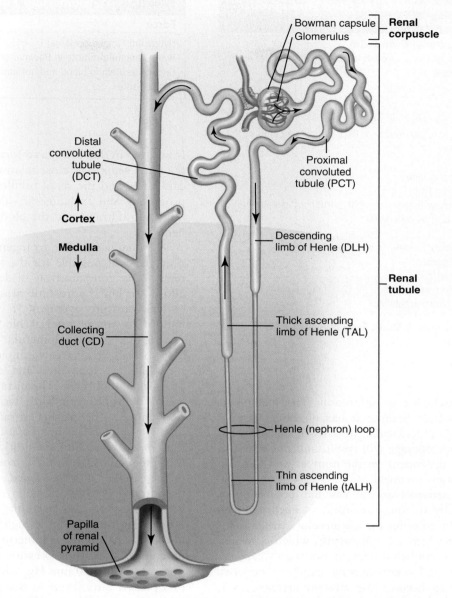

FIGURE 4-2 A diagram of a nephron. *(Modified from Patton KT, Thibodeau GA: Anatomy and physiology, ed 8, St. Louis, 2013, Mosby.)*

papillary ducts that empty into the calyces of the renal pyramids and finally into the renal pelvis. From the renal pelvis, the urine passes to the bladder to await excretion through the urethra.

RENAL CIRCULATION

The kidneys require a rich blood supply to execute their primary function of regulating the internal environment of the body. In fact, despite their mass of only 300 g, or 0.5% of the total body mass, the kidneys receive 25% of the total cardiac output. This high degree of perfusion reflects the direct relationship of the kidney's functional ability to its blood supply.

Each kidney is supplied by a single renal artery that originates from the aorta. As the renal artery successively divides, it forms a distinct vascular arrangement, unique to and specifically adapted for the functions of the kidney. The kidney is the only human organ in which an arteriole subdivides into a capillary bed, becomes an arteriole again, and then for a second time subdivides into a capillary network. In addition, the renal arterioles are primarily end arteries that supply specific areas of renal tissue and do not interconnect.

Therefore disruption in the supply of blood at the afferent arteriole or the glomerulus will dramatically and detrimentally alter the functioning of the associated nephron. Consequently, renal tissue is particularly

BOX 4-1	**Outline of the Nephron and Its Components (As Used Throughout This Text)**

Glomerulus (or Renal Corpuscle)
1. Capillary tuft or glomerulus: often interchanged for entire entity
2. Bowman's capsule

Tubules
1. Proximal tubule
   a. Convoluted portion: pars convoluta
   b. Straight portion: pars recta (or thick descending limb of the loop of Henle)
2. Loop of Henle
   a. Thin descending limb
   b. Thin ascending limb
   c. Thick ascending limb or straight portion of distal tubule; terminates with macula densa
3. Distal tubule
   a. Straight portion; terminates with macula densa
   b. Convoluted portion
4. Collecting tubule (duct)
   a. Cortical collecting tubules
   b. Medullary collecting tubules

Modified from Koushanpour E, Kriz W: Renal physiology, ed 2, New York, 1986, Springer-Verlag.

TABLE 4-1	**Forces Involved in Glomerular Filtration**

Force	Magnitude
Hydrostatic (blood pressure)	+55 mm Hg
Hydrostatic (ultrafiltrate in Bowman's space)	−15 mm Hg
Oncotic (protein in blood and not in ultrafiltrate)	−30 mm Hg
Net pressure	+10 mm Hg

susceptible to ischemia or infarction. The medulla is especially susceptible because it has no direct arterial blood supply. Should vascular stenosis or an occlusion occur, renal tissue damage will result, and the extent of damage will be dependent on the number and location of the blood vessels involved.

An **afferent arteriole** at the vascular pole supplies blood individually to the glomerulus of each nephron (Figure 4-3). On entering the glomerulus, the afferent arteriole branches into a capillary tuft, which is related intimately to the epithelial cells of Bowman's capsule. This branching and anastomosing capillary network comes together to become the **efferent arteriole** as it leaves the glomerulus. Subsequently, the efferent arteriole branches for a second time into a capillary plexus. The type of nephron that the efferent arteriole services determines the vascular arrangement of this second capillary plexus. The outer cortical nephrons have short loops of Henle, and the efferent arteriole branches into a fine capillary plexus—the **peritubular capillaries**—that encompasses the outer cortical tubules entirely. The mid and deep juxtamedullary nephrons have long loops of Henle. The efferent arterioles of these nephrons first branch into a peritubular capillary bed, which enmeshes the cortical portions of the tubules, and then divide into a series of long, U-shaped vessels, the **vasa recta,** which descend deep into the renal medulla close to the loops of Henle. The corresponding ascending vasa recta form the beginnings of the venous renal circulation, emerging

from deep in the medulla to form venules and drain into the renal veins. The close relationship of the peritubular capillaries and the renal tubules enables the sequential processing and exchange of solutes between the lumen fluid (ultrafiltrate) and the bloodstream throughout the nephron.

The unique vascular arrangement of the renal circulation makes it possible for the kidney to function optimally. The comparatively wide-bore afferent arteriole allows for high hydrostatic pressure at the glomerulus.

This pressure averages 55 mm Hg, approximately half of the mean arterial blood pressure, and is the driving force behind glomerular filtration. All other capillary beds have a narrower lumen, which causes greater resistance to blood flow and consequently low blood pressure within them. The ultrafiltrate itself also affects the resultant filtration force across the glomerular filtration barrier. The plasma ultrafiltrate already in Bowman's space exerts a hydrostatic pressure of 15 mm Hg that opposes filtration. In addition, the ultrafiltrate is low in protein and high in water compared with the plasma in the capillary lumen. Hence, water that freely passed the filtration barrier seeks to reenter the plasma from Bowman's space. As a result, an oncotic pressure of 30 mm Hg caused by the higher protein concentration in the plasma opposes glomerular filtration as well. The outcome of these three pressure differences is a net filtration pressure of 10 mm Hg, which favors the formation of a plasma ultrafiltrate in Bowman's space (Table 4-1). Note that the filtration barrier expends no energy in forming the plasma ultrafiltrate, rather the cardiac output provides the glomerular capillary blood pressure that drives plasma ultrafiltration.

The afferent and efferent arterioles exit Bowman's capsule at the vascular pole in proximity to each other. The vascular pole is also the site of the **juxtaglomerular apparatus.** The morphologically distinct structures that compose the juxtaglomerular apparatus are portions of the afferent and efferent arterioles, the extraglomerular mesangial cells (which are continuous with the supporting mesangium of the glomerulus), and the specialized area of the distal convoluted tubule (known as the *macula densa*). Characteristically, large quantities of secretory granules containing the enzyme renin are present in the smooth muscle cells of the afferent

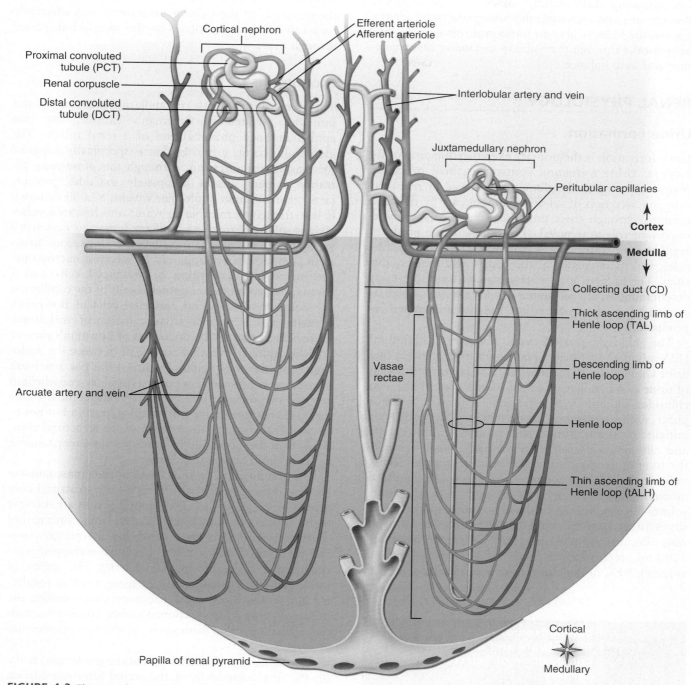

FIGURE 4-3 The vascular circulation of a cortical and juxtamedullary nephron. *(Modified from Patton KT, Thibodeau GA: Anatomy and physiology, ed 8, St. Louis, 2013, Mosby.)*

arteriole located in the juxtaglomerular apparatus. The juxtaglomerular apparatus, which is essentially a small endocrine organ, is the principal producer of renin in the kidney. **Renin** is an enzyme that when released into the bloodstream in response to decreased blood volume, decreased arterial pressure, sodium depletion, vascular hemorrhage, or increased potassium ultimately forms angiotensin and causes the secretion of aldosterone.

Aldosterone secretion stimulates the kidneys to actively retain sodium and passively retain water. As a result, the volume of extracellular fluid expands, the blood pressure increases, and normal potassium levels, as well as normal renal perfusion, are restored. Conversely, an increase in blood volume, an acute increase in blood pressure, or the loss of potassium inhibits renin secretion and enhances sodium excretion (also see "Renal

Concentrating Mechanism," later in this chapter). Because of renin secretion, the juxtaglomerular apparatus and the kidneys play an important role in body fluid homeostasis through their ability to modify blood pressure and fluid balance.

RENAL PHYSIOLOGY

Urine Formation

Urine formation is the primary excretory function of the kidneys. Urine formation consists of three processes: plasma filtration at the glomeruli followed by reabsorption and secretion of selective components by the renal tubules. Through these processes, the kidneys play an important role in removal of metabolic waste products, regulation of water and electrolytes (e.g., sodium, chloride), and maintenance of the body's acid-base equilibrium. The kidneys are the true regulators of the body, determining which substances to retain and which to excrete, regardless of what has been ingested or produced.

The kidneys process approximately 180,000 mL (125 mL/min) of filtered plasma each day into a final urine volume of 600 to 1800 mL. The largest component of urine is water. The principal solutes present are urea, chloride, sodium, and potassium, followed by phosphate, sulfate, creatinine, and uric acid. Other substances initially in the ultrafiltrate, such as glucose, bicarbonate, and albumin, are essentially completely reabsorbed by the tubules. Consequently, the urine of normal healthy individuals does not contain these solutes in significant amounts. Table 4-2 presents a comparison of selected solutes initially filtered by the glomerulus and the quantity actually excreted after passage through the nephrons. Because normal urine output is approximately 1200 mL (approximately 1% of the filtered plasma volume), 99% of the ultrafiltrate that initially collects in

Bowman's space is actually reabsorbed. In addition, the nephrons of the kidneys extensively and selectively reabsorb and secrete solutes as the ultrafiltrate passes through them.

Glomerulus

The glomerulus is a tuft of capillaries encircled by and intimately related to Bowman's capsule, the thin epithelium-lined proximal end of a renal tubule. The glomerulus forms a barrier that is specifically designed for plasma ultrafiltration. Although this *glomerular filtration barrier* almost completely excludes proteins larger than albumin (molecular weight, 67,000 daltons), it is extremely permeable to water and low-molecular-weight solutes. From the capillary lumen to Bowman's space, where the plasma filtrate first collects, four structural components are apparent by electron microscopy: the mesangium, consisting of mesangial cells and a matrix; the fenestrated endothelial cells of the capillaries; the podocytes or visceral epithelial cells of Bowman's capsule; and a distinct trilayer basement membrane sandwiched between the podocytes of Bowman's capsule and the capillary endothelial cells, or between the podocytes and the mesangium (Figure 4-4). No basement membrane is present between the capillary endothelium and the mesangium; this provides evidence of the role the basement membrane has in ultrafiltration but not in structural anchoring. Knowledge of the structural composition of the glomerulus is important in understanding its function in health and disease.

The **mesangium**, located within the anastomosing lobules of the glomerular tuft, forms the structural core tissue of the glomerulus. The mesangial cells are thought to be of smooth muscle origin, retaining contractility characteristics and a large capability for phagocytosis and pinocytosis, which helps to remove entrapped macromolecules from the filtration barrier. The ability of mesangial cells to contract also suggests a role in regulating glomerular blood flow. The matrix surrounding the mesangial cells is, as mentioned earlier, continuous with the extraglomerular mesangium of the juxtaglomerular apparatus.

The capillary endothelial cells of the glomerulus make up the first component of the actual filtration barrier. The endothelium is fenestrated, that is, it has large, open pores 50 to 100 nm in diameter. When viewed from the lumen of the capillary, these openings give the endothelium a dotted swiss appearance (Figure 4-5). In addition, the capillary endothelium possesses a negatively charged coating that repels anionic molecules. The size of the pores and the negative charge of the endothelium play an important role in solute selectivity during plasma ultrafiltration.

The second component of the filtration barrier is the **basement membrane**, which separates the epithelium of the urinary space from the endothelium of the

TABLE 4-2	Comparison of the Initial Ultrafiltrate and the Final Urine Composition of Selected Solutes per Day		
Component	**Initial Ultrafiltrate, mmol**	**Final Urine, mmol**	**Percent Reabsorbed**
Water (1.2 L*)	9,500,000.00	67,000.00	99.3
Urea	910.00	400.00	44.0
Chloride	37,000.00	185.00	99.5
Sodium	32,500.00	130.00	99.6
Potassium	986.00	70.00	92.9
Glucose†	900.00	0.72	100.0
Albumin	0.02	0.001	95.0

*Average 24-hour urine volume; glomerular filtration rate of 125 mL/min.
†Represents average glucose values.

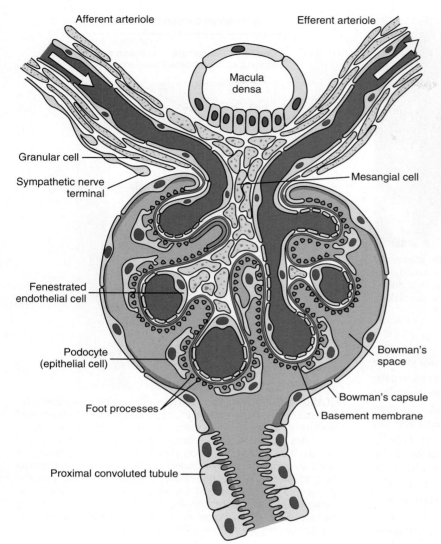

Afferent arteriole

Efferent arteriole

Macula densa

Granular cell

Sympathetic nerve terminal

Mesangial cell

Fenestrated endothelial cell

Podocyte (epithelial cell)

Foot processes

Bowman's space

Bowman's capsule

Basement membrane

Proximal convoluted tubule

FIGURE 4-4 A schematic overview of a glomerulus. The afferent arteriole enters the glomerulus and the efferent arteriole exits the glomerulus at the vascular pole. Also at the vascular pole, a portion of the thick ascending limb of the distal tubule, the macula densa, is in contact with the glomerular mesangium. Bowman's space is formed from specialized epithelial cells (Bowman's capsule) at the end of a renal tubule. At the urinary pole, Bowman's space becomes the tubular lumen of the proximal tubule. Podocytes are the epithelial cells that cover the glomerular capillaries and derive their name from their characteristic footlike processes. The glomerular capillaries are lined with fenestrated endothelial cells (i.e., epithelium with pores). The basement membrane, which separates the capillary endothelium and the podocytes (the epithelium of Bowman's space), is continuous throughout the glomerulus. The basement membrane is absent between the capillary endothelium and the mesangium. The mesangial cells of the glomerular tuft form the structural core of the glomerulus and are continuous with the extraglomerular mesangial cells located at the vascular pole between the afferent and efferent arterioles. The secretory granules of the granular cells contain large amounts of renin. The afferent arteriole is innervated by sympathetic nerves.

glomerular capillaries. The basement membrane has three layers: the lamina rara interna lies adjacent to the capillary endothelium, the lamina densa (electron dense by electron micrograph) is located centrally, and the lamina rara externa is adjacent to the epithelium of Bowman's space (Figure 4-6). The basement membrane consistently courses below the epithelium of Bowman's space and is absent between the capillary endothelium and the supporting mesangium. As mentioned previously, this trilayer structure is not the basement membrane of the glomerular capillaries, rather it contributes specifically to the permeability characteristics of the filtration barrier. Composed principally of collagenous and noncollagenous proteins, the basement membrane of the filtration barrier is a matrix with hydrated interstices. Nonpolar collagenous components are concentrated in the lamina densa. An important polar noncollagenous component, heparan sulfate (a polyanionic proteoglycan), is located primarily in the outer lamina rara layers, endowing the layers with their strongly anionic character.

On the tubule side of the glomerulus, lining Bowman's space, are the **podocytes.** Attached to the glomerular basement membrane, the podocytes constitute the third component of the filtration barrier. The name *podocyte* means foot cell and relates to their footlike appearance when viewed in cross-section (see Figure 4-6). The podocytes completely cover the glomerular capillaries with extending finger-like processes and interdigitate with neighboring podocytes (Figure 4-7, *A*). However, their processes actually do not touch each other, rather a consistent space of 20 to 30 nm separates them, forming a snakelike channel that zigzags across the surface of the glomerular capillaries.[1] This snakelike channel is called the *filtration slit* and covers only about 3% of the total glomerular basement membrane area. The slit is lined with a distinct extracellular structure known as the *slit diaphragm.* The substructure of the slit diaphragm consists of regularly arranged subunits with rectangular open spaces about the size of an albumin molecule. Often the slit diaphragm is considered part of the basement membrane, although it is distinctly separate and

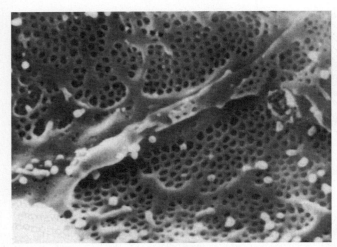

FIGURE 4-5 A scanning electron micrograph of the glomerular capillary endothelium as viewed from the capillary lumen. The openings or fenestrations of the endothelium resemble a dotted swiss pattern. *(From Boron W, Boulpeep E: Medical physiology, updated version, ed 1, Philadelphia, 2005, Saunders.)*

Glomerular capsular membrane

Capillary   Basement   Slit diaphragm
endothelium membrane   (visceral wall of
                        Bowman's capsule)

CL   CB

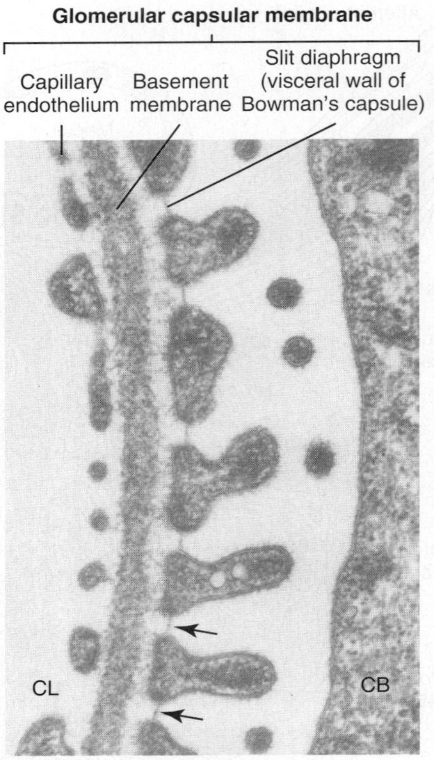

FIGURE 4-6 A transmission electron micrograph of a glomerular filtration barrier. From left to right, capillary lumen (CL), fenestrated capillary endothelium, basement membrane, foot processes of podocytes separated by slit diaphragms, Bowman's space, and portion of an overarching podocyte cell body (CB). The basement membrane consists of three distinct layers: the lamina rara interna (next to the capillary endothelium), the lamina densa, and the lamina rara externa (next to the epithelium or podocytes). The arrows indicate slit diaphragms that lie between the interdigitating foot processes. *(From Boron W, Boulpeep E: Medical physiology, updated version, ed 1, Philadelphia, 2005, Saunders.)*

actually lies on the basement membrane. Podocytes are metabolically active cells. They contain numerous organelles and extensive lysosomal elements that correlate directly with their extensive phagocytic ability. Macromolecules that are unable to proceed through the slit diaphragm or return to the capillary lumen are rapidly phagocytized by podocytes to prevent occlusion of the filtration barrier. Similar to the capillary endothelium, all surfaces of the podocytes, filtration slits, and slit diaphragms that line the urinary space are covered with a thick, negatively charged coating.

In review, the three distinct structures that compose the **glomerular filtration barrier** are (1) the capillary endothelium with its large open pores, (2) the trilayer basement membrane, and (3) the filtration diaphragms located between the podocytes (epithelium) of Bowman's space. Each component maintains an anionic charge on its cellular surface or within it, and each component is essential for proper functioning of the filtration barrier.

The selectivity of the filtration barrier is based on the molecular size and charge of the solute. Water and small solutes rapidly pass through the filtration barrier with little or no resistance. In contrast, larger plasma molecules must overcome the negative charge present on the endothelium and must be able to pass through the endothelial pores, which are 50 to 100 nm in diameter.[1] The **shield of negativity** of the endothelium successfully repels most plasma proteins, thereby preventing the filtration barrier from becoming congested with them. However, neutral and cationic molecules readily pass through the filtration barrier if they do not exceed the size restriction imposed by the basement membrane. To penetrate the basement membrane and the slit diaphragm, neutral and cationic molecules must possess an effective molecular radius of less than 4 nm. The successful passage of

molecules with diameters larger than 4 nm decreases with increasing size. However, molecules with diameters greater than 8 nm typically are not capable of glomerular filtration.[2] Albumin has an effective radius of 3.6 nm and a molecular weight of approximately 67,000 daltons.[3] If the shield of negativity that permeates the basement membrane and the filtration slits is not present, albumin would readily pass through the filtration barrier. This is evidenced in glomerular diseases in which loss of the shield of negativity (e.g., lipoid nephrosis) or an alteration in the filtration barrier structure (e.g., glomerulonephritis) results in proteinuria and hematuria.

The initial ultrafiltrate present in Bowman's space differs from the plasma in that it lacks the blood cells and plasma proteins larger than albumin (including any protein-bound substances). The normal filtration rate of approximately 125 mL/min depends on body size and is discussed at length in the section on glomerular filtration tests. Any condition that modifies glomerular blood flow, hydrostatic or oncotic pressures across the glomerular filtration barrier, or the structural integrity of

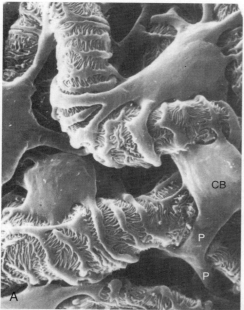

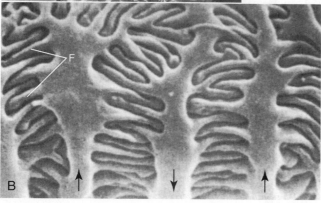

FIGURE 4-7 A scanning electron micrograph of podocytes and their interdigitating foot processes on glomerular capillaries as viewed from Bowman's space. **A,** Epithelial or podocyte cell body (CB) and podocyte foot processes (P) on glomerular capillaries. **B,** An enlargement of interdigitating foot processes (F) of adjacent epithelial cells (podocyte). The arrows indicate primary processes and show the alternating pattern between epithelial cells. (*A, From Boron W, Boulpeep E: Medical physiology, updated version, ed 1, Philadelphia, 2005, Saunders; **B,** From Koushanpour E, Kriz W: Renal physiology, ed 2, New York, 1986, Springer-Verlag. Used by permission.*)

the glomerulus will affect the glomerular filtration rate and ultimately the amount of urine produced.

Tubules

The epithelium that lines the renal tubules changes throughout the five distinct areas of the nephron. Looking at the diverse and specialized epithelial characteristics of each segment aids in understanding the various processes that take place.

Once the glomerular ultrafiltrate has been formed in Bowman's space, hydrostatic pressure alone moves the ultrafiltrate through the remaining tubular portions of

the nephrons. Each tubular portion has distinctively different epithelium, which relates directly to the unique processes that occur there. The first section, the **proximal tubule,** consists of a large convoluted portion (pars convoluta) followed by a straight portion (pars recta). The cells of the proximal tubule are tall and extensively interdigitate with each other (Figure 4-8). These intercellular interdigitations serve to increase the overall cellular surface area and are characteristic of salt-transporting epithelia. The luminal surfaces of these cells have a brush border because of the abundant number of microvilli present (typical of absorbing epithelia as in the small intestine). These densely packed microvilli, by greatly increasing the luminal surface area, provide a maximal area for filtrate reabsorption. In addition, the proximal tubular cells have numerous mitochondria (evidence of their high metabolic activity) and are abundant in the enzymes necessary for active transport of various solutes.

When the straight portion of the proximal tubule enters the outer medulla to become the thin descending limb of the loop of Henle, the tubular epithelium changes. At this point, the epithelium consists of flat, noninterdigitating cells that are simply organized (see Figure 4-8). Depending on the length of the loop of Henle, the cellular organization varies. The longest limbs that reach deep into the medulla have increased cellular complexity. Regardless of the length of the limb, the epithelium changes again at the hairpin turn of the loop of Henle. These epithelial cells, although remaining flat, extensively interdigitate with each other. The interdigitating epithelium found at the hairpin turn continues throughout the thin ascending limb of the loop of Henle.

The thick ascending limb of the loop of Henle (or the straight portion of the distal tubule) is characterized primarily by tall, interdigitating cells (see Figure 4-8). As in the proximal tubular epithelium, large numbers of mitochondria reside, and a high level of enzymatic activity is present. In contrast to proximal tubular cells, only the basal two-thirds of distal tubular cells interdigitate. The topmost or luminal portion of these cells have a simple polygonal shape and maintain a smooth border with neighboring cells. Following the macula densa or the juxtamedullary apparatus is the **distal convoluted tubule.** The amount of tubular convolution is less than that exhibited by the proximal tubule, and the distal convoluted tubule proceeds to a collecting duct after only two to three loops of convolution.

The **collecting duct** traverses the renal cortex and medulla and is the site of final urine concentration. The epithelium of the collecting ducts primarily consists of polygonal cells with some small, stubby microvilli and no intercellular interdigitations (see Figure 4-8). These cells have intercellular junctions or spaces between them that span from their luminal surfaces to their bases. In the presence of antidiuretic hormone (ADH; also known as *arginine vasopressin*), the spaces between the cells

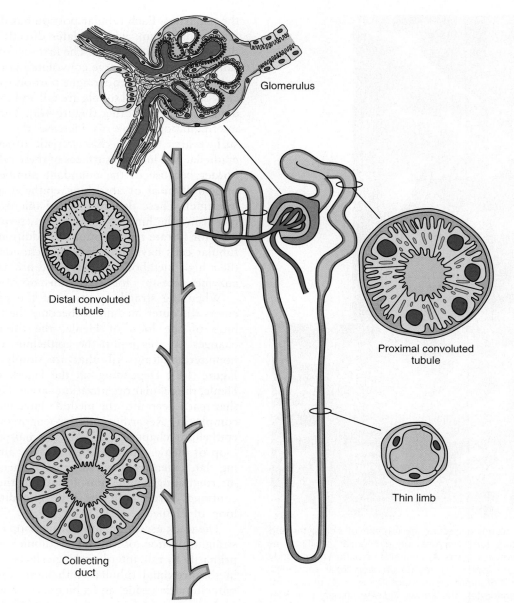

Glomerulus

Distal convoluted
tubule

Proximal convoluted
tubule

Thin limb

Collecting
duct

FIGURE 4-8 The general histologic characteristics of the renal tubular epithelium. Representative cross-sections of the various tubular segments roughly indicate their cellular morphology and the relative size of the cells, the tubules, and the tubular lumens.

dilate, rendering the epithelium highly permeable to water. In contrast, when ADH is absent, the spaces are joined tightly (Figure 4-9). As the collecting duct approaches a papillary tip, the epithelium changes again to cells that are taller and more columnar.

Tubular Function

The fact that only 1% (approximately 1200 mL) of the original plasma ultrafiltrate presented to the renal tubules is excreted as urine is evidence of the large amount of reabsorption that takes place within the renal tubules. In addition to this substantial volume change, the resultant solute makeup of the urine excreted differs dramatically from that of the original ultrafiltrate, underscoring the

dynamic processes carried out by the tubules. By virtue of this renal tubular ability to adjust the excretion of water and solutes, the kidney is the most important organ involved in fluid exchanges. The mechanisms effecting these changes, namely, **tubular reabsorption** and **tubular secretion,** are the same; it is the direction of substance movement that differs, with the substance moved from the tubular lumen into the peritubular capillary blood and interstitium (reabsorption), or from the peritubular capillary blood and interstitium into the tubular lumen (secretion).

Transport. The tubular transport mechanisms (i.e., reabsorption and secretion) are active or passive. **Active transport** is the movement of a substance across a membrane against a gradient. In other words, the

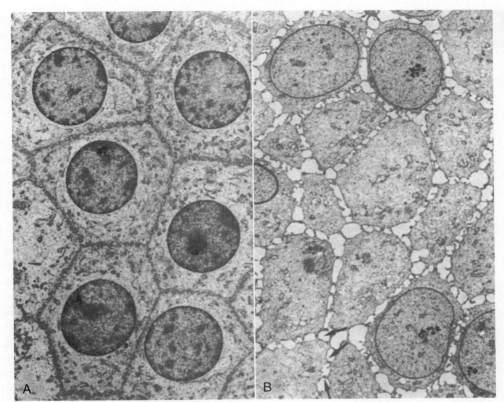

FIGURE 4-9 A transmission electron micrograph of cross-sections of the medullary collecting duct epithelium. **A,** The intercellular spaces are narrow. **B,** The intercellular spaces are dilated. The observed dilation is probably due to the effect of antidiuretic hormone on the epithelium, enabling the passive reabsorption of water. *(From Koushanpour E, Kriz W: Renal physiology, ed 2, New York, 1986, Springer-Verlag. Used by permission.)*

compartments separated by the membrane differ in their chemical or electrical composition. Such transport requires an expenditure of energy, directly or indirectly.

When energy is required to actively transport a substance, as in the exchange of potassium for sodium driven by adenosine triphosphate hydrolysis (the sodium pump), this is called *direct active transport*. When the movement of one substance is coupled with the movement of another substance down a gradient, this is called *indirect active transport* or *cotransport* (e.g., the indirect absorption of glucose with sodium in the proximal tubules).

Active transport occurs across the cell (transcellularly) and involves specific protein-binding sites that span the cell membrane. In active transport, the substance (1) binds to its specific membrane-binding site, (2) is passed through the cell membrane, and (3) is released inside or outside the cell as the binding site undergoes a conformational change.

Passive transport, however, requires no energy and is characterized by the movement of a substance along a gradient, or, in other words, from an area of higher concentration to one of lower concentration, as in the movement of urea. This type of transport may be transcellular or paracellular—between cells by way of junctions and intercellular spaces.

Each solute has a specific transport system. Cellular protein-binding sites may be unique for a particular solute, transporting only that solute across the membrane, or they may transport several solutes, often exhibiting preferential transport of one analyte over another. In addition, the mode of transport, whether active or passive, is not always the same and can differ depending on the tubular location. For example, chloride is reabsorbed actively in the ascending loop of Henle but passively in the proximal tubule (Table 4-3).

Reabsorption. Tubular function is selective, reabsorbing the substances necessary for the maintenance of body homeostasis and function, such as water, salts, glucose, amino acids, and proteins, while excreting waste products such as creatinine and metabolic acids. Table 4-3 summarizes some important ultrafiltrate components according to the location of their tubular reabsorption. The table also indicates the primary mode of transport for each substance. Note that this summary refers to the major overall transport of the substance; in reality, reabsorption of some solutes actually involves several mechanisms. The following section discusses the principal interactions of the major solutes and their transport processes.

Secretion. As with tubular reabsorption, tubular secretion takes place throughout the nephron. The principal

TABLE 4-3	Summary of Tubular Reabsorption of Ultrafiltrate Components	
Location	**Mode of Reabsorption**	**Substance**
Proximal tubule (convoluted and straight portions)	Passive	H_2O, Cl^-, K^+, urea
	Active	Na^+, HCO_3^-, glucose, amino acids, proteins, phosphate, sulfate, Mg^{2+}, Ca^{2+}, uric acid
Loop of Henle		
Thin descending limb	Passive	H_2O, urea
U-turn and thin ascending limb	Passive	Na^+, Cl^-, urea
Thick ascending limb (medullary and cortical)	Passive	Urea
	Active	Na^+, Cl^-
Distal tubule (convoluted portion)	Active	*Na^+, Cl^-, sulfate, uric acid
	Passive	†H_2O
Collecting Tubules		
Cortical	Passive	†H_2O, Cl^-
	Active	*Na^+
Medullary	Passive	H_2O, urea

*Reabsorption under aldosterone control by the renin-angiotensin-aldosterone system.
†Reabsorption under the control of antidiuretic hormone.

TABLE 4-4	Summary of Tubular Secretion of Important Ultrafiltrate Components
Location	**Substance**
Proximal tubule	H^+, NH_3, weak acids and bases
Loop of Henle	Urea
Distal tubule	H^+, NH_3, K^+, uric acid (some drugs)
Collecting tubule	H^+, NH_3, K^+ (some drugs)

roles of the renal secretory process are (1) to eliminate metabolic wastes and those substances not normally present in the plasma, and (2) to adjust the acid-base equilibrium of the body. These two functions overlap in that many metabolic by-products and foreign substances are weak acids and bases, thereby directly affecting the acid-base status of the body. Table 4-4 summarizes some of the important secreted ultrafiltrate solutes and the locations of their tubular secretion.

Most of the substances secreted, other than hydrogen ions, ammonia, and potassium, are weak acids or bases. These weak acids and bases originate from metabolic or exogenous sources. They are (1) substances incompletely metabolized by the body (e.g., thiamine), (2) substances not metabolized at all and secreted unchanged

(e.g., radiopaque contrast media and mannitol), or (3) substances not normally present in the plasma (e.g., penicillin, salicylate). Some of these substances simply cannot pass through the glomerular filtration barrier for excretion because they are bound to plasma proteins, primarily albumin (e.g., unconjugated bilirubin, drugs). As a result, their overall size is dramatically increased, and their original molecular charge may be modified. Tubular secretion, however, provides a means for their elimination. As these relatively large and protein-bound substances flow through the peritubular capillaries, they interact with endothelium-binding sites, are transported into renal tubular cells, and are ultimately secreted into the tubular lumen.

Regulation of Acid-Base Equilibrium. To better understand the role of tubular secretion in the regulation of the body's acid-base equilibrium, basic knowledge of the endogenous production of acids and bases is needed. In health, normal blood pH is alkaline, ranging from 7.35 to 7.45. However, in pathologic disease states, the pH can be as low as 7.00 or as high as 7.80. Blood is alkaline, and its pH is constantly threatened by the endogenous production of acids from normal dietary metabolism. These endogenous acids are formed (1) from the production of carbon dioxide owing to oxidative metabolism of foods that create carbonic acid, (2) from the catabolism of dietary proteins and phospholipids, or (3) from the production of acids in certain pathologic or physiologic conditions, such as acetoacetic acid in uncontrolled diabetes mellitus or lactic acid with exercise.

Three body systems are involved in maintaining the blood pH at a level compatible with life: (1) the blood-buffer system, which involves hemoglobin, bicarbonate, proteins, and inorganic phosphates, (2) the pulmonary system, and (3) the renal system. Although all three systems work together to maintain homeostasis, the blood-buffer and pulmonary systems are able to respond immediately, although only partially, to pH changes. The renal system, however, despite its comparatively slow response, is capable of completely correcting deviations in blood pH.

In response to changes in blood pH, the kidneys selectively excrete acid or alkali in the urine. Whereas excess alkali is eliminated by the excretion of sodium salts, such as disodium phosphate and sodium bicarbonate, excess acids are eliminated by the excretion of titratable acids (monosodium phosphate) and ammonium salts (e.g., NH_4Cl, $[NH_4]_2SO_4$).

Three secretory mechanisms maintain the blood pH, and each relies directly or indirectly on the tubular secretion of H^+ ions. In acidotic conditions, H^+ ions (acids) are secreted by renal tubular cells in exchange for sodium and bicarbonate ions (alkali). In alkalotic conditions, tubular secretion of H^+ ions is minimized which assists in the elimination of excess alkali from the body.

In the first secretory mechanism, H^+ ions are secreted into the proximal tubular lumen, directly preventing

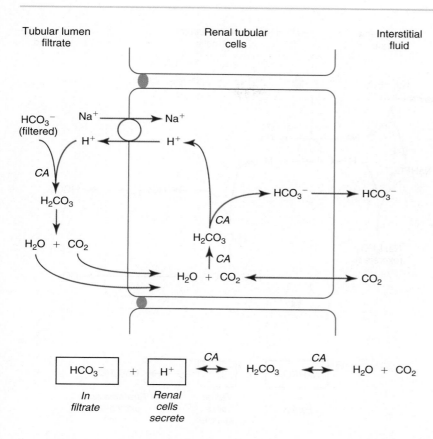

Tubular lumen filtrate   Renal tubular cells   Interstitial fluid

FIGURE 4-10 Hydrogen ion secretion and the mechanism of filtered bicarbonate reabsorption in the proximal tube. *CA*, Carbonic anhydrase.

the loss of bicarbonate, a vital component of the blood-buffer system. In Figure 4-10, bicarbonate ions (HCO_3^-), which readily pass the glomerular filtration barrier, react with the secreted H^+ to form carbonic acid (H_2CO_3) in the tubular lumen. This carbonic acid, however, is rapidly catalyzed to carbon dioxide and water because of the high concentration of the enzyme carbonic anhydrase present in the brush border of the proximal tubular cells. The carbon dioxide diffuses into the proximal cell, where once again, by the action of intracellular carbonic anhydrase, it is converted to HCO_3^- and H^+. As a result, H^+ ions are available once more for tubular secretion and for reabsorption of HCO_3^- ions from the tubular lumen. The reabsorbed bicarbonate diffuses into the interstitial fluid and peritubular capillaries, thereby resupplying the blood-buffer system.

The second secretory mechanism, illustrated in Figure 4-11, depends on the amount of phosphate present in the ultrafiltrate. Phosphoric acids produced by dietary metabolism are converted rapidly in the blood to neutral salts (e.g., Na_2HPO_4) and are transported to the kidney. In the tubular lumen of the nephrons, secreted hydrogen ions exchange with the sodium ions, and disodium phosphate (Na_2HPO_4) becomes monosodium phosphate (NaH_2PO_4) (Equation 4-1). These monobasic phosphates—specifically combined with hydrogen ions and excreted in the urine—are referred to as *titratable acids*. The name derives from the ability to titrate urine to a pH of 7.4 (pH of normal plasma) using a standard

base (e.g., NaOH), to determine the amount of acid present as a result of these monobasic phosphates. Note that hydrogen ions combined with other solutes are not measured by this titration.

As a direct result of these phosphates in the ultrafiltrate, acid is removed from the body and the urine is acidified; in addition, sodium and bicarbonate ions are returned to the peritubular capillary blood.

The third secretory mechanism for acid removal, as illustrated in Figure 4-12, depends on ammonia secretion and the subsequent exchange of sodium ions for ammonium ions. Ammonia (NH_3) is produced in the renal tubular cells by the action of the enzyme glutaminase on the substrate glutamine, obtained from the peritubular capillary blood. Because NH_3 is not ionized, it is lipid soluble and readily diffuses across tubular cell membranes into the tubular lumen. Once in the lumen, NH_3 rapidly combines with H^+ ions to form ammonium ions (NH_4^+). These ions, essentially nondiffusible because of their charge, remain in the tubular lumen and may combine with neutral salts such as sodium chloride or sodium sulfate, a metabolic by-product. Equations 4-2 and 4-3 depict the chemical reactions that take place in the tubular lumen.

Equation 4-1

In blood	$H_3PO_4 + 6Na^+ \rightarrow 3Na_2HPO_4$
In ultrafiltrate	$Na_2HPO_4 + H^+ \rightarrow NaH_2PO_4 + Na^+$
	$Na^+ + HCO_3^- \rightarrow NaHCO_3$ (reabsorbed)

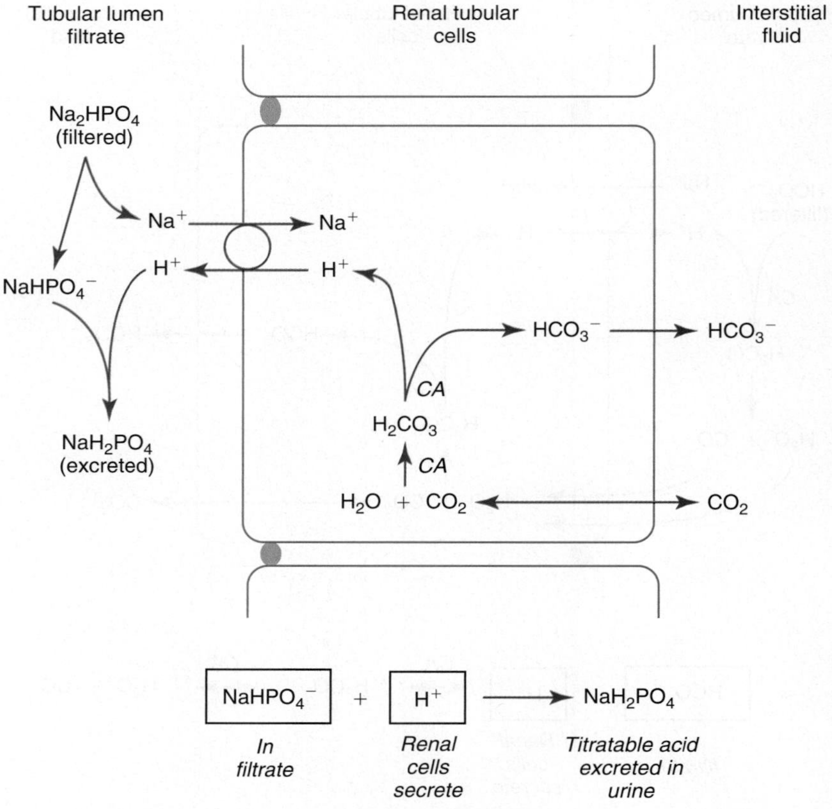

Tubular lumen filtrate   Renal tubular cells   Interstitial fluid

FIGURE 4-11 Hydrogen ion secretion and the formation of titratable acids. This is a mechanism of urine acidification in the collecting ducts. *CA*, Carbonic anhydrase.

$$NaHPO_4^- \quad + \quad H^+ \longrightarrow NaH_2PO_4$$

In filtrate   Renal cells secrete   Titratable acid excreted in urine

Equation 4-2

$$NH_3 + H^+ \rightarrow NH_4^+$$

$$NH_4^+ + NaCl + HCO_3^- \rightarrow NH_4Cl \text{ (excreted)} + NaHCO_3 \text{ (reabsorbed)}$$

Equation 4-3

$$NH_3 + H^+ \rightarrow NH_4^+$$

$$2NH_4^+ + Na_2SO_4 + 2HCO_3^- \rightarrow (NH_4)_2SO_4 \text{ (excreted)} + 2NaHCO_3 \text{ (reabsorbed)}$$

Note that in both reactions, bicarbonate and sodium are replenished and are available for tubular reabsorption.

The ammonia excreted in urine is derived primarily from renal tubular synthesis. Both the proximal and collecting duct cells are responsible for ammonia production, and final urine acidification principally occurs in the collecting ducts. However, the rate of ammonia synthesis is regulated in direct response to the body's acid-base status. For example, the production of ammonia increases in response to acidotic conditions.

In summary, the kidney regulates the acid-base equilibrium of the body using three renal secretory mechanisms: (1) H^+ ion secretion to recover bicarbonate; (2) H^+ ion secretion to yield urine titratable acids (e.g., monosodium phosphate); and (3) H^+ ion and NH_3 secretion to yield ammonium salts (e.g., ammonium chloride,

ammonium sulfate). By each of these mechanisms, hydrogen ion secretion (i.e., the loss of acid) results in sodium or bicarbonate reabsorption (i.e., the gain of alkali). Therefore the kidney modulates its secretion of hydrogen ions and ammonia according to the dynamic acid-base needs of the body.

Tubular Transport Capacity. The capacity of the renal tubules for reabsorption and secretion varies depending on the substance involved. For some substances, as the amount of solute presented to the renal tubules increases, the rate of tubular reabsorption also increases until a maximal rate of reabsorption is attained. This maximal reabsorptive rate remains constant despite any further increases in the solute's concentration. Consequently, excess solute that is not reabsorbed appears in the urine. This reabsorptive characteristic of the renal epithelium is known as the *maximal tubular reabsorptive capacity*. Denoted T_m, it represents the amount of solute (milligrams) reabsorbed per minute. The T_m varies depending on the specific solute and on other factors, such as the glomerular filtration rate. Glucose, amino acids, proteins, phosphate, sulfate, and uric acid are a few of the solutes that exhibit a T_m- limited tubular reabsorptive capacity. These solutes also have a blood concentration, known as the *renal threshold level,* which specifically relates to their T_m. For example, the T_m for glucose is approximately 350 mg/min (when corrected to 1.73 m²

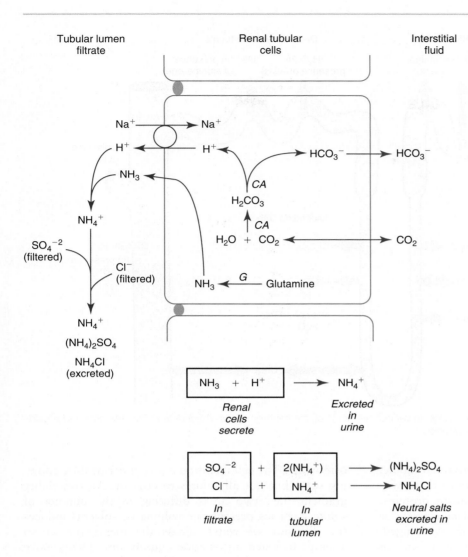

Tubular lumen filtrate

Renal tubular cells

Interstitial fluid

FIGURE 4-12 Hydrogen ion secretion and the formation of ammonium ions. This is a mechanism of urine acidification in the collecting ducts. *CA*, Carbonic anhydrase; *G*, glutaminase.

$$NH_3 + H^+ \longrightarrow NH_4^+$$

Renal cells secrete   *Excreted in urine*

$$SO_4^{-2} + 2(NH_4^+) \longrightarrow (NH_4)_2SO_4$$
$$Cl^- + NH_4^+ \longrightarrow NH_4Cl$$

In filtrate   *In tubular lumen*   *Neutral salts excreted in urine*

body surface area), which corresponds to a plasma renal threshold level for glucose of 160 to 180 mg/dL. Stated another way, regardless of the amount of glucose present in the renal tubular lumen, a maximum of 350 mg can be reabsorbed per minute. When the plasma glucose level exceeds 160 to 180 mg/dL, the ultrafiltrate glucose concentration is greater than the ability of the tubules to reabsorb (T_m), and glucose is excreted in the urine.

Similarly, some solutes secreted by the tubules have a maximal tubular secretory capacity, also denoted T_m (e.g., *p*-aminohippurate, a weak organic acid). The same designation, T_m, is appropriate because both processes refer to the maximum capacity for the active transport of a substance, and the direction of movement—whether into or out of the tubular lumen—is immaterial.

In contrast, some solutes are not limited in the amount that can be reabsorbed (e.g., sodium) or secreted (e.g., potassium). For these substances, other factors influence their rate of transport, such as the tubular flow rate, the amount of time the solute is in contact with the renal epithelium, the concentrations of other solutes in the

filtrate, the presence of transport inhibitors, and changes in hormone levels (e.g., ADH).

Proximal Tubular Reabsorption. The proximal tubule reabsorbs more than 66% of the filtered water, sodium, and chloride. In addition, essentially 100% of glucose, amino acids, and proteins is reabsorbed by a cotransport mechanism that is coupled to sodium. Other solutes such as bicarbonate, phosphate, sulfate, magnesium, calcium, and uric acid are also reabsorbed in the proximal tubule (see Table 4-3). Although these reabsorptive processes significantly reduce the volume and the concentrations of specific solutes, the fluid exiting the proximal tubule remains osmotically unchanged. In other words, despite substantial reabsorption of solutes and water in the proximal tubule, the absolute number of solute particles (osmoles) present per kilogram of water remains identical to that of the original ultrafiltrate, which is identical to the plasma (if made protein-free) in the peritubular capillaries. The solute particles in this filtrate also differ significantly (e.g., less sodium and more chloride) from those in the original ultrafiltrate.

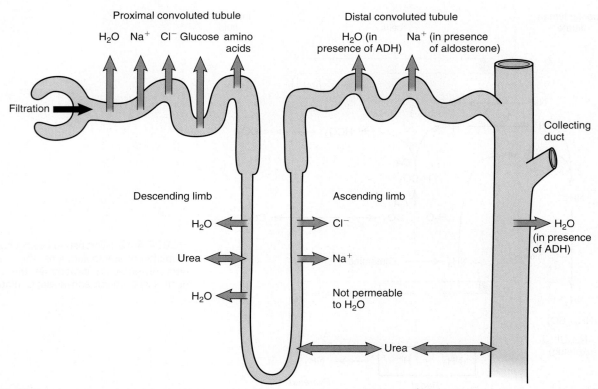

FIGURE 4-13 Tubular reabsorption of solutes and water in various segments of the nephron. *(From Applegate E: The anatomy and physiology learning system, ed 4, Philadelphia, 2011, Saunders.)*

In summary, as the filtrate leaves the proximal tubule, the fluid volume has been reduced by more than two-thirds; significant reabsorption of salts, glucose, proteins, and other important solutes has taken place actively or passively; and the fluid's osmolality remains unchanged. Osmolality—a measurable physical characteristic of urine used to evaluate the ability of the renal tubules to concentrate urine—is discussed further in Chapter 5.

Water Reabsorption. Water is reabsorbed throughout the nephron except in the ascending limbs (thin and thick) of the loops of Henle, located in the renal medulla (Figure 4-13). In the ascending limbs, the tubular epithelium is selectively impermeable to water, despite a large osmotic gradient that exists between the tubular lumen fluid and the medullary interstitium. In all other areas of the nephron, osmosis in synergy with the tubular epithelium is responsible for water reabsorption. The epithelium provides the membrane or barrier retarding the diffusion of water into the interstitium (paracellularly) or into the cells themselves (transcellularly). The anatomic structure of the tubular epithelium—specifically, the characteristics of its intercellular spaces—changes throughout the nephron (as was previously discussed). These epithelial characteristics, regulated by bodily needs and hormonal control, dictate how much water is ultimately reabsorbed by the nephron and where and when this absorption takes place.

Osmosis is the movement of water across a membrane from a solution of low osmolality to one of higher osmolality. The cell membrane is semipermeable, allowing some but not all solutes to cross it. An osmolality gradient (i.e., two areas differing in the number of solute particles present per volume of solvent) induces the diffusion of water across the membrane in an attempt to reach an osmotic equilibrium. This passive mechanism is solely responsible for the massive reabsorption of water by the renal tubules. Critical to this process is the high solute concentration or hypertonicity of the renal medulla, which establishes the necessary osmotic gradient.

Renal Concentrating Mechanism. The only tissue in the body that is hypertonic with respect to normal plasma (i.e., its osmolality is greater than 290 mOsm/kg) is the renal medulla. In medullary tissue, hypertonicity progressively increases; it is lowest at its border with the **isosmotic** cortex and greatest in the papillary tips of the renal pyramids. This increasing hypertonicity is shared by all components in the medullary interstitium, including tissue cells, interstitial fluid, blood vessels, and blood.

The gradient hypertonicity of the medullary interstitium is established and maintained by two countercurrent mechanisms: (1) an "active" countercurrent multiplier mechanism that occurs in the loops of Henle, and (2) a "passive" countercurrent exchange mechanism involving the vasa recta. The loops of Henle and the vasa recta are ideally configured—they are parallel structures that lie close to each other with fluid in the ascending and descending segments flowing in opposite directions, hence the name *countercurrent mechanism*. The ascending limb of the loop of Henle actively reabsorbs sodium and chloride into the medullary interstitium, and this limb is essentially impermeable to water (see Figure 4-13). As this active process occurs, the interstitium increases in tonicity (i.e., the solute concentration increases), and the lumen fluid decreases in tonicity. At the same time in the descending limb, water readily passes into the interstitium, whereas solutes (with the exception of urea) are not reabsorbed. Consequently, the osmolality of the interstitium and that of the descending limb fluid become equal and greater than the osmolality of the fluid in the ascending limb (Figure 4-14, *A*). As this process continues, a gradient of hypertonicity develops, with the descending limb fluid and the interstitium becoming progressively more concentrated. Note that the intratubular osmolality difference in the lumen fluid from cortex to medulla is significantly greater than that seen laterally (i.e., at the same level in descending and ascending tubules). Essentially, the osmotic gradient within the tubule from cortex to medulla has been "multiplied" because of countercurrent processes in which sodium and chloride are actively reabsorbed in the ascending limb while water is passively reabsorbed in the descending limb.

Initially, the countercurrent multiplier mechanism appears to have accomplished little because the lumen fluid in the loop of Henle becomes concentrated in the descending limb only to become diluted (by solute removal) in the ascending limb. The net result is a tubular lumen fluid slightly hypotonic to that originally presented to the loop of Henle (Table 4-5). However, the primary purpose of the countercurrent multiplier mechanism is not to concentrate the lumen fluid but to establish and maintain the gradient hypertonicity in the medullary interstitium. Subsequently, when the lumen fluid enters the collecting tubules, which traverse all areas of the renal cortex and the medulla, the fluid becomes concentrated or diluted to form the final urine.

In contrast, the second countercurrent mechanism is a "passive" exchange process that occurs in the vascular bed deep in the renal medulla. Here, reabsorbed solutes and water in the medullary interstitium are passively moved by diffusion into the vasa recta. Similar to the countercurrent mechanism in the tubular lumens, the blood osmolality is progressively concentrated as it flows toward the papillary tips but progressively diluted when it ascends to the renal cortex. This vascular countercurrent mechanism provides a means to supply nutrients to medullary tissue, as well as remove reabsorbed water for distribution elsewhere in the body. Consequently, these actions also maintain the hypertonicity of the renal medulla.

Despite the substantial exchanges of solutes and water in the tubules up to this point, the lumen fluid leaving the distal tubules is isosmotic (see Table 4-5). In the collecting tubules (or ducts), the last tubular segment of the nephron, the last osmolality change occurs—the final urine is concentrated, is diluted, or remains unchanged. It is important to note that water is never secreted by the tubules; instead, it is selectively not reabsorbed.

In the collecting tubules, processes involving solute exchange and water reabsorption occur simultaneously and under hormonal control. As the isosmotic lumen fluid enters the cortical collecting tubules, sodium and water reabsorption is hormonally controlled by two distinct and independent processes. The renin-angiotensin-aldosterone system is responsible for sodium reabsorption. As is briefly described in the renal circulation section and depicted in Figure 4-15, the juxtaglomerular apparatus releases renin into the bloodstream in response to decreased sodium, blood volume, or blood pressure. Angiotensin II forms rapidly, which stimulates the adrenal cortex to secrete the hormone aldosterone. Subsequently, aldosterone activates sodium reabsorption by the distal and cortical collecting tubules.

Water reabsorption in the collecting tubules requires the presence of ADH (arginine vasopressin). ADH is a hormone produced in the hypothalamus and transferred via the neuronal stalk to the posterior pituitary (neurohypophysis), where it is released into the bloodstream. Vascular baroreceptors located in the heart monitor arterial blood pressure. When an increase in arterial blood pressure occurs, the hypothalamus is signaled, and the release of ADH into the bloodstream is inhibited. This interactive process is called a *negative feedback mechanism* and is outlined in Figure 4-16. As the plasma level of ADH decreases, the epithelium of collecting tubules changes (see Figure 4-9) in such a way that movement of water from the lumen fluid into the medullary tissue decreases. Consequently, water is retained in the lumen fluid, resulting in a dilute (hypotonic or hypo-osmotic) urine. Conversely, when a decrease in blood pressure is sensed by baroreceptors, ADH release is increased. Under ADH stimulation, the collecting tubule epithelium changes and increased water reabsorption occurs as a result of the high medullary osmolality, and a concentrated (hypertonic or hyperosmotic) urine is produced. Note that ADH secretion does not alter sodium and chloride reabsorption.

The osmolality difference between the medullary interstitium and the fluid within the tubules progressively increases as the lumen fluid proceeds to the papillary tips deep in the medulla. It is because of this tremendous gradient that an initial ultrafiltrate osmolality of 290 mOsm/kg in Bowman's space can be concentrated in the final urine to as high as 900 to 1400 mOsm/kg. Note that the final urine excreted is formed in equilibrium with the renal interstitium, hence, urine osmolality can never exceed that of the medullary interstitium.

Normally, the countercurrent multiplier mechanism accounts for about 50% of the solutes concentrated in the renal medulla. The other 50% of the solutes are due to the high medullary concentration of urea

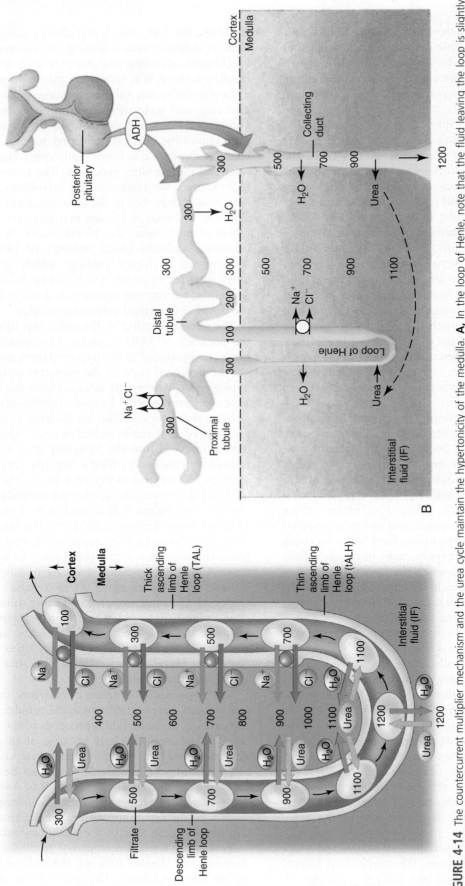

FIGURE 4-14 The countercurrent multiplier mechanism and the urea cycle maintain the hypertonicity of the medulla. **A,** In the loop of Henle, note that the fluid leaving the loop is slightly hypo-osmotic (100) compared with the fluid entering the loop (300). Numbers indicate osmolality in milliosmoles per kilogram H_2O. **B,** Countercurrent mechanisms in an entire nephron. As H_2O leaves the collecting duct (under antidiuretic hormone [ADH] regulation), the solutes become concentrated in the remaining filtrate, and osmolality increases. At the same time, a urea concentration gradient causes it to passively diffuse from the collecting duct into the interstitial fluid (IF) of the medulla. Some urea is eventually secreted back into the tubular lumen by the descending limb of the loop of Henle—the urea cycle *(dashed line).* The hypertonicity of the medulla enables the formation of hypertonic (concentrated) urine, with a maximum urine osmolality of 1200 to 1400 mOsm/kg (i.e., the same osmolality as is seen in the medullary interstitial fluid). *(A, From Patton KT, Thibodeau GA: Anatomy and physiology, ed 8, St. Louis, 2013, Mosby; B, From Thibodeau GA, Patton KT: Anatomy and physiology, ed 5, St Louis, 2003, Mosby.)*

Tubule Segment	Osmolality Change
TABLE 4-5	**Tubular Lumen Fluid Osmolality* Throughout the Nephron**
Proximal tubule	Enters: isosmotic Exits: isosmotic
Loop of Henle Thin descending limb U-turn Thick ascending limb (medullary and cortical)	Enters: isosmotic Becomes progressively hyperosmotic Maximally hyperosmotic Becomes progressively hypo-osmotic Exits: slightly hypo-osmotic
Distal tubule (convoluted portion)	Enters: slightly hypo-osmotic Exits: isosmotic
Collecting tubules	Enters: isosmotic Exits: varies, under ADH control; can be hyperisosmotic, hypo-osmotic, or isosmotic

ADH, Antidiuretic hormone.
*Isosmotic: urine osmolality equals the plasma osmolality (i.e., approximately 290 mOsm/kg).

maintained by a process called the *urea cycle* (see Figure 4-14). Urea, a by-product of protein catabolism, freely penetrates the glomerular filtration barrier, passing into the tubules as part of the ultrafiltrate. Despite the fact that urea is a metabolic waste product and the body has no use for it, 40% to 70% of urea is reabsorbed passively into the medullary interstitium. Urea subsequently diffuses along its concentration gradient into the lumen fluid in the loops of Henle. When the lumen fluid enters the cortical collecting tubules, water is reabsorbed in the presence of ADH, whereas urea is not. Any water reabsorption serves to concentrate further the amount of urea present in the lumen fluid. When the lumen fluid reaches the medullary collecting tubules, water (under ADH influence) and urea readily diffuse into the interstitium. In other words, the cortical epithelium of the collecting tubule is never permeable to urea, whereas the medullary epithelium is readily permeable. Therefore in the medullary collecting tubules, urea diffuses along its concentration gradient from the

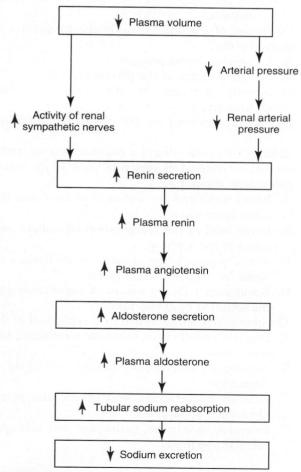

FIGURE 4-15 A schematic representation of the renin-angiotensin-aldosterone system and its role in the tubular reabsorption of sodium.

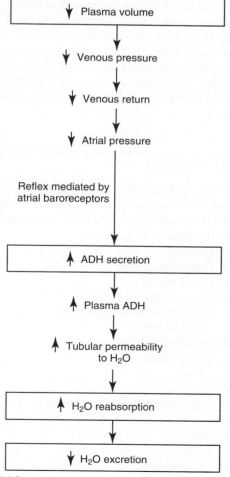

FIGURE 4-16 A schematic representation of the mechanism controlling antidiuretic hormone secretion.

concentrated lumen fluid into the interstitium until the urea concentration in both of these areas is equal. As a result of this urea equilibrium, (1) the sodium salts in the hypertonic medulla osmotically balance the nonurea solutes in the final urine, and (2) the concentration of urea in the final urine is actually determined by urea itself. Another factor affecting urea concentration in the final urine is the urine flow rate. Slow urine flow rates of less than 2 mL/min cause a larger amount of urea to be reabsorbed, whereas flow rates exceeding 2 mL/min allows a constant but minimal amount of urea reabsorption.

In summary, the hypertonicity of the medullary interstitium results from the countercurrent multiplier mechanism and the urea cycle. The hypertonic medulla established by these two processes provides a massive osmotic force for water reabsorption from the collecting tubules and is regulated by the presence of ADH in response to bodily needs. Despite the fact that solutes such as sodium (under aldosterone control) can be selectively reabsorbed or excreted in the distal and collecting tubules, regulation of water content by the collecting tubules ultimately determines the concentration of the final urine excreted. Stated another way, as isosmotic fluid from the distal tubule enters the collecting tubule, solute exchange may occur; however, the total number of solutes (i.e., osmoles) remains constant. It is the volume of water in which these solutes are excreted that varies. Therefore, reabsorption of water by the collecting tubules under ADH control determines whether a concentrated (hypertonic) or a dilute (hypotonic) final urine is produced.

STUDY QUESTIONS

1. Beginning with the glomerulus, number the following structures in the order in which the ultrafiltrate travels for processing and excretion in the kidney.
   __ A. Bladder
   __ B. Calyces
   __ C. Collecting tubule
   __ D. Distal tubule
   __ E. Glomerulus
   __ F. Juxtaglomerular apparatus
   __ G. Loop of Henle
   __ H. Proximal tubule
   __ I. Renal pelvis
   __ J. Ureter
   __ K. Urethra
2. How many nephrons are found in the average kidney?
   A. 13,000
   B. 130,000
   C. 1.3 million
   D. 13 million

3. Ultrafiltration of plasma occurs in glomeruli located in the renal
   A. cortex.
   B. medulla.
   C. pelvis.
   D. ureter.
4. Which component of the nephron is located exclusively in the renal medulla?
   A. Collecting tubule
   B. Distal tubule
   C. Loop of Henle
   D. Proximal tubule
5. Which of the following is not a vascular characteristic of the kidney?
   A. The afferent arteriole has a narrower lumen than the efferent arteriole.
   B. The arteries are primarily end arteries, supplying specific areas of tissue, and they do not interconnect.
   C. The arterioles subdivide into a capillary network, rejoin as an arteriole, and subdivide into a second capillary bed.
   D. The vasa recta vessels deep in the renal medulla form the beginning of the venous renal circulation.
6. Formation of the ultrafiltrate in the glomerulus is driven by the
   A. hydrostatic blood pressure.
   B. oncotic pressure of the plasma proteins.
   C. osmotic pressure of the solutes in the ultrafiltrate.
   D. pressures exerted by the glomerular filtration barrier.
7. Which of the following is a characteristic of renin, an enzyme secreted by specialized cells of the juxtaglomerular apparatus?
   A. Renin stimulates the diffusion of urea into the renal interstitium.
   B. Renin inhibits the reabsorption of sodium and water in the nephron.
   C. Renin regulates the osmotic reabsorption of water by the collecting tubules.
   D. Renin causes the formation of angiotensin and the secretion of aldosterone.
8. The glomerular filtration barrier is composed of the
   A. capillary endothelium, basement membrane, and podocytes.
   B. mesangium, basement membrane, and shield of negativity.
   C. capillary endothelium, mesangium, and juxtaglomerular apparatus.
   D. basement membrane, podocytes, and juxtaglomerular apparatus.

9. The ability of a solute to cross the glomerular filtration barrier is determined by its
   1. molecular size.
   2. molecular radius.
   3. electrical charge.
   4. plasma concentration.
   A. 1, 2, and 3 are correct.
   B. 1 and 3 are correct.
   C. 4 is correct.
   D. All are correct.

10. The epithelium characterized by a brush border owing to numerous microvilli is found in the
    A. collecting tubules.
    B. distal tubules.
    C. loops of Henle.
    D. proximal tubules.

11. The kidneys play an important role in the
    1. excretion of waste products.
    2. regulation of water and electrolytes.
    3. maintenance of acid-base equilibrium.
    4. control of blood pressure and fluid balance.
    A. 1, 2, and 3 are correct.
    B. 1 and 3 are correct.
    C. 4 is correct.
    D. All are correct.

12. What percent of the original ultrafiltrate formed in the urinary space actually is excreted as urine?
    A. 1%
    B. 10%
    C. 25%
    D. 33%

13. What differentiates tubular reabsorption from tubular secretion in the nephron?
    A. The direction of movement of the substance being absorbed or secreted is different.
    B. Reabsorption is an active transport process, whereas secretion is a passive transport process.
    C. Cell membrane–binding sites are different for the reabsorption and secretion of a solute.
    D. The location of the epithelium in the nephron determines which process occurs.

14. During tubular transport, the movement of a solute against a gradient
    A. is called *passive transport*.
    B. requires little to no energy.
    C. involves specific cell membrane–binding sites.
    D. may occur paracellularly, that is, between cells through intercellular spaces.

15. Substances bound to plasma proteins in the blood can be eliminated in the urine by
    A. glomerular secretion.
    B. glomerular filtration.
    C. tubular secretion.
    D. tubular reabsorption.

16. Which statement characterizes the ability of the renal system to regulate blood pH?
    A. The renal system has a slow response with complete correction of the pH to normal.
    B. The renal system has a fast response with complete correction of the pH to normal.
    C. The renal system has a slow response with only partial correction of the pH toward normal.
    D. The renal system has a fast response with only partial correction of the pH toward normal.

17. The kidneys excrete excess alkali (base) in the urine as
    A. ammonium ions.
    B. ammonium salts.
    C. sodium bicarbonate.
    D. titratable acids.

18. Which of the following substances is secreted into the tubular lumen to eliminate hydrogen ions?
    A. Ammonia (NH_3)
    B. Ammonium ions (NH_4^+)
    C. Disodium phosphate (Na_2HPO_4)
    D. Monosodium phosphate (NaH_2PO_4)

19. Urine titratable acids can form when the ultrafiltrate contains
    A. ammonia.
    B. bicarbonate.
    C. phosphate.
    D. sodium.

20. The renal threshold level for glucose is 160 to 180 mg/dL. This corresponds to the
    A. rate of glucose reabsorption by the renal tubules.
    B. concentration of glucose in the tubular lumen fluid.
    C. plasma concentration above which tubular reabsorption of glucose occurs.
    D. plasma concentration above which glucose is excreted in the urine.

21. When too much protein is presented to the renal tubules for reabsorption, it is excreted in the urine because
    A. the renal threshold for protein has not been exceeded.
    B. the maximal tubular reabsorptive capacity for protein has been exceeded.
    C. protein is not normally present in the ultrafiltrate and cannot be reabsorbed.
    D. the glomerular filtration barrier allows only abnormal proteins to pass.

22. More than 66% of filtered water, sodium, and chloride and 100% of filtered glucose, amino acids, and proteins are reabsorbed in the
    A. collecting tubules.
    B. distal tubules.
    C. loops of Henle.
    D. proximal tubules.

23. Water reabsorption occurs throughout the nephron except in the
    A. cortical collecting tubules.
    B. proximal convoluted tubules.
    C. ascending limb of the loops of Henle.
    D. descending limb of the loops of Henle.

24. The process solely responsible for water reabsorption throughout the nephron is
    A. osmosis.
    B. the urea cycle.
    C. the countercurrent exchange mechanism.
    D. the countercurrent multiplier mechanism.

25. Hypertonicity of the renal medulla is maintained by
    1. the countercurrent multiplier mechanism.
    2. the countercurrent exchange mechanism.
    3. the urea cycle.
    4. osmosis.
    A. 1, 2, and 3 are correct.
    B. 1 and 3 are correct.
    C. 4 is correct.
    D. All are correct.

26. Which of the following is not a feature of the renal countercurrent multiplier mechanism?
    A. The ascending limb of the loop of Henle is impermeable to water.
    B. The descending limb of the loop of Henle passively reabsorbs water.
    C. The descending limb of the loop of Henle actively reabsorbs sodium and urea.
    D. The fluid in the ascending and descending limbs of the loop of Henle flows in opposite directions.

27. The purpose of the renal countercurrent multiplier mechanism is to
    A. concentrate the tubular lumen fluid.
    B. increase the urinary excretion of urea.
    C. preserve the gradient hypertonicity in the medulla.
    D. facilitate the reabsorption of sodium and chloride.

28. Which vascular component is involved in the renal countercurrent exchange mechanism?
    A. Afferent arteriole
    B. Efferent arteriole
    C. Glomerulus
    D. Vasa recta

29. Antidiuretic hormone regulates the reabsorption of
    A. water in the collecting tubules.
    B. sodium in the collecting tubules.
    C. sodium in the distal convoluted tubule.
    D. water and sodium in the loop of Henle.

30. Which of the following describes the tubular lumen fluid that enters the collecting tubule compared with the tubular lumen fluid in the proximal tubule?
    A. Hypo-osmotic
    B. Isosmotic
    C. Hyperosmotic
    D. Counterosmotic

31. The final concentration of the urine is determined within the
    A. collecting ducts.
    B. distal convoluted tubules.
    C. loops of Henle.
    D. proximal convoluted tubules.

REFERENCES

1. Koushanpour E, Kriz W: Renal physiology, ed 2, New York, 1986, Springer-Verlag.
2. Longmire M, Choyke PL, Kobayashi H: Clearance properties of nano-sized particles and molecules as imaging agents: considerations and caveats. Nanoscience 3:703–717, 2008.
3. Cotran RS, Kumar V, Robbins SL: Robbins pathological basis of disease, ed 4, Philadelphia, 1989, WB Saunders.

BIBLIOGRAPHY

Alpern RJ, Hebert SC, editors: Seldin and Giebisch's the kidney physiology and pathophysiology, ed 4, Amsterdam, 2008, Academic Press/Elsevier.

Anderson SC, Cockayne S: Clinical chemistry: concepts and applications, New York, 2003, McGraw-Hill.

Burtis CA, Ashwood ER, editors: Tietz textbook of clinical chemistry, ed 3, Philadelphia, 1999, WB Saunders.

Cotran RS, Kumar V, Collins T: Robbins pathologic basis of disease, ed 6, Philadelphia, 1999, WB Saunders.

Cotran RS, Leaf A: Renal pathophysiology, ed 3, New York, 1985, Oxford University Press.

First MR: Renal function. In Kaplan LA, Pesce AJ, Kazmierczak SC, editors: Clinical chemistry: theory, analysis, correlation, ed 4, St. Louis, 2003, Mosby.

Goldman L, Bennett JC, editors: Cecil textbook of medicine, ed 21, Philadelphia, 2000, WB Saunders.

Klahr S, Weiner ID: Disorders of acid-base metabolism. In Chan JCM, Gill JR Jr, editors: Kidney electrolyte disorders, New York, 1990, Churchill Livingstone.

Patton KT, Thibodeau GA: Urinary system. In Anatomy and physiology, ed 7, St Louis, 2010, Mosby/Elsevier.

Pincus MR, Preuss HG, Henry JB: Evaluation of renal function, water, electrolytes, acid-base balance, and blood gases. In Henry JB, editor: Clinical diagnosis and management by laboratory methods, ed 20, Philadelphia, 2001, WB Saunders.

Rose BD, Rennke HG: Renal pathophysiology, Baltimore, 1994, Williams & Wilkins.

Schrier RW, Gottschalk CW: Diseases of the kidney and urinary tract, ed 7, 2001, Lippincott Williams & Wilkins.

number of solute particles present and the mass of particles present relates directly to osmolality and specific gravity measurements, respectively. Osmolality and specific gravity measurements are used to assess the quantity of solutes present in urine, which reflects the ability of the kidneys to produce a concentrated urine.

MEASUREMENTS OF SOLUTE CONCENTRATION

Osmolality

Osmolality is the concentration of a solution expressed in osmoles of solute particles per kilogram of solvent. An osmole (Osm) is the amount of a substance that dissociates to produce 1 mole of particles (6.023×10^{23} particles, Avogadro's number) in a solution. When solute concentrations in body fluids are discussed, the term milliosmole (mOsm) predominates. A mOsm is 1 millimole (mmol) of particles "in solution." For example, urea in solution does not dissociate; therefore 1 mmol of urea (60 mg) equals 1 mOsm. In contrast, NaCl in solution dissociates into two particles, Na^+ ions and Cl^- ions; therefore 1 mmol of NaCl (58 mg) equals 2 mOsm. In other words, the osmolality of a 1 mmol/L NaCl solution is approximately two times greater (owing to dissociation) than that of a 1 mmol/L urea solution. In urine, the solvent is water and the solute particles are those that pass the filtration barrier and are not reabsorbed, plus additional solutes secreted by the renal tubules.

The ultrafiltrate in Bowman's space has the same solute composition as the plasma but lacks albumin and other high-molecular-weight solutes present in the bloodstream. Consequently, the osmolality of this initial filtrate is the same as that of the plasma and is described by the term *isosmotic*. As was discussed in Chapter 4, the solute composition (concentration and type) in the filtrate changes continuously throughout its passage through the tubules of the nephron. In contrast, the osmolality remains unchanged (isosmotic at ≈300 mOsm) until the filtrate reaches the thin descending limb of the loop of Henle (Figure 5-1). The countercurrent multiplier mechanism causes the filtrate in the loops of Henle to become progressively hyperosmotic in the descending limb and then hypo-osmotic in the ascending limb. When the filtrate enters the distal tubules, it is slightly hypo-osmotic (≈100 mOsm).

The final osmolality of urine is determined in the distal tubules and collecting ducts. The surrounding medullary interstitium has a hypertonic concentration gradient that facilitates the reabsorption of water when antidiuretic hormone (ADH) is present. In the distal tubules with ADH present, the filtrate again becomes isosmotic (≈300 mOsm), matching the hypertonicity of the cortical interstitium (see Figure 5-1). As the filtrate passes through the collecting tubules, the osmolality of the filtrate can continue to increase (as water is absorbed)

until it matches that of the surrounding hypertonic medullary interstitium, provided ADH is present. Note that the maximum urine osmolality possible—1200 to 1400 mOsm/kg—is determined by the osmolality of the medullary interstitium. The collecting tubules do not exchange solutes and can only passively reabsorb water until an osmotic equilibrium is attained.

The osmolality of a random urine specimen can be as low as 50 mOsm/kg or as high as 1400 mOsm/kg. Under normal circumstances, urine osmolality ranges from one to three times (275 to 900 mOsm/kg) that of serum (275 to 300 mOsm/kg). The urine-to-serum osmolality ratio (U/S) is a good indicator of the ability of the kidneys to concentrate the urine. In normal individuals with an average fluid intake, the U/S ratio is between 1.0 and 3.0.

The kidneys change the urine osmolality by adjusting the volume of water in which solutes are excreted. With a typical American diet, an individual needs to eliminate 100 to 1200 mOsm of solutes each day. However, diets high in salt and protein require a larger volume of urine to excrete the increased solute load. Some disorders (e.g., diabetes mellitus) can produce as much as 5000 mOsm/day of solutes for elimination. Consequently, a large volume of water is required to excrete them in the urine. Because the kidneys have no direct means of replacing excessive water loss, adequate fluid intake is mandatory. Hence, these individuals experience intense thirst, known as **polydipsia**, to maintain water homeostasis and to excrete the solutes necessary.

Specific Gravity

Specific gravity (SG) is another expression of solute concentration that relates the density of urine to the density of an equal volume of pure water. Because specific gravity is a ratio comparing the mass of the solutes present in urine to pure water, urine specific gravity measurements are always greater than 1.000. As with osmolality, the specific gravity of the initial ultrafiltrate in Bowman's space is the same as that of protein-free plasma, which has an SG of 1.010. As the filtrate passes through the tubules and solute exchange occurs, the specific gravity of the filtrate also changes. Urine specific gravity values normally range from 1.002 to 1.035. The SG value indicates whether the filtrate was ultimately concentrated (SG >1.010) or diluted (SG <1.010) during its passage through the nephrons. Urine specific gravity, like osmolality, depends on the amount of solutes and water eliminated; this is dependent on an individual's fluid intake and state of hydration.

Because density depends on the number of solute particles present and their relative mass, the relationship of specific gravity to osmolality is close but not linear (Figure 5-2). This relationship is relatively constant in health; however, in some conditions this relationship is nonexistent because of the excretion of high-molecular-weight solutes such as glucose, urea, or proteins.

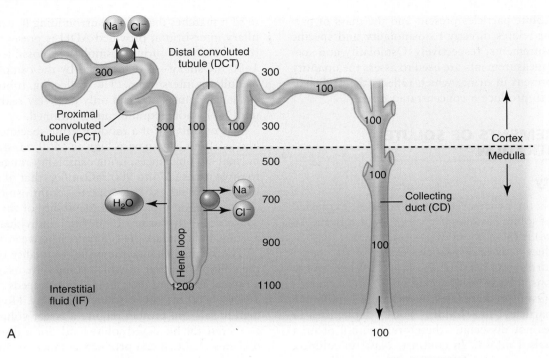

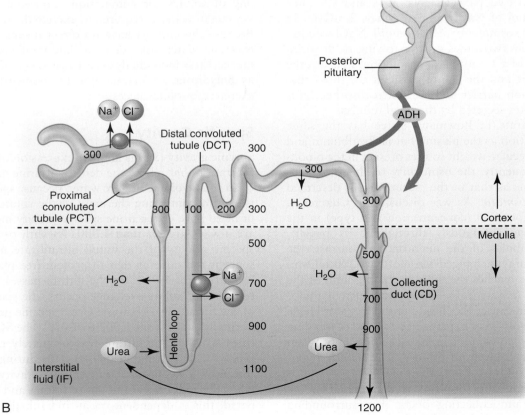

FIGURE 5-1 A, Production of hypotonic urine. Hypotonic urine is produced by a nephron by the mechanism shown here. The isotonic (300 mOsm) tubule fluid that enters the Henle loop becomes hypotonic (100 mOsm) by the time it enters the distal convoluted tubule. The tubule fluid remains hypotonic as it is passes through remaining portions of the nephron, where the walls of the distal tubule and collecting duct are impermeable to H_2O, Na^+, and Cl^-. Values are expressed in milliosmoles. **B,** Production of hypertonic urine. Hypertonic urine can be formed when antidiuretic hormone (ADH) is present. ADH, a posterior pituitary hormone, enables water reabsorption by the distal tubule and collecting duct. Thus hypotonic (100 mOsm) tubule fluid leaving the Henle loop can equilibrate first with the isotonic (300 mOsm) interstitial fluid (IF) of the cortex, then with the increasingly hypertonic (400 to 1200 mOsm) IF of the medulla. As H_2O leaves the collecting duct by osmosis, the filtrate becomes more concentrated with the solutes left behind. The concentration gradient causes urea to diffuse into the IF, where some of it is eventually picked up by tubule fluid in the descending limb of the Henle loop *(long arrow)*. This countercurrent movement of urea helps maintain a high solute concentration in the medulla. Values are expressed in milliosmoles. *(From Patton KT, Thibodeau GA: Anatomy and physiology, ed 8, St. Louis, 2013, Mosby.)*

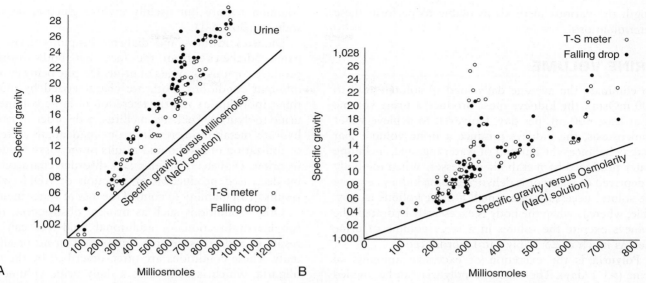

FIGURE 5-2 A comparison of urine specific gravity and urine osmolality. Specific gravity measurements were determined by a direct method (falling drop) and an indirect method (refractometry). The straight lines represent the specific gravity and osmolality results obtained with solutions of varying sodium chloride concentrations. **A,** A comparison of urines obtained from healthy medical students. **B,** A comparison of urines obtained from patients on renal service. (*From Holmes JH: Workshop on urinalysis and renal function studies, Chicago, 1962, American Society of Clinical Pathologists. Used with permission.*)

TABLE 5-2	Comparison of Specific Gravities of Different Solutions				
	Solute Characteristics			**Specific Gravity**	
Solution	**Number of Solute Particles Added**	**Amount of Solute, mol/L**	**Density**	**Refractive Index**	**Ionic (Reagent Strip)**
Water	0.0	0.0	1.000	1.000	1.000
Water and NaCl	5.2×10^{23}	0.43	1.017	1.012	1.005
Water and urea	5.2×10^{23}	0.86	1.021	1.020	1.000
Water and glucose	5.2×10^{23}	0.86	1.056	>1.050	1.000

Table 5-2 shows specific gravity values of water with NaCl, urea, and glucose added. Each solute addition represents essentially the same number of particles added to the solution—approximately 5.2×10^{23} particles. Note that the specific gravity value differs despite the presence of the same number of particles. This occurs because of the effect that solute mass has on some methods used to determine specific gravity. The urinometer (a historical method) is a direct measure of density, whereas refractive index and reagent strip determinations measure density indirectly. Note that regardless of the method used, the presence of large-molecular-weight solutes such as glucose, urea, or protein will dramatically increase the "actual" specific gravity of urine as compared with small solutes such as sodium or chloride ions.

Occasionally, urine specimens can have an extremely high specific gravity value (≥1.050), which exceeds those that are physiologically possible (≈1.040). The excretion of a high-molecular-weight substance, such as radiopaque contrast media (x-ray dye) or mannitol, should be suspected in these specimens. These exogenous substances are infused into patients and excreted in the urine. They are considered a contaminant in urine and do not indicate a disorder or disease process. Note that although these urine specimens have specific gravity results that are physiologically impossible, their osmolality values are normal. This is because osmolality values are only affected by the "number" of solutes present, and the number of these high-molecular-weight solutes is too few compared with the total number of other solutes in the urine (e.g., sodium, urea). In other words, the mass of solutes present is significant and affects the urine specific gravity, but their number is too small to significantly affect the urine osmolality. These urine specimens are considered contaminated and unacceptable for analysis. A new specimen should be collected after an appropriate time has passed and the exogenous substance is no longer being excreted.

In summary, specific gravity and osmolality are physical properties used to assess urine concentration. A specific gravity measurement indicates the collective number and mass of solutes in the urine, whereas a urine osmolality measurement indicates only the number of solutes present, regardless of solute type. Chapter 6 discusses at length the various methods available to perform these determinations.

URINE VOLUME

To eliminate the average daily load of solutes (600 to 700 mOsm), the kidneys must produce a urine volume of at least 500 mL per day. However, to achieve water homeostasis, the kidneys produce a urine volume that exactly balances the amount of water ingested, including water produced by metabolic processes. When the body is deprived of water or is dehydrated, the kidneys excrete the solutes necessary in as small a urine volume as possible, whereas when the body is excessively hydrated, the kidneys excrete the solutes in a large volume of urine (i.e., as much as 25 L/day can be produced).

Polyuria is the excretion of excessive amounts of urine (>3 L/day). The causes of polyuria can be divided diagnostically into two types: (1) conditions with water diuresis (urine osmolality <200 mOsm/kg) and (2) conditions with solute diuresis (urine osmolality ≥300 mOsm/kg).[1] Figure 5-3 provides a flowchart for evaluating polyuria. Conditions characterized by water diuresis have a common link—ADH. With these disorders, ADH secretion is inadequate, or the action of ADH on the renal receptors is ineffective. In contrast, conditions characterized by solute diuresis have no

common feature but usually involve glucose, urea, or sodium (Box 5-1).

Diabetes mellitus and diabetes insipidus derive the name "diabetes" from the fact that both disorders produce copious amounts of urine. Despite being entirely different conditions, both are characterized by intense thirst (polydipsia) and the excretion of large volumes of urine (polyuria). Diabetes mellitus, a disorder of carbohydrate metabolism, results from inadequate secretion or utilization of insulin and results in the loss of glucose in urine. Diabetes insipidus is a disorder characterized by decreased production or function of ADH, which results in an inability to control the loss of water in urine.

Other conditions such as urinary obstruction, renal tubular dysfunction, or additional fluid loss can also result in a decrease in the amount of urine produced daily. These conditions are often described by the term **oliguria**, which is defined as a daily urine volume less than 400 mL/day. This urine volume does not allow the elimination of a normal daily solute load and, if prolonged, death will occur. When no urine is excreted, the term **anuria** applies, and death is imminent unless intervention occurs. In progressive renal disease, anuria usually develops gradually after an initial presentation of oliguria. Anuria can occur suddenly as a result of a dramatic decrease in renal perfusion (e.g., hemorrhage) or because of sudden extensive renal damage.

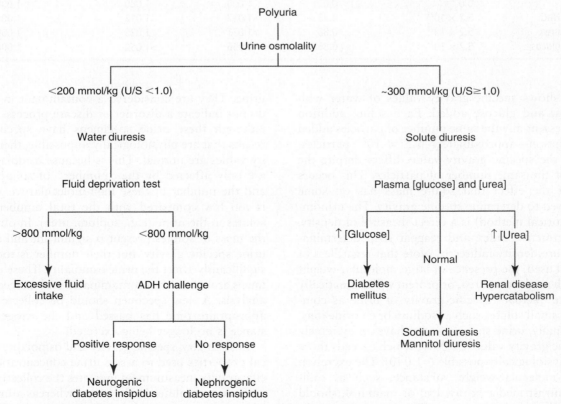

FIGURE 5-3 A flowchart for the evaluation of polyuria. *ADH,* Antidiuretic hormone; *U/S,* urine-to-serum osmolality ratio. (*Redrawn from Walmsley RN, White GH: A guide to diagnostic clinical chemistry, Melbourne, 1983, Blackwell Science.*)

BOX 5-1 | Differentiation of Polyuria

I. Water diuresis (urine osmolality less than 200 mOsm/kg)
  A. Decreased antidiuretic hormone (ADH) secretion
    1. Excessive fluid intake (physiologic)
    2. Neurogenic diabetes insipidus
  B. Ineffective response by kidney to ADH—nephrogenic
    1. Congenital nephrogenic diabetes insipidus
    2. Acquired nephrogenic diabetes insipidus
      a. Renal diseases
      b. Drugs
II. Solute diuresis (urine osmolality 300 ± 50 mOsm/kg)
  A. Sodium
    1. Increased intake
    2. Diuretic therapy
    3. Renal salt-losing disorders
  B. Urea
    1. Hypercatabolic states
    2. Chronic renal failure
    3. Postobstructive nephropathy
    4. Postacute tubular necrosis
  C. Glucose
    1. Diabetes mellitus

Modified from Walmsley RN, White GH: A guide to diagnostic clinical chemistry, Melbourne, 1988, Blackwell Scientific.
ADH, Antidiuretic hormone.

In conclusion, the volume of urine excreted daily (24 hours) can vary from approximately 500 to 1800 mL/day. This total daily volume reflects the quantity of solutes ingested, the fluid intake, and the activity of ADH, as discussed in Chapter 4. However, when renal and metabolic diseases are present, urine volume can decrease to zero output (anuria) or can increase to as much as 15 times normal.

ASSESSMENT OF RENAL CONCENTRATING ABILITY/TUBULAR REABSORPTIVE FUNCTION

Osmolality Versus Specific Gravity

Osmolality and specific gravity are measurements that express the concentrations of solutes in a fluid. With urine, these parameters vary depending on the quantity of water and solutes that is eliminated. Therefore an easy test to assess the renal capacity or ability to conserve water (i.e., tubular reabsorptive function) is to demonstrate that the tubules can produce a concentrated urine specimen, that is, a urine specimen with an osmolality greater than 800 mOsm/kg or a specific gravity greater than 1.025.

Although specific gravity determinations are easier and require less time to perform, osmolality determinations are preferred for the evaluation of renal concentrating ability. Osmolality measurements are considered a more accurate assessment because, as was previously discussed, each solute particle contributes equally to the osmolality value. In contrast, specific gravity measurements are a density comparison that is affected by some solutes more than others. Recall from Table 5-1 that the three most prevalent urine solutes are urea, chloride, and sodium. Chloride and sodium are reabsorbed *selectively* throughout the nephrons by active and passive tubular transport mechanisms. Therefore monitoring the concentration of chloride and sodium in urine reveals the kidney's ability to process and concentrate the ultrafiltrate. In contrast, urea is not an accurate indicator of the kidney's ability to concentrate urine because it is only passively processed in the nephrons (i.e., urea cycle), and the magnitude of this exchange varies owing to several factors (e.g., tubular flow rate).

Another reason that osmolality determinations are better than specific gravity determinations for assessing the concentrating ability of the kidneys is that small quantities of high-molecular-weight solutes (e.g., glucose, protein) will affect specific gravity measurements but do not affect osmolality measurements. Glucose and protein are solutes that are actively and essentially completely reabsorbed in the proximal tubules. Their presence in urine indicates a disease process, not a change in the kidney's ability to concentrate the urine. In contrast to specific gravity measurements, the osmolality of a urine that contains glucose and protein remains relatively constant. In such a urine, the density is significantly increased because of the high molecular weight of glucose and protein, but the actual increase in particle numbers is small compared with the total solutes present (see Figure 5-2). Note that a change in specific gravity indicates a change in solute density, which does not necessarily indicate a change in the ability of the kidney to concentrate urine. In addition, osmolality is preferred over specific gravity measurements because its value increases in direct proportion to an increase in solute number, regardless of the solute type.

With some chronic renal diseases, the tubular concentrating ability slowly diminishes until the urine specific gravity and osmolality are fixed or unchanging. Because the tubules are no longer able to actively reabsorb and secrete selected solutes from the ultrafiltrate as it passes through the nephron, the solute concentration of the ultrafiltrate remains the same. Consequently, urine osmolality and specific gravity are the same as those of the initial ultrafiltrate in Bowman's space—namely, a specific gravity of 1.010 and an osmolality of approximately 300 mOsm/kg (i.e., the same as protein-free plasma). This fixation of the urine solute composition is a common feature of chronic renal diseases that causes polyuria and **nocturia**—excessive urination at night.

Although nocturia is a classic feature of renal disease, it also occurs with conditions characterized by reduced bladder capacity (e.g., pregnancy, bladder stones, prostate enlargement) or simply following excessive fluid intake at night.

Specific gravity and osmolality are nonspecific tests used to determine the concentration of urine. They can only indicate or support a suspected decrease in renal function. The underlying problem—whether it be renal disease, diabetes insipidus, or the effect of diuretic therapy—cannot be discerned by using these tests.

Fluid Deprivation Tests

As outlined in Figure 5-3, polyuria due to water diuresis can result from excessive water intake or from disorders involving ADH (vasopressin). When ADH production or secretion is defective, this indicates *neurogenic* diabetes insipidus. When the problem is lack of renal response to ADH, it is called *nephrogenic* diabetes insipidus. To differentiate the cause of water diuresis, a fluid deprivation test can be performed.

A fluid deprivation test evaluates the ability of renal tubular cells to selectively absorb and secrete solutes. In other words, it assesses the renal concentrating ability of the kidneys. During this test, water consumption by the patient is restricted, and the concentration of the urine is evaluated at timed intervals. In a typical protocol, the patient eats a normal evening meal, and then from 6 PM until 8 AM the next day, he or she drinks no water or other fluids. At 8 AM, a urine specimen is collected and the osmolality determined. If the urine osmolality is greater than 800 mOsm/kg, the renal concentrating ability of the kidneys is considered normal, and the test is ended.

If the osmolality is less than 800 mOsm/kg, fluid deprivation continues. At 10 AM, both serum and urine specimens are collected for osmolality determinations. If the urine osmolality is greater than 800 mOsm/kg or the ratio of urine osmolality to serum osmolality (U/S) is greater than 3.0, normal renal concentrating ability is demonstrated, and the test is ended. If neither condition is met, ADH (vasopressin) is administered subcutaneously, and at 2 PM and 6 PM, serum and urine specimens are collected for osmolality testing. Note that regardless of a patient's response, the test is terminated at 6 PM (i.e., after 24 hours). A positive response to ADH administration is a urine osmolality greater than 800 mOsm/kg or a U/S ratio of 3.0 or greater. These results indicate that the patient's kidneys can respond to ADH, but that inadequate ADH is produced by the patient (i.e., a neurogenic problem). In contrast, a negative response to ADH indicates a nephrogenic problem—the renal receptors for ADH are dysfunctional (see Figure 5-3).

Other tests that assess renal concentrating ability use urine specific gravity measurements. In the Fishberg concentration test, the patient undergoes the same fluid deprivation regimen as was previously described. At each timed interval, a urine specimen is collected and the specific gravity determined. If the urine specific gravity becomes 1.025 or greater, renal concentrating ability is normal, and the test ends.

Differing from the tests already discussed, Mosenthal's test allows patients to maintain their normal diet and fluid intake and requires a special 24-hour urine collection. The 24-hour collection is unique in that it is collected as two separate 12-hour urine collections—a 12-hour day portion and a 12-hour night portion. The volume and specific gravity of each 12-hour urine collection are determined. A normal Mosenthal's test is indicated by a daytime urine volume that exceeds the nighttime volume, and by a nighttime urine specific gravity that is 1.020 or greater.

Osmolar and Free-Water Clearance

Just as simultaneous measurement of serum and urine osmolality can aid a clinician in the differential diagnoses of disease (e.g., neurogenic diabetes insipidus versus nephrogenic diabetes insipidus), determining the quantity of water and solutes not reabsorbed by the kidneys has diagnostic value. This is done by measuring the renal clearance of "solutes" and comparing it with the renal clearance of "solute-free" water. To do so requires the osmolality from a timed urine collection and a corresponding serum specimen. The ratio of urine osmolality to serum osmolality multiplied by the timed urine volume gives the **osmolar clearance,** designated C_{Osm}:

Equation 5-1

$$C_{Osm} \text{ (mL plasma per minute)} = \frac{U_{Osm} \text{ (mOsm/kg)}}{S_{Osm} \text{ (mOsm/kg)}} \times V \text{ (mL/min)}$$

where U is the urine osmolality, V is the volume of urine excreted per minute, and S_{Osm} is the serum osmolality. The osmolar clearance (C_{Osm}) is the volume of plasma water (in mL) cleared by the kidneys each minute. Fasting osmolar clearance values normally vary from 2 to 3 mL/min and do not depend on urine flow.[2]

The total volume (V) of urine excreted by the kidneys actually consists of two separate volumes: osmolar clearance water (C_{Osm}) and solute-free water (C_{H_2O}).

Equation 5-2

$$V \text{ (mL/min)} = C_{Osm} \text{ (mL/min)} + C_{H_2O} \text{ (mL/min)}$$

The osmolar clearance water (C_{Osm}) is the volume of water required to eliminate the solutes from the plasma, whereas the solute-free water (C_{H_2O}) is additional water that exceeds bodily needs, is retained in the tubules, and is eliminated in the urine.

From Equation 5-1, it is evident that for urine to be isosmotic with the plasma ($U_{Osm} = S_{Osm}$), the total urine volume (V) must equal the osmolar clearance volume (V $= C_{Osm}$). When this occurs, the solute-free water clearance (C_{H_2O}) is zero. The solute-free or **free-water clearance** (C_{H_2O}) can be determined by rearrangement.

Equation 5-3

$$C_{H_2O} \text{ (mL/min)} = V \text{ (mL/min)} - C_{Osm} \text{ (mL/min)}$$

When urine is dilute because of water diuresis, the U_{Osm} is less than the S_{Osm} and the total urine volume (V) cleared is greater than the osmolar clearance water (C_{Osm}). Consequently, the solute-free water clearance (C_{H_2O}) is a positive number, indicating that excess water is eliminated and the urine is hypo-osmotic or hypotonic. When the U_{Osm} is greater than the S_{Osm}, as occurs with dehydration, the total urine volume (V) cleared is less than the osmolar clearance water, and the solute-free water clearance is a negative number. A negative free-water clearance indicates that the kidneys are reabsorbing water and are producing urine that is hyperosmotic or hypertonic.

It is important to keep in mind that the solute principally responsible for the osmolality of urine is urea, whereas in serum it is primarily due to sodium and chloride ions. Therefore the applicability of osmolar and free-water clearances is limited to indicating urine solute concentration and volume. These clearances have no value in determining the cause of polyuria or diuresis.[3]

In summary, to maintain the body's overall fluid homeostasis, the kidneys manipulate the amount of water excreted. A required amount of water is needed to eliminate unwanted solutes, and any additional water can be eliminated or reabsorbed. The ultimate goal of the kidneys—to maintain a normal plasma osmolality—is achieved by the selective elimination and reabsorption of solutes and water.

ASSESSMENT OF GLOMERULAR FILTRATION

Renal Clearance

For the kidneys to remove metabolic wastes and selectively reabsorb solutes and water, they require adequate **renal plasma flow** (RPF) through the glomeruli. The RPF determines the amount of plasma ultrafiltrate processed by the nephrons of the kidneys. The volume of renal plasma filtered by the glomeruli directly affects the volume and composition of the urine excreted. The portion of the plasma that does not pass the glomerular filtration barriers flows into the peritubular capillaries, where the renal tubules actively and selectively remove some plasma solutes for excretion. When a solute is filtered but is not secreted or absorbed by the nephrons, its concentration in the urine can be correlated with the renal processing of a volume of plasma. Referred to as **renal clearance,** this is the volume of plasma in milliliters that is completely cleared of a substance per unit of time.

Because renal disease is often a slow process and significant amounts of renal tissue can become nonfunctional before detection of disease, renal clearance tests provide a rapid and relatively easy way to assess a patient's renal status. By measuring the concentration of a substance in the plasma and in a timed urine specimen, the ability of the kidneys to remove the substance from the blood can be determined. This capacity is termed renal clearance (C) and is determined as follows:

Equation 5-4

$$C\,(mL/min) = \frac{U\,(mg/dL) \times V\,(mL/min)}{P\,(mg/dL)}$$

V is the volume of urine excreted in the timed collection (mL/min), *U* is the urine concentration of the substance (e.g., mg/dL) in the timed collection, *P* is the plasma (or serum) concentration of the substance (e.g. mg/dL) collected during the timed interval, and *C* is the renal clearance of the substance (mL/min). Note that the units for the urine and plasma concentrations *must be the same* to cancel each other out in the renal clearance equation. A 24-hour timed collection is preferred for most substances and is mandatory for those analytes or physiologic functions that demonstrate a diurnal variation.

Clearance Tests

A clearance test can aid in the evaluation of glomerular filtration, tubular reabsorption, and tubular secretion, and in determining renal blood flow. Evaluating each of these renal functions requires the use of substances with known and strictly limited modes of renal excretion. For example, substances that are removed exclusively by glomerular filtration (e.g., inulin) can be used to determine the **glomerular filtration rate** (GFR). Whereas substances removed solely by renal tubular secretion (e.g., *p*-aminohippurate, phenolsulfonphthalein) are used to assess the ability of the nephrons to process solutes.

In the clinical laboratory, most clearance tests are performed to evaluate GFR. Hypothetically, any substance that (1) maintains a constant plasma level, (2) is excreted solely by glomerular filtration, and (3) is not reabsorbed or secreted by the tubules can be used to determine GFR. However, the search for the ideal substance for GFR measurement remains an ongoing challenge.

Clearance tests can be performed using endogenous (e.g., urea, creatinine) or exogenous substances. A variety of exogenous agents have been evaluated in the quest for a safe, simple, and accurate method by which to measure GFR. These exogenous substances can be divided into two categories: those with a radioisotope label (^{125}I-iothalamate, ^{125}I-diatrizoate, ^{51}Cr-EDTA [chromium ethylenediaminetetraacetic acid], and ^{99}Tc-DTPA [technetium diethylenetriaminepentaacetic acid]) and those without (inulin and iohexol iothalamate). Newer approaches using exogenous agents have eliminated the need for a continuous intravenous infusion, replacing it with a single (bolus) intravenous injection or a subcutaneous injection. Whereas exogenous substances provide a more accurate measurement of GFR, these clearance tests are often more labor intensive, expensive, and inconvenient for the patient.

Inulin Clearance. The inulin clearance test, although rarely performed for clinical purposes, remains the reference method for GFR determination. Inulin, an exogenous nontoxic fructopolysaccharide (molecular weight, 5200) is not absorbed by the gastrointestinal tract and must be administered intravenously before and throughout the performance of this test. Inulin is not modified by the body and readily passes the glomerular filtration barriers, where it is neither reabsorbed nor secreted by the renal tubules. Although inulin is an ideal substance for determining GFR, performing an inulin clearance test is not practical for routine or periodic GFR measurements.

Creatinine Clearance. To eliminate the disadvantages inherent with exogenous agents, an endogenous substance with a renal clearance that approximates that of inulin has been sought. Urea and creatinine, because of their large urinary concentrations and ease of measurement, have been evaluated extensively. Urea, however, is reabsorbed by the tubules, and its concentration is directly affected by the urine flow rate. In addition, diet affects plasma urea levels. As a result, urea clearances are imprecise and inaccurate, and are rarely performed. In contrast, creatinine is not reabsorbed by the renal tubules, nor is it affected by the urine flow rate, and plasma levels are not altered by a normal diet. Hence, the **creatinine clearance test** is the most commonly used clearance test for routine assessment of GFR. Because the most accurate creatinine clearance is obtained using a 24-hour urine collection, this test is inconvenient for patients. In recent years, studies have demonstrated the value and clinical usefulness of calculating an "estimated" GFR (eGFR) to detect and monitor kidney disease.[3]

Since 1938, it has been known that the creatinine clearance closely approximates that of inulin.[4] Creatinine is a by-product of muscle metabolism, formed from creatine and phosphocreatine (Figure 5-4). It is produced at a steady rate, resulting in a constant plasma concentration and a constant urine excretion rate. Because creatinine production depends directly on muscle mass, production varies with the patient's gender, physical activity, and age: Males and muscular athletes (male and female) produce more creatinine than do nonathletic females, children, or the elderly. Because of this dependence on individual muscle mass, creatinine clearance values are normalized to the external body surface area of an average individual: 1.73 m². In the calculation for the normalized creatinine clearance (C) (Equation 5-5), the factor 1.73 m²/SA denotes the body surface area of the average individual divided by the calculated body surface area of the patient.

Equation 5-5

$$C\,(mL/min) = \frac{U \times V}{P} \times \frac{1.73\,m^2}{SA}$$

where U is the urine concentration of creatinine, V is the volume of urine excreted in milliliters per minute, P is the plasma concentration of creatinine, and SA is the patient's body surface area.

The body surface area of an individual is determined by using the patient's height and weight. It can be obtained from a nomogram[15] or can be calculated using the following equation.

Equation 5-6

$$\log SA = (0.425 \times \log W) + (0.725 \times \log H) - 2.144$$

where SA is the body surface area in square meters, W is the patient's weight (mass) in kilograms, and H is the patient's height in centimeters.

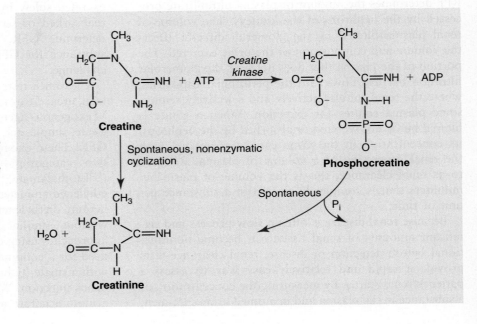

FIGURE 5-4 The formation of creatinine from creatine and phosphocreatine. *ADP,* Adenosine diphosphate; *ATP,* adenosine triphosphate.

TABLE 5-3	Variation in Reference Intervals for Serum Creatinine and Creatinine Clearance According to Age and Gender*		
	Age, yr	Serum Creatinine, mg/L	Creatine Clearance, mL/min/1.73 m²
Males	10	5-8	60-130
	20	8-13	80-135
	40	9-14	75-130
	60	10-14.5	45-100
	80	7-14	30-80
Females	10	5-8	60-130
	20	7-11	70-120
	40	8-12	60-110
	60	8-12.5	45-95
	80	8-13	30-80

From Lente FV: "Creatinine" in analytes, Clin Chem News 16:8, 1990.
*The factor 1.73 m² normalizes clearance for average body surface area.

Normalization of the creatinine clearance test enables the comparison of clearance results (i.e., GFR) with those of other individuals, regardless of the patient's body surface area. Table 5-3 lists typical reference intervals for serum creatinine and creatinine clearance tests based on age and gender.

Advantages and Disadvantages. The measurement of creatinine in urine and serum (or plasma) is rapidly and easily performed; in addition, the precision and reliability of each measurement method are known and well documented. Despite its advantages, the creatinine clearance test has several shortcomings that must be addressed to ensure the correct interpretation of results. In reality, a small amount of creatinine is secreted by the renal tubules (≈7% to 10%).[5] This secretion results in an elevated urine excretion concentration (U in Equation 5-4), which would result in an overestimation of the GFR. This increase is offset, however, when the popular, nonspecific alkaline picrate method (Jaffe reaction) is used for creatinine measurement. Because of the reaction of plasma noncreatinine chromogens by this method, the plasma creatinine result (P in Equation 5-4) also is overestimated. Fortunately, these two factors offset each other, and the creatinine clearance correlates well with the inulin clearance. When more specific creatinine methods (e.g., enzymatic) are used, these factors do not offset each other. In the latter case, the measured plasma creatinine is not overestimated but the urine creatinine is overestimated because of the tubular secretion. As a result, the creatinine clearance (C in Equation 5-4) is overestimated, and the clearance results do not compare as well with the inulin clearance.

Patients with diminished renal function (i.e., their plasma creatinine concentration is increased) can be difficult to evaluate using the creatinine clearance. In these patients, the renal tubular secretion of creatinine (a process limited by maximal tubular secretory capacity) is increased because of the elevated plasma concentration; this results in an increased concentration in the urine (U in Equation 5-4), and again an erroneous GFR is obtained. Other factors known to interfere with the renal secretion of creatinine are exogenous agents such as salicylate, trimethoprim, and cimetidine. These drugs inhibit the tubular secretion of creatinine, thereby lowering the urine creatinine concentration and causing a falsely low creatinine clearance or GFR.

In summary, several factors affect the tubular secretion of creatinine, and the method used for creatinine quantitation can directly affect the creatinine clearance result obtained. Despite these shortcomings, the creatinine clearance continues to provide health care providers with a useful measurement of the GFR. Because creatinine methods have been extensively researched and have proven reliability, the periodic performance of a creatinine clearance provides valuable diagnostic and prognostic information about a patient's ongoing renal status.

Importance of Time Interval. To perform a creatinine clearance test, a timed urine specimen must be obtained. The time interval over which the urine collection takes place must be provided with the specimen. Because of diurnal variation in the GFR, a 24-hour urine collection is considered the specimen of choice for creatinine clearance determinations. The plasma specimen for the clearance determination can be obtained anytime during the 24-hour period. Shorter collection intervals (e.g., 12-hour or 2-hour intervals) may be used, especially with patients requiring repeated GFR determinations to monitor their renal status. In these cases, the patient must be kept well hydrated throughout the test, the urine collection should be performed at the same time of day for comparison purposes, and the plasma sample is usually obtained midway through the collection. Because creatinine clearance results can vary by as much as 15% to 20% within a single individual, 24-hour collections are preferable.[5] Collections taken over a shorter time interval can increase this variability even more. See Chapter 3 for more detailed information regarding the collection of timed urine specimens.

The importance of the urine collection and its timing cannot be overemphasized. By using the time interval and the total volume of urine collected, the amount of urine excreted in milliliters per minute is calculated for insertion into the clearance equation. From Equation 5-5, it is evident that the volume of urine (V) and its creatinine concentration (U) directly affect the magnitude of clearance results.

It is important to look at some factors that can affect the parameters of the clearance equation. Improper storage of the urine specimen with subsequent bacterial proliferation can result in creatinine breakdown to creatine (because of pH changes) or degradation of creatinine by bacterial creatinases. Either situation leads to a falsely decreased urine creatinine value (U).

However, if the urine volume (V) used for the clearance determination is incorrect, the clearance results are also invalid. Practically speaking, it is almost impossible to evaluate the acceptability of information (urine volume, collection interval) submitted with a specimen for a creatinine clearance. However, evaluating individual plasma and urine creatinine results and determining what they indicate about renal status and the clearance equation can alert the laboratorian to inconsistencies in the information provided. The example provided in Box 5-2 highlights the importance of (1) evaluating the individual plasma and urine creatinine results used in the clearance equation, and (2) being aware of potential preanalytical problems that can occur, such as incomplete specimen collection and inaccurate recording of information (e.g., urine volume).

Despite its disadvantages, the creatinine clearance test remains an important diagnostic tool to evaluate renal function, specifically glomerular filtration. Pathologic conditions that cause alterations in the glomerular filtration barrier or changes in renal blood flow to glomeruli will be reflected in the GFR. For example, if a decreased amount of blood plasma is presented to the glomeruli for processing, the GFR decreases. Note that the kidney does not adjust the GFR; rather, the afferent and efferent arterioles modify blood flow to the glomeruli in response to changes in renal hemodynamics. Consequently, a constant blood flow maintains a constant GFR. Because of this close relationship between the GFR and renal blood flow, the creatinine clearance test provides valuable information about renal function.

Alternate Approaches to Assessing Glomerular Filtration Rate

Estimated GFR (eGFR). It is recommended that laboratories calculate the eGFR whenever a serum creatinine test is performed on patients age 18 years and older. The eGFR is a simple and effective tool that can be used to assist health care providers in detecting chronic kidney disease, particularly in high-risk individuals, such as those with diabetes, hypertension, cardiovascular disease, or a family history of kidney disease. The GFR can be estimated using a calculation based on the serum creatinine level and the patient's age, gender, and ethnicity. The recommended formula was developed and validated by the Modification of Diet in Renal Disease (MDRD) Study.[3,6] The equation varies, depending on the method used to measure serum creatinine. Equation 5-7 shows the original MSRD equation, which is used when the creatinine method is not calibrated to an isotope dilution mass spectrometry (IDMS) reference method.

Equation 5-7   Original

$$GFR (mL/min/1.73\,m^2) = 186 \times (S_{cr})^{-1.154} \times (Age, in years)^{-0.203}$$
$$\times (0.742\ \textit{if female})$$
$$\times (1.212\ \textit{if African American})$$

Equation 5-8 is the equation used when the creatinine method is calibrated to an IDMS reference method.

Equation 5-8   IDMS–traceable

$$GFR (mL/min/1.73\,m^2) = 175 \times (S_{cr})^{-1.154} \times (Age, in years)^{-0.203}$$
$$\times (0.742\ \textit{if female})$$
$$\times (1.212\ \textit{if African American})$$

Although other formulas have been proposed to calculate the eGFR, the MDRD equation is the most extensively validated in Caucasian and African American populations.[3] In addition, studies comparing it with other equations such as the Cockcroft-Gault, and with 24-hour creatinine clearance results, have demonstrated its superiority.[3-7]

When the MDRD equation is used, the most accurate values are obtained when the eGFR is less than or equal to 60 mL/min per 1.73 m² body surface area. Therefore,

---

BOX 5-2 | Creatinine Clearance

Example

The laboratory received a 24-hour urine collection from a 26-year-old male (6'4" or body surface area = 2.34 m²; 230 lb), and the total urine collection volume measured 800 mL. After creatinine determinations were performed by the alkaline picrate method, clearance results were calculated:

Plasma creatinine (P):   1.2 mg/dL
Urine creatinine (U):   150 mg/dL
Urine volume (V):   800 mL/24 hr

$$C = \frac{U \times V}{P}$$
$$= \frac{(150\,mg/dL) \times (800\,mL/24\,hr \times 1\,hr/60\,min)}{1.2\,mg/dL}$$

C = 69 mL/min (abnormally low clearance result despite a normal plasma level)

$$C_{corrected} = 69\,mL/min \times \frac{1.73\,m^2}{2.34\,m^2}$$

$$C_{corrected} = 51\,mL/min$$

Discussion

From these data, the normalized creatinine clearance is extremely low compared with a reference range of 80 to 125 mL/min/1.73 m². Even correction for the patient's height and weight does not bring the glomerular filtration rate closer to "normal." This abnormally low glomerular filtration rate is unusual because the patient's plasma creatinine is normal (reference range, 0.8 to 1.3 mg/dL). All specimen identifications were checked, and the creatinine determinations were repeated, with the same results obtained. The plasma creatinine value agreed with previous determinations on this patient.

The best explanation points to a problem with the urine collection. Most likely, (1) some urine was lost or discarded during the 24-hour collection, (2) the time interval for the collection is incorrect, or (3) the specimen was preserved improperly and creatinine has degraded.

the National Kidney Disease Education Program (NKDEP) guidelines recommend that only eGFR values less than or equal to 60 should be reported numerically. Values for eGFR above this range should be reported simply as "greater than 60."[8] For additional discussion of the clinical utility of eGFR measurements, a clinical chemistry text should be consulted.

β₂-Microglobulin and Cystatin C. In renal disease, the remaining functional nephrons of the kidneys compensate for their decreasing numbers by increasing their functional capacity. Consequently, loss of 50% to 60% of the nephrons must occur before creatinine results indicate a reduction in renal function, with a significantly decreased GFR. This "creatinine blind" phase has led to the search for better markers of renal function and to the evaluation of low-molecular-weight proteins such as β_2-microglobulin and cystatin C. Neither of these proteins is the ideal marker of renal function in all patient populations; however, studies have indicated that in certain clinical situations, they can be more sensitive and specific endogenous markers of renal function (i.e., GFR) than creatinine.

β_2-Microglobulin is a single polypeptide chain with a molecular weight of 11,800 daltons. As the β-chain of the human leukocyte antigens, β_2-microglobulin resides on the surface of all nucleated cells. Therefore its concentration in plasma and in all body fluids is essentially constant. In health, β_2-microglobulin readily passes the glomeruli and is reabsorbed completely (99.9%) by the proximal tubular cells, where it is catabolized. Therefore with normal renal function, the concentration of β_2-microglobulin in plasma remains constant, and its excretion in urine is low (e.g., 0.03 to 0.37 mg/day).

β_2-Microglobulin is a better marker of reduced renal tubular function than of glomerular function (i.e., GFR). When tubular reabsorptive function is reduced or lost, the β_2-microglobulin concentration in serum remains essentially normal, whereas its concentration in urine increases significantly. Simultaneous measurements of serum and urine β_2-microglobulin levels can accurately indicate this alteration in renal processing and are clinically useful in (1) identifying allograft rejection in kidney transplant recipients, and (2) differentiating glomerular and tubular renal diseases.

Increased plasma concentrations of β_2-microglobulin accompany a reduction in GFR. Unfortunately, β_2-microglobulin is also elevated in numerous disorders associated with increased cell turnover such as inflammatory conditions, autoimmune disorders, viral infections, amyloidosis, and multiple myeloma. In addition, therapies such as hemodialysis and corticosteroid medications cause an increase in the serum β_2-microglobulin concentration.

A technically related disadvantage of β_2-microglobulin is its susceptibility to degradation in acidic environments. Although this is not a problem with serum specimens, degradation is an issue when urine specimens are collected. Precautions must be taken when collecting and processing urine specimens for β_2-microglobulin analysis to ensure that the urine is alkalinized during collection, or that patients are medicated in such a way that the excreted urine is alkaline. In summary, β_2-microglobulin can be a useful marker of renal tubular function, whereas its use as a marker of GFR is limited.

Cystatin C is a low-molecular-weight protein (13,000 daltons) that has potential as a marker for long-term monitoring of renal function. It is a cysteine proteinase inhibitor produced by all nucleated cells at a constant rate. Like β_2-microglobulin, cystatin C readily passes the glomeruli, is reabsorbed by the proximal tubular cells, and is catabolized, hence cystatin C does not return to the blood circulation. Serum levels of cystatin C are essentially constant and are independent of the individual's age, gender, and muscle mass. As the GFR decreases, levels of cystatin C in the blood increase. Several studies have suggested that cystatin C analysis provides equivalent and in some patient populations enhanced detection of adverse early changes in GFR compared with a serum creatinine or creatinine clearance test.[9,10] However, disadvantages of cystatin C include its higher analysis costs and possibly high intraindividual variation.

The need for long-term monitoring of renal function is important for a variety of patient groups. These include individuals with known renal disease, as well as those who have the potential to develop renal disease, such as individuals with diabetes, hypertension, or autoimmune disease, and those taking nephrotoxic medications (e.g., chemotherapeutic agents, transplant antirejection drugs, certain antibiotics). Because early detection of adverse changes in renal function enables early intervention, the quest for a better marker than creatinine continues. The ultimate role that β_2-microglobulin and cystatin C levels will play in long-term monitoring of renal function remains to be elucidated.

Screening for Albuminuria

Proteinuria of glomerular origin appears early in the course of diabetic nephropathy. Therefore monitoring of urine albumin excretion in individuals with diabetes mellitus aids in the detection and treatment of early nephropathy. Albuminuria is also a marker of increased cardiovascular morbidity and mortality in diabetic individuals. Early detection of low levels of increased urine albumin excretion (microalbuminuria) signals the need for additional screening for possible vascular disease and aggressive intervention to reduce cardiovascular risk factors.[11]

Although the exact mechanism of this proteinuria is not understood clearly, the increased glomerular permeability results from changes in the glomerular filtration barrier. The single most important factor associated with the development of this glomerular proteinuria is hyperglycemia. Because glucose is capable of nonenzymatic binding with various proteins, it apparently combines with proteins of the glomerular filtration barrier, causing glomerular permeability changes and stimulating the growth of the mesangial matrix.

Glomerular changes are evidenced by a urine albumin excretion that exceeds 30 mg/day (or 20 µg/min). Screening for microalbuminuria can be performed using a random, timed, or 24-hour urine collection. Whereas a 24-hour urine collection provides accurate information and allows simultaneous determination of creatinine clearance, it is not the easiest specimen to collect. In contrast, a random urine specimen, which is readily obtainable, can provide accurate albumin excretion information. To use a random urine specimen, the amount of albumin present must be normalized against the creatinine concentration, hence the albumin-to-creatinine ratio is determined. Daily excretion of albumin can be highly variable; therefore at least two of three urine collections analyzed during a 3- to 6-month period should demonstrate increased albumin concentrations before an individual is identified as having microalbuminuria. The definition of microalbuminuria using a random urine specimen is excretion of greater than 30 mg of albumin per gram of creatinine (>30 mg albumin/g creatinine).[11] See Chapter 7 for a discussion of several sensitive tests that are used to rapidly and economically screen urine specimens for low-level increases in urine albumin.

ASSESSMENT OF RENAL BLOOD FLOW AND TUBULAR SECRETORY FUNCTION

Determination of Renal Plasma Flow and Renal Blood Flow

Normal renal function depends on adequate renal blood flow (RBF). If blood flow to the kidneys changes for any reason, glomerular filtration and the ability of the nephrons to reabsorb and secrete solutes and water also change. The glomeruli produce an ultrafiltrate from the plasma portion of the circulating blood. Note that the portion of blood plasma that is not filtered proceeds into the peritubular capillaries and is processed by the tubules. Not all the blood that flows into the kidney is processed. In fact, approximately 8% of the RBF never comes into contact with functional renal tissue.[12] Renal plasma flow (RPF) is different from RBF. RPF and RBF are related to each other as described in Equation 5-9, in which Hct denotes the hematocrit.[2]

Equation 5-9

$$RBF = \frac{RPF}{1 Hct}$$

The ideal clearance substance used to measure RPF and subsequently RBF must (1) reside exclusively in the plasma portion of the blood, (2) be removed from the plasma primarily by renal tubular secretion, and (3) be removed completely from the plasma in its first pass through the kidney, resulting in essentially zero concentration in the venous renal blood. When a substance is completely removed from the plasma after passage through the glomeruli and the peritubular capillaries, the actual plasma flow in milliliters per minute can be determined using the traditional clearance equation (see Equation 5-4). Note that to evaluate the secretory function of the renal tubules, the RPF must be normal. Conversely, to evaluate RPF, the tubular secretory function must be normal.

Clearance tests using p-aminohippurate and phenolsulfonphthalein assess renal tubular secretory function. Both substances are secreted actively by the renal tubules; however, phenolsulfonphthalein is not completely removed as it passes through the kidney and is unsatisfactory for assessing the RPF. Although the RPF can be determined by using the p-aminohippurate clearance test, other techniques using radioactive substances (e.g., ^{131}I-orthoiodohippuran) have also been used. Measurements of secretory function and RPF are not routinely performed because they require intravenous infusion of an exogenous substance.

The most common test used to measure RPF is the p-aminohippurate clearance test. p-Aminohippurate is an exogenous, nontoxic, weak organic acid that is secreted almost exclusively by the proximal tubules (a small amount is filtered through the glomerulus). At certain plasma levels, p-aminohippurate is secreted completely during its first pass through the kidneys, hence the p-aminohippurate clearance test provides not only an excellent indicator of renal tubular secretory function but also a means of determining the RPF and the RBF when normal secretory function is known. Although the p-aminohippurate clearance test is the reference method for measurement of the RPF, current methods used for analysis of p-aminohippurate in urine and plasma are difficult and time-consuming. Because p-aminohippurate is an exogenous substance, it must be infused—another drawback to its routine clinical use.

A normal RPF as determined by the p-aminohippurate clearance test ranges from 600 to 700 mL/min. Assuming an average normal hematocrit of 0.42 (42%) and by using Equation 5-7, normal values for the RBF range from approximately 1000 to 1200 mL/min. By using this information and a normal resting cardiac output of approximately 6 L/min, one can calculate that the kidneys receive approximately 16% to 20% of the total cardiac output. This measurement does not account for the 8% of the RBF that never contacts functioning renal tissue. Adding in the 8%, the kidneys receive approximately 25% of the total cardiac output.

Assessment of Tubular Secretory Function for Acid Removal

As described in Chapter 4, the renal tubules actively secrete acids in response to changes in the acid-base equilibrium of the body. The metabolism of proteins and phospholipids results in the formation of sulfuric and phosphoric acids. These acids are neutralized rapidly by bicarbonate into CO_2 and the neutral salts Na_2SO_4 and Na_2HPO_4. The CO_2 is excreted by the lungs, whereas the neutral salts are passed into the ultrafiltrate at the kidneys. As the renal tubules secrete ammonia and hydrogen ions, the neutral salts are further modified into ammonium salt (e.g., $[NH_4]_2SO_4$) or titratable acid (i.e., NaH_2PO_4) for excretion, hence evaluation of the renal tubular ability to produce an acid urine involves the measurement of ammonium salts and titratable acids. Normally, 50 to 100 mmol of acid is excreted in the urine each day.[13]

Measurement of Titratable Acid Versus Urinary Ammonia. In urine, the amount of acid (H^+) combined with ammonia is normally twice that excreted as titratable acid. Titratable acid formation is limited by the concentration of phosphate ions in the ultrafiltrate. Because the plasma concentration of phosphate ions is normally small, the ultrafiltrate concentration is also small. However, ammonia is produced and secreted by the renal tubules in direct response to the need to eliminate acid from the body. Ammonia production is not limited, and healthy renal tubules increase production to remove additional amounts of metabolic acids. For example, in patients experiencing diabetic ketoacidosis, ammonium salt excretion can reach as much as 400 mmol/day, whereas their titratable acid excretion increases to only 100 to 200 mmol/day. In contrast, diseased tubules lose the ability to produce and secrete ammonia, as well as to secrete hydrogen ions. In these cases, the quantity of total acids excreted daily may decrease to 3 to 35 mmol/day. At the same time, the amount of ammonium salts excreted compared with titratable acids may also decrease to the point where more acid is excreted as free titratable acid than is combined with ammonia.

Because the kidneys play a crucial role in maintaining a normal acid-base balance, systemic acidosis occurs if the tubular secretory function is compromised. In fact, renal failure usually is associated with acidosis. Therefore, valuable information regarding tubular secretory function can be obtained by measuring the total hydrogen ion excretion in urine (titratable acid and ammonium salts).

Oral Ammonium Chloride Test. The oral ammonium chloride test involves the oral administration of ammonium chloride, which metabolizes to urea and HCl. To adjust for the increased acid, the kidneys excrete increased quantities of titratable acid and ammonium salts, and the urine becomes more acidic. Plasma bicarbonate measurements are made before and midway through the test to monitor the depletion of the body's bicarbonate pool. If the initial plasma bicarbonate is low (<20 mmol/L), the test should not be performed. An initial morning 2-hour urine specimen is collected before the test. If the pH of the specimen is below 5.3, acid excretion is normal and the test need not be performed. During the test, urine is collected every 2 hours for 8 to 10 hours. Each 2-hour collection is measured for pH, titratable acid, and ammonium excretion.

Normal individuals are able to reduce the urine pH to below 5.3, with a total hydrogen ion excretion (titratable acid plus ammonium salts) greater than 60 mmol/min. The titratable acid and the ammonium salt excretion should exceed 25 mmol per minute. At the same time, the plasma bicarbonate level should fall to below 26 mmol/L. Failure to excrete an acidic urine following this challenge test supports a diagnosis of renal tubular acidosis. Renal tubular acidosis is a condition characterized by defective tubular hydrogen ion secretion, defective tubular ammonia production, or defective bicarbonate reabsorption in the proximal tubules. Regardless of the specific defect involved, patients with renal tubular acidosis excrete alkaline urine despite a systemic acidosis.

Measurement of titratable acids is performed by titrating a well-mixed aliquot of urine with 0.1 N NaOH to an endpoint pH of 7.4 using a pH meter. This endpoint corresponds to a blood pH of 7.4 and a urine pH of 4.4.[14] Subsequently, the ammonium concentration is calculated as the difference between the total acidity of the urine and the acids present as titratable acids.

In conclusion, although measurements of localized functions of the nephron are possible, they are not performed routinely in a clinical setting. Instead, the most common and practical urine tests used to evaluate renal function routinely are the creatinine clearance test for assessment of GFR; a urine osmolality determination for tubular concentrating ability; and a urine protein electrophoresis to evaluate glomerular permeability to plasma proteins. In addition, plasma creatinine levels and eGFR calculations provide ongoing indications of compromised or changing renal function.

STUDY QUESTIONS

1. Which of the following solutes are present in the largest molar amounts in urine?
   A. Urea, chloride, and sodium
   B. Urea, creatinine, and sodium
   C. Creatinine, uric acid, and ammonium
   D. Urea, uric acid, and ammonium

2. Renal excretion is not involved in the elimination of
   A. electrolytes and water.
   B. normal by-products of fat metabolism.
   C. soluble metabolic wastes (e.g., urea, creatinine).
   D. exogenous substances (e.g., drugs, x-ray contrast media).

3. The concentration of which substances provides the best means of distinguishing urine from other body fluids?
   A. Creatinine and urea
   B. Glucose and protein
   C. Uric acid and ammonia
   D. Water and electrolytes

4. What is the definition of the *osmolality* of a solution?
   A. The density of solute particles per liter of solvent
   B. The mass of solute particles per kilogram of solvent
   C. The number of solute particles per kilogram of solvent
   D. The weight of solute particles per liter of solvent

5. The osmolality of a solution containing 1.0 mole of urea is equal to that of a solution containing
   A. 1.0 mole of HCl.
   B. 1.0 mole of H_2PO_4.
   C. 0.5 mole of NaCl.
   D. 0.5 mole of glucose.

6. The maximum osmolality that urine can achieve is determined by the
   A. quantity of solutes ingested in the diet.
   B. presence of antidiuretic hormone in the collecting tubules.
   C. osmolality of the medullary interstitium.
   D. osmolality of fluid entering the collecting tubules.

7. Serum osmolality remains relatively constant, whereas the urine osmolality ranges from
   A. one-third to one-half that of serum.
   B. one-third to equal that of serum.
   C. one to three times that of serum.
   D. three to five times that of serum.

8. Another name for excessive thirst is
   A. polydipsia.
   B. polyuria.
   C. hydrophilia.
   D. hydrostasis.

9. Specific gravity measurements are not affected by
   A. temperature.
   B. solute charge.
   C. solute mass.
   D. solute number.

10. Osmolality is a measure of solute
    A. density.
    B. mass.
    C. number.
    D. weight.

11. Which of the following solutes, if added to pure water, affects the specific gravity more than it affects its osmolality?
    A. Sodium
    B. Chloride
    C. Potassium
    D. Glucose

12. Occasionally the specific gravity of a urine specimen exceeds that physiologically possible (i.e., >1.040). Which of the following substances when found in urine could account for such a high value?
    A. Creatinine
    B. Glucose
    C. Mannitol
    D. Protein

13. The excretion of large volumes of urine (>3 L/day) is called
    A. glucosuria.
    B. hyperuria.
    C. polydipsia.
    D. polyuria.

14. The daily volume of urine excreted normally ranges from
    A. 100 to 500 mL/day.
    B. 100 to 1800 mL/day.
    C. 500 to 1800 mL/day.
    D. 1000 to 3000 mL/day.

15. When the body is dehydrated, the kidneys
    A. excrete excess solutes in a constant volume of urine.
    B. excrete solutes in as small a volume of urine as possible.
    C. decrease the quantity of solutes excreted and decrease the urine volume.
    D. increase the quantity of solutes excreted while holding the urine volume constant.

16. The excretion of less than 400 mL of urine per day is called
    A. anuria.
    B. hypouria.
    C. nocturia.
    D. oliguria.

17. The ultrafiltrate in the urinary space of the glomerulus has a specific gravity of
    A. 1.005 and a lower osmolality than the blood plasma.
    B. 1.010 and the same osmolality as the blood plasma.
    C. 1.015 and a higher osmolality than the blood plasma.
    D. 1.035 and a higher osmolality than the blood plasma.

18. All of the following conditions may produce nocturia except
    A. anuria.
    B. pregnancy.
    C. chronic renal disease.
    D. fluid intake at night.
19. Which renal function is assessed using specific gravity and osmolality measurements?
    A. Concentrating ability
    B. Glomerular filtration ability
    C. Tubular excretion ability
    D. Tubular secretion ability
20. A fluid deprivation test is used to
    A. determine renal plasma flow.
    B. investigate the cause of oliguria.
    C. assess renal concentrating ability.
    D. measure the glomerular filtration rate.
21. A fluid deprivation test involves the measurement of serum and urine
    A. density.
    B. osmolality.
    C. specific gravity.
    D. volume.
22. The volume of plasma cleared per minute in excess of that required for solute elimination is called the
    A. creatinine clearance.
    B. free-water clearance.
    C. osmolar clearance.
    D. renal clearance.
23. A free-water clearance value of −1.2 would be expected from a patient experiencing
    A. polyuria.
    B. dehydration.
    C. water diuresis.
    D. excessive fluid intake.
24. Calculate the osmolar and free-water clearances using the following patient data.
    Serum osmolality: 305 mOsm/kg
    Urine osmolality: 250 mOsm/kg
    Urine volume: 300 mL/2 hours
    A. Is this individual excreting more water than is necessary for solute removal? Yes/No
    B. Is the osmolar clearance "normal" (i.e., 2.0 to 3.0 mL/min)? Yes/No
    C. From the free-water clearance result obtained, is the urine hypo-osmotic or hyperosmotic?
25. Which of the following is an endogenous substance used to measure glomerular filtration rate?
    A. Urea
    B. Inulin
    C. Creatinine
    D. *p*-Aminohippurate

26. Renal clearance is defined as the volume of
    A. urine cleared of a substance per minute.
    B. plasma cleared of a substance in a time interval.
    C. plasma flowing through the kidney per minute.
    D. plasma containing the same amount of substance in 1 mL of urine.
27. Creatinine is a good substance to use for a renal clearance test because it
    A. is exogenous.
    B. is reabsorbed.
    C. is affected by fluid intake.
    D. has a constant plasma concentration.
28. Which of the following groups would be expected to have the greatest 24-hour excretion of creatinine?
    A. Infants
    B. Children
    C. Women
    D. Men
29. Creatinine clearance results are "normalized" using an individual's body surface area to account for variations in the individual's
    A. age.
    B. sex.
    C. dietary intake.
    D. muscle mass.
30. The following data are obtained from a 60-year-old female who is 4′8″ tall and weighs 88 lb:
    Plasma creatinine: 1.2 mg/dL
    Urine creatinine: 500 mg/L
    Urine volume: 1440 mL/24 hr
    A. Calculate the creatinine clearance.
    B. Calculate the normalized creatinine clearance. (Determine the body surface area using Equation 5-6.)
    C. Are these results normal for this patient? (Use reference intervals provided in Table 5-3.)
31. A 24-hour urine collection is preferred for determination of creatinine clearance because of diurnal variation in the
    A. glomerular filtration rate.
    B. plasma creatinine.
    C. creatinine excretion.
    D. urine excretion.
32. Which of the following situations results in an erroneous creatinine clearance measurement?
    A. A 24-hour urine collection from an individual on a vegetarian diet
    B. A 24-hour urine collection maintained at room temperature throughout the collection
    C. A plasma sample drawn at the beginning instead of during the 24-hour urine collection
    D. Creatinine determinations made using the nonspecific alkaline picrate method (Jaffe reaction)

33. A 45-year-old female African American had her serum creatinine determined using a creatinine method that is NOT calibrated to an IDMS reference method. Her serum creatinine was 1.5 mg/dL; what is her eGFR using the appropriate MDRD equation?
   A. 40 mL/min/1.73 m^2
   B. 48 mL/min/1.73 m^2
   C. 51 mL/min/1.73 m^2
   D. 54 mL/min/1.73 m^2

34. The glomerular filtration rate is controlled by
   A. the renal blood flow.
   B. the renal plasma flow.
   C. the countercurrent mechanism.
   D. hormones (e.g., aldosterone, antidiuretic hormone).

35. For measurement of renal plasma flow, *p*-aminohippurate is an ideal substance to use because it
   A. is easily measured in urine and plasma.
   B. is endogenous and does not require an infusion.
   C. is secreted completely in its first pass through the kidneys.
   D. maintains a constant plasma concentration throughout the test.

36. What percentage of the total cardiac output is received by the kidneys?
   A. 8%
   B. 15%
   C. 25%
   D. 33%

37. Measuring the quantity of hydrogen ion excreted as titratable acids and ammonium salts in urine provides a measure of
   A. tubular secretory function.
   B. tubular reabsorptive function.
   C. glomerular filtration ability.
   D. renal concentrating ability.

38. The oral ammonium chloride test evaluates the ability of the tubules to secrete
   A. ammonium and chloride.
   B. phosphate and sodium.
   C. bicarbonate and chloride.
   D. ammonia and hydrogen.

CASE 5-1	A 52-YEAR-OLD FEMALE WITH A 25-YEAR HISTORY OF TYPE 1 DIABETES MELLITUS SUBMITS A 24-HOUR URINE COLLECTION FOR TESTING. A BLOOD SAMPLE WAS ALSO COLLECTED WHEN SHE BROUGHT THE URINE SPECIMEN TO THE LABORATORY. THE FOLLOWING INFORMATION AND RESULTS ARE OBTAINED:

Patient Information
Height: 5'5" (165 cm)
Weight: 160 lb (72.7 kg)

Results		Reference Intervals
Creatinine, serum:	2.3 mg/dL	0.8-1.3 mg/dL
Urine volume, 24-hour:	1000 mL	600-1800 mL/day
Creatinine, urine:	190 mg/dL	Varies with hydration
Albumin, urine:	9.5 mg/dL	Varies with hydration

1. Calculate this patient's body surface area using Equation 5-6.
2. Calculate the normalized creatinine clearance result using the data provided.
3. Calculate the albumin excretion in milligrams per day (mg/day).
4. Calculate the albumin excretion in micrograms per minute (µg/min).
5. Calculate the urine albumin-to-creatinine ratio in micrograms albumin per milligram of creatinine (µg albumin/mg creatinine).

CASE 5-2 **A 24-YEAR-OLD MAN WHO HAD PREVIOUSLY SUSTAINED A SEVERE HEAD INJURY IN A CAR ACCIDENT IS SEEN BY HIS PHYSICIAN. HE COMPLAINS OF POLYDYPSIA AND POLYURIA. NEUROGENIC DIABETES INSIPIDUS IS SUSPECTED, AND TESTS ARE PERFORMED TO RULE OUT COMPULSIVE WATER INGESTION. THE FOLLOWING ROUTINE URINALYSIS IS OBTAINED.**

Results:

Physical Examination
Color: colorless
Clarity: clear
Odor: —

Chemical Examination
SG: 1.005
pH: 6.0
Blood: negative
Protein: negative
LE: negative
Nitrite: negative
Glucose: negative
Ketones: negative
Bilirubin: negative
Urobilinogen: normal
Ascorbic acid: —

1. Explain briefly the cause of polyuria in patients with diabetes insipidus.
2. Without fluid restrictions, this patient's urine osmolality most likely is
   A. less than 200 mOsm/kg.
   B. greater than 200 mOsm/kg.
3. This patient's polyuria should be classified as
   A. oncotic diuresis.
   B. psychosomatic diuresis.
   C. solute diuresis.
   D. water diuresis.

4. In patients with neurogenic diabetes insipidus, if antidiuretic hormone is given intravenously, the urine osmolality should
   A. remain unchanged.
   B. decrease.
   C. increase.
5. Which of the following tests should be used to evaluate this patient?
   A. Free-water clearance test
   B. Fluid deprivation test
   C. Glucose tolerance test
   D. Osmolar clearance test
   Indicate whether each of the following statements is true (T) or false (F).
6. Patients with diabetes insipidus often have glucose present in the urine.
7. Patients with diabetes insipidus often have a high urine specific gravity.
8. Patients with diabetes insipidus often have urinary ketones present because of an inability to use the glucose present in the blood.
9. Diabetes is a general term referring to disorders characterized by copious production and excretion of urine.

LE, Leukocyte esterase; *SG,* specific gravity.

REFERENCES

1. Walmsley RN, White GH: A guide to diagnostic clinical chemistry, ed 2, Melbourne, 1988, Blackwell Scientific.
2. Koushanpour E, Kriz W: Renal physiology, ed 2, New York, 1986, Springer-Verlag.
3. Poggio ED, Wang X, Greene T, et al: Performance of the modification of diet in renal disease and Cockcroft-Gault equations in the estimation of GFR in health and in chronic kidney disease. J Am Soc Nephrol 16:459–466, 2005.
4. Miller BF, Winkler AW: The renal excretion of endogenous creatinine in man: comparison with exogenous creatinine and inulin. J Clin Invest 17:31–40, 1938.
5. Rock RC, Walker WG, Jennings CD: Nitrogen metabolites and renal function. In Tietz NW, editor: Fundamentals of clinical chemistry, ed 3, Philadelphia, 1987, WB Saunders.
6. Myers GL, Miller WG, Coresh J, et al, National Kidney Disease Education Program Laboratory Working Group: Recommendations for improving serum creatinine measurement: a report from the Laboratory Working Group of the National Kidney Disease Education Program. Clin Chem 52:5–18, 2006.
7. Coresh J, Stevens LA: Kidney function estimating equations: where do we stand? Curr Opin Nephrol Hypertens 15:276–284, 2006.
8. Levey AS, Coresh J, Balk E, et al: National Kidney Foundation practice guideline for chronic kidney disease evaluation, classification, and stratification. Ann Intern Med 139:137–147, 2003.
9. Laterza OF, Price CP, Scott MG: Cystatin C: an improved estimator of glomerular filtration rate? Clin Chem 48:699–707, 2002.
10. Pucci L, Triscornia S, Lucchesi D, et al: Cystatin C and estimates of renal function: searching for a better measure of kidney function in diabetes patients. Clin Chem 53:480–488, 2007.
11. American Diabetics Association: Nephropathy in diabetes (position statement). Diabetes Care 27(Suppl 1):S79–S83, 2004.
12. Duston H, Corcoran A: Functional interpretation of renal tests. Med Clin North Am 39:947–956, 1955.
13. Lennon EJ, Lemann J, Litzow JR: The effect of diet and stool composition on the net external acid balance of normal subjects. J Clin Invest 45:1601–1607, 1966.
14. First MR: Renal function. In Kaplan LA, Pesce AJ, editors: Clinical chemistry: theory, analysis, and correlation, ed 2, St Louis, 1989, Mosby.
15. Boothby WM: Nomogram to determine body surface area. Boston Med Surg J 185:337, 1921.

BIBLIOGRAPHY

Alpern RJ, Hebert SC, editors: Seldin and Giebisch's The kidney physiology and pathophysiology, ed 4, Amsterdam, 2008, Academic Press/Elsevier.

Anderson SC, Cockayne S: Clinical chemistry: concepts and applications, New York, 2003, McGraw-Hill.

Burtis CA, Ashwood ER, editors: Tietz textbook of clinical chemistry, ed 3, Philadelphia, 1999, WB Saunders.

Kumar V, Abbas A, Aster J: Robbins and Cotran pathologic basis of disease, ed 8, Philadelphia, 2010, Saunders.

Goldman L, Schafer AI, editors: Goldman's Cecil medicine, ed 24, Philadelphia, 2011, Saunders.

Hall JE: Guyton and Hall textbook of medical physiology, ed 12, Philadelphia, 2011, Saunders.

Kaplan LA, Pesce AJ, Kazmierczak SC, editors: Clinical chemistry: theory, analysis, correlation, ed 4, St Louis, 2003, Mosby.

Oh MS: Evaluation of renal function, water, electrolytes, and acid-base balance. In McPherson RA, Pincus MR, editors: Clinical diagnosis and management by laboratory methods, ed 21, Philadelphia, 2007, Saunders.

Patton KT, Thibodeau GA: Anatomy and physiology, ed 7, Philadelphia, 2010, Saunders.

Schrier RW, Gottschalk CW: Diseases of the kidney and urinary tract, ed 7, Philadelphia, 2001, Lippincott Williams & Wilkins.

Physical Examination of Urine

KEY TERMS

clarity (also called *turbidity*) The transparency of a urine specimen. Clarity varies with the amount of suspended particulate matter in the urine specimen.

colligative property A characteristic of a solution that depends only on the number of solute particles present, regardless of the molecular size or charge. The four colligative properties are freezing point depression, vapor pressure depression, osmotic pressure elevation, and boiling point elevation. These properties form the basis of methods and instrumentation used to measure the concentration of solutes in body fluids (e.g., serum, urine, fecal supernates). (See *freezing point osmometer* and *vapor pressure osmometer.*)

density An expression of concentration in terms of the mass of solutes present per volume of solution.

diuresis An increase in urine excretion. Various causes of diuresis include increased fluid intake, diuretic therapy, hormonal imbalance, renal dysfunction, and drug ingestion (e.g., alcohol, caffeine).

freezing point osmometer An instrument that measures osmolality based on the freezing point depression of a solution compared with that of pure water. An osmometer consists of a mechanism to supercool the sample below its freezing point. Subsequently, freezing of the sample is induced, and as ice crystals form, a sensitive thermistor monitors the temperature until an equilibrium is attained between solid and liquid phases. This equilibrium temperature is the freezing point of the sample, from which the osmolality of the sample is determined. One osmole of solutes per kilogram of solvent (1 Osm/kg) depresses the freezing point of water by 1.86° C.

ionic specific gravity The density of a solution based on ionic solutes only. Nonionizing substances such as urea, glucose, protein, and radiographic contrast media are not detectable using ionic specific gravity measurements (e.g., specific gravity by commercial reagent strips).

refractive index The ratio of light refraction in two differing media (n). The refractive index is expressed mathematically using light velocity (V) or the angle of refraction (sin Ø) in the two media, as $n_2/n_1 = V_1/V_2$ or $n_2/n_1 = \sin Ø_1 / \sin Ø_2$. The refractive index is affected by the wavelength of light used, the temperature of the solution, and the concentration of the solution.

refractometry An indirect measurement of specific gravity based on the refractive index of light.

urobilin An orange-brown pigment derived from the spontaneous oxidation of colorless urobilinogen.

urochrome A lipid-soluble yellow pigment that is produced continuously during endogenous metabolism. Present in plasma and excreted in the urine, urochrome gives urine its characteristic yellow color.

uroerythrin A pink (or red) pigment in urine that is thought to derive from melanin metabolism. Uroerythrin deposits on urate crystals to produce a precipitate described as "brick dust."

vapor pressure osmometer An instrument that measures osmolality based on the vapor pressure depression of a solution compared with that of pure water. The dew point of the air in a closed chamber containing a small amount of a sample is measured and compared with that obtained using pure water. A calibrated microprocessor converts the change in the dew point observed into osmolality, which is read directly from the instrument readout.

The study of urine is the oldest clinical laboratory test still performed. Historically, only the physical characteristics of urine were evaluated—color, clarity, odor, and taste. The latter characteristic—taste—has not been performed for centuries because of chemical methods that can be used to assess the "sweetness" of urine. The physical characteristics of urine continue to play an important part in a routine urinalysis. The presence of disease processes and abnormal urine components can be evident during the initial physical examination of urine.

COLOR

Urine color, which is normally various shades of yellow, can range from colorless to amber to orange, red, green, blue, brown, or even black. These color variations can indicate the presence of a disease process, a metabolic abnormality, or an ingested food or drug. However, color variations can simply result from excessive physical activity or stress. It is important to note that a change in urine color is often the initial or only reason why an individual seeks medical attention.

The characteristic yellow color of normal urine is principally due to the pigment **urochrome**.[1] A product of endogenous metabolism, urochrome is a lipid-soluble pigment that is present in plasma and excreted in urine. Patients in chronic renal failure, with decreased excretion of urochrome, may exhibit a characteristic yellow pigmentation of their skin caused by deposition of urochrome in their subcutaneous fat. Because urochrome production and excretion are constant, the intensity of the color of urine provides a crude indicator of urine concentration and the hydration state of the body. A concentrated urine is dark yellow, whereas a dilute urine is pale yellow or colorless. Urochrome, similar to other lipid-soluble pigments, darkens on exposure to light.[2] This characteristic darkening is often observed in urine specimens that are improperly stored. Small amounts of **urobilin** (an orange-brown pigment) and **uroerythrin** (a pink pigment) also contribute to urine color. Urobilin and uroerythrin are normal urine constituents; uroerythrin is most evident when it deposits on urate crystals, producing a precipitate often described as brick dust.

The terminology used to describe urine colors often differs among laboratories. Regardless of the terminology used, an established list of terms should be available and used by all personnel in the laboratory. These terms should reduce ambiguity in color interpretation and improve consistency in the reporting of urine colors.[3] Terms such as *straw* and *beer brown* should be replaced with *light yellow* and *amber*. The term *bloody* should be avoided. Although *bloody* is descriptive, it is not a color; *red* or *pink* would be more appropriate. Table 6-1 lists some appropriate urine color terms and the substances that can cause these colors.

An abnormal urine, that is, one that reflects a pathologic process, may not have an abnormal color, whereas a normally colored urine may contain significant pathologic elements. For example, a normal yellow or colorless urine can actually contain large amounts of glucose or porphobilinogen. In contrast, a red urine, often an indicator of the presence of blood, can result from ingestion of beets by genetically disposed individuals. Nevertheless, urine color is valuable in the preliminary assessment of a urine specimen.

Many substances are capable of modifying the normal color of urine. The same substance can impart a different color to urine depending on (1) the amount of the substance present, (2) the urine pH, and (3) the structural form of the substance, which can change over time. Red blood cells provide an excellent example. In fresh acidic urine, red blood cells can be present despite a typical yellow-colored urine, or the urine color may appear pink or red. The color of the urine varies with the quantity of

TABLE 6-1	Urine Color Terms and Common Causes*		
Color		**Substance**	**Comments and Clinical Correlation**
Colorless to pale yellow		Dilute urine	Fluid ingestion; polyuria due to diabetes mellitus or diabetes insipidus
Yellow		Normal urine	Due to the normal pigment, urochrome (as well as uroerythrin and urobilin)
Dark yellow to amber		Concentrated urine, excessive urobilin	Limited fluid intake—dehydration, strenuous exercise, first morning specimen, fever; excessive conversion of urobilinogen to urobilin with time
		Bilirubin	If shaken, foam is yellow
Dark yellow-green		Biliverdin	Greenish coloration due to bilirubin that oxidized to biliverdin upon standing or improper storage
Orange	Foods	Carotene	High consumption of vegetables and fruits that contain carotene
	Drugs	Phenazopyridine (Pyridium, Azo-Gantrisin)	Medication—urinary analgesic; bright color at acid pH
		Warfarin (Coumadin)	Medication—anticoagulant
		Rifampin	Medication—tuberculosis treatment
Bright yellow	Foods	Riboflavin	Multivitamins, B-complex vitamins
Yellow-brown	Drugs	Nitrofurantoin	Medication—antibiotic
Pink	Blood	Hemoglobin, red blood cells (RBCs)	Blood in urine from urinary tract or from contamination (e.g., menstrual bleeding)
	Inherited	Porphobilin	Oxidized porphobilinogen (colorless); caused by improper handling and storage of urine specimens; associated with acute intermittent porphyria (a rare genetic disorder)
Red	Blood	RBCs	Intact RBCs observed microscopically; urine cloudy
		Hemoglobin	Urine clear, if no intact RBCs present (e.g., intravascular hemolysis); hemolysis evident in plasma/serum
	Foods	Beet ingestion	In acidic urine of genetic disposed individuals; alkaline urine is yellow
	Drugs	Senna	Over-the-counter laxatives (e.g., Ex-Lax)
Red-purple	Inherited	Porphyrins	Excessive oxidation of colorless porphyrinogens and porphobilinogen to colored compounds (rare conditions); caused by improper handling and storage of these specimens
Brown		Myoglobin	Rhabdomyolysis—urine clear; plasma/serum normal yellow appearance
	Blood	Methemoglobin	Oxidized hemoglobin
	Drugs	Metronidazole (Flagyl)	Medication—treatment for trichomoniasis, *Giardia*, amebiasis; darkens the urine
Dark brown to black		Melanin	Oxidized melanogen (colorless); develops upon standing and associated with malignant melanoma
	Inherited	Homogentisic acid	Color develops upon standing in alkaline urine; associated with alkaptonuria (a genetic metabolic disorder)
Blue or green	Infection	*Pseudomonas*	Urinary tract infection with *Pseudomonas*
		Indican	Infection of the small intestine
	Dyes	Methylene blue (dye) containing	Urinary analgesics (e.g., TracTabs, Urised, Uro blue, Mictasol blue); excessive use of mouthwashes
		Chlorophyll containing	Breath deodorizers (Clorets), excessive use of mouthwashes
	Drugs	Amitriptyline (Elavil)	Medication—antidepressant
		Indomethacin (Indocin)	

*Note that numerous medications, foods, and dyes can cause changes in urine color. This list is limited and focuses on those most commonly encountered in the clinical laboratory.

red blood cells present. As red blood cells disintegrate, hemoglobin is released and oxidizes to methemoglobin, which causes the urine color to become brown or even black. Alkaline urine with red blood cells present is often red-brown in color. In such specimens, disintegration of cellular components is enhanced by the alkaline pH and

hemoglobin oxidation promoted. When glomerular or tubular damage of nephrons occur, blood enters the urinary tract and the hemoglobin becomes oxidized before it collects in the bladder. In this case, the urine appears brownish rather than the typical red color that is associated with the presence of blood.

A fresh brown urine can indicate the presence of blood, hemoglobin, or myoglobin. Distinguishing among these substances is difficult, particularly between hemoglobin and myoglobin, because all three produce a positive chemical test for blood. Red blood cells are confirmed by microscopic examination, whereas the discrimination between hemoglobin and myoglobin requires additional urine chemical testing and possibly an evaluation of the blood plasma. Chapter 7 provides further discussion on the differentiation of hemoglobin and myoglobin in urine.

Bilirubin is another substance that can contribute to urine color. It is a by-product of hemoglobin catabolism and has a characteristic yellow color. When present in sufficient amounts in urine or plasma, bilirubin imparts a distinctive amber coloration. However, upon standing or improper storage, bilirubin oxidizes to biliverdin, causing the urine to take on a greenish hue. Bilirubin is also susceptible to photo-oxidation by artificial light or sunlight; therefore specimens must be stored properly to avoid degradation of this component. This photosensitivity is temperature dependent; optimal specimen stability is obtained by storing the specimens at low temperatures in the dark.

Some substances are colorless and normally do not contribute to urine color. However, upon standing or improper storage, they convert to colored compounds. Urobilinogen, a normal constituent in urine, is colorless, whereas its oxidation product urobilin is orange-brown. Porphobilinogen, a colorless and chemically similar (tetrapyrroles) substance, is a solute found in the urine of patients with abnormal porphyrin metabolism (heme synthesis). Porphobilin, the oxidation product of porphobilinogen, can impart a pink color to urine. As a result, urine that contains these substances can change color over time; this may alert the laboratorian to its presence and the need for additional testing. However, these color changes are often subtle and take hours to develop.

A multitude of urine colors result from ingested substances, and often the colors have no clinical significance. Highly pigmented foods such as fresh beets, breath fresheners containing chlorophyll, candy dyes, and vitamins A and B can impart distinctive colors to urine. Included in this group of ingested substances are numerous medications, some of which are used specifically to treat urinary tract infection. Other medications are present because they are eliminated from the body in the urine. Table 6-2 lists commonly encountered drugs and the colors they impart to the urine. It is worth noting that phenazopyridine, a urinary analgesic often encountered in the clinical laboratory, imparts a distinctive yellow-orange coloration (similar to orange soda pop) with a thick consistency to the urine. This drug-produced color frequently interferes with the color interpretation of chemical reagent strip tests; alternative chemical testing methods must be used with these urine specimens.

Pathologic conditions can be indicated by the presence of certain analytes and components that color the

TABLE 6-2	Urine Color Changes With Some Commonly Used Drugs
Drug	**Color**
Alcohol, ethyl	Pale yellow or colorless (diuresis)
Amitriptyline (Elavil)	Blue-green
Anthraquinone laxatives (senna, cascara)	Reddish, alkaline; yellow-brown, acid
Chlorzoxazone (Paraflex) (muscle relaxant)	Red
Deferoxamine mesylate (Desferal) (chelates iron)	Red
Ethoxazene (Serenium) (urinary analgesic)	Orange, red
Fluorescein sodium (given intravenously)	Yellow
Furazolidone (Furoxone) (Tricofuron) (an antibacterial, antiprotozoal nitrofuran)	Brown
Indigo carmine dye (renal function, cytoscopy)	Blue
Iron sorbitol (Jectofer) (possibly other iron compounds forming iron sulfide in urine)	Brown on standing
Levodopa (L-dopa) (for parkinsonism)	Red then brown, alkaline
Mepacrine (Atabrine) (antimalarial) (intestinal worms, *Giardia*)	Yellow
Methocarbamol (Robaxin) (muscle relaxant)	Green-brown
Methyldopa (Aldomet) (antihypertensive)	Darken; if oxidizing agents present, red to brown
Methylene blue (used to delineate fistulas)	Blue, blue-green
Metronidazole (Flagyl) (for *Trichomonas* infection, amebiasis, *Giardia*)	Darkening, reddish brown
Nitrofurantoin (Furadantin) (antibacterial)	Brown-yellow
Phenazopyridine (Pyridium) (urinary analgesic), also compounded with sulfonamides (Azo-Gantrisin)	Orange-red, acid pH
Phenindione (Hedulin) (anticoagulant) (important to distinguish from hematuria)	Orange, alkaline; color disappears on acidifying
Phenol poisoning	Brown; oxidized to quinones (green)
Phenolphthalein (purgative)	Red-purple, alkaline pH
Phenolsulfonphthalein (PSP, also BSP)	Pink-red, alkaline pH
Rifampin (Rifadin, Rimactane) (tuberculosis therapy)	Bright orange-red
Riboflavin (multivitamins)	Bright yellow
Sulfasalazine (Azulfidine) (for ulcerative colitis)	Orange-yellow, alkaline pH

From Henry B: Clinical diagnosis and management by laboratory methods, ed 18, Philadelphia, 1991, WB Saunders.

urine. Substances such as melanin, homogentisic acid, indican, porphyrins, hemoglobin, and myoglobin or components such as red blood cells provide evidence of a pathologic process. In each case, urine suspected of containing these components requires additional chemical testing and investigation. Many of these substances are discussed individually along with the metabolic diseases that produce them in Chapters 7 and 9.

However, contaminants—substances not produced in the urinary tract—can also color the urine; these include fecal material, menstrual blood, and hemorrhoidal blood.

In summary, the color of urine is actually a combination of the colors imparted by each constituent present. To evaluate urine color consistently, the criteria outlined in Box 6-1 are necessary. Without attention to these details and to the use of established terminology, consistent reporting of urine color is not possible.

FOAM

If a normal urine specimen is shaken or agitated sufficiently, a white foam can be forced to develop at its surface that readily dissipates on standing. The characteristics of urine foam, namely, its color, ease of formation, and the amount produced, are modified by the presence of protein and bilirubin.

Moderate to large amounts of protein (albumin) in urine cause a stable white foam to be produced when the urine is poured or agitated (Figure 6-1, *B*). Similar to egg albumin, the foam that develops is thick and long lasting. In addition, a larger volume of foam is easily produced by agitation of this urine compared with urine in which protein is not present.

When bilirubin is present in sufficient amounts, the foam if present will be characteristically yellow (Figure 6-1, *A*). This coloration may be noticed when the urine is being processed and the physical characteristics recorded. Although not definitive, this distinctive yellow coloration of the foam provides preliminary evidence for the presence of bilirubin.

Most substances that intensify or change the color of urine do not alter the color or characteristics of the urine foam. In other words, despite significant changes in urine color, the foam, if forced to form by agitation, remains white and readily dissipates.

Foam characteristics noted in the physical examination are not reported in a routine urinalysis; instead, they

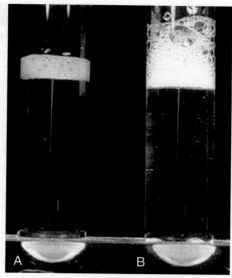

FIGURE 6-1 A, Distinctive coloration of urine foam due to the high bilirubin concentration in the urine specimen. **B,** Large amount of urine foam due to a high concentration of protein, specifically albumin, in the urine specimen.

serve as preliminary and supportive evidence for the presence of bilirubin and abnormal amounts of protein in the urine. These suspected substances must be detected and confirmed during the chemical examination before either substance is reported.

CLARITY

Clarity, along with color, describes the overall visual appearance of a urine specimen. It is assessed at the same time as urine color and refers to the transparency of the specimen. Often called turbidity, **clarity** describes the cloudiness of the urine caused by suspended particulate matter that scatters light. The criteria outlined in Box 6-1 for assessing urine color also apply when evaluating urine clarity. An established list of descriptive terms for clarity used by all laboratory personnel ensures consistency in reporting and eliminates ambiguity. Table 6-3 defines common clarity terminology and provides a list of substances that produce these characteristics.

In health, a freshly voided "clean catch" urine specimen is usually clear. If precautions are not taken, particularly with female patients, to eliminate potential contamination from the skin or from vaginal secretions, a normal specimen can appear cloudy. Likewise, if a specimen is handled improperly after collection, bacterial growth can cause the specimen to become cloudy.

Precipitation of solutes dissolved in urine, most commonly amorphous urates and phosphates, can cause a normal urine specimen to appear cloudy. Amorphous phosphates and carbonates produce a white or beige precipitate and are present only in alkaline urine. In acidic urine, a pinkish precipitate ("brick dust") results from the deposition of uroerythrin on amorphous urate

TABLE 6-3 | Clarity Terms

Term	Definition	Possible Causes
Clear	No (or rare) visible particles; transparent	All solutes present are soluble. *Note:* The possibility of an abnormal solute such as glucose, proteins (albumin, hemoglobin, myoglobin), or bilirubin is not ruled out.
Hazy or Slightly cloudy	Visible particles present; newsprint can be read when viewed through urine tube	Clarity varies with the substance and the amount present: • Blood cells—red blood cells (RBCs), white blood cells (WBCs)
Cloudy	Significant particulate matter; newsprint is blurred or difficult to read when viewed through urine tube	• Crystals of normal or abnormal solutes • Epithelial cells • Fat (lipids, chyle) • Microbes—bacteria, yeast, trichomonads
Turbid	Newsprint cannot be seen when viewed through urine tube	• Mucus, mucin, pus • Radiographic contrast media • Semen, spermatozoa, prostatic fluid • Contaminants: feces, powders, talc, creams, lotions

Modified from Schweitzer SC, Schumann JL, Schumann GB: Quality assurance guidelines for the urinalysis laboratory. J Med Technol 3:11, 1986.

BOX 6-2 | Classification of Substances Causing Urine Turbidity

Pathologic
- RBCs
- WBCs
- Bacteria (fresh urine)
- Yeast
- Trichomonads
- Renal epithelial cells
- Fat (lipids, chyle)
- Abnormal crystals
- Semen, spermatozoa, prostatic fluid*
- Feces (fistula)*
- Calculi
- Pus

Nonpathologic
- Normal solute crystals (e.g., urates, phosphates, calcium oxalate)
- Squamous epithelial cells
- Mucus, mucin
- Radiographic contrast media
- Semen, spermatozoa, prostatic fluid*
- Contaminants: feces,* powders, talc, creams, lotions

*Indicates that substance could be nonpathologic or pathologic, depending on the cause of its presence in the urine.

and uric acid crystals. Indirectly, the color of the precipitate indicates whether a urine pH is acid (pink) or alkaline (white, beige).

On close inspection of the particulate matter in urine, a specific component may be evident. Most often noted are red blood cells and small blood clots. Similarly, the excretion of fat or lymph, although rare, should be suspected in urine that appears opalescent or milky. Urine clarity provides a rapid quality check for the microscopic examination, that is, a cloudy urine specimen should have significant numbers of components present when viewed microscopically.

Substances that cause urine turbidity can be pathologic or nonpathologic (Box 6-2). Principally, those substances considered nonpathologic are contaminants or normal urine components. Spermatozoa and prostatic fluid are considered to be urine contaminants because they are not derived from the urinary tract, rather, they use it as a conveyance. Radiographic contrast media

present in the urine following an x-ray procedure are iatrogenic and are not indicative of disease. The presence of fecal material and many squamous epithelial cells usually indicates improper collection of the urine specimen. Pathologic conditions, however, such as a fistula between the bladder and the colon can also result in the presence of fecal material in urine, which causes a persistent urinary tract infection.

Pathologic substances in urine indicate (1) deterioration of the barrier normally separating the urinary tract from the blood, (2) a disease process, or (3) a metabolic dysfunction. For example, the presence of red blood cells in urine indicates damage to the urinary tract. At times the site of injury can be localized, as with the presence of dysmorphic red blood cells, which are highly indicative of glomerular damage, or with the presence of red blood cells in casts, which indicate glomerular or tubular origin. White blood cells in urine indicate an inflammatory process somewhere in the urinary system. Although bacteria are the most common cause of urinary tract infection, other agents can produce inflammation without bacteriuria (see Chapter 9). In fresh urine, the presence of bacteria, white blood cells, and casts indicates an infection of the upper urinary tract (e.g., renal pelvis, interstitium), whereas the presence of bacteria and white blood cells "without casts" implies a lower urinary tract infection (e.g., bladder, urethra). In contrast, yeast and trichomonads, although agents of infection, commonly originate from a vaginal infection and often are contaminants when present in the urine specimen of a female. Regardless of their origin, these organisms are reported routinely when observed in the microscopic examination of a urine specimen.

In summary, clear urine is not necessarily normal. Abnormal amounts of glucose, protein, lysed red blood cells, or white blood cells can be present in a clear, negative-appearing urine. Note that these components are detectable by a chemical examination. However, a freshly voided cloudy urine requires further investigation to determine the substance causing the turbidity.

ODOR

Historically, urine odor led to the research and discovery of the metabolic disease phenylketonuria. Currently, urine odors, unless remarkably strong or different, are not detected in a routine urinalysis. Because urine contains many organic and inorganic substances (by-products of metabolism), normal urine has a characteristic aromatic odor. This odor is normally faint and unremarkable; however, if normal urine is allowed to stand at room temperature and age, it becomes particularly odorous and ammoniacal because of the conversion of urea to ammonia by bacteria. Normally, urine in the urinary tract is sterile. When it passes out of the body via the urethra, it can easily become contaminated by normal bacterial flora on the skin surface. In an improperly stored urine specimen, these contaminating organisms can proliferate. Because of this, urine odor may indicate that a specimen is old and is not suitable for testing because of the many changes that occur in unpreserved urine (see Chapter 3). However, a patient with a urinary tract infection can produce an ammonia-smelling urine owing to bacterial metabolism that is occurring within the urinary tract. The distinguishing factor is that in the latter case, the urine smells distinctly ammoniacal even when it has been freshly voided. Severe urinary tract infection can cause a strongly pungent or fetid aroma from pus, protein decay, and bacteria. Before proceeding with testing, it is imperative to determine that urines with strong odors are fresh specimens, and that they have been properly stored.

Ingestion of certain foods or drugs can cause urine to have a noticeably different odor. Foods such as asparagus and garlic or intravenous medications containing phenolic derivatives can result in urine with an unusual or distinct aroma. Several metabolic disorders may cause urine to have an unusual odor (Table 6-4). For example, conditions of increased fat metabolism with formation and excretion of aromatic ketone bodies produce a sweet- or fruity-smelling urine. Of these conditions, the most common disorder is diabetes mellitus, in which glucose present in the blood (see Box 6-2) cannot be used, and body fat is metabolized to compensate. Table 6-4 lists numerous amino acid disorders that produce noticeably odd urine odors. Patients with these disorders exhibit clinical signs of metabolic dysfunction, and their diagnoses do not rely on the detection of urine odor (see Chapter 9). Various urine tests play an important role in the differential diagnosis of these metabolic disorders.

On occasion, a urine specimen can smell strongly of bleach or other cleaning agents. Sometimes the agent was added to the urine specimen intentionally (i.e., the

TABLE 6-4	Causes of Urine Odors
Odor	**Cause**
Aromatic, faintly	Normal urine
Ammoniacal	"Old" urine—improperly stored
Pungent, fetid	Urinary tract infection
Sweet, fruity	Ketone production due to: • Diabetes mellitus • Starvation, dieting, malnutrition • Strenuous exercise • Vomiting, diarrhea

Unusual odor:
  Mousy, barny
  Maple syrup
  Rancid
  Rotting/old fish
  Cabbage, hops
  Sweaty feet
  Distinctive
 	
  Menthol-like
	Associated amino acid disorder:
	  Phenylketonuria
	  Maple syrup urine disease
	  Tyrosinemia
	  Trimethylaminuria
	  Methionine malabsorption
	  Isovaleric and glutaric acidemias
	  Ingested substances: asparagus, garlic, onions
	  Phenol-containing medications

Bleach	Adulteration of the specimen or container contamination

specimen was adulterated) to interfere with testing, particularly when a urine specimen was collected for detection of prescription or illicit drugs. However, if a household container is used to collect a specimen, a cleaning agent may be present by accident (i.e., the container was contaminated before collection). Regardless of the cause of contamination, the specimen is not acceptable for urinalysis.

TASTE

Although historically (circa 1674) urine was tasted to detect the presence of urinary sugars, urine is no longer tasted. The terms mellitus, meaning "sweet," and insipidus, meaning "tasteless," were assigned to the disease diabetes because of the taste of the urine produced by these two different diseases. Both disorders produce copious amounts of urine, hence the name diabetes; however, the causes of these disorders are entirely different.

CONCENTRATION

Another physical characteristic of urine is concentration, that is, the quantity of solutes present in the volume of water excreted. As discussed in Chapter 5, urine is normally 94% water and 6% solutes; the amount and type of solutes excreted vary with the patient's diet, physical activity, and health. A dilute urine has fewer solute particles present per volume of water, whereas a concentrated urine has more solute particles present per volume of water. As was previously mentioned, color provides a crude indicator of urine concentration. Dilute urine contains fewer of the solutes that impart color and therefore is light yellow or even colorless. Similarly, a concentrated normal urine is dark yellow because of an increase in pigmented solutes without a corresponding increase in the water volume of the urine.

Urine concentration in the clinical laboratory most often is expressed as specific gravity or osmolality. As was discussed in Chapter 5, these expressions of solute composition are similar and yet different. In a healthy individual, good correlation is maintained between urine specific gravity and urine osmolality; however, with disease, this relationship may not exist (see Figure 5-1). In addition, methods available for determining specific gravity and osmolality differ with respect to instrumentation, complexity, and the time required to perform the determination. As a result, specific gravity is used most often to rapidly assess urine concentration, whereas osmolality is used when more accurate and specific information is required.

Specific Gravity

Specific gravity (SG) is an expression of urine concentration in terms of **density** (i.e., the mass of solutes present per volume of solution). It is a ratio of urine density to the density of an equal volume of pure water under specific conditions. As a density measurement, the number of solutes in the urine, as well as their molecular size, affects SG. Equation 6-1 shows that as the density of urine approaches the density of pure water, the specific gravity approaches unity (1.000).

Equation 6-1

$$SG = \frac{\text{Density of urine}}{\text{Density of equal volume of pure water}}$$

The greater the urine density, the larger the specific gravity value. It is physiologically impossible for the body to excrete pure water (1.000), and the lowest urine specific gravity obtainable is approximately 1.002. Conversely, the maximum specific gravity that urine can attain is a value equal to that of the hyperosmotic renal medulla, which is approximately 1.040.

Urine specific gravity methods can be categorized as direct or indirect measurements of urine density. This distinction is important because the molecular size of solutes does not affect indirect SG measurements to the same degree as direct methods. Methods include urinometry and harmonic oscillation densitometry, which now are only of historical interest. Today in the clinical laboratory, indirect specific gravity measurements such as refractometry and the reagent strip chemical method are used.

Direct specific gravity methods determine the actual or true density of urine, regardless of the solutes present. In other words, all solutes are detected and measured, including those that are always in urine such as urea and electrolytes, as well as those that can be present as the result of disease (glucose, protein) or for iatrogenic

reasons (radiographic media). Note that the presence of the latter high-molecular-weight solutes does not reflect renal concentrating ability. These solutes are present because of other abnormal processes unrelated to concentrating ability. Historically, when direct specific gravity methods were used, the presence of glucose and protein was identified, and when present, corrections were made to eliminate their contributions to the specific gravity measurement. In contrast, radiographic contrast media cannot be corrected for, and after a suitable time that allows for complete elimination of the imaging agent, a new urine specimen should be obtained. Note that if high-molecular-weight solutes are not recognized as present when direct and some indirect (refractometry) SG methods are used, erroneous conclusions regarding renal concentrating ability may be made.

Temperature affects density. Therefore when historical *direct* specific gravity methods were used, urine temperature was controlled during measurement (harmonic oscillation densitometry), or a correction factor was used when urine temperature deviated from a predetermined value (urinometry).

Urinometry. The urinometer, also known as a hydrometer (Figure 6-2), is no longer considered an accurate device for determination of urine specific gravity.[4] The urinometer is a weighted glass float with a long, narrow, calibrated stem. When placed in pure (distilled or deionized) water at a specific temperature, the urinometer sinks, displacing a volume of water equal to its weight. The meniscus of the water intersects the calibrated stem

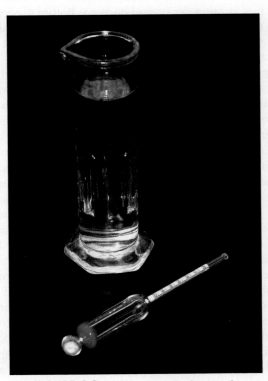

FIGURE 6-2 A urinometer (hydrometer).

of the urinometer at the value 1.000. When placed in a solution of greater density than water (i.e., solutes are present), the urinometer displaces a smaller volume of liquid (it does not sink as deep), and the specific gravity read off the calibrated stem is greater than 1.000.

Many disadvantages are associated with using a urinometer, in particular, (1) a large volume (10 to 15 mL) of urine is required, (2) the urinometer must be calibrated daily, (3) temperature corrections are needed for specimens with temperature differences greater than 3° C from the calibrated temperature, and (4) corrections are required when glucose or protein is present. For each gram per deciliter (g/dL) of protein present, the specific gravity is increased by 0.003; for each gram per deciliter (g/dL) of glucose, the specific gravity is increased by 0.004. A urinometer can be cumbersome and temperamental. For example, inaccurate readings are obtained when the float touches the sides of the container, or when wetting of the calibrated stem above the water line is excessive.

Harmonic Oscillation Densitometry. Harmonic oscillation densitometry (HOD) is rarely used today despite its ability to accurately and precisely determine urine specific gravity with linearity up to 1.080. This method was initially used on a semiautomated urinalysis workstation known as the Yellow IRIS (IRIS Diagnostics Division, Chatsworth, CA). HOD is a direct SG method that uses sound waves to measure urine density. During testing, a portion of the urine sample is held in a U-shaped glass tube that has an electromagnetic coil on one end and a motion detector on the other end. An electrical current applied to the coil generates a sound wave of fixed frequency. This sonic oscillation is transmitted through the specimen, and the frequency attenuation is measured. The frequency (the oscillating cycle period) observed is directly proportionate to the sample density, and a microprocessor converts the frequency to a corresponding specific gravity value. Because temperature affects density, a thermistor monitors the sample temperature in the tube and provides this information to the microprocessor for correction, when necessary.

Refractometry. Refractometry, an indirect measure of specific gravity, is based on the refractive index of light. When light passes from air into a solution at an angle, the direction of the light beam is refracted and its speed is decreased (Figure 6-3). The ratio of light refraction in the two differing media is called the **refractive index.** The refractive index (n) of the solution can be expressed mathematically using the velocity of the incident and refracted light beams or their respective angles as follows.

Equation 6-2

$$\frac{n_2}{n_1} = \frac{V_1}{V_2} \quad or \quad \frac{n_2}{n_1} = \frac{\sin\theta_1}{\sin\theta_2}$$

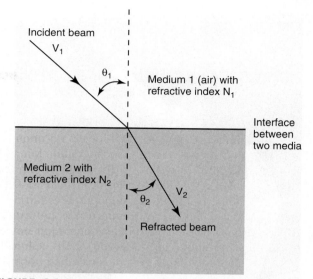

FIGURE 6-3 A schematic diagram illustrates the refraction (or bending) of light as it passes from one medium to another of differing density. The velocity of the light beam also changes.

In Equation 6-2, n_1 is the refractive index of air, which by convention equals 1.0; n_2 is the refractive index of the solution being measured; V_1 is the velocity of light in air; V_2 is the velocity of light in the solution; $\sin\theta_1$ is the angle of the incident beam of light; and $\sin\theta_2$ is the angle of the refracted beam of light. Although the velocity or the angles of refraction can be used to determine the refractive index, measurement of angles is the principle routinely used by refractometers.

Three factors affect the refractive index of a solution: (1) the wavelength of light used, (2) the temperature of the solution, and (3) the concentration of the solution. The temperature and the concentration of a solution affect its refractive index because they produce changes in the density of the solution. This direct relationship to solution density allows use of the refractive index to measure specific gravity. Stated another way, as the temperature changes or the quantity of solutes in a solution changes, so does its density, hence, the refractive index changes. Refractometry measures all the solutes in a solution, including any glucose and protein present.

Routinely, white light provides the radiant light beam used in refractometers. Isolation of a monochromatic light beam from polychromatic white light is managed by the design of the refractometer. Within the refractometer, a prism, a liquid compensator, and the chamber cover work together to direct a single wavelength of light onto the calibrated scale. Refractive index measurements can differ depending on the wavelength used. Refractometers using a wavelength of 589 nm are most common. Figure 6-4 shows a manual refractometer widely used in the clinical laboratory.

The calibration of a refractometer is checked daily, or whenever it is in use. Calibration assessment is easy and

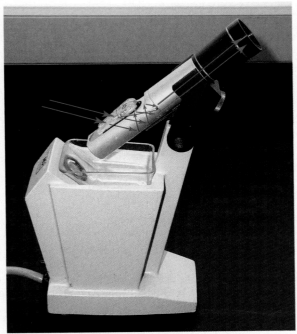

FIGURE 6-4 A refractometer with the pathway of light superimposed.

TABLE 6-5	Calibration Solutions for Refractometry
SG	**Solution**
1.000	Water, distilled
1.015	NaCl, 0.513 mol/L (3% w/v)
1.022	NaCl, 0.856 mol/L (5% w/v)
1.034	Sucrose, 0.263 mol/L (9% w/v)

involves determining the SG of distilled water, which has an SG of 1.000. After the SG of distilled water is confirmed, one or two additional solutions are analyzed to ensure calibration across the range of possible urine SG values (Table 6-5). SG calibrators are typically sodium chloride or sucrose solutions of known concentration; they are available commercially or can be prepared by the laboratory. In addition, urine controls at low, medium, and high SG values should be routinely analyzed and results recorded. Should the refractometer require calibration adjustment, a set-screw is available on the body of the instrument. However, before any adjustments are made, the glass surface and the coverplate of the refractometer should be thoroughly cleaned and all calibration solutions rechecked.

Use of refractometry to measure urine specific gravity has several advantages, most notably the small sample required and the ability to automatically make temperature compensations for specimens between 15° C and 38° C. One to two drops of urine placed between the coverplate and the prism cover glass rapidly equilibrate in temperature with the instrument. Within the refractometer is a liquid reservoir with a refractive index that varies with temperature. As the refracted light beam from the sample passes through this reservoir, the light beam is corrected to the value that would be obtained at a temperature of 20° C. The refracted light beam makes several passes through the measuring prism before the lens focuses it onto the calibrated scale. In the viewing field, a distinct edge between light and dark areas is evident. This boundary is the point at which the specific gravity value is read from the scale (Figure 6-5). The scale is calibrated for urine testing at the factory. Similarly, refractometers are available that have a second calibrated scale in the viewing field for determination of serum or plasma protein concentration based on the refractive index.

In summary, refractometry compares the velocity or angle of refraction of light in a solution versus that of light in air. In a solution, as the number of solutes increases, the velocity of light decreases and the angle of light refraction decreases. Refractometers automatically compensate for temperatures ranging from 15° C to 38° C; they are calibrated for urine specific gravity and serum protein determinations, and they require a small sample volume. As with direct specific gravity measurements, refractometer results are increased by the presence of high molecular weight solutes such as glucose, protein, mannitol, or radiographic media. By refractometry, for each gram per deciliter (g/dL) of protein present, the specific gravity is increased by 0.003; whereas for each gram per deciliter (g/dL) of glucose, the specific gravity is increased by 0.002.[5] Radiographic contrast media in urine can cause very high SG results that are physiologically impossible (e.g., 1.050 or higher). Currently, clinical laboratories rarely make corrections to urine refractometer results when protein and glucose are present.

Reagent Strip Method. The reagent strip SG method is an indirect colorimetric estimation of urine density based on the quantity of ionic or charged solutes (Na^+, Cl^-, K^+, NH_4^+) present. Note that nonionic solutes are not measured. Hence this method can be referred to as **ionic specific gravity** (SG_{ionic}). In health, the ability of the kidneys to selectively reabsorb and secrete ionic solutes and water determines the concentration (density) of the urine excreted. Excretion of nonionic solutes such as urea, glucose, protein, or radiographic media does not reflect the status of this renal function. Glucose in urine usually indicates a metabolic disorder (diabetes mellitus), whereas protein often indicates a renal condition such as a change in the glomerular filtration barrier (glomerulonephritis, nephrotic syndrome). No other SG method is able to eliminate the effects of nonionic large-molecular-weight solutes on SG results. Therefore, reagent strip SG

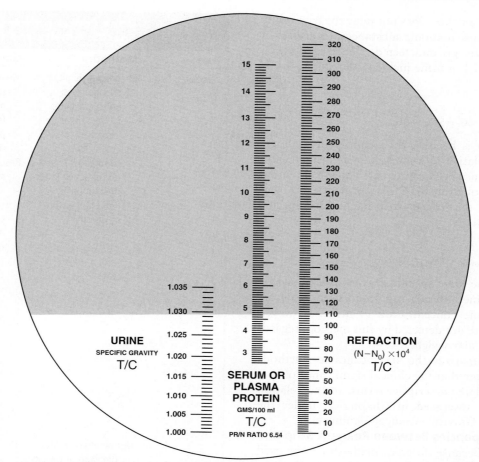

FIGURE 6-5 A schematic representation of the viewing field and scale in the refractometer. (*Courtesy Leica, Inc., Buffalo, NY. Reprinted with permission.*)

results are uniquely valuable in assessing the ability of the kidneys to handle water and ionic solutes when glucose or protein is also present in the urine. In summary, although reagent strip SG results may not indicate the true density of urine when nonionic solutes are present, they do reflect the renal concentrating ability to selectively handle ionic solutes and water. Note however that reagent strip SG measurements are affected by urine pH with the most accurate results obtained when the urine pH is 7.0-7.5.[5] Acid urine causes falsely increased SG results; whereas more alkaline urine causes falsely decreased results. When reagent strips are read by a reagent strip reader, the SG reading is automatically corrected by the instrument.

This chemical SG method consists of a reagent test pad adhered to an inert plastic strip. The test pad is impregnated with a polyelectrolyte, a pH indicator, and is maintained at an alkaline pH. When the strip is immersed in urine, the pK_a (which is the negative

logarithm of the ionization constant of an acid) of the polyelectrolyte decreases proportionately to the ionic concentration of the specimen. As the pH of the test pad decreases, the bromthymol blue indicator changes color from dark blue-green (SG_{ionic} 1.000) to yellow-green (SG_{ionic} 1.030). Stated another way, as the number of ions present in the urine is increased, more protons are released from the polyelectrolyte, resulting in a decrease in the test pad pH and a change in the indicator.

Equation 6-3

$$
\begin{array}{c}
\overset{\diagup\diagdown\diagup\diagdown}{\underset{\substack{\text{O O O}\\ \text{O O O}\\ \text{H H H}}}{\text{C C C}}}
\quad + \quad
\overset{\overline{}\;\overline{}\;\overline{}}{\underset{\substack{+ \; + \; + \; +\\ \text{(urine ions)}}}{}}
\quad \rightarrow \quad
\overset{\diagup\diagdown\diagup\diagdown}{\underset{\substack{\text{O O O}\\ \text{O}^-\ \text{O}\ \text{O}^-\\ \text{H}}}{\text{C C C}}}
\quad + \quad H^+
\end{array}
$$

This indirect SG method does not relay the true solute concentration because nonionic substances, regardless of their molecular size, go undetected. The true or total specific gravity (SG_T) of urine includes all solutes—ionic and nonionic.

Equation 6-4

$$SG_T = SG_{ionic} + SG_{nonionic}$$

When a person is healthy, the quantity of nonionic solutes in urine relative to ionic solutes is insignificant. As a result, the ionic specific gravity is equal to the total specific gravity (Equation 6-5). This provides the basis for the efficacy of the reagent strip method for specific gravity determinations.

Equation 6-5

$$\text{If } SG_{nonionic} <<< SG_{ionic}, \text{ then } SG_T = SG_{ionic}$$

In summary, the ionic specific gravity determined by the reagent strip method is a rapid and useful tool for evaluating the ionic concentration of urine. However, nonionic solutes are not detected by this method, regardless of their molecular weight.

Table 6-6 summarizes the specific gravity methods discussed here. Note that the clinical significance of specific gravity, associated descriptive terms, and correlation with disease, are discussed in Chapter 7, under the heading "Specific Gravity—Clinical Significance."

SG Result Discrepancies Between Reagent Strip and Refractometry. Because different methods can be used to determine specific gravity, it is imperative that the limitations of each method are known to ensure proper interpretation of results. Similarly, the range of SG values that are physiologically possible must be recognized (i.e., 1.002 to 1.040). When urine produces an abnormally high SG value (>1.040) by refractometry but a normal SG result by reagent strip, radiographic contrast media or another large-molecular-weight solute (e.g., mannitol) should be suspected. Note that the kidneys cannot produce urine with an SG greater than 1.040. A discrepancy (i.e., a difference greater than 0.005) between these SG methods alerts the laboratorian to the presence of a solute that is detected by refractometry but is not ionic, and hence is not detected by the reagent strip method. In these cases, the reagent strip method provides a more accurate assessment of the ability of the kidney to concentrate the urine.

As has been discussed, the presence of large quantities of glucose or protein can falsely increase the SG result by refractometry, whereas the reagent strip SG result is not affected.

Osmolality

As was described in Chapter 5, osmolality is the concentration of a solution expressed in terms of osmoles of solute particles per kilogram of water. An *osmole* is defined as the amount of a substance that dissociates to produce 1 mole of particles in a solution. For example, glucose in a solution does not dissociate; therefore 1 mole of glucose equals 1 mole of particles, or 1 osmole. In contrast, sodium chloride (NaCl) dissociates into two particles: Na^+ ions and Cl^- ions, hence 1 mole of NaCl produces 2 osmoles of particles in solution. Molecular weight does not play a role in osmolality. Despite the

TABLE 6-6	Urine Concentration Assessment: Specific Gravity and Osmolality	
Test	**Method**	**Limitations**
Specific gravity	Reagent strip: pK_a change of an polyelectrolyte; indirect measure of density	Measures only ionic (charged) solutes; nonionic solutes (e.g., glucose, protein) are not detected
	Refractometry: based on refractive index of solution; indirect measure of density	Results affected by molecular size and structure; large solutes (e.g., protein, glucose, mannitol, radiographic contrast media) contribute more to value than small solutes (e.g., sodium, chloride); correction calculation can be performed when high concentrations of protein and glucose are present, but they are rarely done
	Urinometry—a direct measure of density	Historical; unacceptable accuracy for urine measurements[4]
	Harmonic oscillation densitometry—a direct measure of density	No limitations—very accurate and precise; no longer available on urinalysis analyzers
Osmolality	Freezing point depression	No limitations; all solutes contribute equally to result obtained; time-consuming compared with SG methods
	Vapor pressure depression	Does not detect volatile solutes (e.g., ethanol, methanol, ethylene glycol); time-consuming compared with SG methods

relatively large molecular weight of glucose (MW 180), when sodium chloride (MW 58) is present in an equal molar amount, an osmolality approximately double that of glucose is produced.

Because the osmolality of biological fluids such as urine and serum is very low, the *milliosmole* (mOsm) is the unit of choice. Osmolality (mOsm *per kilogram of* H_2O) is considered more precise than its counterpart, osmolarity (mOsm *per liter of solution*) because osmolality does not vary with temperature. In contrast, because the volume of a solution varies with temperature, so does its osmolarity. In urine, the solvent is water and the solutes are those that pass the glomerular filtration barrier and are not reabsorbed by the tubules, plus additional substances secreted by the tubules into the ultrafiltrate as it passes through the nephrons.

Normal serum osmolality values range from 275 to 300 mOsm/kg, whereas urine osmolality values are one to three times greater at 275 to 900 mOsm/kg. The kidneys excrete unwanted solutes in the volume of water that the body does not need. As a result, urine osmolality can vary greatly, depending on diet, fluid intake, health, and physical activity, whereas serum osmolality remains relatively constant.

Osmolality measurements are used principally (1) to evaluate the renal concentrating ability of the kidneys, (2) to monitor renal disease, (3) to monitor fluid and electrolyte balance, and (4) to differentially diagnose the cause of polyuria. For a discussion of osmolality and specific gravity measurements in the evaluation of renal function, see "Assessment of Renal Concentrating Ability/Tubular Reabsorptive Function" in Chapter 5.

Osmolality is determined by measuring a **colligative property** of the sample. Colligative properties of a solution depend only on the number of solute particles present. Particle size and ionic charge have no effect; only the number of particles present as ions or as undissociated molecules in the solution affects colligative properties. The four colligative properties are (1) depression of freezing point, (2) depression of vapor pressure, (3) elevation in osmotic pressure, and (4) elevation of boiling point. These properties are interrelated, and the value of one can be used to calculate each of the others. In the clinical laboratory, freezing point depression osmometry predominates for several reasons. This method can be used to detect the presence of volatile solutes (e.g., ethanol, methanol, ethylene glycol), and results are accurate even with lipemic serum samples.[6]

Freezing Point Osmometry. A contemporary **freezing point osmometer** consists of four principal components: (1) a mechanism to supercool the sample slowly to about −7° C, (2) a thermistor to monitor the temperature of the sample, (3) a means to initiate freezing (or "seeding") of the sample, and (4) a direct readout display.

The specimen, urine or serum, in a sample chamber is placed into the osmometer. The instrument begins the cooling sequence depicted in Figure 6-6. The initial

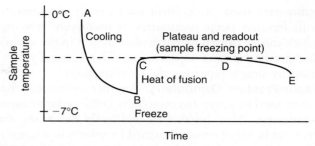

FIGURE 6-6 A time-temperature curve during freezing point depression osmometry.

supercooling process (segment AB, Figure 6-6) proceeds slowly to prevent premature freezing of the sample. As the sample temperature approaches −7° C, freezing of the sample is induced ("seeded") by the instrument (point B). As ice crystals form, the heat of fusion released to the sample (segment BC) is detected by a thermistor. The sample temperature increases until an equilibrium between the solid (ice) and liquid phases is reached, which by definition is the freezing point (segment CD). This temperature plateau is maintained for approximately 1 minute or longer before it again decreases (segment DE). Using the freezing point obtained, the instrument calculates and then displays the osmolality of the sample using the proportionality formula given in Equation 6-6.

Equation 6-6

$$\frac{1000\,\text{mOsm particles}}{-1.86°\,\text{C}} = \frac{x\,\text{mOsm particles}}{measured\,\text{freezing point of sample}}$$

Measurement of freezing point depression is based on the fact that pure water freezes at 0° C, and that adding 1 mole (1000 mOsm) of solute particles to 1 kg pure water causes the freezing point to decrease by 1.86° C. This relationship is constant and enables the use of a simple proportionality formula. For example, assume that the thermistor probe measures the freezing point of a urine specimen as −1.20° C. By inserting this value into the equation and solving for x, the osmolality of the urine sample is found to be 645.2 mOsm/kg. To achieve the precision of ±2 mOsm/kg, as is seen with freezing point osmometers, accurate temperature measurements are crucial. The thermistor obtains these temperature measurements accurately and rapidly.

For osmolality results to be read directly from the instrument readout, the microprocessor of the osmometer must be calibrated using sodium chloride standard solutions of known osmolality. These sodium chloride solutions are available commercially in concentrations ranging from 50 to 1500 mOsm or are prepared by the laboratory. Following calibration, the osmometer measures the freezing point, converts it to the corresponding osmolality value, and displays it on the direct readout.

The sample size necessary for osmolality determinations varies from 20 µL to 2.0 mL, depending on the osmometer used. A problem occasionally encountered with freezing point osmometry is premature freezing, which can be caused by particulate matter in the sample that prevents proper supercooling. This is usually overcome by simply repeating the determination.

Vapor Pressure Osmometry. Another instrument that can be used to determine osmolality is the **vapor pressure osmometer**. This instrument indirectly measures the decrease in vapor pressure caused by solutes in a sample. The smaller sample size (7 mL) is advantageous; however, because of its inability to detect volatile solutes, vapor pressure osmometers are usually not used in clinical laboratories.

In conclusion, osmolality and specific gravity are expressions of urine concentration. Heavy molecules such as glucose, protein, and radiographic media significantly affect specific gravity measurements but do not affect osmolality measurements because the amount of these substances is insignificant compared with the total number of other solutes present. Because all solutes contribute equally to osmolality, regardless of their molecular size, osmolality is considered a better and more accurate assessment of solute concentration in serum and urine. Table 6-6 gives a summary of each of the methods discussed in the evaluation of urine concentration.

VOLUME

Although the amount or volume of urine excreted per day is a physical characteristic of urine, urine samples are not routinely assessed for volume alone. Normally, urine volume varies from 600 to 1800 mL/day, with less than 400 mL excreted at night. When an individual excretes more than 500 mL of urine at night, the condition is termed *nocturia* and is a feature associated with chronic progressive renal failure. In chronic renal failure, the kidneys lose their ability to concentrate urine. Consequently, the specific gravity of the urine excreted is unchanged and is the same as that of the initial plasma ultrafiltrate, namely, 1.010. The term *isosthenuria* is used to describe this inability of the kidneys to alter the specific gravity of the ultrafiltrate as it passes through the nephrons (i.e., the ultrafiltrate remains isosmotic with plasma).

A person's diet, health, and exercise directly affect daily urine volume. The kidneys maintain a balance between fluid intake and excretion; however, their control is one-sided. Any excess fluid ingested but not needed can be excreted as urine, but the kidneys have a limited ability to compensate for lack of adequate fluid intake. As the quantity of metabolic solutes that need elimination from the body increases, so does the volume of water required to excrete them. If the body lacks adequate hydration, these solutes accumulate in the body despite the best efforts of the kidneys to eliminate them.

Polyuria is the excretion of 3 L or more of urine each day (>3 L/day). Any increase in urine excretion is termed

TABLE 6-7	Urine Volume Terms, Definitions, and Clinical Correlations	
Term	**Definition**	**Clinical Correlations**
Diuresis	Increased urine excretion (>1800 mL/day)	Solute excretion • Diabetes mellitus—glucose • Drugs—diuretic therapy, caffeine, alcohol • Renal disease Water excretion • Excessive fluid intake—IV administration, compulsive water intake • Diabetes insipidus—ability to retain water is lost • Renal disease • Drugs—lithium
Polyuria	Urine exceeds 3 L/day	Same as *Diuresis*
Oliguria	Urine excretion less than 400 mL/day	Decreased renal blood flow • Dehydration, water deprivation • Shock, hypotension Renal disease • Urinary tract obstruction • Renal tubular dysfunction • End-stage renal disease • Nephrotic syndrome Edema
Anuria	No urine excreted	Acute renal failure • Ischemic causes—shock, heart failure • Nephrotoxic causes—drugs, toxic agents Urinary tract obstruction Hemolytic transfusion reactions

diuresis and can be due to excessive water intake (polydipsia), diuretic therapy, hormonal imbalance, renal dysfunction, or drug ingestion (e.g., alcohol, caffeine). Table 6-7 summarizes conditions of water and solute diuresis that result in polyuria.

Oliguria is a decrease in urine excretion (<400 mL/ day) that can be caused by simple water deprivation, excessive sweating, diarrhea, or vomiting. Any condition that decreases the blood supply to the kidneys can cause oliguria and eventually anuria if not corrected. Oliguric urines have an elevated specific gravity (≈1.030) because the kidneys maximally excrete solutes into the decreased water available. When plasma protein is lost and water shifts from the intravascular to the extravascular compartment, as in conditions of edema, oliguria can result. Oliguria also develops with various renal diseases, ranging from urinary tract obstruction to end-stage renal disease.

Anuria is the complete lack of urine excretion. Anuria is fatal if not immediately addressed because of the accumulation of toxic metabolic by-products in the body. Any condition or disease, chronic or acute, that destroys functioning renal tissue can result in anuria. Principal among these are conditions that decrease the blood supply to renal tissue, such as hypotension, hemorrhage, shock, and heart failure. Toxic chemicals and nephrotoxic antibiotics can induce acute tubular necrosis, leading to loss of functional renal tissue and anuria (or oliguria). In addition, hemolytic transfusion reactions and urinary tract obstructions can result in anuria.

In conclusion, urine volume measurements are not performed routinely. Although this information can serve as a valuable diagnostic aid, urine volume is usually determined with a timed urine collection and is used to calculate the concentration of specific urine solutes, or to assess renal function (e.g., the glomerular filtration rate). Chapter 5 discusses renal function and its effect on urine volume. The terms *polyuria, oliguria,* and *anuria* are usually assigned on the basis of a patient's health history and clinical observation and are not based on timed urine collections. Table 6-7 outlines these urine volume terms, their definitions, and their causes.

STUDY QUESTIONS

1. The color of normal urine is due to the pigment
   A. bilirubin
   B. urobilin
   C. uroerythrin
   D. urochrome

2. A single substance can impart different colors to urine depending on the
   1. amount of the substance present.
   2. storage conditions of the urine.
   3. pH of the urine.
   4. structural form of the substance.
   A. 1, 2, and 3 are correct.
   B. 1 and 3 are correct.
   C. 4 is correct.
   D. All are correct.

3. Which of the following urine characteristics provides the best rough indicator of urine concentration and body hydration?
   A. Color
   B. Clarity
   C. Foam
   D. Volume

4. Which of the following pigments deposits on urate and uric acid crystals to form a precipitate described as "brick dust"?
   A. Bilirubin
   B. Urobilin
   C. Uroerythrin
   D. Urochrome

5. Match the colors to the urine pigment/substance. Note that more than one color can be selected for a pigment/substance.

Urine Pigment/Substance	Color of Pigment/Substance
___ A. Bilirubin	1. Colorless
___ B. Biliverdin	2. Yellow
___ C. Hemoglobin	3. Orange
___ D. Myoglobin	4. Red
___ E. Porphobilinogen	5. Pink
___ F. Urobilin	6. Purple
___ G. Urobilinogen	7. Brown
___ H. Urochrome	8. Green
___ I. Uroerythrin	

6. Which of the following criteria should one use to consistently evaluate urine color and clarity?
   1. Mix all specimens well.
   2. Use the same depth or volume of a specimen.
   3. Evaluate the specimens at the same temperature.
   4. View the specimens against a dark background with good lighting.
   A. 1, 2, and 3 are correct.
   B. 1 and 3 are correct.
   C. 4 is correct.
   D. All are correct.

7. Select the urine specimen that does not indicate the possible presence of blood or hemoglobin.
   A. Clear, red urine
   B. Cloudy, brown urine
   C. Clear, brown urine
   D. Cloudy, amber urine

8. A urine that produces a large amount of white foam when mixed should be suspected to contain increased amounts of
   A. bilirubin.
   B. protein.
   C. urobilin.
   D. urobilinogen.

9. Which of the following substances can change the color of a urine and its foam?
   A. Bilirubin
   B. Hemoglobin
   C. Myoglobin
   D. Urobilin

10. The clarity of a well-mixed urine specimen that has visible particulate matter and through which news print can be seen but not read should be described as
   A. cloudy.
   B. flocculated.
   C. slightly cloudy.
   D. turbid.

11. Classify each substance that can be present in urine as indicating a (1) pathologic or (2) nonpathologic condition.
    __ A. Bacteria (fresh urine)
    __ B. Bacteria (old urine)
    __ C. Fat
    __ D. Powder
    __ E. Radiographic contrast media
    __ F. Red blood cells
    __ G. Renal epithelial cells
    __ H. Spermatozoa
    __ I. Squamous epithelial cells
    __ J. Urate crystals
    __ K. White blood cells
    __ L. Yeast

12. Which of the following urine specimens is considered normal?
    A. A freshly voided urine that is brown and clear
    B. A freshly voided urine that is yellow and cloudy
    C. A clear yellow urine specimen that changes color upon standing
    D. A clear yellow urine specimen that becomes cloudy upon refrigeration

13. A white or beige precipitate in a "normal" alkaline urine most likely is caused by
    A. amorphous phosphates.
    B. amorphous urates.
    C. uric acid crystals.
    D. radiographic contrast media.

14. Match the urine odor to the condition or substance that can cause it. You may select more than one odor for a condition.

Condition/Substance	Urine Odor
__ A. Diabetes mellitus	1. Ammonia-like
__ B. Normal urine	2. Bleach
__ C. Old, improperly stored urine	3. Faintly aromatic
__ D. Specimen adulteration	4. Pungent, fetid
__ E. Starvation	5. Sweet, fruity
__ F. Urinary tract infection	

15. Which of the following methods used to determine the specific gravity of urine does not detect the presence of urine protein or glucose?
    A. Harmonic oscillation densitometry
    B. Reagent strip
    C. Refractometry
    D. Urinometry

16. A small ion and a large uncharged molecule have the same effect when urine concentration is determined by
    A. urinometry.
    B. osmolality.
    C. reagent strip.
    D. refractometry.

17. Which of the following specific gravity values is physiologically impossible?
    A. 1.000
    B. 1.010
    C. 1.020
    D. 1.030

18. Match the principle to the appropriate specific gravity method. A principle can be used more than once.

Specific Gravity Method	Principle of Method
__ A. Harmonic oscillation densitometry	1. Density
__ B. Reagent strip	2. Refractive index
__ C. Refractometry	3. pK_a changes
__ D. Urinometry	

19. Which of the following methods is an indirect measure of specific gravity?
    1. Reagent strip
    2. Urinometry
    3. Refractometry
    4. Harmonic oscillation densitometry
    A. 1, 2, and 3 are correct.
    B. 1 and 3 are correct.
    C. 4 is correct.
    D. All are correct.

20. The refractive index of a solution is affected by the
    1. wavelength of light used.
    2. size and number of the solutes present.
    3. concentration of the solution.
    4. temperature of the solution.
    A. 1, 2, and 3 are correct.
    B. 1 and 3 are correct.
    C. 4 is correct.
    D. All are correct.

21. Refractometry is preferred for specific gravity measurements because it
    1. uses a small amount of sample.
    2. is fast and easy to perform.
    3. automatically compensates for temperature.
    4. measures only ionic solutes.
    A. 1, 2, and 3 are correct.
    B. 1 and 3 are correct.
    C. 4 is correct.
    D. All are correct.

22. The principle of the reagent strip method for measuring specific gravity is based on
    A. the pK_a of a polyelectrolyte decreasing in proportion to the ionic concentration of the specimen.
    B. the pH of a polyelectrolyte decreasing in proportion to the ionic concentration of the specimen.
    C. the pK_a of a polyelectrolyte increasing in proportion to the ionic concentration of the specimen.
    D. the pH of a polyelectrolyte increasing in proportion to the ionic concentration of the specimen.

23. Ionic specific gravity (SG_{ionic}) measurements obtained using reagent strips provide useful clinical information because
   A. all of the urinary solutes present are measured.
   B. the quantity of nonionic solutes in urine relative to ionic solutes is significant.
   C. excretion of nonionic solutes (e.g., urea, glucose, protein) does not reflect renal dysfunction.
   D. the ability of the kidneys to concentrate urine is reflected in the reabsorption and secretion of ionic solutes.

24. Which of the following as described is not a colligative property?
   A. Boiling point elevation
   B. Freezing point depression
   C. Osmotic pressure depression
   D. Vapor pressure depression

25. An advantage of freezing point osmometry over vapor pressure osmometry is its
   A. increased turnaround time.
   B. use of a smaller volume of sample.
   C. ability to detect volatile substances.
   D. decreased interference from plasma lipids.

26. Osmolality measurements are considered to be a more accurate assessment of solute concentration in body fluids than are specific gravity measurements because
   A. all solutes contribute equally.
   B. heavy molecules do not interfere.
   C. they are not temperature dependent.
   D. they are less time-consuming to perform.

27. The freezing point of a urine specimen is determined to be $-0.90°$ C. What is the osmolality of the specimen?
   A. 161 mOsm/kg
   B. 484 mOsm/kg
   C. 597 mOsm/kg
   D. 645 mOsm/kg

28. Which of the following will not influence the volume of urine produced?
   A. Diarrhea
   B. Exercise
   C. Caffeine ingestion
   D. Carbohydrate ingestion

CASE 6-1

A routine urinalysis on a urine specimen collected from a hospitalized patient revealed a specific gravity greater than 1.050 with the use of refractometry.

1. The best explanation for this specific gravity result is that the urine specimen
   A. is old and has deteriorated.
   B. contains radiographic contrast media.
   C. is concentrated because the patient is ill and dehydrated.
   D. contains abnormally high levels of sodium and other electrolytes because the patient is taking diuretics.

2. Which of the following actions should be taken?
   A. Report the urinalysis results; no further action is needed.
   B. Report the urinalysis results and suggest that the patient be instructed to increase fluid intake.
   C. Contact the patient care unit to determine whether the patient is taking a diuretic; if so, report the urinalysis results.
   D. Do not report the urinalysis results; request that a urine specimen be recollected after several hours.

CASE 6-2

A prenatal examination including a routine urinalysis is performed on a 28-year-old female. Her physical examination is unremarkable. When asked about her health, she states that it is generally good, except for several urinary tract infections in the past. In fact, she thinks she might be getting one now and has been taking an over-the-counter product that lessens her discomfort. The following urinalysis results are obtained:

   Color: bright orange (like soda pop)
   Clarity: clear

1. Which of the following statements best explains the orange color of the urine?
   A. She has a liver disorder and bilirubin is present in the urine.
   B. The urine is concentrated, which can be confirmed by the urine specific gravity.
   C. She has recently eaten fresh beets and is genetically disposed to produce this abnormally colored urine.
   D. The over-the-counter product contains phenazopyridine, which imparts this characteristic color to urine.

2. The urine specimen was placed in a refrigerator while the laboratory determined whether the physician wanted a microscopic examination performed (i.e., the request slip was not appropriately completed). When the specimen was later removed to prepare an aliquot for microscopic analysis, the specimen was still orange but was now cloudy. Which of the following statements best explains this increase in urine turbidity?
   A. The delay in analysis has allowed bacteria to proliferate.
   B. Squamous epithelial cells in the urine have degenerated.
   C. Because of the temperature change, normal urine solutes have precipitated.
   D. The specimen was contaminated with vaginal fluids, and yeast has propagated.

REFERENCES

1. Drabkin DL: The normal pigment of urine: the relationship of urinary pigment output to diet and metabolism. J Biol Chem 75:443–479, 1927.
2. deWardner HE: The kidney, ed 5, New York, 1985, Churchill Livingstone.
3. Schweitzer SC, Schumann JL, Schumann GB: Quality assurance guidelines for the urinalysis laboratory. J Med Technol 3:569, 1986.
4. Clinical and Laboratory Standards Institute (CLSI): Urinalysis and collection, transportation, and preservation of urine specimens; approved guideline, ed 2, NCCLS document GP-16-A2, Wayne, PA, 2001, CLSI.
5. Chadha V, Garg U, Alon U: Measurement of urinary concentration: a critical appraisal of methodologies, Pediatr Nephrol 16:374–382, 2001.
6. Tietz NW, Pruden EL, Siggaard-Andersen O: Electrolytes, blood gases, and acid-base balance. In Tietz NW, editor: Fundamentals of clinical chemistry, ed 3, Philadelphia, 1987, WB Saunders.

BIBLIOGRAPHY

Alpern RJ, Hebert SC, editors: Seldin and Giebisch's The kidney physiology and pathophysiology, ed 4, Amsterdam, 2008, Academic Press/Elsevier.
Burtis CA, Ashwood ER, editors: Tietz textbook of clinical chemistry, ed 3, Philadelphia, 1999, WB Saunders.
Kumar V, Abbas A, Aster J: Robbins and Cotran pathologic basis of disease, ed 8, Philadelphia, 2010, Saunders.
Ben-Ezra J, Zhao S, McPherson RA: Basic examination of urine. In McPherson RA, Pincus MR, editor: Clinical diagnosis and management by laboratory methods, ed 21, Philadelphia, 2007, Saunders.
Goldman L, Schafer AI, editors: Goldman's Cecil medicine, ed 24, Philadelphia, 2011, Saunders.
Ringsrud KM, Linne JJ: Urinalysis and body fluids: a color text and atlas, St Louis, 1995, Mosby-Year Book.
Schrier RW, Gottschalk CW: Diseases of the kidney and urinary tract, ed 7, Philadelphia, 2001, Lippincott Williams & Wilkins.
Strasinger SK, Di Lorenzo MS: Urinalysis and body fluids, ed 4, Philadelphia, 2001, FA Davis.

Chemical Examination of Urine

LEARNING OBJECTIVES

After studying this chapter, the student should be able to:

1. State the proper care and storage of commercial reagent strip and tablet tests and cite at least three potential causes of their deterioration.
2. Describe quality control procedures for commercial reagent strip and tablet tests.
3. Discuss appropriate specimen and testing techniques used with commercial reagent strip and tablet tests.
4. State the chemical principle used on reagent strips for measurement of the following:
   * Specific gravity
   * pH
5. Summarize the clinical significance of the following substances when present in urine and describe the chemical principles used on reagent strips to measure them:
   * Blood
   * Leukocyte esterase
   * Nitrite
   * Protein
   * Glucose
   * Ketones
   * Bilirubin
   * Urobilinogen
   * Ascorbic acid
6. Compare and contrast the sensitivity, specificity, and potential interferences of each commercial reagent strip and tablet test.
7. Differentiate between hematuria and hemoglobinuria.
8. Discuss the clinical significance of myoglobin. Compare and contrast myoglobinuria and hemoglobinuria.
9. Discuss the limitations of leukocyte esterase and nitrite reagent strip tests for the detection of leukocyturia and bacteriuria.
10. Compare and contrast the mechanisms for and the clinical significance of the following types of proteinuria:
    * Overflow proteinuria
    * Glomerular proteinuria
    * Postural proteinuria
    * Tubular proteinuria
    * Postrenal proteinuria
11. Discuss the clinical features of the nephrotic syndrome and Fanconi's syndrome, including the specific renal dysfunctions involved.
12. Compare and contrast the chemical principle, sensitivity, and specificity of the following tests for the detection of proteins in the urine:
    * Reagent strip protein test
    * Sulfosalicylic acid precipitation test
    * Sensitive albumin tests (i.e., microalbumin)
13. Describe two physiologic mechanisms that result in glucosuria.
14. Compare and contrast the glucose reagent strip test and the copper reduction test for the measurement of sugars in urine.
15. Describe three conditions that result in ketonuria.
16. Briefly explain the metabolic pathway that results in ketone formation, state the relative concentrations of the three ketones formed, and discuss the reagent strip and tablet tests used to detect them.
17. Summarize the formation of bilirubin and urobilinogen, discuss their clinical significance, and describe three physiologic mechanisms that result in altered bilirubin metabolism.
18. Compare and contrast the principle, sensitivity, specificity, and limitations of the following methods for detection of bilirubin in urine:
    * Physical examination
    * Reagent strip test
    * Tablet test
19. Describe two chemical principles used by reagent strip tests to detect urine urobilinogen and compare their sensitivity, specificity, and limitations.
20. Summarize the formation of porphobilinogen, discuss its clinical significance, and compare the principle, sensitivity, specificity, and limitations of the following porphobilinogen screening methods:
    * Physical examination
    * Hoesch test
    * Watson-Schwartz test
21. State the importance of ascorbic acid detection in urine; describe methods used to detect ascorbic acid; identify reagent strip tests that are affected adversely by ascorbic acid; and explain the mechanism of interference in each reagent strip test.

CHAPTER OUTLINE

KEY TERMS

albuminuria Increased urinary excretion of the protein albumin.

ascorbic acid (also called *vitamin C*) A water-soluble vitamin that is a strong reducing agent that readily oxidizes to its salt, dehydroascorbate.

ascorbic acid interference Inhibition of a chemical reaction by the presence of ascorbic acid. As a strong reducing agent, ascorbic acid readily reacts with diazonium salts or hydrogen peroxide, removing these chemicals from intended reaction sequences. As a result, colorless dehydroascorbate is formed, causing no or a reduced color change.

bacteriuria The presence of bacteria in urine.

bilirubin A yellow-orange pigment resulting from heme catabolism. Bilirubin causes a characteristic discoloration of urine, plasma, and other body fluids when present in the fluid in significant amounts. When exposed to air, bilirubin oxidizes to biliverdin, a green pigment.

Ehrlich's reaction The development of a red or magenta chromophore as a result of the interaction of a substance (e.g., urobilinogen, porphobilinogen) with *p*-dimethylaminobenzaldehyde (also called *Ehrlich's agent*) in an acid medium.

Fanconi's syndrome A complication of inherited and acquired diseases characterized by generalized proximal tubular dysfunction resulting in aminoaciduria, proteinuria, glucosuria, and phosphaturia.

glomerular proteinuria Increased quantities of protein in urine caused by a compromised or

diseased glomerular filtration barrier.

glucosuria The presence of glucose in urine.

glycosuria See *glucosuria*.

hematuria The presence of red blood cells in urine.

heme moiety A tetrapyrrole ring (protoporphyrin IX) with a single, centrally bound iron atom.

hemoglobinuria The presence of hemoglobin in urine.

hemosiderin An insoluble form of storage iron. When renal tubular cells reabsorb hemoglobin, the iron is catabolized into ferritin (a major storage form of iron). Ferritin subsequently denatures to form insoluble hemosiderin granules (micelles of ferric hydroxide) that appear in the urine 2 to 3 days after a hemolytic episode.

isosthenuria Excretion of urine that has the same specific gravity (and osmolality) as the plasma. Because the specific gravity of protein-free plasma and the original unltrafiltrate is 1.010, the inability to excrete urine with a higher or lower specific gravity indicates significantly impaired renal tubular function.

jaundice Yellowish pigmentation of skin, sclera, body tissues, and body fluids caused by the presence of increased quantities of bilirubin. Jaundice appears when plasma bilirubin concentrations reach approximately 2 to 3 mg/dL, that is, two to three times normal bilirubin levels.

ketonuria The presence of ketones (i.e., acetoacetate, hydroxybutyrate, and acetone) in urine.

leukocyturia The presence of leukocytes, that is, white blood cells, in the urine. Compare pyuria.

myoglobinuria The presence of myoglobin in urine.

nephrotic syndrome A complication of numerous disorders characterized by the presentation of proteinuria, hypoalbuminemia, hyperlipidemia, lipiduria, and generalized edema.

overflow proteinuria An increased amount of protein in urine caused by increased quantities of plasma proteins passing through a healthy glomerular filtration barrier.

porphobilinogen An intermediate compound formed in the production of heme and a porphyrin precursor.

porphyrinuria The presence of increased quantities of porphyrins or porphyrin precursors in urine.

postrenal proteinuria An increased amount of protein in urine resulting from a disease process that adds protein to urine after its formation by renal nephrons.

postural (orthostatic) proteinuria Increased protein excretion in urine only when an individual is in an upright (orthostatic) position.

protein error of indicators A phenomenon characterized by several pH indicators. These pH indicators undergo a color change in the presence of protein despite a constant pH. Described originally by Sorenson in 1909, the protein error of indicators serves as the basis of the protein screening tests used on reagent strips.

proteinuria The presence of an increased amount of protein in urine.

pseudoperoxidase activity The action of heme-containing compounds (e.g., hemoglobin, myoglobin) to mimic true peroxidases by catalyzing the oxidation of some substrates in the presence of hydrogen peroxide.

pyuria The presence of pus, a protein-rich fluid that contains white blood cells and cellular debris, in urine. Compare leukocyturia.

renal proteinuria Increased quantities of protein in urine as a result of impaired renal function.

tubular proteinuria Increased quantities of protein in urine caused by impaired or altered renal tubular function.

urinary tract infection The invasion and proliferation of microorganisms in the kidney or urinary tract.

urobilinogen A colorless tetrapyrrole derived from bilirubin.

Urobilinogen is produced in the intestinal tract by the action of anaerobic bacteria and later is reabsorbed partially. Most reabsorbed urobilinogen is reprocessed by the liver and reexcreted in the bile; the rest passes to the kidneys for excretion in the urine. The portion of urobilinogen that is not reabsorbed becomes oxidized to the orange-brown pigment urobilin in the large intestine; this accounts for the characteristic color of feces.

REAGENT STRIPS

Commercial reagent strips are routinely used for chemical analysis of urine. Reagent strips enable rapid screening of urine specimens for pH, protein, glucose, ketones, blood, bilirubin, urobilinogen, nitrite, and leukocyte esterase. In addition, specific gravity and ascorbic acid can be determined by reagent strip, depending on the brand of strip used. Four commonly used brands of commercial reagent strips are Multistix (Siemens Healthcare Diagnostics Inc., Deerfield, IL), Chemstrips (Roche Diagnostics, Indianapolis, IN), vChem Strips (Iris Diagnostics, Chatsworth, CA), and Aution Sticks (Arkray Inc., Kyoto, Japan). Most commercial reagent strips are available with single or multiple test pads on a reagent strip, which allows flexibility in test selection and cost containment.

A reagent strip is an inert plastic strip onto which reagent-impregnated test pads are bonded (Figure 7-1). Chemical reactions take place after the strip is wetted with urine. Each reaction results in a color change that can be assessed visually or mechanically. By comparing the color change observed with the color chart supplied by the strip manufacturer, qualitative results for each reaction are determined. See Appendix A for samples of the color charts and reporting formats provided by manufacturers on reagent strip containers. Depending on the test performed, results are reported (1) in concentration (milligrams per deciliter); (2) as small, moderate, or large; (3) using the plus system (1+, 2+, 3+, 4+); or (4) as positive, negative, or normal. The specific gravity and the pH are exceptions; these results are *estimated* in their respective units. Manufacturers currently do not consistently use the same reporting terminology. For example, Multistix strips report glucose values less than 100 mg/dL as negative, whereas Chemstrip and vChem strips report these glucose results as normal. These minor inconsistencies between products can be confusing.

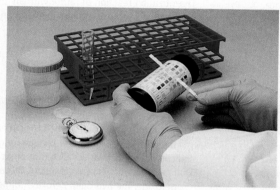

FIGURE 7-1 A commercial reagent strip or dipstick consists of reagent-impregnated test pads that are fixed to an inert plastic strip. After the strip has been appropriately wetted in a urine sample, chemical reactions cause the reaction pads to change color. At the appropriate "read time," results are determined by comparing the color of each reaction pad with the appropriate analyte on the color chart. *(From Young AP, Proctor DB: Kinn's The medical assistant: an applied learning approach, ed 11, St Louis, 2011, Saunders.)*

Therefore, laboratorians must be aware of the reporting format, the chemical principles involved, and the specificity and sensitivity of each test included on the reagent strips used in their laboratory.

The chemical principles used on reagent strips are basically the same, with manufacturers usually differing only in the determination of urobilinogen (Table 7-1). Reagent strips are available with a single test pad (e.g., Albustix, a single protein test pad) or with a variety of test pad combinations. These combinations vary from 2 to 10 test pads per reagent strip and enable health care providers to selectively screen urine specimens for only those constituents that interest them (e.g., Chemstrip 2 LN and Multistix 2 have only two pads: leukocyte esterase and nitrite tests). Some manufacturers also include a pad to account for urine color when automated reagent strip readers (i.e., reflectance photometers) are used.

TABLE 7-1	Comparison of Reagent Strip Principles
Test	**Principle**
Specific gravity	Ionic solutes present in the urine cause protons to be released from a polyelectrolyte. As protons are released, the pH decreases and produces a color change of the bromthymol blue indicator from blue-green to yellow-green. Chemstrip and Multistix reagent strips only Polyelectrolyte used: • Chemstrip: ethylene glycol-bis tetraacetic acid • Multistix: polymethylvinyl ether/maleic acid
pH	Double-indicator system. Indicators methyl red and bromthymol blue are used to give distinct color changes from orange to green to blue (pH 5.0 to 9.0)
Blood	Pseudoperoxidase activity of the heme moiety. The chromogen reacts with a peroxide in the presence of hemoglobin or myoglobin to become oxidized and produce a color change from yellow to green. Chromogen used: tetramethylbenzidine
Leukocyte esterase	Action of leukocyte esterases to cleave an ester and form an aromatic compound is followed by an azocoupling reaction of the aromatic amine formed with a diazonium salt on the reagent pad. The azo dye produced causes a color change from beige to violet. Ester used: • Chemstrip and vChem: indoxylcarbonic acid ester • Multistix: derivatized pyrrole amino acid ester
Nitrite	Diazotization reaction of nitrite with an aromatic amine to produce a diazonium salt is followed by an azocoupling reaction of this diazonium salt with an aromatic compound on the reagent pad. The azo dye produced causes a color change from white to pink. Amine used: • Chemstrip: sulfanilamide • Multistix and vChem: p-arsanilic acid Aromatic compound: • Chemstrip and Multistix: tetrahydrobenzoquinolinol • vChem: naphthylethylenediamine
Protein	Protein error of indicators. When the pH is held constant by a buffer (pH 3.0), indicator dyes release H^+ ions because of the protein present. Color change ranges from yellow to blue-green. Indicator used: derivatives of tetrabromophenol blue
Glucose	Double-sequential enzyme reaction. Glucose oxidase on reagent pad catalyzes the oxidation of glucose to form hydrogen peroxide. The hydrogen peroxide formed in the first reaction oxidizes a chromogen on the reagent pad. The second reaction is catalyzed by a peroxidase provided on the pad. The color change differs with the chromogen used. Chromogen used: • Chemstrip: tetramethylbenzidine • Multistix: potassium iodide • vChem: tolidine hydrochloride
Ketones	Legal's test—nitroprusside reaction. Acetoacetic acid in an alkaline medium reacts with nitroferricyanide to produce a color change from beige to purple. The Chemstrip and vChem reagent strips include glycine in the reaction pad, which enables the detection of acetone; Multistix strips do not.
Bilirubin	Azocoupling reaction of bilirubin with a diazonium salt in an acid medium to form an azo dye. Color changes from light tan to beige or light pink are observed. Diazonium salt used: • Chemstrip: 2,6-dichlorobenzene diazonium tetrafluoroborate • Multistix: 2,4-dichloroaniline diazonium salt • vChem: 2,4- dichlorobenzene diazonium tetrafluoroborate
Urobilinogen	Chemstrip and vChem strips: azocoupling reaction of urobilinogen with a diazonium salt in an acid medium to form an azo dye. Color changes from light pink to dark pink are observed. Diazonium salt used: • Chemstrip: 4-methoxybenzene-diazonium-fluoroborate • vChem: 3,2-dinitro-4-fluoro-4-diazonium-diphenylamine tetrafluoroborate • Multistix strips: modified Ehrlich's reaction. Urobilinogen present reacts with Ehrlich's reagent (p-dimethylaminobenzaldehyde) to form a red compound. Color changes from light orange-pink to dark pink are observed.
Ascorbic acid	Ascorbic acid reduces a dye impregnated in the reagent pad, causing a color change from blue to orange. Dye used: Chem: 2,6-dichlorophenolindophenol

Because reducing agents such as ascorbic acid have the potential to adversely affect several reagent strip test results, it is important that these and other potential interferences are detected or eliminated. In this regard, vChem strips include a test pad to detect ascorbic acid, whereas Chemstrip reagent strips use an iodate overlay on the blood test pad to eliminate ascorbic acid interference. The presence of interferences must be known to enable alternative testing, when possible, or appropriate modification of the results to be reported. Common interferences encountered in the chemical examination of urine and the effects these interferences have on urinalysis results are discussed for each specific reagent strip test in this chapter.

Care and Storage

Chemical reagent strips ,which are sometimes called dipsticks, are examples of state-of-the-art technology. Before the development of the first dry chemical dipstick test for glucose in the 1950s, all chemical tests were performed individually in test tubes. Reagent strips have significantly reduced the time required for testing and have reduced costs (e.g., reagents, personnel) with enhanced test sensitivity and specificity and decreased the amount of urine required for testing.

To ensure the integrity of reagent strips, their proper storage is essential and the manufacturer's directions must be followed. Each manufacturer provides a comprehensive product insert that outlines the chemical principles, reagents, storage, use, sensitivity, specificity, and limitations of its reagent strips. All reagent strips must be protected from moisture, chemicals, heat, and light. Any strips showing evidence of deterioration, contamination, or improper storage should be discarded. Tight-fitting lids, along with desiccants or drying agents within the product container, help eliminate test pad deterioration due to moisture. Fumes from volatile chemicals, acid, and alkaline can adversely affect the test pads and should be avoided. All reagent strip containers protect the reagent strips from ultraviolet rays and sunlight; however, the containers themselves must be protected to prevent fading of the color chart located on the label of the container. Reagent strips should be stored in their original containers at temperatures below 30° C (86° F); they are stable until the expiration date indicated on the label. To ensure accurate test results, all reagent strips—whether from a newly opened container or from one that has been opened for several months—must be periodically tested using appropriate control materials.

Quality Control Testing

Quality control testing of reagent strips not only ensures that the reagent strips are functioning properly but also confirms the acceptable performance and technique of the laboratorian using them. Multiconstituent controls at two distinct levels (e.g., negative and positive) for each reaction must be used to check the reactivity of reagent strips. New containers or lot numbers of reagent strips must be checked "at a frequency defined by the laboratory, related to workload, suggested by the manufacturer, and in conformity with any applicable regulations."[1]

Commercial or laboratory-prepared materials can serve as acceptable negative controls. Similarly, positive controls can be purchased commercially or prepared by the laboratory. Because of the time and care involved in making a multiconstituent control material that tests each parameter on the reagent strip, most laboratories purchase control materials. When control materials are tested, acceptable test performance is defined by each laboratory. Regardless of the control material used, care must be taken to ensure that analyte values are within the critical detection levels for each parameter. For example, a protein control concentration of 1 g/dL would be inappropriate as a control material because it far exceeds the desired critical detection level of 10 to 15 mg/dL.

An additional quality check on chemical and microscopic examinations, as well as on the laboratorian, involves aliquoting a well-mixed urine specimen from the daily workload and having a different laboratory (interlaboratory) or a technologist on each shift (intralaboratory) analyze the specimen. Interlaboratory duplicate testing checks the entire urinalysis procedure and detects innocuous changes when manual urinalyses are performed, such as variations in the speed of centrifugation and in centrifuge brake usage. Intralaboratory duplicate testing can be used to evaluate the technical competency of laboratorians.

TABLET AND CHEMICAL TESTS

Care and Storage

Commercial tablet tests (e.g., Ictotest, Clinitest, Acetest [all from Siemens Healthcare Diagnostics Inc., Deerfield, IL]) must be handled and stored according to the inserts provided by the manufacturers. These products are susceptible to deterioration from exposure to light, heat, and moisture. Therefore they should be visually inspected before each use and discarded if any of the following changes have occurred: tablet discolored, contamination or spoilage evident, incorrect storage, or past the expiration date. Note that the stability of the reaction tablets can decrease after opening because of repeated exposure to atmospheric moisture. To ensure tablet integrity, an appropriate quality control program must be employed.

Chemical tests such as the sulfosalicylic acid (SSA) precipitation test, the Hoesch test, the Watson-Schwartz test, or any other tests, require appropriately made and tested reagents. When new reagents are prepared, they should be tested in parallel with current "in-use" reagents to ensure equivalent performance. Chemical tests must also be checked according to the laboratory's quality control program to ensure the reliability and reproducibility of test results obtained.

Quality Control Testing

As with reagent strips, tablet or chemical tests performed in the urinalysis laboratory must have quality control materials run to ensure the integrity of the reagents and the technique used in testing. Some commercial controls for reagent strips can also be used to check the integrity of Clinitest, Ictotest, and Acetest tablets. In addition, lyophilized chemistry controls or laboratory-made control materials can be used. For example, a chemistry albumin standard at an appropriate concentration (approximately 30 to 100 mg/dL) serves as a satisfactory control for performance of the SSA protein precipitation test.

Positive and negative quality control materials must be analyzed according to the frequency established in the laboratory's policy. New tablets and reagents should be checked before they are placed into use and periodically thereafter.

CHEMICAL TESTING TECHNIQUE

Reagent Strips

Although reagent strips are easy to use, proper technique is imperative to ensure accurate results. The manufacturer's instructions provided with reagent strips and tablet tests should be followed. Note that these instructions can vary among different manufacturers. Box 7-1 summarizes an appropriate manual reagent strip testing technique.

A fresh, well-mixed, uncentrifuged specimen is used for testing. If the specimen is maintained at room temperature, it must be tested within 2 hours after collection

---

BOX 7-1	Appropriate Manual Reagent Strip Testing Technique

Room Conditions: Good lighting, preferably fluorescent; avoid direct sunlight
Urine specimen: At room temperature
Technique:
1. Using *uncentrifuged* urine, mix specimen well.
2. Dip reagent strip *briefly* into urine wetting all reaction pads and start timing device.
3. Remove excess urine by drawing edge of strip against rim of container or by blotting strip edge on absorbent paper.
4. At the appropriate times, read results of each reaction pad using the color chart on the container.
5. Discard strip into biohazard waste.

---

to avoid erroneous results caused by changes that can occur in unpreserved urine[1] (see Table 3-1). If the urine specimen has been refrigerated, it should be allowed to warm up to room temperature before testing with reagent strips to avoid erroneous results. The specimen can be tested in the original collection container or after an aliquot is poured into a labeled centrifuge tube. The reagent strip should be *briefly* dipped into the urine specimen, wetting all test pads. Excess urine should be drained from the strip by drawing the edge of the strip along the rim of the container or by placing the strip edge on an absorbent paper. Inadequate removal of excess urine from the strip can cause contamination of one test pad with the reagents from another, whereas prolonged dipping of the strip causes the chemicals to leach from the test pad into the urine. Both of these actions can produce erroneous test results.

When reagent strips are read, the time required before full color development varies with the test parameter. To obtain reproducible and reliable results, the timing instructions provided by the manufacturer must be followed. Timing intervals can differ among reagent strips from the same manufacturer and among different manufacturers of the same test. For example, when a Multistix strip is used, the ketone test pad is read at 40 seconds; however, when Ketostix strips are used, the test area is read at 15 seconds. Some reagent strips have the flexibility of reading all test pads, except leukocytes, at any time between 60 and 120 seconds (e.g., Chemstrip, VChem strips), whereas others require the exact timing of each test pad for semiquantitated results (e.g., Multistix strips).

Visual interpretation of color varies slightly among individuals; therefore reagent strips should be read in a well-lit area with the strip held close to the color chart. The strip must be properly oriented to the chart before results are determined. Because of similar color changes by several of the test pads, improper orientation of the strip to the color chart is a potential source of error. (See Appendix A, Reagent Strip Color Charts.) Note that color changes appearing only along the edge of a reaction pad or after 2 minutes are diagnostically insignificant and should be disregarded. When reagent strips are read by automated instruments, the timing intervals are set by the factory. The advantage of automated instruments in reading reagent strips is their consistency in timing and color interpretation regardless of room lighting or testing personnel. Some instruments, however, are unable to identify and compensate for urines that are highly pigmented owing to medications. This can lead to false-positive reagent strip test results because the true color reaction is masked by the pigment present. Laboratorians should identify highly pigmented urine specimens and manually test them using reagent strips or alternative methods. Table 7-2 summarizes the sensitivity and specificity of three brands of commercial reagent strips.

TABLE 7-2	Comparison of the Sensitivity and Specificity of Reagent Strips	
Test	**Sensitivity**	**Specificity**
Specific gravity	Chemstrip: 1.000 to 1.030 Multistix: 1.000 to 1.030	Detects only ionic solutes; provides "estimate" in 0.005 increments *Falsely low*: • Glucose and urea >1 g/dL (Chemstrip) • pH ≥6.5; add 0.005 (Multistix) *Falsely high*: • Protein approximately equal to 100 to 500 mg/dL • Ketoacidosis
pH	Chemstrip: 5.0 to 9.0, in 1.0 pH increments Multistix: 5.0 to 8.5, in 0.5 pH increments vChem: 5.0 to 9.0, in 1.0 pH increments	pH; hydrogen ion concentration No interferences known; unaffected by protein concentration

Blood	Chemstrip: 0.02 to 0.03 mg/dL Hgb (5 to 10 RBCs/μL)
	Multistix: 0.02 to 0.06 mg/dL Hgb (6 to 20 RBCs/μL)
	vChem: 0.02 to 0.03 mg/dL Hgb (5 to 10 RBCs/μL)
		Equally specific for hemoglobin and myoglobin
		Intact RBCs are lysed on reagent pad
		False-positive results:
		• Menstrual contamination
		• Peroxidases (e.g., microbial)
		• Strong oxidizing agents (e.g., hypochlorite in detergents)
		False-negative or *decreased* results:
		• Ascorbic acid:
		  • Multistix (≥9 mg/dL)
		  • vChem (≥5 mg/dL)
		  • Chemstrip unaffected
		• High specific gravity
		• Captopril (Multistix)
		• Formalin
		• High nitrite (>10 mg/dL)

Leukocyte esterase	Chemstrip: approximately 10 WBCs/μL Multistix: approximately 5 to 15 WBCs/per high-power field (~10 to 25 WBCs/μL) vChem: approximately 20 WBCs/μL in 90% of urines tested	Detects only granulocytic leukocytes *False-positive* results: • Highly colored substances that mask results, such as drugs (phenazopyridine), beet ingestion • Vaginal contamination of urine • Formalin *False-negative* results: • Lymphocytes are not detected • Increased glucose (>3 g/dL) or protein (>500 mg/dL) • High specific gravity • Strong oxidizing agents (soaps, detergents) • Drugs such as gentamicin, cephalosporins, tetracycline
Nitrite	Chemstrip: 0.05 mg/dL nitrite ion in 90% of urines tested Multistix: 0.06 mg/dL nitrite ion vChem: 0.05 mg/dL nitrite ion in 90% of urines tested	*False-positive* results: • Highly colored substances that mask results, such as drugs (phenazopyridine), beet ingestion • Improper storage with bacterial proliferation *False-negative* results: • Ascorbic acid (≥25 mg/dL) interference • Various factors that inhibit or prevent nitrite formation despite bacteriuria
Protein	Chemstrip: 6.0 mg/dL in 90% of urines tested Multistix: 15 to 30 mg/dL vChem: 15 mg/dL in 90% of urines tested	More sensitive to albumin than globulins, hemoglobin, myoglobin, immunoglobulin light chains, mucoproteins, or others *False-positive* results: • Highly buffered or alkaline urine (pH ≥9), such as alkaline drugs, improperly preserved specimen, contamination with quaternary ammonium compounds • Highly colored substances that mask results, such as drugs (phenazopyridine), beet ingestion *False-negative* results: • Presence of proteins other than albumin • Highly colored substances that mask results, such as drugs (phenazopyridine, nitrofurantoin), beet ingestion

Continued

TABLE 7-2	Comparison of the Sensitivity and Specificity of Reagent Strips—cont'd	
Test	**Sensitivity**	**Specificity**
Glucose	Chemstrip: 40 mg/dL, in 90% of urines tested Multistix: 75 to 125 mg/dL vChem: 45 mg/dL in 90% of urines tested	Specific for glucose Affected by high specific gravity and low temperatures *False-positive* results: • Strong oxidizing agents, such as bleach • Peroxide contaminants *False-negative* results: • Ascorbic acid ($\geq$50 mg/dL) • Improperly stored specimens (i.e., glycolysis)
Ketones	Chemstrip: 9.0 mg/dL acetoacetate and 70 mg/dL acetone, in 90% of urines tested Multistix: 5.0 to 10 mg/dL acetocetate vChem: 8.0 mg/dL acetoacetate and 50 mg/dL acetone, in 90% of urines tested	Does not detect β-hydroxybutyrate *False-positive* results: • Compounds containing free-sulfhydryl groups, such as MESNA, captopril, *N*-acetylcysteine • Highly pigmented urines • Atypical colors with phenylketones and phthaleins • Large quantities of levodopa metabolites *False-negative* results: • Improper storage, resulting in volatilization and bacterial breakdown
Bilirubin	Chemstrip: 0.5 mg/dL conjugated bilirubin in 90% of urines tested Multistix: 0.4 to 0.8 mg/dL conjugated bilirubin vChem: 0.5 mg/dL conjugated bilirubin in 90% of urines tested	*False-positive* results: • Drug-induced color changes, such as phenazopyridine, indican- indoxyl sulfate • Large quantities of chlorpromazine metabolites *False-negative* results: • Ascorbic acid ($\geq$25 mg/dL) • High nitrite concentrations • Improper storage or light exposure, which oxidizes or hydrolyzes bilirubin to nonreactive biliverdin and free bilirubin

Urobilinogen	Chemstrip: 0.4 mg/dL urobilinogen
	Multistix: 0.2 mg/dL urobilinogen
	vChem: 1.0 mg/dL urobilinogen
		The total absence of urobilinogen cannot be determined. Reactivity
		increases with temperature, optimum 22° C to 26° C
		False-positive results:
		• Multistix
		  • Any other Ehrlich's reactive substance
		  • Atypical colors caused by sulfonamides, *p*-aminobenzoic acid,
		    p-aminosalicylic acid
		  • Substances that induce color mask results, such as drugs
		    (phenazopyridine), beet ingestion
		• Chemstrip and vChem
		  • Highly colored substances that mask results, such as drugs
		False-negative results:
		• Formalin (>200 mg/dL), a urine preservative
		• Improper storage, resulting in oxidation to urobilin

Ascorbic acid	vChem: 20 mg/dL, in 90% of urines tested	*False-positive* results: • Free-sulfhydryl drugs (e.g., MESNA, captopril, *N*-acetylcysteine)

Tablet and Chemical Tests

With each tablet test, the manufacturer's directions must be followed exactly to ensure reproducible and reliable results. All chemical tests, such as the SSA precipitation test for protein or the Watson-Schwartz test for urobilinogen and porphobilinogen, must be performed according to established written laboratory procedures. As with reagent strips, the laboratorian should know the sensitivity, specificity, and potential interferences for each test. Chemical and tablet tests are generally performed (1) to confirm results already obtained by reagent strip testing; (2) as an alternative method for highly pigmented urine; (3) because they are more sensitive for the substance of interest than the reagent strip test (e.g., Ictotest tablets); or (4) because the specificity of the test differs from that of the reagent strip test (e.g., SSA test, Hoesch test).

CHEMICAL TESTS

Specific Gravity

Specific gravity is a physical property of urine and an expression of solute concentration. Chapters 5 and 6 discuss specific gravity at length. Following is a discussion of the indirect chemical method used on reagent strips to measure specific gravity.

Clinical Significance. The ultrafiltrate that enters the Bowman space of the glomeruli has the same specific gravity as protein-free plasma (SG = 1.010). As the ultrafiltrate passes through the nephrons, solutes and water are selectively absorbed and secreted. If the tubules are unable to perform these functions, the specific gravity of the urine excreted will always be identical to that of the original ultrafiltrate. This condition, termed **isosthenuria**, implies significant renal tubular dysfunction and is a feature of "end-stage" renal disease. Patients who excrete urine with a fixed specific gravity of 1.010, regardless of their hydration, will also present with nocturia, because the kidneys are unable to selectively retain solutes and water adequately. Urine specimens with a specific gravity less than 1.010 can be termed *hyposthenuric*, whereas those with a specific gravity greater than 1.010 are termed *hypersthenuric*. These terms are simply descriptive regarding urine solute concentration and, unlike isosthenuria, do not imply renal dysfunction.

The kidneys excrete the solutes necessary in the amount of water that is not needed by the body. Because solute and water intake varies, so does the specific gravity of the urine. Normally, the specific gravity of urine ranges from 1.002 to 1.035. Values less than or greater than this range require further investigation because a urine specific gravity equal to 1.000 or greater than approximately 1.040 is physiologically impossible. Urine specimens with values of approximately 1.000 must be checked by a second method (e.g., refractometry). To make sure that the specimen is truly urine, a creatinine or urea determination could be performed. In addition, the laboratorian should verify that quality control materials have been analyzed and documented to ensure the integrity of the reagent strip results obtained. Note that specimens with an extremely high specific gravity of 1.040 or greater owing to the excretion of radiographic contrast media or mannitol can be accurately assessed by osmometry or by using the specific gravity reagent strip method.

Despite a full range of possible values, the specific gravity of most random urine specimens varies between 1.010 and 1.025. During excessive sweating, dehydration, or fluid restriction, urine specific gravity values often exceed 1.025. Box 7-2 summarizes the clinical significance associated with urine specific gravity results.
Principle. The reagent strip specific gravity test does not measure the total solute content but only those solutes that are ionic. Keep in mind that only ionic solutes indicate the renal concentrating and secreting ability of the kidneys and have diagnostic value. Because of the diversity of methods available for measuring specific gravity and for detecting and measuring solutes, it is important that health care providers are informed of the test method used in the laboratory and its principles, sensitivity, specificity, and limitations. All methods available for specific gravity determination are discussed at length in Chapter

BOX 7-2	Clinical Significance of Urine Specific Gravity Results
Specific Gravity	**Indication or Cause**
1.000	Physiologically impossible–same as pure water; suspect adulteration of urine specimen
1.001–1.009	Dilute urine; associated with increased water intake or water diuresis (e.g., diuretics, inadequate secretion/action of ADH*)
1.010–1.025	Indicates average solute and water intake and excretion
1.025–1.035 (1.040 maximum)	Concentrated urine; associated with dehydration, fluid restriction, profuse sweating, osmotic diuresis
>1.040	Physiologically impossible; indicates presence of iatrogenic substance (e.g., radiographic contrast media, mannitol)

*Antidiuretic hormone (ADH), also known as *arginine vasopressin* (AVP).

6 and summarized in Table 6-6. For a brief summary of the reagent strip principle, refer to Table 7-1.

pH

Clinical Significance. The kidneys play a major role in regulating the acid-base balance of the body, as was discussed in Chapter 4. The renal system, the pulmonary system, and blood buffers provide the means for maintaining homeostasis at a pH compatible with life. Normal daily metabolism generates endogenous acids and bases; in response, the kidneys selectively excrete acid or alkali. Normally, the urine pH varies from 4.5 to 8.0. The average individual excretes a slightly acidic urine of pH 5.0 to 6.0 because endogenous acid production predominates. However, during and after a meal, the urine produced is less acidic. This observation is known as the *alkaline tide*.

Urine pH can affect the stability of formed elements in urine. An alkaline pH enhances lysis of cells and degradation of the matrix of casts. Because pH values greater than 8.0 and less than 4.5 are physiologically impossible, they require investigation when obtained. The three most common reasons for a urine pH greater than 8.0 are (1) a urine specimen that was improperly preserved and stored, resulting in the proliferation of urease-producing bacteria, (2) an adulterated specimen (i.e., an alkaline agent was added to the urine after collection), and (3) the patient was given a highly alkaline substance (e.g., medication, therapeutic agent) that was subsequently excreted by the kidneys. In the latter situation, efforts should be made to ensure adequate hydration of the patient to prevent in vivo precipitation of normal urine solutes (e.g., ammonium biurate crystals), which can cause renal tubular damage.

TABLE 7-3	Clinical Correlation of Urine pH Values
pH	**Indication or Cause**
<4.5	Physiologically impossible; suspect adulteration of urine specimen
4.5–6.9	**Acid urine**; associated with • Diet: high protein, cranberry ingestion • Sleep • Metabolic acidosis (e.g., ketoacidosis, starvation, severe diarrhea, uremia, poisons—ethylene glycol, methanol) • Respiratory acidosis (e.g., emphysema, chronic lung disease) • Urinary system disorders: UTI* with acid-producing bacteria (*Escherichia coli*), chronic renal failure, uremia • Medications used to induce: ammonium chloride, ascorbic acid, methionine, mandelic acid
7.0–7.9	**Alkaline urine**; associated with • Diet: vegetarian, citrus fruits, low carbohydrate • Metabolic alkalosis (e.g., vomiting, gastric lavage) • Respiratory alkalosis (e.g., hyperventilation) • Urinary system disorders: UTI* with urease–producing bacteria (*Proteus* sp., *Pseudomonas* sp.), renal tubular acidosis • Medications used to induce: sodium bicarbonate, potassium citrate, acetazolamide
>8.0	Physiologically impossible; indicates: • presence of an iatrogenic alkaline substance (intravenous medication or agent) • improperly stored urine specimen • contamination with an alkaline chemical (preservative)

*UTI, Urinary tract infection.

Because the kidneys constantly maintain the acid-base balance of the body, ingestion of acids or alkali or any condition that produces acids or alkali directly affects the urine pH. Table 7-3 lists urine pH values and common causes associated which them. This ability of the kidneys to manipulate urine pH has many applications. An acid urine prevents stone formation by alkaline-precipitating solutes (e.g., calcium carbonate, calcium phosphate) and inhibits the development of urinary tract infection. An alkaline urine prevents the precipitation of and enhances the excretion of various drugs (e.g., sulfonamides, streptomycin, salicylate) and prevents stone formation from calcium oxalate, uric acid, and cystine crystals.

The urine pH provides valuable information for assessing and managing disease and for determining the suitability of a specimen for chemical testing. Correlation of urine pH with a patient's condition aids in the diagnosis of disease (e.g., production of an alkaline urine despite a metabolic acidosis is characteristic of renal tubular acidosis). Individuals with a history of stone formation can monitor their urine pH and can use this information to modify their diets if necessary. Highly alkaline urine of pH 8.0 to 9.0 can also interfere with chemical testing, particularly in protein determination.

Methods

Reagent Strip Tests. All commercial reagent strips, regardless of the manufacturer, are based on a double-indicator system using bromthymol blue and methyl red. This indicator combination produces distinctive color changes from orange (pH 5.0) to green (pH 7.0) to blue (pH 9.0) (Equation 7-1).

Equation 7-1

$$\underset{\substack{\text{Oxidized dye}\\ \text{(yellow)}}}{\text{Ind}^-} + \text{H}^+\text{ions} \rightarrow \underset{\substack{\text{Reduced dye}\\ \text{(green to blue)}}}{\text{H}-\text{Ind}}$$

The range provided on the strips is from pH 5.0 to pH 9.0 in 0.5 or 1.0 pH increments, depending on the manufacturer. No interferences with test results are known, and the results are not affected by protein concentration. However, erroneous results can occur from pH changes caused by (1) improper storage of the specimen with bacterial proliferation (a falsely increased pH); (2) contamination of the specimen container before collection (a falsely increased or decreased pH depending on the agent); or (3) improper reagent strip technique, causing the acid buffer from the protein test pad to contaminate the pH test area (a falsely decreased pH).

pH Meter. Although the accuracy provided by a pH meter is not usually necessary, a pH meter is an alternative method for determining the urine pH. Various pH meters are available; the manufacturer's operating instructions supplied with the instrument must be followed to ensure proper use of the pH meter and valid results. Nevertheless, the components involved in and the principle behind all pH meters are basically the same.

A pH meter consists of a silver–silver chloride indicator electrode with a pH-sensitive glass membrane connected by a salt bridge to a reference electrode (usually a calomel electrode, $Hg-Hg_2Cl_2$). When the indicator electrode is placed in urine, a difference in H^+ activity develops across the glass membrane. This difference causes a change in the potential difference between the indicator and the reference electrodes. This voltage difference is registered by a voltmeter and is converted to a pH reading. Because pH measurement is temperature dependent and pH decreases with increasing temperature, it is necessary that the pH measurement be adjusted for the temperature of the urine during measurement. Newer pH meters perform this temperature compensation automatically.

A pH meter is calibrated with the use of two or three commercially available standard buffer solutions. Accurate pH measurements require that the pH meter be calibrated using at least two different standards in the pH range of the test solution, and that adjustment for the temperature of the test solution be made manually or automatically. In addition, the pH-sensitive glass electrode must be clean and maintained to prevent protein buildup or bacterial growth.

pH Test Papers. Various indicator papers with different pH ranges and sensitivities are commercially available. The indicator papers do not add impurities to the urine. In use, they produce sharp color changes for comparison with a supplied color chart of pH values.

Blood

Clinical Significance. As was discussed in Chapter 6, blood in urine can result in various presentations of color or may not be visually evident. Historically, color and clarity or microscopic viewing was used to detect the presence of blood in urine. Chemical methods now provide a rapid and sensitive means of detecting the presence of blood. Blood can enter the urinary tract anywhere from the glomeruli to the urethra or can be a contaminant in the urine as a result of the collection procedure used. Lysis of red blood cells with the release of hemoglobin is enhanced in alkaline or dilute urine (e.g., SG ≤ 1.010). Without current chemical methods, the presence of free hemoglobin in urine would go undetected. True hemoglobinuria—free hemoglobin from plasma passing the glomerular filtration barriers into the ultrafiltrate—is uncommon. Most often, intact red blood cells enter the urinary tract and then undergo lysis to varying degrees. **Hematuria** is the term used to describe an abnormal quantity of red blood cells in the urine, whereas **hemoglobinuria** indicates the urinary presence of hemoglobin.

Even small increases in the quantity of red blood cells in urine are diagnostically significant. The chemical methods used detect the **heme moiety**—the tetrapyrrole ring (protoporphyrin IX) of a hemoglobin molecule with its centrally bound iron (Fe^{+2}) atom. Note, however, that substances other than hemoglobin also contain a heme moiety such as myoglobin and cytochromes. Of particular interest is myoglobin (MW 17,000), an intracellular protein of muscle that will be increased in the bloodstream when muscle tissue is damaged by trauma or disease. Because of its small size, myoglobin readily passes the glomerular filtration barriers and is excreted in the urine. As a result, a positive chemical test for blood is nonspecific, indicating the presence of hemoglobin, red blood cells, or myoglobin. Whether one or all of these substances are present requires confirmation and differentiation. Correlation with urine microscopic examination results, the appearance of the patient's plasma, and the results of plasma chemical tests may be necessary to confirm which substances are present.

Hematuria and Hemoglobinuria. A feature that helps distinguish between hematuria and hemoglobinuria is urine clarity. Hematuria is often evident by a cloudy or smoky urine specimen, whereas with true hemoglobinuria, the urine is clear. Urine colors for both are similar, and color variations range from normal yellow to pink, red, or brown, depending on the amount of blood or hemoglobin present. In addition, urine pH can affect the appearance of these specimens. For example, an alkaline pH promotes red blood cell lysis and hemoglobin oxidation.

Numerous diseases of the kidneys or urinary tract, trauma, drug therapy, or strenuous exercise can result in hematuria and hemoglobinuria (Box 7-3). The detection of hematuria or hemoglobinuria is an early indicator of disease that is not always visually evident and when present always requires further investigation. The amount of blood in a urine specimen has no correlation with disease severity, nor can the amount of blood alone identify the location of the bleed. In combination with a microscopic examination, however, when red blood cells are present in casts, a glomerular or tubular origin is indicated.

As was previously stated, true hemoglobinuria is uncommon. Any condition resulting in intravascular hemolysis has the potential for producing hemoglobinuria. However, free hemoglobin in the bloodstream is bound rapidly by plasma haptoglobin. This hemoglobin-haptoglobin complex is too large to pass through the glomerular filtration barriers, so it remains in the plasma

BOX 7-3	Clinical Significance of Positive Blood Reaction
Finding	**Possible Cause**
Hematuria	Kidney and urinary tract disease: • glomerulonephritides • pyelonephritis • cystitis (bladder infection) • renal calculi (stones) • tumors (benign and cancerous) Trauma Hypertension Strenuous exercise, normal exercise, smoking Medications (cyclophosphamide, anticoagulants) and chemical toxicity
Hemoglobinuria	Intravascular hemolysis—transfusion reactions, hemolytic anemia, paroxysmal nocturnal hemoglobinuria Extensive burns Infections: malaria, *Clostridium perfringens*, syphilis, mycoplasma Chemical toxicity: copper, nitrites, nitrates Exertional hemolysis: marching, karate, long distance running
Myoglobinuria	Muscle trauma: crushing injuries, surgery, contact sports Muscle ischemia: carbon monoxide poisoning, alcohol-induced, or after illicit drug use Muscle infections (myositis): viral, bacterial Myopathy due to medications Seizures/convulsions Toxins: snake venoms, spider bites

TABLE 7-4	Comparison of Selected Urine and Plasma Components in Mild and Severe Hemolytic Episodes		
		Intravascular Hemolysis	
Test	Normal Values	Mild (chronic)	Severe (acute)
Urine			
Bilirubin, conjugated	Absent	Absent	Absent
Bilirubin, unconjugated	Absent	Absent	Absent
Urobilinogen	Normal (≤1.0 mg/dL)	Normal to increased	Increased
Blood (hemoglobin)	Absent	Absent	Present
Hemosiderin	Absent	Absent	Present
Plasma			
Bilirubin, conjugated	Up to 0.2 mg/dL	Normal	Normal
Bilirubin, unconjugated	0.8-1.0 mg/dL	Increased	Increased
Haptoglobin	83-267 mg/dL	Decreased	Absent
Free hemoglobin	1.0-5.0 mg/dL	Normal	Increased

and is removed from the circulation by the liver, where it is metabolized. If all available plasma haptoglobin is bound, any additional free hemoglobin readily passes through the glomeruli with the ultrafiltrate. As dissociated dimers (MW ≈38,000), hemoglobin is reabsorbed principally by the proximal renal tubules and is catabolized to ferritin. Within the renal cells, ferritin is denatured to form **hemosiderin,** a storage form of iron that is insoluble in aqueous solutions. Hemosiderin usually appears in urine 2 to 3 days after a hemolytic episode and appears as yellow-brown granules (1) within sloughed renal tubular cells, (2) as free-floating granules, or (3) within casts. A Prussian blue–staining test (Rous test) performed on a concentrated urinary sediment aids in visualization and identification of hemosiderin. The presence of urinary hemosiderin is intermittent and should not be solely relied on to confirm a hemolytic episode or a chronic hemolytic condition. Table 7-4 compares urine and plasma values of analytes that can be used to monitor chronic and acute hemolytic episodes.

Myoglobinuria. Myoglobin is a monomeric heme-containing protein involved in the transport of oxygen in muscles. Skeletal or cardiac muscle damage caused by a crushing injury, vigorous physical exercise, or ischemia causes the release of myoglobin into the blood. Because of its small molecular size (MW 17,000), myoglobin readily passes the glomerular filtration barrier. Its adverse renal effects are related to catabolism of the heme moiety and formation of free radicals during this process. Nontraumatic disorders such as alcohol overdose, toxin ingestion, and certain metabolic disorders can result in **myoglobinuria** (see Box 7-3). In fact, nontraumatic myoglobinuria with acute renal failure is common in patients with an alcohol overdose or a history of cocaine or heroin addiction.[2] Myoglobinuria may be obvious based on the patient's medical history and presenting symptoms such as a crushing injury; however, nontraumatic rhabdomyolysis (muscle damage) has vague symptoms (nausea, weakness, swollen, tender muscles), and chemical analysis is often required for diagnosis.

Differentiation of Hemoglobinuria and Myoglobinuria. Myoglobin appears to be more toxic to renal tubules than hemoglobin. The reason for this is unclear but may be related to their difference in glomerular clearance and to other factors such as hydration, hypotension, and aciduria. Differentiating between hemoglobinuria and myoglobinuria can be difficult but is important (1) for diagnosis, (2) for predicting a patient's risk for acute renal failure, and (3) for treatment.

Visual inspection of urine and plasma can help distinguish between hemoglobinuria and myoglobinuria, but these gross observations are of limited value. Urine colors can be similar—hemoglobinuria causes a red or brown urine, whereas myoglobinuria causes a pink, red, or brown urine. Hemoglobin is not cleared as rapidly from the plasma as myoglobin; therefore with hemoglobinuria, the plasma often shows various degrees of hemolysis. In contrast, myoglobin is rapidly cleared by glomerular filtration, and the plasma appears normal.

Historically, the differentiation of hemoglobin and myoglobin in clinical laboratories has relied on the ammonium sulfate precipitation method. This method was based on the different solubility characteristics of hemoglobin and myoglobin when saturated with 80% ammonium sulfate. At this salt concentration, hemoglobin precipitates out of solution, whereas myoglobin remains soluble in the supernatant. Only red or brown urine is tested, and an assessment is made by observing whether the urine color precipitates out of or remains in the supernate after 80% saturation with ammonium sulfate. Because of reliance on visual observation, this method does not detect low levels of hemoglobinuria (<30 mg/dL). At these low levels, false-negative results for hemoglobin would be reported because no visible precipitation is observed.[2] With the availability of sensitive and specific immunoassays and high-performance liquid chromatography methods, the ammonium sulfate precipitation method for differentiation is no longer clinically useful.

TABLE 7-5	Differentiation of Hemoglobinuria and Myoglobinuria	
Parameter	**Hemoglobinuria**	**Myoglobinuria**
Urine color:	Pink, red, brown	Pink, red, brown
Blood reagent strip test:	Positive	Positive
Serum color:	Pink to red (hemolysis)	Pale yellow (normal)
Serum chemistry tests:		
Haptoglobin	Decreased to absent	Normal
Myoglobin	Normal	Increased
Free hemoglobin	Increased	Normal
Creatine kinase (CK)	Increased, but <10 times upper reference limit	Increased, but >10 times upper reference limit

The following approach to differentiating between hemoglobin and myoglobin is similar to a protocol recommended by Shihabi, Hamilton, and Hopkins in 1989 for development of a "rhabdomyolysis/hemolysis profile."[2] Normally, myoglobin excretion is less than 0.04 mg/dL; however, during extreme exercise, it can increase to 40 times the normal rate without adverse renal effects. Only urine myoglobin concentrations exceeding 1.5 mg/dL are associated with a patient's risk of developing acute renal failure. Because available blood reagent strip tests are sensitive and capable of detecting approximately 0.04 mg/dL of myoglobin, urine from patients suspected of having rhabdomyolysis should be diluted 1:40 before testing for myoglobin. If the blood reagent strip test is negative when testing the diluted urine sample, no significant rhabdomyolytic process is occurring. However, if the test is positive, the creatine kinase level should be determined using the patient's plasma. A rhabdomyolytic process will cause the plasma creatine kinase concentration to exceed the normal upper reference limit by 40 times or greater. This will occur because of the high concentration of creatine kinase in muscle cells. If the diagnosis of hemoglobinuria versus myoglobinuria is still questionable, test the patient's plasma for myoglobin. Rhabdomyolysis will cause a markedly elevated plasma myoglobin level. Table 7-5 compares laboratory findings that aid in the differential diagnosis of hemoglobinuria and myoglobinuria.

Method. Despite various manufacturers, reagent strip tests for blood detection are based on the same chemical principle: the **pseudoperoxidase activity** of the heme moiety. The reagent pad is impregnated with the chromogen tetramethylbenzidine and a peroxide. Through pseudoperoxidase activity of the heme moiety, peroxide is reduced and the chromogen becomes oxidized, producing a color change on the reaction pad from yellow to green (Equation 7-2). Depending on the manufacturer, intact red blood cells may be lysed on the reaction pad; this results in release of hemoglobin and the development of a mottled or dotted pattern.

Equation 7-2

$$H_2O_2 + \text{Chromogen*} \xrightarrow[Mb]{Hb} \text{Oxidized chromogen} + H_2O$$

*Tetramethylbenzidine. *Hb*, Hemoglobin; *Mb*, myoglobin.

Color charts are provided on the labels of reagent strip containers for visual assessment of the reaction pads. A homogeneous color change results from hemoglobin, whereas a mottled pattern can occur when intact red blood cells are lysed and their hemoglobin is released. Test results can be reported as negative, trace, small, moderate, or large, or the plus (1+, 2+, 3+) system can be used.

Because intact red blood cells are not "dissolved" in urine, they can settle out or can be removed from the urine by centrifugation. Therefore it is important that urine specimens are well mixed and tested for blood before centrifugation. In contrast, hemoglobin is dissolved in the urine and will not settle out. In other words, it is detectable in the urine before centrifugation and in the supernatant afterward.

Because proteins other than hemoglobin, such as myoglobin, contain the heme moiety, blood reagent strip tests can detect their presence. All reagent strips, regardless of their manufacturer, are equally specific for hemoglobin and myoglobin. Other heme-containing substances, such as mitochondrial cytochromes, are present in quantities too small to be detected. See Table 7-2 for the sensitivities of several available reagent strips. To relate the sensitivity for hemoglobin to that for red blood cells, assume that approximately 30 picograms of hemoglobin is contained in each red blood cell; then 10 lysed red blood cells is the equivalent of approximately 0.03 mg/dL hemoglobin.[3]

Blood reagent strips are one of several reagent strip chemistry tests susceptible to **ascorbic acid interference.** Whenever red blood cells are observed in microscopic examination of the urine sediment, but the chemical examination is negative for blood, ascorbic acid (vitamin C) should be suspected. Ascorbic acid is a strong reducing substance that reacts directly with peroxide (H_2O_2) impregnated on the blood reagent pad and removes it from the intended reaction, thereby preventing oxidation of the chromogen. As a result, false-negative or falsely low reagent strip results for blood can be obtained from specimens that contain ascorbic acid. Chemstrip reagent strips have successfully eliminated this interference through the use of an "iodate scavenger pad." On Chemstrip reagent strips, a proprietary iodate-impregnated mesh overlies the blood reagent pad and oxidizes any ascorbic acid before it can interfere in the chemical reaction. vChem reagent strips take a different approach. These strips include a separate ascorbic acid test pad to detect and alert the laboratorian to the presence of ascorbic acid. Excretion and detection of ascorbic acid in urine, as well as a summary of the reagent strip tests affected by ascorbic acid, are discussed later in this section.

False-positive results for blood can be obtained when menstrual or hemorrhoidal blood contaminates the urine. Other causes include strong oxidizing agents such as sodium hypochlorite or hydrogen peroxide that directly oxidize the chromogen or microbial peroxidases produced by certain bacterial strains (e.g., *Escherichia coli*) that can catalyze the reaction in the absence of the intended pseudoperoxidase, hemoglobin. Refer to Table 7-2 and the manufacturer's insert for other substances that can affect blood reagent strip results.

Leukocyte Esterase

Clinical Significance. Normally, a few white blood cells (leukocytes) are present in urine: 0 to 8 per high-power field or approximately 10 white blood cells per microliter. The number of white blood cells per microliter varies slightly depending on the standardized procedure used to prepare the sediment for microscopic examination. Increased numbers of leukocytes in urine indicate inflammation, which can be present anywhere in the urinary system—from the kidneys to the lower urinary tract (bladder, urethra). The presence of approximately 20 or more white blood cells per microliter is a good indication of a pathologic process. Increased numbers of white blood cells are found more often in urine from women than from men, in part because of the greater incidence of urinary tract infection in women, but also because of the increased potential for a woman's urine to be contaminated with vaginal secretions.

Before the development of reagent strip tests that detect leukocyte esterase, the presence of white blood cells was determined solely by microscopic examination of urine sediment. The chemical detection of leukocyte esterase provides a means to determine the presence of white blood cells even when they are no longer viable or visible. Remember, white blood cells are particularly susceptible to lysis in hypotonic and alkaline urine, as well as from bacteriuria, high storage temperatures, and centrifugation. Therefore, the presence of significant numbers of white blood cells or a large quantity of leukocyte esterase in urine may indicate an inflammatory process within the urinary tract or, in urine from women, could indicate contamination with vaginal secretions.

Increased numbers of white blood cells in urine can be present with or without **bacteriuria** (bacteria in the urine) (see Box 7-4). However, the most commonly encountered cause of **leukocyturia** is a bacterial infection involving the kidneys (pyelonephritis) or the lower

BOX 7-4 | **Diagnostic Utility of Positive Leukocyte Esterase Reaction**

Condition	Possible Cause
Infection in kidneys or urinary tract	Bacteria Nonbacterial: yeast, *Trichomonas vaginalis*, *Chlamydia trachomatis*
Inflammation in kidneys or urinary tract	Acute interstitial nephritis Trauma

urinary tract, such as cystitis or urethritis. In these conditions, leukocyturia is usually accompanied by bacteriuria of varying degrees. In contrast, kidney and urinary tract infections involving trichomonads, mycoses (e.g., yeast), chlamydia, mycoplasmas, viruses, or tuberculosis cause leukocyturia or **pyuria** without bacteriuria.

Methods. Reagent strip tests detect leukocyte esterases that are found in the azurophilic granules of granulocytic leukocytes. These granules are present in the cytoplasm of all granulocytes (neutrophils, eosinophils, and basophils), monocytes, and macrophages. Therefore the reagent strip method does not detect lymphocytes. Several advantages of the leukocyte esterase screening test are its ability (1) to detect the presence of intact and lysed white blood cells, and (2) to serve as a screening test for white blood cells that is independent of procedural variations for sediment preparation.

All reagent strip tests for leukocyte esterase detection are based on the action of the leukocyte esterase to cleave an ester, impregnated in the reagent pad, to form an aromatic compound. Immediately following hydrolysis of the ester, an azocoupling reaction takes place between the aromatic compound produced and a diazonium salt provided on the test pad. The end result is an azo dye with a color change of the reagent pad from beige to violet (Equations 7-3 and 7-4).

Equation 7-3 Esterhydrolysis Reaction

$$\underset{\text{(on pad)}}{\text{Ester}} \xrightarrow[\text{esterases}]{\text{leukocyte}} \underset{\text{Aromatic compound}}{\text{Ar}'}$$

Equation 7-4 Azocoupling Reaction

$$\underset{\text{Diazonium salt (on pad)}}{\text{Ar}-\text{N}^{+}\equiv\text{N}} + \underset{\text{Aromatic compound}}{\text{Ar}'} \xrightarrow{\text{Acid}} \underset{\text{Azo dye}}{\text{Ar}-\text{N}=\text{N}-\text{Ar}'}$$

This screening test for leukocyte esterase initially detects about 10 to 25 white blood cells per microliter. However note that a negative result does not rule out the presence of increased numbers of white blood cells; it only indicates that the amount of leukocyte esterase present is insufficient to produce a positive test. This can occur despite increased numbers of white blood cells when (1) the white blood cells present are lymphocytes, or (2) the urine is significantly dilute (hypotonic). Results for this chemical test often are reported as negative or positive. The quantitative evaluation of white blood cells in urine sediment is part of the microscopic examination; however, lysis of these cells may have occurred.

Therefore this reagent strip test provides a means to identify urine specimens that require further evaluation because of increased quantities of leukocyte esterases (i.e., increased numbers of granulocytic leukocytes).

False-positive results for leukocyte esterase are most often obtained on urine specimens contaminated with vaginal secretions. Other potential sources of false-positive results are drugs or foodstuffs that color the urine red or pink in an acid medium. These substances (e.g., phenazopyridine, nitrofurantoin, beets) mask the reagent pad so that its color resembles that of a positive reaction.

Substances that can reduce the sensitivity of the leukocyte esterase reaction and cause false-negative results include increased protein (500 mg/dL), increased glucose (≥3 g/dL), and high specific gravity. Antibiotics such as gentamicin or cephalosporin and strong oxidizing agents (interfere with reaction pH) can also produce false-negative results.

Note that oxalic acid is not an interferent with the leukocyte esterase reaction when urine is tested. In human urine (without an acid preservative), oxalic acid cannot exist but is present exclusively as its salt—oxalate. This is because human urine always has a pH greater than 4.5. However, if acidifying agents are added to a urine specimen after collection to reduce the pH to 4.4 or lower, oxalate can be converted (reduced) to oxalic acid. If this acidified urine is tested, a falsely low or negative result for leukocyte esterase could be obtained.

Nitrite

Clinical Significance. Routine screening for urine nitrite provides an important tool to identify urinary tract infection. A **urinary tract infection** (UTI) can involve the bladder (cystitis), the renal pelvis and tubules (pyelonephritis), or both. Two pathways for the development of UTI are possible: (1) the movement of bacteria up the urethra into the bladder (ascending infection), and (2) the movement of bacteria from the bloodstream into the kidneys and urinary tract. Ascending infections represent the more prevalent type of UTI. The microorganisms involved are usually gram-negative bacilli that are normal flora of the intestinal tract. The most common infecting microorganism is *Escherichia coli*, followed by *Proteus* species, *Enterobacter* species, and *Klebsiella* species. Urinary tract infection occurs eight times more often in females than in males. In addition, catheterized individuals, regardless of gender, have a high incidence of infection. Various factors involved in the incidence of UTI are discussed under "Tubulointerstitial Disease" and "Urinary Tract Infections" in Chapter 9.

Normally, the bladder and the urine are sterile. This sterility is maintained by the constant flushing action when urine is voided. A UTI can begin as the result of urinary obstruction (e.g., tumor), bladder dysfunction, or urine stasis. Once bacteria have established a bladder infection (cystitis), ascension to the kidneys is possible but is not inevitable. Urinary tract infections can be asymptomatic (asymptomatic bacteriuria), particularly in the elderly, and the nitrite test provides a means of identifying these patients. With early intervention, the spread of infection to the kidneys and the potential to develop renal complications can be prevented.

Screening urine for nitrite and leukocyte esterase provides a means of identifying patients with bacteriuria. Normally, nitrates are consumed in the diet (e.g., in green vegetables) and are excreted in the urine without nitrite formation. When nitrate-reducing bacteria are infecting the urinary tract and adequate bladder retention time is allowed, these bacteria convert dietary nitrate to nitrite. However, not all bacteria contain the enzyme (nitrate reductase) necessary to reduce dietary nitrates to nitrite. Factors that affect nitrite formation and detection include the following: (1) The infecting microbe must be a nitrate reducer, (2) adequate time (a minimum of 4 hours) must be allowed between voids for bacterial conversion of nitrate to nitrite, and (3) adequate dietary nitrate must be consumed and available for conversion. In addition, nitrite detection can be reduced by subsequent conversion by bacteria of nitrite to nitrogen, or by antibiotic therapy that inhibits bacterial conversion of nitrate to nitrite. To appropriately screen for nitrite, the urine specimen of choice is a first morning void or a specimen collected after the urine has been retained in the bladder for at least 4 hours. This latter requirement can be difficult because frequent micturition is a common presenting symptom of UTI.

Note that the screening test for urine nitrite does not replace a traditional urine culture, which can also specifically identify and quantify the bacteria present. The nitrite test simply provides a rapid, indirect means of identifying the presence of nitrate-reducing bacteria in urine at minimal expense. In doing so, the test also helps identify patients with asymptomatic bacteriuria that might otherwise go undiagnosed. See Box 7-5 for diagnostic uses of the nitrite test alone or in combination with the leukocyte esterase.

Methods. Reagent strip tests for nitrite are based on the same principle: the diazotization reaction of nitrite with an aromatic amine to form a diazonium salt, followed by an azocoupling reaction (Equations 7-5 and 7-6). The aromatic amine for the first reaction and the aromatic compound for the second reaction are impregnated in the reagent pad. The azo dye produced from these reactions causes a color change from white to pink.

Equation 7-5

$$\underset{\substack{\text{Aromatic amine}\\\text{(on pad)}}}{Ar-NH_2} + \underset{\text{Nitrite}}{NO_2^-} \xrightarrow{\text{acid}} \underset{\text{Diazonium salt}}{Ar-N^+=N}$$

Equation 7-6

$$\underset{\text{Diazonium salt}}{Ar-N^+=N} + \underset{\substack{\text{Aromatic compound}\\\text{(on pad)}}}{Ar'} \xrightarrow{\text{acid}} \underset{\text{Azo dye}}{Ar-N=N-Ar'}$$

BOX 7-5	Diagnostic Utility of Nitrite* Reaction

Use	Findings
Screening for UTI*	• Positive test indicates possible UTI • Bladder—cystitis • Kidney—pyelonephritis • Urethra—urethritis • In combination with the leukocyte esterase (LE) test, identifies urine specimens that should proceed to urine culture
Monitor treatment effectiveness	Repeat testing after antibiotic therapy to screen for on-going presence of *nitrate-reducing bacteria*

UTI, Urinary tract infection.
*Organisms that do not reduce nitrate to nitrite are not detected, such as non-nitrate reducing bacteria, yeast, trichomonads, and Chlamydia.

Results for nitrite are reported as negative or positive. Any degree of pink color is considered to be a positive result; however, no correlation exists between a positive result and the quantity of bacteria present. In fact, a negative test does not rule out the possibility of bacteriuria because of the factors previously discussed. The sensitivity of the reagent strip test is such that the presence of approximately 1×10^5 organisms or more produces a positive result in most cases. Table 7-2 shows the sensitivity and specificity characteristics of several brands of reagent strips.

Substances that color the urine red or pink in an acid medium (e.g., phenazopyridine, beets) can cause false-positive nitrite results. The color induced from these substances masks the reagent pad and interferes with visual interpretation. In these cases, microscopic examination of urine sediment or a urine culture is the only means of identifying bacteriuria. Improper handling and storage of urine specimens can cause bacterial proliferation and in vitro nitrite formation. These unacceptable specimens could produce positive nitrite results, when in fact no in vivo bacteriuria exists.

High concentrations of ascorbic acid in urine can cause false-negative nitrite results. Ascorbic acid directly reacts with the diazonium salt produced in the diazotization reaction (see Equation 7-5) to form a colorless end product. Consequently, the azocoupling reaction cannot occur and the reaction pad remains negative despite the presence of adequate nitrite. Any factor that inhibits nitrite formation can also cause false-negative results, despite bacteriuria with nitrate-reducing bacteria.

In conclusion, nitrite reagent strips provide a rapid, economical means of detecting significant bacteriuria caused by nitrate-reducing bacteria. The test is a screening test only and is limited by various factors, including microorganism characteristics, dietary factors, bladder retention time, and specimen storage. Despite these disadvantages, the test remains an important part of a routine urinalysis.

Protein

Clinical Significance. Normal urine contains up to 150 mg (1 to 14 mg/dL) of protein each day. This protein originates from the ultrafiltration of plasma and from the urinary tract itself. Proteins of low molecular weight (<40,000) readily pass through the glomerular filtration barriers and are reabsorbed. Because of their low plasma concentration, only small quantities of these proteins appear in the urine. In contrast, albumin, a moderate-molecular-weight protein, has a high plasma concentration. This fact, combined with its ability (although limited) to pass through the filtration barriers, accounts for the small amount of albumin present in normal urine. Actually, less than 0.1% of plasma albumin enters the ultrafiltrate, and 95% to 99% of all filtered protein is reabsorbed. High-molecular-weight proteins (>90,000) are unable to penetrate a healthy glomerular filtration barrier. The end result is that the proteins in normal urine consist of about one-third albumin and two-thirds globulins. Among proteins that originate from the urinary tract itself, three are of particular interest: (1) uromodulin (also known as Tamm-Horsfall protein), which is a mucoprotein synthesized by the distal tubular cells and involved in cast formation, (2) urokinase, which is a fibrinolytic enzyme secreted by tubular cells, and (3) secretory immunoglobulin A, which is synthesized by renal tubular epithelial cells.[4]

The presence of an increased amount of protein in urine, termed **proteinuria**, is often the first indicator of renal disease. For most patients with proteinuria (prerenal and renal), the protein present at an increased concentration is albumin, although to varying degrees. Protein reabsorption by the renal tubules is a nonselective, competitive, and threshold-limited (T_m) process. Basically, when an increased amount of protein is presented to the tubules for reabsorption, the tubules randomly reabsorb the protein in a rate-limited process. As the quantities of proteins other than albumin increase and compete for tubular reabsorption, the amount of albumin excreted in the urine also increases. Proteinuria results from (1) an increase in the quantity of plasma proteins that are filtered, or (2) filtering of the normal quantity of proteins but with a reduction in the reabsorptive ability of the renal tubules. Early detection of proteinuria (i.e., albumin) aids in identification, treatment, and prevention of renal disease. However, protein excretion is not an exclusive feature of renal disorders, and other conditions can also present with proteinuria.

Proteinuria can be classified into four categories: prerenal or overflow proteinuria, glomerular proteinuria, tubular proteinuria, and postrenal proteinuria. This differentiation is based on a combination of protein origination and renal dysfunction; together, they determine the types and sizes of proteins observed in the urine (Box 7-6).

Overflow proteinuria results from increased quantities of plasma proteins in the blood readily passing through theglomerular filtration barriers into the urine. As soon as the level of plasma proteins returns to normal, the proteinuria resolves. Conditions that result in this increased urine excretion of low-molecular-weight plasma proteins include septicemia, with spilling of acute phase reactant proteins; hemoglobinuria, after a hemolytic episode; and myoglobinuria, which follows muscle injury. Immunoglobulin paraproteins (κ and λ monoclonal light chains) are also low-molecular-weight proteins that are abnormally produced in multiple myeloma and macroglobulinemia. These light chain diseases account for approximately 12% of monoclonal gammopathies. Historically, the presence of immunoglobulin light chains, also known as Bence Jones proteins, was identified in urine by their unique solubility as related to temperature. An aliquot of the urine specimen would be heated, and if the urine coagulated at 40° C to 60° C and redissolved at 100° C, this indicated the presence of immunoglobulin light chains, that is, Bence Jones protein. Today, electrophoretic techniques are available to specifically identify and quantitate these light chain proteins.

Renal proteinuria can present with a glomerular pattern, a tubular pattern, or a mixed pattern. Disease can cause changes to glomerular filtration barriers such that increased quantities of plasma proteins are allowed to pass with the ultrafiltrate. In *glomerular proteinuria,* the tubular capacity for protein reabsorption (T_m) is exceeded and an increased amount of protein is excreted in the urine. As stated in Chapter 4, albumin would readily pass through the glomerular filtration barriers if not for its negative charge, which allows only a small amount of albumin to pass. Consequently, any disorder that alters the negativity of glomerular filtration barriers will (1) enable an increased amount of albumin to freely pass, and (2) allow other moderate-molecular-weight proteins of similar charge to pass, such as α_1-antitrypsin, α_1-acid glycoprotein, and transferrin (Box 7-7). The glomeruli are considered to be *selective* if they are able to retard the passage of high-molecular-weight proteins (>90,000) and *nonselective* if discrimination is lost and high-molecular-weight proteins are allowed into the ultrafiltrate.

Glomerular proteinuria occurs in primary glomerular diseases or disorders that cause glomerular damage. It is the most common type of proteinuria encountered and is the most serious clinically. The proteinuria is usually heavy, exceeding 2.5 g/day of total protein, and can be as much as 20 g/day. lists some of the Conditions that can result in glomerular proteinuria are listed in Box 7-6. Glomerular proteinuria can develop into a clinical condition termed the **nephrotic syndrome**. This syndrome is characterized by proteinuria exceeding approximately 3.5 g/day, hypoalbuminemia, hyperlipidemia, lipiduria,

and generalized edema. The nephrotic syndrome is a complication of numerous disorders and is discussed more fully in Chapter 9.

The detection of what seem to be minor increases in urine albumin excretion has particular merit in patients with diabetes, hypertension, or peripheral vascular disease. Although the exact mechanism of proteinuria is not clearly understood in each of these disorders, increased glomerular permeability appears to result from changes in glomerular filtration barriers. With diabetic individuals, the most important factor associated with the development of glomerular proteinuria is hyperglycemia. Because glucose is capable of nonenzymatic binding with various proteins, it apparently combines with proteins of the glomerular filtration barriers, causing glomerular permeability changes and stimulating growth of the mesangial matrix. In health, urine albumin excretion is less than 30 mg/day; when glomerular changes occur in a diabetic individual, urine albumin excretion increases to 30 to 300 mg/day. Because rigorous treatment in the early stages of disease can reverse these changes, chemical methods for the detection of low levels of albumin play an important role. See "Sensitive Albumin Tests" later in this chapter and Chapter 5.

Several conditions, termed *functional proteinurias,* induce a mild glomerular or mixed pattern of proteinuria in the absence of renal disease. Changes in glomerular blood flow (e.g., renal vasoconstriction) and enhanced glomerular permeability appear to be the primary mechanisms involved. Strenuous exercise, fever, extreme cold exposure, emotional distress, congestive heart failure, and dehydration are associated with this type of proteinuria. The amount of protein excreted is usually less than 1 g/day. Functional proteinurias are transitory and resolve with time and with supportive treatment.

Postural (orthostatic) proteinuria is considered to be a functional proteinuria. This condition is characterized by the urinary excretion of protein only when the individual is in an upright (orthostatic) position. A first morning urine specimen is normal in protein content, whereas specimens collected during the day contain elevated quantities of protein. It is theorized that when the patient is in the upright position, increased renal venous pressure causes renal congestion and glomerular changes. Although this condition is considered to be benign, persistent proteinuria may develop, and evidence of glomerular abnormalities has been found by renal biopsy in a few patients.[5] Urine protein excretion in postural proteinuria is usually less than 1.5 g/day. Individuals suspected of having postural proteinuria collect two urine specimens: a first morning specimen and a second specimen collected after the patient has been in an upright position for several hours. If the first specimen is negative for protein and the second is positive, a tentative diagnosis of postural proteinuria can be made. These individuals should be monitored every 6 months and reevaluated as necessary.

BOX 7-6 | **Classification of Proteinuria**

Proteinuria Classification	Proteinuria Description	Proteins Present	Causes
Pre-Renal	Overflow proteinuria: increase *in plasma* low MW proteins leads to increased excretion in urine	Normal proteins: • Myoglobin • Hemoglobin • Acute phase reactants Abnormal proteins: • Ig light chains (Bence Jones protein)	Muscle injury Intravascular hemolysis Infection Inflammation Multiple myeloma
Renal	Glomerular proteinuria: *GFB is defective* allowing plasma proteins to enter ultrafiltrate	*Selective*: Increase in albumin and moderate MW <u>plasma</u> proteins or *Nonselective*: Increase in all proteins, including high MW plasma proteins	Primary glomerular diseases: • Glomerulonephritis • Glomerulosclerosis • Minimal change disease Glomerular *damage* due to: • Poststreptococcal glomerulonephritis • Diabetes mellitus • Lupus erythematosus • Amyloidosis • Sickle cell anemia • Transplant rejection • Infectious disease (malaria, hepatitis B, bacterial endocarditis) • Preeclampsia • Cancers (leukemia, lymphoma) • Drugs (penicillamine, lithium) and toxins (heavy metals) Transitory glomerular *changes*: • Strenuous exercise • Fever, dehydration • Hypertension • Postural (orthostatic) proteinuria • Postpartum period • Extreme cold exposure
	Tubular proteinuria: *defective tubular reabsorption of* protein	Increase in the low MW proteins *normally present* in the ultrafiltrate including albumin	Acute/chronic pyelonephritis Interstitial nephritis Renal tubular acidosis Renal tuberculosis Fanconi's syndrome Systemic diseases—sarcoidosis, lupus erythematosus, cystinosis, galactosemia, Wilson's disease Hemoglobinuria—hemolytic disorders Myoglobinuria—muscle injury Drugs (aminoglycosides, sulfonamides, penicillins, cephalosporins) Toxins and poisons (heavy metals) Transplant rejection Strenuous exercise
Post-Renal	Urine includes proteins produced by the urinary tract or the urine is contaminated with proteins during excretion	Pus Menstrual and hemorrhoidal blood Vaginal secretions Prostatic secretions	Inflammation Malignancy Injury/trauma Contamination during urination

GFB, Glomerular filtration barrier; Ig, immunoglobulin; MW, molecular weight.

BOX 7-7	Principal Proteins in Glomerular Proteinuria

Albumin
Transferrin
α_1-Antitrypsin
α_1-Acid glycoprotein

BOX 7-8	Principal Proteins in Tubular Proteinuria

Albumin
β_2-Microglobulin
Retinol-binding protein
α_2-Microglobulin
α_1-Microglobulin
Lysozyme

Proteinuria that occurs during pregnancy is usually transient and sometimes is associated with delivery, toxemia, or renal infection. A wide range in the amount of protein excreted has been noted. Protein excretion associated with preeclamptic toxemia approaches 3 g/day, whereas minor increases up to 300 mg/day occur with normal pregnancy.

Tubular proteinuria occurs when normal tubular reabsorptive function is altered or impaired. When either occurs, plasma proteins that normally are reabsorbed—such as β_2-microglobulin, retinol-binding protein, α_2-microglobulin, or lysozyme—will be increased in the urine. The urine total protein concentration is usually less than 2.5 g/day, with low-molecular-weight proteins predominating (Box 7-8). Although albumin is found in increased amounts, it does not approach the level found in glomerular proteinuria. In light of this, chemical testing methods that detect predominantly albumin (e.g., reagent strip tests) are limited in their ability to detect increased urine protein.

When tubular proteinuria is suspected, a quantitative urine total protein method should be employed, or a protein precipitation method sensitive to all proteins can be used for screening (e.g., SSA precipitation test). Tubular proteinuria, originally discovered in workers exposed to cadmium dust (a heavy metal), can result from a variety of disorders (see Box 7-6). It can occur alone or with glomerular proteinuria, as in chronic renal disease or renal failure, in which case the urine proteins excreted result in a mixed pattern.

A condition particularly characterized by proximal tubular dysfunction is **Fanconi syndrome.** This syndrome has the following distinctive urine findings: aminoaciduria, proteinuria, glycosuria, and phosphaturia. Associated with inherited and acquired diseases, this syndrome of altered tubular transport mechanisms

retains normal glomerular function. Heavy metal poisoning and the hereditary disease cystinosis are common causes of Fanconi syndrome.

Postrenal proteinuria can result from an inflammatory process anywhere in the urinary tract—in the renal pelves, ureters, bladder (cystitis), prostate, urethra, or external genitalia. Another cause can be the leakage of blood proteins into the urinary tract as a result of injury and hemorrhage. In addition, contamination of urine with vaginal secretions or seminal fluid can result in a positive protein test or proteinuria.

In summary, an increase in urine protein results from (1) increased plasma proteins overflowing into the urine (prerenal); (2) renal changes—glomerular, tubular, or both; or (3) inflammation and postrenal sources. Table 7-6 compares various proteins present in normal urine with urine characteristic of glomerular and tubular renal disease. Note the relative quantity of total protein present, the sizes of proteins that predominate, and the differences in the percentage of protein reabsorbed.

Methods. Historically, qualitative or semiquantitative screening tests for urine protein relied on protein precipitation techniques. Proteins denature upon exposure to extremes of pH or temperature, and the most visible evidence of this is a decrease in solubility. In clinical laboratories, sulfosalicylic acid at room temperature may be used to detect urine protein. This protein precipitation method detects all proteins—albumin and globulins. False-positive precipitation results can be obtained when x-ray contrast media and certain drugs (e.g., penicillins) are present in high concentrations; this can require additional testing before protein results are reported.

Positive urine protein results should be evaluated and correlated with urine specific gravity results. Large volumes of urine (polyuria) can produce a negative protein reaction despite significant proteinuria because the protein present is being excessively diluted. Likewise, a trace amount of protein present in dilute urine indicates greater pathology compared with a trace amount in a concentrated urine. Note that an abnormally high specific gravity (>1.040) is a strong indicator that radiographic contrast media is present. It can be excreted in the urine for up to 3 days after the radiographic procedure and can produce a delayed positive protein precipitation test[3] (see "Sulfosalicylic Acid Precipitation Test").

Once the presence of an increased amount of urine protein has been established, accurate methods are available to differentiate and quantify the proteins. Electrophoresis, nephelometry, turbidimetry, and radial immunodiffusion methods are used and are discussed at length in clinical chemistry textbooks. Despite the qualitative or semiquantitative nature of the protein tests discussed in this chapter, they remain vital tools in the detection and monitoring of diseases that cause proteinuria.

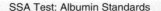

SSA Test: Albumin Standards

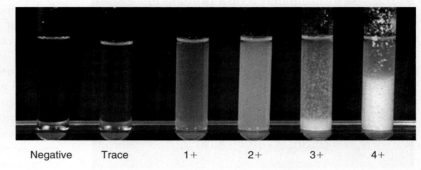

Negative   Trace   1+   2+   3+   4+

FIGURE 7-3 A series of albumin standards analyzed using the sulfosalicylic acid precipitation test.

TABLE 7-6	Characterization of Renal Proteinuria		
	Normal	Glomerular Disease	Tubular Disease
Total protein, g/day	<0.15	>2.5	<2.5
Albumin, mg/day	50	>500	<500
β_2-Microglobulin, mg/day	0.150	0.150	20
Tubular reabsorption of filtered proteins, %	95	3	50

Modified from Waller KV, Ward MW, Mahan JD, et al: Current concepts in proteinuria, Clin Chem 35:755-765, 1989.

Sulfosalicylic Acid Precipitation Test. Various procedures are available for performance of the SSA test; these methods differ in terms of the volume of centrifuged urine used (3 mL vs. 11 mL) and the concentration of the SSA reagent (3.0% vs. 7.0%). Despite these differences, the final solution concentration (urine plus reagent) is the same: 0.015 g of SSA per milliliter of total solution.

Because particulate matter suspended in urine can interfere with turbidity assessment, the SSA test is performed on clear supernatant urine following centrifugation. The urine supernate and the reagent are added together and mixed by inversion. After a 10-minute, room temperature incubation, the tube is inverted and evaluated. With the use of ordinary room light, the precipitation reaction is graded as negative, trace, 1+, 2+, 3+, or 4+ according to a predetermined protocol (Figure 7-3 and Table 7-7). Some institutions replace the plus grading system with concentration values (milligrams per deciliter) corresponding to the standards used or the albumin values obtained when reagent strips are used. The SSA method is sensitive to 5 to 10 mg/dL of protein, regardless of the type of protein present.

If the presence of radiographic contrast media is suspected in a specimen because of an abnormally high specific gravity result, or if lack of correlation is noted between the SSA method and the reagent strip method, the SSA precipitate should be viewed microscopically.

Drugs (e.g., penicillins) and contrast media form crystalline precipitates, whereas protein precipitates are amorphous. When the SSA result is crystalline, protein results obtained by using the reagent strip can be reported. When the SSA precipitate is amorphous, the discrepancy between the SSA and the reagent strip method is highly indicative of the presence of urinary proteins other than albumin (e.g., globulins, Bence Jones proteins), and further investigation (e.g., protein electrophoresis) is required.

Although a rare occurrence, false-negative or decreased SSA results for protein can be obtained with highly buffered or extremely alkaline (pH ≥9.0) urine. In the latter case, the precipitating reagent (acid) is neutralized, leading to erroneous results. Because urine specimens exceeding pH 8.0 are not physiologically possible and indicate contamination or improper storage, they should not be used. However, if highly alkaline urine is acidified to approximately pH 5.0 and is retested using SSA, an accurate protein result can be obtained.[6]

Note that the SSA test should not be used to confirm a protein result obtained by reagent strip because it lacks protein specificity, and its sensitivity varies with the proteins present.

Reagent Strip Tests. Commercial reagent strips available for routine protein screening use the same principle, originally described by Sorenson in 1909, and termed the **protein error of indicators.** When the pH is held constant by a buffer, certain indicator dyes release hydrogen ions as a result of the presence of proteins (anions), causing a color change. The reaction pad is impregnated with a buffer that maintains the test area at pH 3.0. If protein is present, it acts as a hydrogen receptor, accepting hydrogen ions from the pH indicator and thereby causing a color change (Equation 7-7).

Equation 7-7

$$\underset{\text{dye}}{\text{Indicator}} + \underset{\text{(albumin)}}{\text{Protein}} \xrightarrow{\text{pH 3.0}} \underset{\text{(blue-green)}}{\text{H}^+ \text{ ions released from indicator}}$$

The intensity of the color change is directly related to the amount of protein present. Protein reagent strip results are reported as concentrations in milligrams per deciliter (mg/dL) by matching the resultant reaction pad

TABLE 7-7	Sulfosalicylic Acid Precipitation Grading Guideline	
Result	Observations	Appropriate Protein Concentration*
Negative	No turbidity or increase in turbidity • When the tube is viewed from the top, a circle is visible in the bottom of the test tube†	<5 mg/dL
Trace	Perceptible turbidity • When the tube is viewed from the top, a circle is *not* visible in the test tube bottom • Can read newsprint through mixture	5-20 mg/dL
1+	Distinct turbidity *without* discrete granulation • *Cannot* read newsprint through mixture	30 mg/dL
2+	Turbidity with granulation; *no* flocculation‡	100 mg/dL
3+	Turbidity with granulation *and* flocculation	300 mg/dL
4+	Large clumps of precipitate or a solid mass	≥500 mg/dL

*This value correlates with the reagent strip result if the only protein present is albumin.

†While holding a test tube filled with a clear solution vertically, view the bottom of the tube looking through the solution from the top. A circle formed by the tube bottom is visible. As a solution increases in turbidity, this circle will no longer be evident.

‡Flocculation is the association of particulates or precipitates to form small clumps or aggregates called *floc*.

TABLE 7-8	Comparison of Reagent Strip and SSA Protein Test Results	
Reagent Strip Result	SSA Result	Possible Explanations
Positive	Negative	• Highly alkaline or buffered urine *with no albumin present* – False positive reagent strip test • Highly alkaline or buffered urine *with albumin present* – False negative SSA test • To differentiate, acidify urine to pH ~5.0 and retest.
Negative	Positive*	• Protein other than albumin present • Radiographic contrast media present • Drugs and/or drug metabolites present

*Examine precipitate microscopically—drugs and radiographic media form crystalline precipitates; whereas, protein precipitates are amorphous.

color with the color chart provided on the reagent strip container.

This method is more sensitive to albumin than to any other protein, and negative results will occur despite the presence of other proteins. Table 7-8 provides a comparison of the reagent strip protein test to the SSA precipitation method. Globulins, myoglobin, hemoglobin, immunoglobulin light chains (Bence Jones proteins), and mucoproteins are usually not detected by the reagent strip test because the concentration of these proteins are usually insufficient to cause a color change. For example, when the reagent strip blood result is *less than* large (i.e., trace, small, or moderate), the concentration of hemoglobin is not high enough to contribute to the protein result.

Extremely alkaline (pH ≥9.0) or highly buffered urine can overwhelm the buffering capacity of the reaction pad to produce false-positive results. As with protein precipitation methods, adjusting the urine with acid to approximately pH 5.0 and retesting using the reagent strip test will produce an accurate protein result.

Tubular reabsorption of protein is a nonselective, competitive process. When an increased amount of protein is presented to the tubules for reabsorption, the tubules randomly reabsorb protein through a rate-limited process. As a result, the amount of albumin in urine increases as other proteins, which are normally not present, compete for reabsorption. Hence the reagent strip detection of albumin is often capable of detecting most instances of proteinuria.

Sensitive Albumin Tests. Identification and management of patients at risk for kidney disease are enhanced greatly by the detection and monitoring of urine albumin excretion. Routine reagent strip methods are unable to detect the low levels of albumin excretion (10 to 20 mg/L *or* 1 to 2 mg/dL) that are clinically significant; hence sensitive albumin screening tests were developed. Periodic monitoring of urine for low-level albumin excretion greatly benefits individuals with diabetes, hypertension, or peripheral vascular disease. These patients have been shown to develop low-level **albuminuria** before nephropathy. Studies have demonstrated that early intervention to reduce hyperglycemia in diabetic patients or to normalize blood pressure in hypertensive people can reduce progression to clinical nephropathy.[7-9]

Several commercial reagent strip methods are available to screen urine for low-level increases in albumin; they include the OSOM ImmunoDip urine albumin test (Sekisui Diagnostics Corporation, Framingham, MA), the Micral test (Roche Diagnostics), the Multistix PRO reagent strip test, and the Clinitek Microalbumin reagent strip test (Siemens Healthcare Diagnostics Inc.) (Table 7-9).

TABLE 7-9 | **Sensitive Albumin (Microalbumin) Tests**

Test	Principle	Detection Limit*	Reaction Time	Specificity
Immunodip[10]	Immunochemical; albumin binds antibody-coated blue latex particles; saturated and unsaturated albumin- antibody complexes are isolated and differentiated by migration on strip; intensity comparison of two blue bands determines albumin concentration.	12-18 mg/L (1.2-1.8 mg/dL)	3 minutes; color stable 8 hours	No interferences known
Micral test strips[11,12]	Immunochemical; albumin binds gold-labeled antibody-enzyme conjugate; albumin-bound complex migrates to detection pad, where bound enzyme converts substrate on pad to red chromophore; color intensity increases with albumin concentration.	15-20 mg/L (1.5-2.0 mg/dL)	1 minute; color stable ≤5 minutes	*False-positive results:* • Oxytetracycline • Strong oxidizing agents (e.g., soaps, detergents) *False-negative results:* • Urine specimen temperature <10° C (<50° F)
CLINITEK Microalbumin test strips[13,14,15]	*Albumin test* Dye binding; at a constant pH, albumin causes a sulfonephthalein dye impregnated in the pad to change color. *Note:* Strips can only be read instrumentally; manufacturer permits no visual interpretation.	20-40 mg/dL (2.0-4.0 mg/dL)	≈2 minutes	*Albumin and creatinine tests* *False-positive results:* • Hemoglobin or myoglobin (≥5 mg/dL) • Highly colored substances mask results, such as drugs (phenazopyridine, nitrofurantoin), beet ingestion • Strong oxidizing agents (e.g., soaps, detergents) • Cimetidine (creatinine only)
Creatinine	*Creatinine test* Creatinine reacts with copper to form a complex that possesses peroxidase activity; peroxide on the pad is reduced, tetramethylbenzidine is oxidized, and a chromogen produces a color change; creatinine concentration is determined by comparing the color of the reaction pad to color blocks provided on the container.	100 mg/L (10.0 mg/dL)		
Multistix PRO test strips[14,15]	*Albumin test* Same principle as Clinitek Microalbumin test strips; however, detection limit differs. Results can be interpreted visually (or instrumentally).	80-150 mg/L (8.0-15.0 mg/dL)	≈1 minute	Same as CLINITEK Microalbumin test strips
Protein: low	Visual interpretation: Protein: low (albumin) concentration is determined by comparing color of the reaction pad to color blocks provided on the container.			
Creatinine	*Creatinine test* Same principle as Clinitek Microalbumin test strips. Results can be interpreted visually (or instrumentally). Visual interpretation: Creatinine concentration is determined by comparing color of the reaction pad to color blocks provided on the container.	100 mg/L (10.0 mg/dL)		

*Sensitive albumin tests typically report protein concentration in mg/L. Concentrations in mg/dL are provided to enable rapid comparison with reagent strip and SSA methods.

The ImmunoDip test is an immunochemical-based reagent strip reaction housed in a hard plastic case or stick. The test stick is placed into the urine specimen such that the vent hole located near one end is completely immersed. The unique design of the plastic housing controls the rate of urine flow over the reagent strip and the amount of urine that participates in the reaction. Another benefit of this unique housing is that once the test is completed, the result remains fixed and can be read up to 8 hours after testing without deterioration. Urine enters the vent hole of the test stick, and albumin, if present, binds to monoclonal antibodies that are coupled to blue latex particles on the test pad. The degree of saturation of the latex particles with urine albumin determines the location to which the albumin-antibody-latex particle complex ultimately migrates by capillary action. Unsaturated complexes bind to the lower band or zone on the reagent strip, whereas saturated complexes migrate to the top zone.[10] Comparing the intensity of the two blue bands provides semiquantitative albumin results. A lower band that is darker than the top band indicates an albumin concentration less than 12 mg/L (1.2 mg/dL); bands of equal intensity indicate an albumin level of 12 to 18 mg/L (1.2 to 1.8 mg/dL); and a top band darker than the lower band indicates an albumin concentration of 20 mg/L (2.0 mg/dL) or greater.

The Micral test uses gold-labeled monoclonal antibodies in its immunochemical reagent strip test.In this reaction, albumin in the urine binds with a soluble antibody-enzyme conjugate that is impregnated on the reaction pad. Only the albumin-conjugate immunocomplex, moving by capillary action, passes into the reaction zone of the strip, because an intermediate zone immobilizes any excess, unbound conjugate. Once in the reaction zone, the enzyme (β-galactosidase) bound to the antibody reacts with the substrate (chlorophenol red galactoside) in the reaction zone to produce a red dye.[11,12] Timing and technique are crucial; therefore the manufacturer's instructions must be followed to ensure accurate test results. The Micral Test method is capable of detecting as little as 15 to 20 mg/L (1.5 to 2 mg/dL) of human albumin in urine. A color chart to determine albumin results from 0 to 100 mg/L (0 to 10 mg/dL) is provided on the reagent strip container.

The CLINITEK Microalbumin reagent strip and Multistix PRO reagent strip (Siemens Healthcare Diagnostics Inc.) tests use a dye-binding method to determine low levels of urine albumin.[13,14] A high-affinity sulfonephthalein dye impregnated in the pad changes color when it binds albumin. A buffer also impregnated on the reaction pad maintains a constant pH to ensure optimal protein discrimination and reactivity for albumin.[16] The development of any blue color is due to the presence of albumin, and color changes on the reaction pad range from pale green to aqua blue. The CLINITEK Microalbumin reagent strip test, which must be read

instrumentally, is able to detect albumin concentrations of 20 to 40 mg/L (2 to 4 mg/dL). In contrast, Multistix PRO reagent strips can be read visually or instrumentally, and the lowest level of protein detection is approximately 150 mg/L (15 mg/dL). Although these strips use essentially the identical chemical reaction, their sensitivity and the manufacturer-recommended reporting terminology differ, that is, milligrams per liter (mg/L) of albumin for the CLINITEK Microalbumin reagent strip test and milligrams per deciliter (mg/dL) of protein—low for the Multistix PRO reagent strip test.

Both reagent strips also include a reaction pad that determines semiquantitatively the urine creatinine concentration. Creatinine in the urine reacts with copper sulfate impregnated in the pad to form a copper-creatinine complex that possesses peroxidase activity.[15] The reaction pad also is impregnated with a chromogen (tetramethylbenzidine) and a peroxide. Once the copper-creatinine complex is formed, it causes the peroxide to be reduced and the chromogen to oxidize, producing a color change on the reaction pad from orange to green (Equations 7-8 and 7-9). Note the similarity of this indicator reaction to that universally used in reagent strip tests for blood (see Equation 7-2).

Equation 7-8

$$Cu^{2+} + Creatinine \rightarrow Cu - Creatinine\ complex$$

Equation 7-9

$$H_2O_2 + Chromogen* \xrightarrow{Cu\text{-}creatinine\ complex} Oxidized\ chromogen + H_2O$$

*Tetramethylbenzidine.

The inclusion of 4-hydroxy-2-methylquinoline in the reaction pad reduces interference from ascorbic acid and hemoglobin to greater than 22 mg/dL and 5 mg/dL, respectively.[15] Assessment of albumin (protein) and creatinine on these reagent strips enables the estimation of an albumin-to-creatinine (A/C) or protein-to-creatinine ratio. For the Multistix PRO reagent strips, a table is provided to determine whether the protein-to-creatinine ratio is normal or abnormal. In contrast, the CLINITEK Microalbumin reagent strips, which are read instrumentally, report an estimate of the A/C ratio numerically as "less than 30 mg/g" (normal), "30 to 300 mg/g" (abnormal), or "greater than 300 mg/g" (abnormal). Conversion of results to SI units (i.e., milligrams of albumin per millimoles of creatinine) is also an option.

Note that not all positive sensitive albumin tests provide evidence of abnormality because extremely low levels of urine albumin, that is, concentrations less than 20 mg/L (<2.0 mg/dL), are considered normal. Low-level transient increases in albumin can occur with strenuous exercise, dehydration, and acute illness with fever. Keep in mind that overhydration (dilute urine) can mask increased urine albumin excretion. In these situations, determination of an A/C or protein-to-creatinine ratio reduces the numbers of false-positive and false-negative test results. Simultaneous urine creatinine measurement, as with CLINITEK Microalbumin and Multistix PRO reagent strips, accounts for these hydration effects and results in useful estimates of the A/C ratio or the protein-to-creatinine ratio.[16] For example, concentrated urine that contains a small amount of protein can be correctly identified as "normal," whereas a dilute urine specimen with a small amount of protein can be correctly identified as "abnormal."

In summary, periodic monitoring for low-level urine albumin excretion should be performed for individuals at increased risk for developing kidney disease, such as those with hypertension or diabetes (type 1 or type 2). Early identification of kidney changes enables early intervention. Before a diagnosis of microalbuminuria is made, a positive screening test should be confirmed with a quantitative protein assay.

Glucose

Clinical Significance. The presence of glucose in urine is termed **glucosuria** (or **glycosuria**). Normally, all glucose that passes through the glomerular filtration barrier into the ultrafiltrate is actively reabsorbed by the proximal renal tubules. However, tubular reabsorption of glucose is a threshold-limited process with a maximum reabsorptive capacity (T_m) averaging about 350 mg/min. The T_m for glucose differs with gender and body surface area, ranging from 250 to 360 mg/min in females and from 295 to 455 mg/min in males. When the level of glucose in the blood exceeds its renal threshold level of approximately 160 to 180 mg/dL, the ultrafiltrate concentration of glucose exceeds the reabsorptive ability of the tubules, and glucosuria occurs.

Glucosuria is caused by (1) a prerenal condition (hyperglycemia), or (2) a renal condition (defective tubular absorption). Diabetes mellitus is the most common disease that causes hyperglycemia and glucosuria. This disease is characterized by ineffective glucose utilization caused by inadequate insulin secretion or abnormal insulin action. As a result, patients with undiagnosed or inadequately controlled diabetes have blood glucose concentrations that exceed the renal threshold level, and glucosuria occurs. The clinical presentation of diabetes mellitus varies; often individuals are asymptomatic, and initial detection results from a routine blood or urine test. Because diabetes mellitus is a leading cause of death in the United States, and because early intervention and treatment can prevent or delay the many long-term complications of this disease, routine screening of urine for glucose is an important part of a urinalysis.

Conditions other than diabetes mellitus can cause hyperglycemia with glucosuria. These conditions include various hormonal disorders, liver disease, pancreatic disease, central nervous system damage, and drugs (Box 7-9). The causes, presentation, and treatments of these diseases differ; the common link is inadequate utilization of glucose, which causes glucosuria. Therefore when a

BOX 7-9	Presentations of Glucosuria and Associated Disorders
Findings	**Disorders**
Prerenal: Hyperglycemia with Glucosuria	Diabetes mellitus
	Hormonal disorders
	• Increased thyroid hormone—hyperthyroidism
	• Increased growth hormone—acromegaly
	• Increased epinephrine and glucocorticoids—stress, anxiety, and Cushings disease
	Liver disease
	Pancreatic disease
	Cerebrovascular accident (stroke)
	Drugs—thiazides, corticosteroids, oral contraceptives
	Pregnancy
Renal: Defective tubular reabsorption; glucosuria with normal plasma glucose	Fanconi's syndrome
	End stage renal disease
	Cystinosis
	Heavy metal poisoning
	Genetic disorders
	Pregnancy

patient has glucosuria, further evaluation of the blood and urine is required to identify the specific disease process.

It is possible for an individual to have hyperglycemia without glucosuria. Glucose freely passes through the glomerular filtration barriers; however, if these barriers are compromised because of disease, the glomerular filtration rate can be decreased. In these cases, hyperglycemia can be present, but because of a decreased glomerular filtration rate, only limited amounts of glucose are able to pass into the ultrafiltrate. The tubules are able to reabsorb all the glucose presented to them, and glucosuria is not present. Any disease that decreases the glomerular filtration rate, such as renal arteriosclerosis or low cardiac output, can result in hyperglycemia without glucosuria. Figure 7-2 summarizes glucosuria mechanisms and their relationship to hyperglycemia and renal tubular function.

Sugars other than glucose can appear in the urine, although, like glucose, they are normally not present. Various circumstances can cause the urinary excretion of other sugars such as galactose, fructose, lactose, maltose, or pentose. The most significant of these is the excretion of galactose because it signifies a disease (galactosemia) that has severe and irreversible consequences. Galactosemia is an inherited disorder characterized by an inability to metabolize galactose to glucose. The genetic defect varies, but all forms involve the reduction or absence of an enzyme required for galactose metabolism. Galactose 1-phosphate uridyl

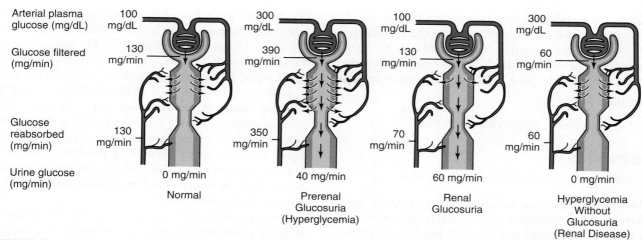

Arterial plasma glucose (mg/dL)	100 mg/dL	300 mg/dL	100 mg/dL	300 mg/dL
Glucose filtered (mg/min)	130 mg/min	390 mg/min	130 mg/min	60 mg/min
Glucose reabsorbed (mg/min)	130 mg/min	350 mg/min	70 mg/min	60 mg/min
Urine glucose (mg/min)	0 mg/min	40 mg/min	60 mg/min	0 mg/min
	Normal	Prerenal Glucosuria (Hyperglycemia)	Renal Glucosuria	Hyperglycemia Without Glucosuria (Renal Disease)

FIGURE 7-2 A schematic diagram comparing the filtration and reabsorption of glucose by proximal tubular cells normally and in conditions of hyperglycemia and renal tubular disease.

transferase (GALT) is the enzyme involved in the most common, classical form (see Chapter 9 for additional discussion of galactosemias). Lactose is a disaccharide of D-galactose and D-glucose. It is present in milk and is the principal dietary source of galactose. Infants born with an enzyme deficiency to metabolize galactose must be recognized at birth, so that milk can be eliminated from their diet. If this deficiency goes undetected, the increased concentration of galactose in the infant's blood causes the formation of toxic intermediate products of metabolism (e.g., galactonate, galactitol), which cause irreversible brain damage. With classical galactosemia (GALT), galactonate accumulates and the infant fails to thrive, vomits, and has diarrhea, hepatomegaly, and jaundice. With rarer enzyme deficiencies, galactitol is formed, which causes cataract formation in newborns. If these conditions are recognized early, galactose can be eliminated from the diet, resulting in normal growth and development. Detection of galactose and other reducing sugars in urine relies on tests for reducing substances. Because galactosemia has serious complications and is life threatening, blood screening (heelstick) of newborn infants for classical galactosemia (GALT) is mandated in the United States. In addition, it is a common practice for laboratories to routinely screen the urine from children younger than 2 years for reducing substances.

Lactose may be found in the urine of pregnant women or of premature infants. Rarely, urine may contain fructose as the result of excessive fruit or honey ingestion; pentoses (xylose and arabinose) from excessive fruit ingestion (e.g., plums, cherries) or from a rare genetic defect; or maltose and glucose together in some diabetic patients. Of the many sugars that can be present in urine, only glucose and galactose signify pathologic conditions.

The diagnostic utility of urine glucose testing is summarized in Box 7-10. Because sugars are not normally

BOX 7-10	Diagnostic Utility of Urine Glucose Testing

Test	Reason
Glucose Reagent Strip test	Screen for diabetes mellitus
Combination of Glucose Reagent Strip test and Clinitest	Screen for inherited metabolic diseases that involve **reducing** sugars • Galactose:* screen urine from children <2 y • Lactose, fructose, maltose, pentose

*Blood testing of newborn infants for "classical" galactosemia (GALT) is mandated by law in the United States.

excreted in the urine, a routine urinalysis should include a screening test for them. The sugar most commonly encountered is glucose; however, in children younger than 2 years, it is important to test for any reducing sugar. Note that other reducing substances can also be present in the urine (e.g., homogentisic acid, ascorbic acid, salicylates). Consequently, urine specimens that produce a positive reduction test require further evaluation to identify the reductant present (see "Copper Reduction Tests").

Methods

Reagent Strip Tests. Urine screening for glucose dates back to the Babylonians and the Egyptians, who tasted urine to detect the presence of urinary sugars. Now urine glucose screening by a reagent strip test is a cost-effective, noninvasive means of identifying individuals with glucosuria. The glucose reagent strip was the first "dip and read" reagent strip developed by Miles, Inc., in 1950. Glucose reagent strip tests use a double sequential enzyme reaction and detect *only* glucose (Equations 7-10 and 7-11). Glucose oxidase impregnated on the reaction pad rapidly catalyzes the oxidation of glucose to form hydrogen peroxide and gluconic acid. The hydrogen peroxide formed oxidizes the chromogen on the pad in the presence of peroxidase. The color change observed depends on the chromogen used in the reaction, which varies with the brand of reagent strips.

Equation 7-10

$$Glucose + O_2 \xrightarrow[oxidase]{glucose} Gluconic\ acid + H_2O_2$$

Equation 7-11

$$H_2O_2 + Chromogen \xrightarrow{peroxidase} Oxidized\ chromogen + H_2O$$

Results are reported as negative (or normal), and positive tests are assessed quantitatively in concentration units of milligrams per deciliter (mg/dL) or grams per deciliter (g/dL). Because virtually all glucose is reabsorbed by the renal tubules, a urine concentration of less than 20 mg/dL is considered normal, and the sensitivity of glucose reagent strips is adjusted to avoid detection of these small amounts of glucose (see Table 7-2). Specific gravity and temperature can modify the sensitivity of the reagent strip for glucose. As the urine specific gravity increases or the temperature of the urine decreases (e.g., refrigeration), the sensitivity of the reagent strip to glucose is decreased. Similarly, high concentrations of urine ketones, that is, ketonuria (≥40 mg/dL), can reduce the sensitivity of the reagent strip to low glucose concentrations (75 to 125 mg/dL). However, ketonuria occurs when glucose is inadequate (starvation), or when the glucose that is present cannot be proper metabolized (diabetes). In the former situation, no glucose is excreted in the urine, and in the latter case, the amount of glucose present in the urine is usually very large. In other words, the possibility of significant ketonuria with low-level glucosuria is rarely encountered.

False-positive reagent strip tests for glucose can be caused by strong oxidizing agents (e.g., sodium hypochlorite) or contaminating peroxides that directly interact with the chromogen. However, because of the specificity of the reagent strip for glucose, false-negative results are common. Ascorbic acid in concentrations of 50 mg/dL or more directly reduces the hydrogen peroxide produced in the first reaction. Consequently, the chromogen is not oxidized and a false-negative result can be obtained. Routine ascorbic acid detection performed simultaneously with glucose screening enables detection of false-negative results.[18] The difference between no glucose and low levels of glucose in urine directly impacts disease management; therefore testing should not be compromised. Improper storage of urine specimens should be avoided because bacterial glycolysis can cause false-negative results.

Copper Reduction Tests. In the 19th century, the copper reduction ability of some sugars in an alkaline medium was discovered, and the term *reducing sugar* was coined. Glucose, fructose, galactose, lactose, maltose,

and pentose are a few of the reducing sugars; common table sugar, sucrose, is not a reducing sugar. The reducing ability of a sugar is determined by the presence of the reducing group ($\!>\!C = O$), which is present in all monosaccharides. In some disaccharides, the reducing group is used in its formation (a glycosidic linkage), and the resultant sugar is nonreducing (e.g., sucrose). As a medical student, Stanley Benedict modified the original, time-consuming copper reduction test into a practical liquid test.[19] A tablet version of Benedict's test is the Clinitest reagent tablet (Siemens Healthcare Diagnostics Inc.), which is widely used in clinical laboratories to detect reducing substances.

Copper reduction tests are based on the ability of reducing substances to convert cupric sulfate to cuprous oxide, which results in a color change from blue to green to orange. Clinitest tablets contain all the reagents necessary for this reaction: anhydrous copper sulfate, sodium hydroxide, citric acid, and sodium bicarbonate. A mixture of approximately 0.25 mL of urine (5 drops) and 0.50 mL of water (10 drops) is prepared in a test tube, and one reagent tablet is added. The tube is allowed to stand undisturbed. During this period, the mixture bubbles as citric acid and sodium bicarbonate react to form carbon dioxide (CO_2). This gas blankets the reaction mixture and prevents room air from participating in the chemical reaction. At the same time, this chemical reaction is promoted by heat generated from the interaction of sodium hydroxide and water. Fifteen seconds *after* the bubbling reaction stops, the tube is shaken, and the color of the mixture is compared to a color chart provided (Figure 7-4). Equation 7-12 depicts the reaction.

Equation 7-12

$$\underset{(blue)}{CuSO_4} + \underset{substance}{Reducing} \xrightarrow{Heat\ and\ alkali} \underset{(yellow)}{CuOH} + \underset{(red)}{Cu_2O} + \underset{substance}{Oxidized} + H_2O$$

Clinitest results must be evaluated immediately, and any color change that occurs after 15 seconds is ignored. When the color change is not read at 15 seconds after bubbling ceases, falsely low results may be reported if the pass-through phenomenon took place. The pass-through phenomenon occurs in the presence of high concentrations of reducing substances and is evidenced by the color of the mixture "passing through" all colors possible. In other words, it becomes orange (the highest concentration) but then proceeds to change back to green-brown (a low concentration). The mechanism for this phenomenon is the reoxidation of the resultant cuprous oxide to cupric oxide and other cupric complexes (green). Reoxidation can occur in the presence of high concentrations of reducing substances or following exposure of the reaction mixture to room air after the protective CO_2 gas blanket disperses. To observe this phenomenon within the 15-second reaction period, very high glucose concentrations must be present. If the reaction mixture is not observed during testing

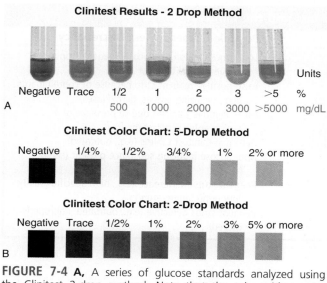

FIGURE 7-4 **A,** A series of glucose standards analyzed using the Clinitest 2-drop method. Note that the tube with greater than 5000 mg/dL glucose has demonstrated the "pass-through" effect (i.e., after reaction, the mixture returns to a greenish color). **B,** Clinitest color charts. Note the subtle differences between the 5-drop and 2-drop color charts. It is essential that reaction mixtures be compared with the proper color chart to obtain accurate results. *Do not use these color charts for diagnostic testing.*

BOX 7-11	Reducing Substances in Urine That Cause Copper Reduction Tests

Sugars
Monosaccharides
Glucose
Fructose
Disaccharides
Galactose
Lactose
Maltose
Pentoses
Arabinose
Ribose

Ascorbic Acid
Vitamins or fruits
Drug preparations (e.g., intravenous tetracycline)

Drugs and Their Metabolites
Salicylates
Penicillin
Cephalosporins
Nalidixic acid
Sulfonamides

Cysteine

Homogentisic Acid

and the 15-second time period is exceeded, the color observed (after the pass-through) may no longer indicate the high glucose concentration, and falsely low results may be reported. Note that adherence to the manufacturer's procedural directions will avoid this potential technical error.

An alternate approach to quantifying high glucose concentrations is to perform the Clinitest method using 2 drops of urine instead of the usual 5 drops. Whereas the 5-drop method can detect 250 mg/dL (0.25 g/dL) glucose, the 2-drop method requires a minimum of 350 mg/dL (0.35 g/dL) to obtain a positive result. An advantage of the 2-drop method is that it enables glucose quantitation up to 5 g/dL and reduces the possibility of the pass-through effect. Semiquantitative results in grams per deciliter are obtained by comparison with the appropriate color chart, with different charts provided for the 5-drop and 2-drop methods.

Copper reduction tests are nonspecific, and reducing substances in urine, other than sugars, can produce positive results when present in significant amounts. Box 7-11 provides a partial listing of these reducing substances. Although creatinine, ketone bodies, and uric acid are reducing substances, the amounts present in urine, even in extreme cases, are usually insufficient to produce a positive Clinitest result. Ascorbic acid is the most commonly encountered agent that produces positive copper reduction tests in the absence of glucose. It can also cause a discrepancy between the results obtained using the glucose reagent strip test and the Clinitest method. Radiographic contrast media can cause

false-negative or decreased results. Urine of low specific gravity appears to increase the sensitivity of the Clinitest method slightly, whereas sulfonamide metabolites or methapyrilene compounds interfere with the reaction, causing decreased results.

As was previously mentioned, the excretion of glucose or galactose is pathologically significant. Therefore urine from children younger than 2 years should be tested with a copper reduction test to screen for reducing substances that are formed as a result of galactosemia. When a reducing sugar other than glucose is determined to be present, and galactosemia is suspected, blood tests are used to definitively identify classical (GALT) and variant forms of galactosemia.

Comparison of the Clinitest Method and Glucose Reagent Strip Tests. Because glucose reagent strip tests have a lower detection limit than the Clinitest method, it is possible to obtain a negative Clinitest result and a positive glucose reagent strip test on a urine specimen. These results would indicate a low concentration of glucose (approximately 40 to 200 mg/dL). If, however, the Clinitest result is positive and the glucose reagent strip result is negative, a reducing substance other than glucose is present. In either case, it is assumed that all reagents and strips are functioning properly. Outdated reagent strips or tablets, as well as contaminating agents, could produce similar result combinations (Table 7-10). Because Clinitest tablets are hygroscopic—they take up and retain water—protecting them from moisture, light,

Glucose Reagent Strip Test	Clinitest Tablet Test	Possible Causes of Test Discrepancy
TABLE 7-10	**Comparison of the Glucose Reagent Strip Test and the Clinitest Tablet Test**	
Positive	Negative	Low concentration of glucose, reagent strip more sensitive than Clinitest False-positive reagent strip because of contaminants (e.g., oxidizing agents, peroxidases) False negative Clinitest due to presence of radiographic contrast media Defective Clinitest tablets (e.g., outdated)
Negative	Positive	Non-glucose reducing substance present (see Box 7-11) Reagent strip interference (e.g., high specific gravity, low urine temperature) Reagent strips defective (e.g., outdated, improperly stored)

and heat is imperative. These tablets should be visually inspected before use to ensure their integrity.

Ketones

Formation. The terms *ketones* and *ketone bodies* identify three intermediate products of fatty acid metabolism: acetoacetate, β-hydroxybutyrate, and acetone (Figure 7-5). Normally, the end products of fatty acid metabolism are carbon dioxide and water, and no measurable ketones are produced. However, when carbohydrate availability is limited, the liver must oxidize fatty acids as its main metabolic substrate. As a result, large amounts of acetyl coenzyme A are formed, and the Krebs cycle becomes overwhelmed. To handle the increased acetyl coenzyme A load, the liver mitochondria begin active ketogenesis. Large quantities of ketones are released into the bloodstream (ketonemia) and provide energy to the brain, heart, skeletal muscles, and kidneys.

The amount of each ketone body in the blood varies with the severity of the condition. However, the average distribution of ketones in serum and urine is 78% β-hydroxybutyrate, 20% acetoacetate, and 2% acetone. When the blood ketone concentration exceeds 70 mg/dL (the renal threshold level), ketones are excreted in the urine.[20] This condition is termed **ketonuria.** Because acetone is also eliminated by the lungs, the breath of patients with ketonemia has a distinctive acetonic or fruity odor.

Clinical Significance. Normally when carbohydrates are available, ketone synthesis is inhibited, blood ketone levels are 3 mg/dL or less, and urine ketone excretion is about 20 mg/day. Any condition that causes increased fat metabolism can result in ketonemia and ketonuria. These conditions can be divided into one of three categories: (1) an inability to use carbohydrates, (2) an inadequate carbohydrate intake, or (3) loss of carbohydrates. Box 7-12 provides a list of conditions that can result in

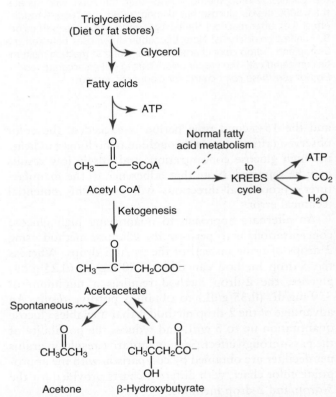

FIGURE 7-5 The formation of ketones from fatty acid metabolism. *ATP,* Adenosine triphosphate; *CoA,* coenzyme A; *SCoA,* succinyl coenzyme A.

significant ketone formation with subsequent ketonemia and ketonuria.

Regardless of the initiating condition, the sequence of ketone formation is the same. By far the most common clinical presentation is seen in patients with uncontrolled diabetes mellitus. In these patients, the body is unable to use carbohydrates, and fat metabolism increases

BOX 7-12 | Causes of Ketonuria

Inability to utilize available carbohydrates
   Diabetes mellitus
Insufficient carbohydrate consumption
   Starvation
   Diet regimens
   Alcoholism
   Severe exercise
   Cold exposure
   Acute febrile illnesses in children
Loss of carbohydrates
   Frequent vomiting (e.g., pregnancy, illness)
   Defective renal reabsorption (e.g., Fanconi's syndrome)
   Digestive disturbances

dramatically. As a result, ketoacids (ketones) accumulate in the patient's plasma, causing the plasma pH and bicarbonate to decrease. To eliminate these ketones and the large amount of glucose present, substantial amounts of body water are excreted (diuresis). Without replenishment or intervention, large quantities of electrolytes are lost in the urine, and a chemical imbalance results in acidosis and potentially diabetic coma. This condition is characteristically preceded by polyphagia, polydipsia, polyuria, and complaints of fatigue, nausea, and vomiting.

The detection of ketones in urine can serve as a valuable monitoring and management tool for patients with type 1 diabetes mellitus. Ketonuria is an early indicator of insulin deficiency, and ketoacidosis can develop slowly and progressively as a result of repeated insufficient insulin doses. In contrast, people with type 2 diabetes mellitus rarely develop ketoacidosis.[21] Chapter 9 further discusses the classification of diabetes and the metabolic derangements encountered.

Methods. As is depicted in Figure 7-5, the first ketone body formed by the liver cells is acetoacetate. A large portion of this acetoacetate is enzymatically reduced to β-hydroxybutyrate, while a minute portion is converted to acetone and carbon dioxide. None of the clinical laboratory tests for ketones detect and measure all three ketones. Although β-hydroxybutyrate is the ketone body of greatest average concentration during ketogenesis, methods for its detection in urine are not available. In contrast, inexpensive and rapid methods that detect acetoacetate and acetone based on the nitroprusside reaction (Legal's test or Rothera's test) are commonplace. These nitroprusside reaction–based tests are 15 to 20 times more sensitive to acetoacetate than they are to acetone, and they do not react with β-hydroxybutyrate.[22]

Before the development of the nitroprusside test, the ferric chloride test (Gerhardt's test, 1865) was used to detect ketones. Unfortunately, many other substances, most notably salicylates, also produce positive results.

The search for a more specific and sensitive method for ketone detection resulted in the nitroprusside test, which was originally developed by Legal in 1883 and was later modified by Rothera in 1908. Although the test is no longer performed routinely in clinical laboratories, Rothera's tube test is more sensitive to acetoacetate (1 to 5 mg/dL) and acetone (10 to 25 mg/dL) than the current test modification available on reagent strips or tablet tests.

Reagent Strip Tests. The ketone reagent strip tests are based on the nitroprusside reaction with sodium nitroprusside (nitroferricyanide) impregnated in the reagent pad. In an alkaline medium, acetoacetate reacts with nitroprusside to produce a color change from beige to purple. β-Hydroxybutyrate is not detected by reagent strip tests; however, Chemstrip and vChem strips include glycine in the reagent pad, which enables detection of acetone, in addition to acetoacetate (Equation 7-13).

Equation 7-13

$$\text{Acetoacetate} + \text{Sodium} \; (+\,\text{GLY}) \xrightarrow{\text{alk}} \underset{\text{color}}{\text{Purple}}$$
$$\text{(and acetone)} \quad \text{nitroprusside}$$

Gly, Glycine.

Ketone results can be reported in a variety of ways: by qualitatively using the plus system (negative, 1+, 2+, 3+); as negative, small, moderate, or large; or semiquantitatively, as a concentration in milligrams per deciliter (negative, 5, 15, 40, 80, 160 mg/dL). All reagent strip tests are sensitive at 5 to 10 mg/dL of acetoacetate, with Chemstrip and vChem strips also detecting acetone concentrations of 50 to 70 mg/dL.

Several agents can produce a false-positive reagent strip test for ketones. Most notable are compounds that contain free sulfhydryl groups. These include 2-mercaptoethane sulfonic acid (MESNA), a rescue drug used in the treatment of cancers; captopril, an antihypertensive drug; N-acetylcysteine, a treatment for acetaminophen overdose; D-penicillamine; and cystine, an amino acid. Because of the increasingly widespread use of these and other agents containing free sulfhydryl groups, it is imperative that laboratorians are aware of these potential interferences, and that they review and confirm positive ketone results. In 1989, less than 1% of participating laboratories correctly reported a negative result for ketones on a College of American Pathologists urine survey specimen that contained only a free sulfhydryl drug.[23]

A rapid and easy means of detecting a false-positive reaction caused by a free sulfhydryl–containing drug when performingthe reagent strip test or the tablet test (Acetest, to be discussed) is possible. In high concentrations, these drugs cause the ketone reaction pad to become immediately positive; however, by the appropriate read time, the color fades dramatically or disappears. In contrast when *true ketones* are present, the purple color of the reaction pad or tablet intensifies.

Because automated reagent strip readers read the strips at shorter intervals than when the strips are read visually, many false-positive results can be obtained. With lower drug concentrations, fading of the strip or tablet color is not always evident, in which case a drop of glacial acetic acid can be added to the reaction pad or to the reagent tablet. If the purple color fades or disappears, *true ketones* are not present. If these drugs are known or are determined to be present (e.g., diabetic patient taking captopril), the detection of ketones by these methods is compromised.

Highly pigmented urine can produce false-positive reagent strip and tablet tests. In addition, positive results or atypical colors can occur when levodopa metabolites, phenylketones, or phthaleins (e.g., bromsulphthalein, phenolsulfonphthalein dyes) are present. These substances react with the alkali in the test medium to produce color.[3]

The primary reason for false-negative ketone tests is improper specimen collection and handling. Because of rapid volatilization of acetone at room temperature and the breakdown of acetoacetate by bacteria, urine specimens should be tested immediately or refrigerated. False-negative tests can alsooccur as the result of deterioration of the nitroprusside reagent in the reaction pads or tablets from exposure to moisture, heat, or light.

Nitroprusside Tablet Test for Ketones (Acetest). A tablet test for the detection of ketones in urine is the Acetest (Siemens Healthcare Diagnostics Inc.). The Acetest uses the same nitroprusside reaction as the ketone reagent strip test and has a detection limit of 5 mg/dL acetoacetate in urine. The tablets contain glycine, which enables the reaction of acetone and lactose, which acts as a color enhancer. An advantage of this tablet test is the flexibility of specimen type: urine, serum, plasma, or whole blood. One drop of a specimen is placed directly on the tablet, and after the appropriate timed interval, the tablet color is compared to a color chart provided (Figure 7-6). Positive results are evidenced by a purple color and are reported as negative, small, moderate, or large. Any pink, tan, or yellow coloration should be ignored.

False-positive and false-negative results can occur for the same reasons as were described in the section on reagent strip tests for ketones. Therefore, regardless of the nitroprusside method used, specimen and reagent integrity and the laboratorian's knowledge of potential interferences are essential for obtaining accurate results.

Bilirubin and Urobilinogen

Formation. **Bilirubin** is an intensely orange-yellow pigment that when present in significant amounts causes a characteristic coloration of plasma and urine. The principal source of bilirubin (85%) is hemoglobin released daily from the breakdown of senescent red blood cells in the reticuloendothelial system. Other normal sources of bilirubin are destroyed red blood cell precursors in the

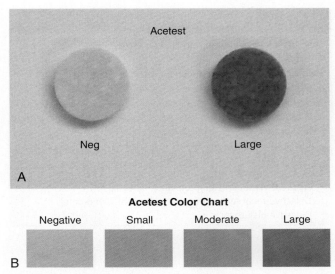

FIGURE 7-6 A, A positive Acetest for ketones. **B,** An Acetest color chart. *Do not use this color chart for diagnostic testing.*

bone marrow and other heme-containing proteins such as myoglobin or cytochromes.

After the heme moiety been released in the peripheral tissues, it undergoes catabolism to form bilirubin. The iron is bound by transferrin and is returned to the iron stores of the liver and bone marrow; the protein is returned to the amino acid pool for reuse; and the α-carbon from the protoporphyrin ring is expired by the lungs as carbon monoxide. This reaction sequence results in the formation of the tetrapyrrole biliverdin, which is rapidly and enzymatically reduced to bilirubin. The conversion of heme to bilirubin requires about 2 to 3 hours.[24] Figure 7-7 provides a schematic representation of heme catabolism to form bilirubin.

Bilirubin released into the bloodstream from the peripheral tissues is water insoluble and becomes reversibly bound to albumin. This association enhances its solubility and prevents bilirubin from crossing cell membranes into tissues where it can be toxic. While bound to albumin, bilirubin is too large and is unable to cross the glomerular filtration barriers to be excreted in urine. When the blood passes through the liver sinusoids, hepatocytes rapidly remove bilirubin from albumin in a carrier-mediated active transport process. Once within hepatocytes, bilirubin is rapidly conjugated with glucuronic acid to produce water-soluble bilirubin monoglucuronide and diglucuronide (collectively termed *conjugated bilirubin*). Normally, all the conjugated bilirubin formed is transported against a concentration gradient into the bile duct and ultimately into the small intestine. Should conjugated bilirubin reenter the bloodstream because of hepatocellular disease, it easily and rapidly passes the glomerular filtration barriers of the kidneys and is excreted in the urine.

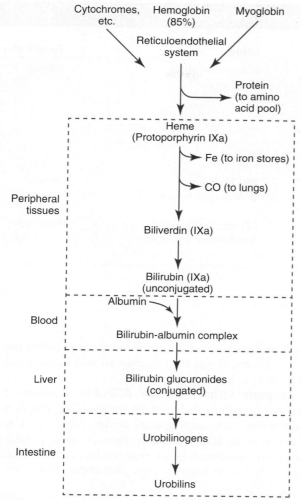

FIGURE 7-7 A schematic diagram of hemoglobin catabolism.

Clinical Significance. Disturbances in any aspect of bilirubin formation, hepatic uptake, metabolism, storage, or excretion are possible in a variety of diseases. Depending on the dysfunction, unconjugated bilirubin, conjugated bilirubin, or both may be produced in abnormally increased amounts, resulting in hyperbilirubinemia and possibly *bilirubinuria*.

In healthy individuals, only trace amounts of bilirubin (0.02 mg/dL) are excreted, and its presence is normally undetectable by routine testing methods. Therefore any detectable amount of bilirubin is considered to be significant and requires further clinical investigation. Its presence indicates the disruption of or an increase in hemoglobin catabolism. An increase in plasma bilirubin and its appearance in urine are early indicators of liver disease and can occur before any other clinical symptoms. Bilirubinemia and bilirubinuria are detectable long before the development of **jaundice**—the yellowish pigmentation of skin, sclera, tissues, and body fluids caused by bilirubin—that appears when plasma bilirubin concentrations reach 2 to 3 mg/dL (approximately two to three times normal).

Three principal mechanisms of altered bilirubin metabolism occur. They can result in an increase in urine bilirubin, urine urobilinogen, or both, as well as changes in fecal color (Table 7-11 and Figure 7-8). The first mechanism is prehepatic, indicating that the abnormality occurs before the handling of bilirubin by the liver. In other words, liver function is normal, and the dysfunction is an overproduction of bilirubin from heme. This overproduction occurs in hemolytic conditions such as hemolytic anemia, sickle cell disease, hereditary spherocytosis, and transfusion reactions, or in ineffective erythropoietic diseases such as thalassemia or pernicious anemia. In each of these conditions, large amounts of heme are catabolized into unconjugated bilirubin in the peripheral tissues. Because the bilirubin is unconjugated and is bound to albumin, it cannot be excreted in the urine. As a result, large amounts of bilirubin are presented to the liver for conjugation and excretion into the bile. The liver has a large capacity for bilirubin conjugation; most unconjugated bilirubin is removed in its first pass through the liver. Because a larger amount of bilirubin is excreted into the intestine, a larger amount of urobilinogen is formed and thus an increased amount of urobilinogen is reabsorbed into the enterohepatic circulation. As a result, the urine remains negative for bilirubin, but the urobilinogen concentration increases to above its normal value of 1 mg/dL or less.

The second mechanism of altered bilirubin metabolism is hepatic in origin and results from hepatocellular disease or disorders. Liver conditions affect the ability of the hepatocytes to perform the tasks of bilirubin uptake, conjugation, and excretion. The severity of the disorder and therefore the amount of bilirubin or urobilinogen present in the urine vary. Depending on the extent of hepatocellular damage, conjugated bilirubin can leak

Once in the intestinal tract, conjugated bilirubin is deconjugated, then reduced by anaerobic intestinal bacteria to form the colorless tetrapyrrole urobilinogen. A portion of the urobilinogen formed is subsequently reduced to stercobilinogen. Normally, about 20% of the urobilinogen is reabsorbed and reenters the liver via the hepatic portal circulation; in contrast, stercobilinogen cannot be reabsorbed. Of the reabsorbed urobilinogen, most is reexcreted by the liver into the bile; however, 2% to 5% of the urobilinogen normally remains in the bloodstream. At the kidneys. plasma urobilinogen readily passes the glomerular filtration barriers and is excreted in the urine (1 mg/dL or less). Spontaneous oxidation of urobilinogen and stercobilinogen in the large intestine results in the formation of urobilin and stercobilin. These compounds are orange-brown and account for the characteristic color of feces. Similarly, oxidation of the urobilinogen in urine to urobilin can contribute to the color observed in a urine specimen.

TABLE 7-11	Diagnostic Utility of Urine Bilirubin, Urobilinogen, and Fecal Color		
Jaundice Classification	**Conditions**	**Urine**	**Fecal Color**
Prehepatic (Increased heme degradation)	**Hemolytic disorders** • Transfusion reactions • Sickle cell disease • Hereditary spherocytosis • Hemolytic disease of newborn **Ineffective erythropoiesis** • Thalassemia • Pernicious anemia	Bilirubin: Negative Urobilinogen: ↑	Normal
Hepatic (Hepatocellular disorder)	Hepatitis Cirrhosis Genetic disorders	Bilirubin: Positive Urobilinogen: Normal to ↑	Normal
Posthepatic (Obstruction)	Gallstones Tumors (carcinoma) Fibrosis	Bilirubin: Positive Urobilinogen: ↓ to absent	Pale, chalky, "acholic"

directly back into the systemic circulation from damaged hepatocytes. Because this bilirubin is conjugated, it readily passes through the glomerular filtration barriers and is excreted in the urine. Hepatocellular damage also affects the reexcretion of intestinally reabsorbed urobilinogen. Because less urobilinogen is removed from the portal circulation by a diseased liver, more urobilinogen reaches the kidneys. The urine urobilinogen concentration can be increased or can remain normal, depending on the extent of hepatocellular damage.

The third mechanism of altered bilirubin metabolism involves posthepatic obstruction of the bile duct or biliary system. In these conditions, the liver functions normally; however, conjugated bilirubin that is transported to the biliary system is unable to pass into the intestine because of an obstruction. In these cases, conjugated bilirubin accumulates in the liver and eventually overflows or backs up into the systemic circulation. The kidneys rapidly clear the conjugated bilirubin, and bilirubinuria occurs. At the same time, little or no bilirubin is passing into the intestine. Consequently, no urobilinogen is formed and none is available for intestinal reabsorption. Because of this, the feces becomes characteristically acholic (pale white or tan) because the customary bile pigments (i.e., stercobilin and urobilin) are severely decreased or absent.

Bilirubin Methods

Physical Examination. Because of the characteristic pigmentation of bilirubin, its presence is often suspected in distinctly dark yellow-brown or amber urine specimens. These specimens are sometimes described as "beer brown." If these urines are agitated or shaken, the foam that forms has the characteristic yellow color that indicates the presence of bilirubin (see Figure 6-1). Note that clinically significant increases in urine bilirubin can be

small and may not appreciably alter urine color; therefore, a chemical test for bilirubin should be included in all routine urinalyses.

Reagent Strip Tests for Bilirubin. Reagent strip tests for bilirubin are based on the coupling reaction of a diazonium salt, impregnated in the reagent pad, with bilirubin in an acid medium to form an azodye: azobilirubin. This azocoupling reaction produces a color change from light tan to beige or pink (Equation 7-14).

Equation 7-14

$$\text{Bilirubin glucuronide} + \underset{\text{(Aromatic compound)}}{Ar-N^+ \equiv N} \xrightarrow{\text{Acid}} \underset{\text{Azo dye (Brown)}}{\text{Azobilirubin}}$$
(Diazonium salt)

Results are reported as negative, small, moderate, or large; or when the plus system is used, as negative, 1+, 2+, or 3+. The lower limit of detection for reagent strip tests is approximately 0.5 mg/dL of conjugated bilirubin. Note that a 25-fold increase in urine bilirubin excretion is necessary before bilirubin is detected by this method. Various drugs that color the urine red in an acid medium, such as phenazopyridine, can cause false-positive reactions. Other drugs, such as large quantities of chlorpromazine metabolites, can react directly with the diazonium salt to produce a false-positive test.

False-negative results are caused by ascorbic acid (≥25 mg/dL) that reacts directly with the diazonium salt to form a colorless end product, in which case bilirubin is unable to participate in the azocoupling reaction. Increased nitrite concentrations that result from urinary tract infections can interfere through the same mechanism described for ascorbic acid. Because bilirubin is unstable, improper specimen storage can cause false-negative bilirubin tests. When exposed to artificial light or sunlight, bilirubin rapidly photo-oxidizes to biliverdin

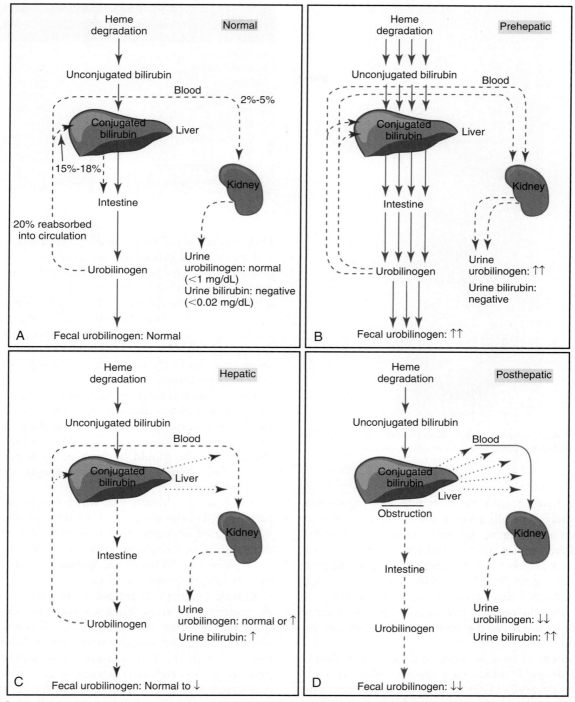

FIGURE 7-8 Bilirubin metabolism and alterations in normal metabolism caused by disease. **A,** Normal bilirubin metabolism. **B,** Prehepatic alteration of bilirubin metabolism. **C,** Hepatic alteration of bilirubin metabolism. **D,** Posthepatic alteration of bilirubin metabolism.

or hydrolyzes to free bilirubin. Because neither of these compounds reacts in the bilirubin reagent strip test, once this bilirubin conversion has taken place, false-negative results will be obtained. The light sensitivity of bilirubin is temperature dependent; it is enhanced at room temperature and is retarded at low or refrigerator temperatures.

Diazo Tablet Test for Bilirubin (Ictotest Method). A tablet test for the detection of bilirubin in urine is the Ictotest method (Siemens Healthcare Diagnostics Inc.). This tablet test is based on the same azocoupling reaction of bilirubin with a diazonium salt on which reagent strips are based. A notable difference is its significantly lower detection limit. Bilirubin concentrations as low as

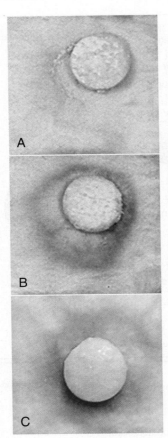

FIGURE 7-9 A, A negative Ictotest. **B,** A positive Ictotest for bilirubin. **C,** A negative Ictotest showing an atypical color.

0.05 to 0.1 mg/dL can be detected. This represents approximately fourfold greater sensitivity to bilirubin than is seen with reagent strip tests. Because of this sensitivity difference, it is not unusual for a urine specimen to produce a positive Ictotest result despite a negative reagent strip test result. When specific requests are made for urine bilirubin determination, or when bilirubin is suspected from the physical examination but the reagent strip result is negative, the Ictotest method should be performed.

The Ictotest method is quick and easy to perform. Urine (10 drops) is added to a special absorbent pad, and an Ictotest tablet is placed atop the urine premoistened pad. Two drops of water are added to the tablet and allowed to flow onto the pad. After 30 seconds, the tablet is removed, and the absorbent pad is observed for the development of any purple or blue coloration, which indicates a positive test (Figure 7-9). Any other colors, such as red or pink, are considered a negative test result for bilirubin. Because the chemical principles of the Ictotest method and the reagent strip tests are similar, the tablet test is subject to the same interferences as have been seen with reagent strip tests.

Urobilinogen Methods. Urobilinogen is normally present in urine in concentrations of 1 mg/dL or less (≈1

Ehrlich unit) or 0.5 to 2.5 mg/day. Although qualitative and quantitative procedures are available for urobilinogen detection, qualitative urine screening tests predominate. Because urobilinogen excretion is enhanced in alkaline urine, the specimen of choice for quantifying or monitoring is a 2-hour collection following the midday meal (i.e., 2 PM to 4 PM). This collection correlates with the typical "alkaline tide" (alkaline pH) observed in the urine after meals. Quantitative urobilinogen procedures are rarely performed.

Urobilinogen is labile in acid urine and easily photooxidizes to urobilin. Because urobilin is nonreactive in these tests, urine collection and handling procedures must be followed to ensure the integrity of the specimen. Urine specimens should be fresh or appropriately preserved and at room temperature during testing (see Chapter 3).

The Watson-Schwartz test, which is used primarily to detect porphobilinogen, can be used to specifically identify increased amounts of urine urobilinogen. It can also differentiate urobilinogen from other Ehrlich's reactive substances. For details of the Watson-Schwartz test, see the "Porphobilinogen" section.

Classic Ehrlich's Reaction. Before the development of reagent strip tests, **Ehrlich's reaction** was used to qualitatively screen for urobilinogen. This test is based on the reaction of urobilinogen with *p*-dimethylaminobenzaldehyde (Ehrlich's reagent) in an acid medium to produce a characteristic magenta or red chromophore. Numerous substances react with Ehrlich's reagent to produce a red color and are often collectively termed *Ehrlich's reactive substances* (Box 7-13). The test is performed by mixing 1 part Ehrlich's reagent with 10 parts urine in a tube and observing the mixture for any pink color after a 5-minute incubation (Equation 7-15).

Equation 7-15

$$\text{Urobilinogen} + \text{Ehrlich's reagent} \xrightarrow{\text{acid}} \text{Red color}$$

Serial dilutions (e.g., 1:10, 1:20, 1:30) of urine can be made and semiquantitative results determined. Any perceptible pink is considered a positive test result; normal urobilinogen concentrations can be positive up to the

1:20 dilution. This tube test is no longer performed for urobilinogen screening because it is time-consuming, nonspecific, and costly. However, various modifications (e.g., Watson-Schwartz test, Hoesch test) can be used to screen for urine porphobilinogen.

Reagent Strip Tests for Urobilinogen

Multistix Reagent Strips. The principles for urobilinogen reagent strip tests, including their sensitivity and specificity, differ depending on the brand used. Multistix reagent strips are based on the classic Ehrlich's reaction. The reagent pad is impregnated with Ehrlich's reagent (*p*-dimethylaminobenzaldehyde), a color enhancer, and an acid buffer. As urobilinogen reacts with Ehrlich's reagent to form a red chromophore, the reagent pad changes from light pink to dark pink (Equation 7-16).

Equation 7-16   Ehrlich's Reaction

$$\underset{\text{Urobilinogen}}{\text{Ehrlich's reactive substance}} + \underset{\text{Ehrlich's reagent}}{\text{p-dimethylamino-benzaldehyde}} \xrightarrow{\text{Acid}} \underset{\text{color}}{\text{Red}}$$

False-positive results can occur because of the presence of other Ehrlich's reactive substances. However, this reaction can vary and should not be relied on to screen for substances other than urobilinogen, such as porphobilinogen.[25] Another problem is seen in substances that mask the reaction pad with a drug-induced or atypical color (e.g., phenazopyridine, red beets, azo dyes). These colors interfere with visual interpretation of the test. Formalin, a urine preservative, and high concentrations of nitrites inhibit or interfere with the reaction. The reactivity of the reaction pad increases with temperature; therefore urine specimens should be at room temperature or warmer when tested.

Chemstrip and vChem Reagent Strips. Chemstrip and vChem reagent strip tests for urobilinogen are based on an azocoupling reaction. A diazonium salt impregnated in the reagent pad reacts with urobilinogen in the acid medium of the reaction pad (Equation 7-17). The azo dye produced causes a color change from white to pink.

Equation 7-17   Azocoupling Reaction

$$\text{Urobilinogen} + \underset{\text{Aromatic compound}}{\text{Ar} - \text{N}^+} \equiv \underset{\text{Diazonium salt}}{\text{N}} \xrightarrow{\text{acid}} \underset{\text{(red)}}{\text{Azo dye}}$$

Unlike Ehrlich's reaction, this reagent strip test is specific for urobilinogen. Pigmented substances that mask the reagent pad (e.g., phenazopyridine, red beets, azo dyes) can interfere with color interpretation and can cause false-positive results. False-negative results can occur from nitrites (>5 mg/dL), from formalin, or from improper storage of the urine specimen.

Regardless of the reagent strip used, urobilinogen results of 1 mg/dL or less are reported as such and are considered normal. Increased urobilinogen values are reported semiquantitatively in milligrams per deciliter (1 mg/dL is approximately equivalent to 1 Ehrlich unit). All reagent strip tests detect normal levels of urobilinogen in urine; see Table 7-1 for their individual sensitivity

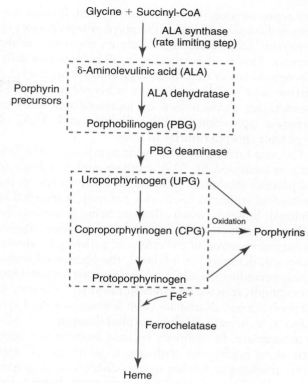

FIGURE 7-10 A schematic diagram of heme synthesis.

limits. Note, however, that the absence of urobilinogen cannot be determined. In other words, these tests cannot clearly or reliably indicate a decrease in or the absence of urine urobilinogen. The absence of urobilinogen formation is best reflected by fecal analysis (acholic stool) or by blood test profiles that include bilirubin analysis.

In summary, urobilinogen results can vary depending on the brand of reagent strips used. Urine specimens that contain significant quantities of other Ehrlich's reactive substances can give higher values using a nonspecific reagent strip test (Multistix) than would be obtained using a specific reagent strip test (Chemstrip or vChem).

Porphobilinogen

Clinical Significance. Porphobilinogen is a porphyrin precursor and an important intermediate compound in the formation of heme (Figure 7-10). Porphobilinogen is formed when two molecules of δ-aminolevulinic acid (ALA) condense in a reaction catalyzed by ALA dehydratase. Subsequently, four molecules of porphobilinogen condense to form the first porphyrinogen, uroporphyrinogen. The porphyrinogens can oxidize spontaneously and irreversibly to form their respective porphyrins. Once this process has taken place, the porphyrin cannot reenter the heme synthetic pathway; it has no biologic function and is excreted. Normally, heme synthesis is regulated so closely that only trace amounts of the porphyrin precursors ALA (at less than approximately 1.4 mg/dL) and porphobilinogen (at less than approximately 0.4 mg/dL) are formed. If heme synthesis is disrupted, however, the porphyrin precursors or porphyrins accumulate, depending on the defect in the pathway. This synthesis occurs in all mammalian cells, although the major sites of heme production are the bone marrow and the liver. Various inherited or induced disorders are characterized by increased quantities of porphyrin precursors (porphobilinogen and ALA) or porphyrins (**porphyrinuria**) in urine.

The rate-limiting step in heme synthesis is the first reaction catalyzed by ALA synthase and is subject to end-product inhibition by heme. In other words, in the presence of sufficient heme, this pathway is retarded or inhibited; however, when adequate heme is lacking, the pathway is stimulated to increase its formation. Should an enzyme required in the synthetic pathway be absent, decreased, defective, or inhibited, the compound immediately preceding the action of that enzyme accumulates. For example, in acute intermittent porphyria, the enzyme porphobilinogen deaminase (also known as UPG I synthase) is deficient, causing porphobilinogen and ALA to accumulate. In addition, because heme is not being formed to inhibit the pathway, it is stimulated even more, resulting in further overproduction of porphyrin precursors. Because porphyrin precursors have a low renal threshold, they are rapidly removed from the bloodstream and appear in urine. Increased amounts can be detected by performing a Hoesch or a Watson-Schwartz test.

Although urine screening and quantitative tests are available for porphobilinogen, no screening procedure for ALA is currently possible. Chapter 9 discusses various inherited and induced disorders that result in the overproduction of porphyrin precursors or porphyrins, as well as their clinical features, diagnosis, and treatment.

Methods

Physical Examination. The porphyrin precursor porphobilinogen is colorless and nonfluorescent. In contrast, its oxidized form, porphobilin, is dark red. Most often, a pink or red urine implies blood or hemoglobin, but when the test for blood is negative, porphyria should be one of several possibilities suspected. Photo-oxidation of porphobilinogen to porphobilin is responsible for the reddish appearance. Keep in mind that the visual observation of a red color depends greatly on the concentration of porphobilin in the urine, which varies with hydration. In addition, other pigments or chromogens normally present in the urine can modify the color observed.

Hoesch Test for Porphobilinogen. The Hoesch test is basically an inverse Ehrlich's reaction. In other words, the ratio of the volume of urine to reagent is reversed. This causes the reaction mixture to be highly acidic, which prevents urobilinogen from reacting, except when present in very high concentrations (i.e., >20 mg/dL). Because the Hoesch test is rapid, easy to perform, and sensitive, it may be used to screen for porphobilinogen.

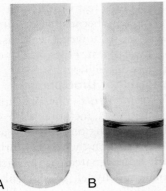

FIGURE 7-11 The Hoesch test (urine + reagent) *before the tube is mixed.* **A,** A negative test. **B,** A positive test.

To perform the Hoesch test, 2 mL of *modified* Ehrlich's reagent (Hoesch reagent) is placed in a tube, and 2 drops of urine is added. When a deep pink or red color develops instantaneously at the interface of the reagent and urine, porphobilinogen is present (Figure 7-11). If the tube is shaken, the color disperses throughout the mixture. The intensity of the color relates directly to the porphobilinogen concentration; however, quantitation is not performed by this method. The Hoesch test can detect porphobilinogen concentrations as low as 2 mg/dL.

Despite its sensitivity and specificity for porphobilinogen, interpretation of the Hoesch test can be difficult because of the development of atypical colors. To resolve questionable results, the Hoesch test can be confirmed using the Watson-Schwartz test. Indoles or drugs (e.g., phenazopyridine) can cause false-positive or questionable results. Methyldopa is also capable of producing false-positive results in both tests. However, the Hoesch test requires the presence of large quantities of these substances to give a false-positive result and therefore is preferred over the Watson-Schwartz test when porphobilinogen is suspected or known to be present.

Watson-Schwartz Test for Porphobilinogen and Urobilinogen. The Watson-Schwartz test is a modification of the original Ehrlich's reaction and can be used as a screening test for urine porphobilinogen. Porphobilinogen can be differentiated from urobilinogen and from other Ehrlich's reactive substances. This test is based on the different solubility characteristics of porphobilinogen and urobilinogen with respect to pH and solvent type. Essentially, Ehrlich's reaction is performed but with solvents of slightly different polarity; the layer in which the red chromophore resides identifies the substance present (Equations 7-18 through 7-20).

Equation 7-18   Modified Ehrlich's Reaction

Porphobilinogen + Ehrlich's reagent + Sodium acetate $\xrightarrow{\text{acid}}$ Red color

TABLE 7-12	Watson-Schwartz Test Result Summary		
Result	Modified Ehrlich Reaction	Chloroform Layer (bottom)	Butanol layer (top)
Negative	No pink color*	—	—
Urobilinogen positive	Pink	Pink	(Pink)†
Porphobilinogen positive	Pink	No color	No color
Positive for *other* Ehrlich reactive substances	Pink	No color	Pink

*The urine mixture is usually colorless or pale yellow; the yellow color from urea varies with urine concentration.

†When sequentially extracting, if urobilinogen remains in the aqueous layer due to insufficient chloroform extraction, it will extract into the butanol layer during the second extraction.

Equation 7-19

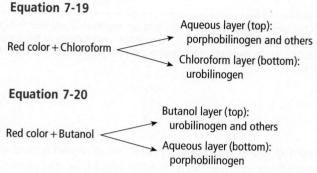

Red color + Chloroform

Aqueous layer (top): porphobilinogen and others

Chloroform layer (bottom): urobilinogen

Equation 7-20

Red color + Butanol

Butanol layer (top): urobilinogen and others

Aqueous layer (bottom): porphobilinogen

To perform a qualitative Watson-Schwartz test, equal parts (≈2 mL each) of urine and Ehrlich's reagent are mixed in a tube. The volume is doubled by adding saturated sodium acetate (≈4 mL), and the solution is mixed again. A positive test results in the development of a characteristic red or magenta color (the aldehyde chromophore) at this step.

When the mixture does not show a red color, or if an orange color develops, the test is negative and no further testing is done. If the mixture develops a red color, an extraction is performed by adding chloroform (≈2 to 5 mL) to the mixture, followed by vigorous shaking. The phases are allowed to separate, which can be hastened by centrifugation. If the red color resides only in the aqueous phase (the top layer), porphobilinogen or another Ehrlich's reactive substance is present, and a butanol extraction must be performed. If the red color resides only in the chloroform phase (the bottom layer), increased amounts of urobilinogen are present. If the red color is noted in both phases, the aqueous layer must be reextracted with chloroform to ensure complete extraction of the red chromophore for proper identification.

To perform the butanol extraction, the aqueous phase (the top layer) is transferred to another tube and an equal volume of butanol is added. The tube is shaken vigorously, and the phases are allowed to separate. If the red color remains in the aqueous phase (now the bottom layer), porphobilinogen is present. If the red color is in the butanol phase (the top layer), urobilinogen or other Ehrlich's reactive substances are present. Table 7-12 provides a summary for interpreting the Watson-Schwartz

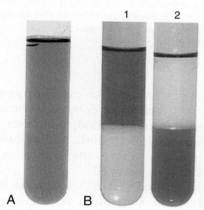

FIGURE 7-12 A, A positive Ehrlich's reaction, which indicates the presence of an Ehrlich reactive substance in the urine. **B,** A modified Watson-Schwartz test using the same urine: *tube 1* is the chloroform extraction; *tube 2* is the butanol extraction. The test is positive for porphobilinogen.

test (Figure 7-12). The Watson-Schwartz test is more sensitive than the Hoesch test and is capable of detecting urine porphobilinogen concentrations greater than 0.6 mg/dL.[26]

Ascorbic Acid

Clinical Significance. Ascorbic acid, also known as vitamin C, is normally present in the diet but is also used as a preservative or a dietary supplement in foods and beverages. Ascorbic acid is a water-soluble vitamin, which means that it does not require fat for absorption, and that any excess vitamin is immediately excreted in the urine as ascorbic acid or its principal metabolite, oxalate. Of the oxalates present in normal urine, approximately 50% are derived from ascorbic acid metabolism. Ascorbic acid functions as an enzyme cofactor in connective tissue proteins. Humans cannot synthesize vitamin C; therefore dietary intake is essential. Major dietary sources include citrus fruits and vegetables (tomatoes, green peppers, cabbage, and leafy greens). Daily supplementation with ingestion of megadoses of vitamin

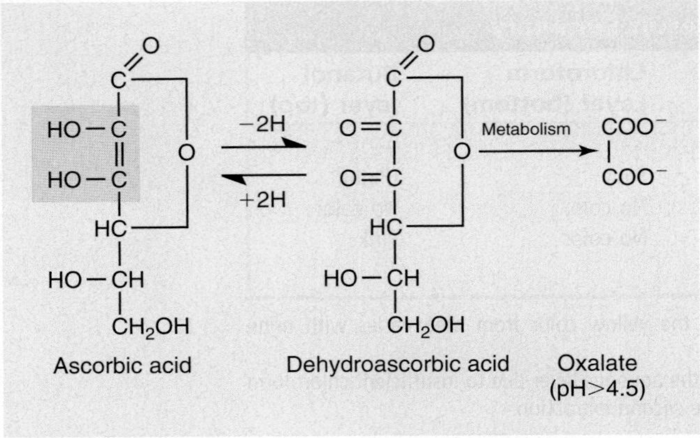

FIGURE 7-13 Ascorbic acid. The highlighted ene-diol group of ascorbic acid is responsible for its strong reducing ability (i.e., as a hydrogen donor). Normally, the principal metabolite of ascorbic acid—oxalate—accounts for approximately 50% of the urinary oxalate excreted daily.

TABLE 7-13		False Negative or Decreased Reagent Strip Results Due to Ascorbic Acid Interference
Test		
Test Affected	**Ascorbic Acid Concentration Needed**	**Mode of Interference**
Blood*	≥9 mg/dL	Reacts with H_2O_2 on reagent pad
Bilirubin	≥25 mg/dL	Reacts with diazonium salt on reagent pad
Nitrite	≥25 mg/dL	Reacts with diazonium salt produced by first reaction
Glucose	≥50 mg/dL	Reacts with H_2O_2 produced by first reaction

*Chemstrip reagent strip tests for blood are significantly resistant to high ascorbic acid concentration. At a hemoglobin concentration of 0.6 mg/dL, positive results were obtained despite the presence of 70 mg/dL ascorbic acid.

C is a common practice, which can cause an increase in the amount of ascorbic acid excreted in the urine. Normally, without supplementation, urine excretion averages less than 5 mg/dL of vitamin C. With supplementation, significant intraindividual variations in urinary vitamin C concentrations are attained.

In an extensive study, 22.8% of routine urine specimens tested positive for ascorbic acid.[18] The mean urine concentration was 37.2 mg/dL (2120 mol/L), with values ranging from 7.1 to 339.5 mg/dL (405 to 19,350 mol/L). The presence of ascorbic acid in urine can compromise the results obtained with several reagent strip tests. Therefore routine urinalysis protocols should include a screening test for ascorbic acid, or, when necessary, reagent strips that are not subject to interference from ascorbic acid should be used.

Mechanisms of Interference. Ascorbic acid is a strong reducing substance because of its ene-diol group (Figure 7-13). As a hydrogen donor, ascorbic acid readily oxidizes to dehydroascorbic acid, a colorless compound. Reagent strip tests that use hydrogen peroxide or a diazonium salt are subject to ascorbic acid interference. Whether these compounds are impregnated in the reaction pad or are produced by a first reaction, they are removed by ascorbic acid, which prevents the intended reaction. As a result, colorless dehydroascorbic acid is produced, no positive color change is observed, and a false-negative or a falsely low result is obtained. Reagent strip tests for blood, bilirubin, glucose, and nitrite are vulnerable to ascorbic acid interference (Table 7-13). However because of reagent strip variations, some brands are more susceptible than others to this interference (see the specific test sections for additional discussion or Table 7-2).

The presence of ascorbic acid in urine most often is suspected when microscopic examination reveals increased numbers of red blood cells but the reagent strip test for blood is negative. The effect of ascorbic acid on decreasing glucose reagent strip results is less obvious and may be suspected only when ketones are positive and glucose negative, or when a discrepancy exists between the copper reduction test and the reagent strip test for glucose. Ascorbic acid remains a source of false-negative or decreased chemical test results when some brands of reagent strips are used, thus highlighting the importance of reading the product inserts provided by each reagent strip manufacturer.

Method. A few reagent strip manufacturers include an ascorbic acid test pad on their reagent strips, for example, vChem (Iris Diagnostics) and Urispec GP + A (Henry Schein Inc., Melville, NY). The reaction principle is based on the action of ascorbic acid to reduce a dye impregnated in the reagent pad. The reduced dye causes a distinct color change from blue to orange (Equation 7-21).

Equation 7-21

$$\text{L-Ascorbic acid} + \text{Oxidized dye} \xrightarrow{\text{buffer}} \text{Reduced dye} + \text{Dehydroascorbic acid}$$

These reagent strip tests produce positive results with ascorbic acid concentrations as low as 7.0 mg/dL and consistently detect 20 mg/dL of ascorbic acid in 90% of urines tested.[18] False-positive results can be obtained when free-sulfhydryl drugs (e.g., MESNA, captopril, N-acetylcysteine) are also present in the urine.[27] Note that these false-positive results may be identified only when the ketone test is also falsely positive, or when the medication history is provided.

Results can be reported semiquantitatively by comparing the color of the reaction pad with the color

TABLE 7-14	Findings That Can Initiate Reflex Testing
Parameter	**"Possible" Components Present Microscopically**
Color: abnormal	Red, brown, pink: suggest RBCs (hematuria)
Clarity: not clear	To identify elements causing turbidity; could be normal or pathologic
Protein	Casts, fat
Blood	RBCs (WBCs)
Leukocyte esterase	WBCs (bacteria)
Nitrite	Bacteria (WBCs)
SG >1.035	Determine whether iatrogenic crystals (e.g., drugs, x-ray contrast media) are causing high result

TABLE 7-15	Correlation Between Chemical and Microscopic Examinations
Chemical Result	**"Possible" Microscopic Findings**
SG >1.040	Suspect excretion of high-molecular-weight solute: x-ray dye crystals (acid pH) or other unusual crystal
Acid (pH <7.0)	Crystals of *normal* solutes: calcium oxalate, amorphous urates, urates (Na, K, Mg, Ca), uric acid (pH ≤5.5) *Pathologic* crystals (pH ≤6.5): bilirubin, cholesterol, cystine, hemosiderin, leucine, tyrosine, drugs (ampicillin, sulfamethoxazole, acyclovir), x-ray contrast media
Neutral (pH 7.0)	Calcium oxalate, urates (Na, K, Mg, Ca), and most alkaline crystals
Alkaline (pH >7.0)	Calcium oxalate, amorphous phosphates, calcium phosphates, triple phosphate, calcium carbonate, ammonium biurate
Blood positive (urine not clear)	RBCs; RBC casts, blood casts, hemosiderin (myoglobin)
Blood positive (urine clear)	Hemoglobin (from lysed RBC), myoglobin
Leukocyte esterase positive	WBCs intact or lysed; WBC casts
Nitrite positive	Bacteria: quantity variable
Protein positive	Increased casts; fat as globules, free-floating, in casts, in oval fat bodies (when protein ≥300 mg/dL or 3+), sperm (seminal fluid contamination)

chart provided, or simply as positive or negative for ascorbic acid.

Another strip test for detection and semiquantitation of ascorbic acid in foodstuffs, such as wine, fruit, and vegetable juices, is manufactured by E. Merck as the Merckoquant ascorbic acid test. These single test reagent strips are based on the same reaction principle cited but use phosphomolybdate as the chromogen. As ascorbic acid reduces this dye to molybdenum blue, a color change from yellow to blue is observed. The lowest level of ascorbic acid detectable is 5 mg/dL, and interference from substances with similar reduction potential is possible.

REFLEX TESTING AND RESULT CORRELATION

In some laboratories, the microscopic examination may not be performed unless specifically requested by the health care provider, or when results from the physical and chemical examinations trigger its performance. Results that trigger reflex testing vary among laboratories based on their patient population, reagent strips in use, and instrumentation. Table 7-14 provides a selected listing of parameters and the microscopic components associated with each.

As was previously stated, it is important to ensure that results obtained from physical, chemical, and microscopic examinations correlate, especially when urinalysis testing is performed manually. The potential for specimen mix-up is primarily due to the centrifugation required for preparation of the urine sediment for microscopic review. Table 7-15 lists chemical examination results and possible findings in the microscopic examination that correlate. When results do not correlate between

TABLE 7-16	Typical Reference Intervals for Chemical Examination of Urine*
Component	**Result**
Bilirubin	Negative
Glucose	Negative
Ketones	Negative
Leukocyte esterase	Negative
Nitrite	Negative
pH	4.5 to 8.0
Protein	Negative
Urobilinogen	≤1 mg/dL

*Using random urine specimens; see Appendix B for reference intervals of a "complete" urinalysis—physical, chemical and microscopic examinations.

physical, chemical, and microscopic examinations, action must be taken to resolve discrepancies before patient results are reported. Table 7-16 provides typical reference intervals for the chemical examination of random urine specimens and Appendix B lists values for a complete urinalysis.

STUDY QUESTIONS

1. To preserve the integrity of reagent strips, it is necessary that they are
   A. humidified adequately.
   B. stored in a refrigerator.
   C. stored in a tightly capped container.
   D. protected from the dark.

2. Using quality control materials, one should check reagent strip performance
   1. at least once daily.
   2. when a new bottle of strips or tablets is opened.
   3. when a new lot number of strips or tablets is placed into use.
   4. once each shift by each laboratorian performing urinalysis testing.
   A. 1, 2, and 3 are correct.
   B. 1 and 3 are correct.
   C. 4 is correct.
   D. All are correct.

3. Which of the following is not checked by quality control materials?
   A. The technical skills of the personnel performing the test
   B. The integrity of the specimen, that is, that the specimen was collected and stored properly
   C. The test protocol, that is, that the procedure was performed according to written guidelines
   D. The functioning of the equipment used, for example, the refractometer and the reagent strip readers

4. Quality control materials used to assess the performance of reagent strips and tablet tests must
   A. be purchased from a commercial manufacturer.
   B. yield the same results regardless of the commercial brand used.
   C. contain chemical constituents at realistic and critical detection levels.
   D. include constituents to assess the chemical and microscopic examinations.

5. Which of the following is not a source of erroneous results when reagent strips are used?
   A. Testing a refrigerated urine specimen
   B. Timing using a clock without a second hand
   C. Allowing excess urine to remain on the reagent strip
   D. Dipping the reagent strip briefly into the urine specimen.

6. Select the primary reason why tablet (e.g., Ictotest) and chemical tests (e.g., sulfosalicylic acid precipitation test) generally are performed.
   A. They confirm results suspected about the specimen.
   B. They are alternative testing methods for highly concentrated urines.
   C. Their specificity differs from that of the reagent strip test.
   D. They are more sensitive to the chemical constituents in urine.

7. In a patient with chronic renal disease, in whom the kidneys can no longer adjust urine concentration, the urine specific gravity would be
   A. 1.000.
   B. 1.010.
   C. 1.020.
   D. 1.030.

8. Urine pH normally ranges from
   A. 4.0 to 9.0.
   B. 4.5 to 7.0.
   C. 4.5 to 8.0.
   D. 5.0 to 6.0.

9. Urine pH can be modified by all of the following except
   A. diet.
   B. increased ingestion of water.
   C. ingestion of medications.
   D. urinary tract infections.

10. The double-indicator system used by commercial reagent strips to determine urine pH uses which two indicator dyes?
    A. Methyl orange and bromphenol blue
    B. Methyl red and bromthymol blue
    C. Phenol red and thymol blue
    D. Phenolphthalein and litmus

11. All of the following can result in inaccurate urine pH measurements *except*
    A. large amounts of protein present in the urine.
    B. double-dipping of the reagent strip into the specimen.
    C. maintaining the specimen at room temperature for 4 hours.
    D. allowing excess urine to remain on the reagent strip during the timing interval.

12. Which of the following aids in the differentiation of hemoglobinuria and hematuria?
    A. Urine pH
    B. Urine color
    C. Leukocyte esterase test
    D. Microscopic examination

13. Select the correct statement(s).
    1. Myoglobin and hemoglobin are reabsorbed readily by renal tubular cells.
    2. Hemosiderin, a soluble storage form of iron, is found in aqueous solutions.
    3. When haptoglobin is saturated, free hemoglobin passes through the glomerular filtration barrier.
    4. Hemosiderin is found in the urine during a hemolytic episode.
    A. 1, 2, and 3 are correct.
    B. 1 and 3 are correct.
    C. 4 is correct.
    D. All are correct.

14. Which statement about hemoglobin and myoglobin is true?
    A. They are heme-containing proteins involved in oxygen transport.
    B. Their presence is suspected when urine and serum appear red.
    C. Their presence in serum is associated with high creatine kinase values.
    D. They precipitate out of solution when the urine is 80% saturated with ammonium sulfate.

15. On the reagent strip test for blood, any heme moiety (e.g., hemoglobin, myoglobin) present in urine catalyzes
    A. oxidation of the chromogen and hydrogen peroxide.
    B. reduction of the chromogen in the presence of hydrogen peroxide.
    C. reduction of the pseudoperoxidase while the chromogen undergoes a color change.
    D. oxidation of the chromogen while hydrogen peroxide is reduced.

16. Which of the following blood cells will not be detected by the leukocyte esterase pad because it lacks esterases?
    A. Eosinophils
    B. Lymphocytes
    C. Monocytes
    D. Neutrophils

17. Microscopic examination of a urine sediment revealed an average of 2 to 5 white blood cells per high-power field, whereas the leukocyte esterase test by reagent strip was negative. Which of the following statements best accounts for this discrepancy?
    A. The urine is contaminated with vaginal fluid.
    B. Many white blood cells are lysed, and their esterase has been inactivated.
    C. Ascorbic acid is interfering with the reaction on the reagent strip.
    D. The amount of esterase present is below the sensitivity of the reagent strip test.

18. Which of the following statements describes the chemical principle involved in the leukocyte esterase pad of commercial reagent strips?
    A. Leukocyte esterase reacts with a diazonium salt on the reagent pad to form an azo dye.
    B. An ester and a diazonium salt combine to form an azo dye in the presence of leukocyte esterase.
    C. An aromatic compound on the reagent pad combines with leukocyte esterase to form an azo dye.
    D. Leukocyte esterase hydrolyzes an ester on the reagent pad, then an azocoupling reaction results in the formation of an azo dye.

19. Which of the following conditions most likely accounts for a negative nitrite result on the reagent strip despite the presence of large quantities of bacteria?
    1. The bacteria present did not have enough time to convert nitrate to nitrite.
    2. The bacteria present are not capable of converting nitrate to nitrite.
    3. The patient is not ingesting adequate amounts of nitrate in the diet.
    4. The urine is dilute and the level of nitrite present is below the sensitivity of the test.
    A. 1, 2, and 3 are correct.
    B. 1 and 3 are correct.
    C. 4 is correct.
    D. All are correct.

20. The chemical principle of the nitrite reagent pad is based on the
    A. pseudoperoxidase activity of nitrite.
    B. diazotization of nitrite followed by an azocoupling reaction.
    C. azocoupling action of nitrite with a diazonium salt to form an azo dye.
    D. hydrolysis of an ester by nitrite combined with an azocoupling reaction.

21. Which of the following substances or actions can produce false-positive nitrite results?
    A. Ascorbic acid
    B. Vaginal contamination
    C. Strong reducing agents
    D. Improper specimen storage

22. Normally, daily urine protein excretion does not exceed
    A. 150 mg/day.
    B. 500 mg/day.
    C. 1.5 g/day.
    D. 2.5 g/day.

23. Which of the following proteins originates in the urinary tract?
    A. Albumin
    B. Bence Jones protein
    C. β_2-Microglobulin
    D. Uromodulin

24. Match each type of proteinuria with its description.

Description	Type of Proteinuria
__ A. Defective protein reabsorption in the nephrons	1. Overflow proteinuria
__ B. Increased urine albumin and mid- to high-molecular-weight proteins	2. Glomerular proteinuria
__ C. Increase in low-molecular-weight proteins in urine	3. Tubular proteinuria
__ D. Immunoglobulin light chains in the urine	4. Postrenal proteinuria
__ E. Proteins originating from a bladder tumor	
__ F. Protein excreted only in an orthostatic position	
__ G. Hemoglobinuria and myoglobinuria	
__ H. Nephrotic syndrome	
__ I. Fanconi's syndrome	

25. Which of the following statements about Bence Jones protein is correct?
    A. The protein consists of κ and λ light chains.
    B. The protein is often found in the urine of patients with multiple sclerosis.
    C. The protein precipitates when urine is heated to 100° C and redissolves when cooled to 60° C.
    D. The protein can produce a positive reagent strip protein test and a negative sulfosalicylic acid (SSA) precipitation test.

26. A urine specimen is tested for protein by reagent strip and by the SSA test. The reagent strip result is negative, and the SSA result is 2+. Which of the following statements best explains this discrepancy?
    A. A protein other than albumin is present in the urine.
    B. The reagent strip result is falsely negative because the urine has a pH of 8.0.
    C. A large quantity of amorphous urates in the urine caused the false-positive SSA result.
    D. The time interval for reading the reagent strip pad was exceeded, causing a false-negative result.

27. Which of the following statements best describes the chemical principle of the protein reagent strip test?
    A. The protein reacts with an immunocomplex on the pad, which results in a color change.
    B. The protein causes a pH change on the reagent strip pad, which results in a color change.
    C. The protein accepts hydrogen ions from the indicator dye, which results in a color change.
    D. The protein causes protons to be released from a polyelectrolyte, which results in a color change.

28. A urine specimen is tested for glucose by a reagent strip and by the Clinitest method. The reagent strip result is 100 mg/dL, and the Clinitest result is 500 mg/dL. Which of the following statements would best account for this discrepancy?
    A. The Clinitest tablets have expired or were stored improperly.
    B. A large amount of ascorbic acid is present in the specimen.
    C. A strong oxidizing agent (e.g., bleach) is contaminating the specimen.
    D. The reagent strip is exhibiting the pass-through phenomenon, which results in a falsely low value.

29. Which of the following substances if present in the urine results in a negative Clinitest?
    A. Fructose
    B. Lactose
    C. Galactose
    D. Sucrose

30. The glucose reagent strip test is more sensitive and specific for glucose than the Clinitest method because it detects
    A. other reducing substances and higher concentrations of glucose.
    B. no other substances and higher concentrations of glucose.
    C. other reducing substances and lower concentrations of glucose.
    D. no other substances and lower concentrations of glucose.

31. Which of the following statements about glucose is false?
    A. Glucose readily passes the glomerular filtration barrier.
    B. Glucose is reabsorbed passively in the proximal tubule.
    C. Glucosuria occurs when plasma glucose levels exceed 160 to 180 mg/dL.
    D. High plasma glucose concentrations are associated with damage to the glomerular filtration barrier.

32. The pass-through phenomenon observed with the Clinitest method when large amounts of glucose are present in the urine is due to
    A. "carmelization" of the sugar present.
    B. reduction of copper sulfate to green-brown cupric complexes.
    C. depletion of the substrate, that is, not enough copper sulfate is present initially.
    D. reoxidation of the cuprous oxide formed to cupric oxide and other cupric complexes.

33. The glucose specificity of the double sequential enzyme reaction used on reagent strip tests is due to the use of
    A. gluconic acid.
    B. glucose oxidase.
    C. hydrogen peroxide.
    D. peroxidase.

34. Which of the following ketones is not detected by the reagent strip or tablet test?
    A. Acetone
    B. Acetoacetate
    C. Acetone and acetoacetate
    D. β-Hydroxybutyrate

35. Which of the following can cause false-positive ketone results?
    A. A large amount of ascorbic acid in urine
    B. Improper storage of the urine specimen
    C. Drugs containing free sulfhydryl groups
    D. A large amount of glucose (glucosuria)

36. Which of the following will not cause ketonemia and ketonuria?
    A. An inability to use carbohydrates
    B. Inadequate intake of carbohydrates
    C. Increased metabolism of carbohydrates
    D. Excessive loss of carbohydrates

37. The ketone reagent strip and tablet tests are based on the reactivity of ketones with
    A. ferric chloride.
    B. ferric nitrate.
    C. nitroglycerin.
    D. nitroprusside.

38. Which of the following statements about bilirubin is true?
    A. Conjugated bilirubin is water insoluble.
    B. Bilirubin is a degradation product of heme catabolism.
    C. Unconjugated bilirubin readily passes through the glomerular filtration barrier.
    D. The liver conjugates bilirubin with albumin to form conjugated bilirubin.

39. The bilirubin reagent strip and tablet tests are based on
    A. Ehrlich's aldehyde reaction.
    B. the oxidation of bilirubin to biliverdin.
    C. the reduction of bilirubin to azobilirubin.
    D. the coupling of bilirubin with a diazonium salt.

40. Which of the following are characteristic urine findings from a patient with hemolytic jaundice?
    A. A positive test for bilirubin and an increased amount of urobilinogen
    B. A positive test for bilirubin and a decreased amount of urobilinogen
    C. A negative test for bilirubin and an increased amount of urobilinogen
    D. A negative test for bilirubin and a decreased amount of urobilinogen

41. Which of the following results show characteristic urine findings from a patient with an obstruction of the bile duct?
    A. A positive test for bilirubin and an increased amount of urobilinogen
    B. A positive test for bilirubin and a decreased amount of urobilinogen
    C. A negative test for bilirubin and an increased amount of urobilinogen
    D. A negative test for bilirubin and a decreased amount of urobilinogen

42. Which of the following conditions can result in false-positive bilirubin results?
    A. Elevated concentrations of nitrite
    B. Improper storage of the specimen
    C. Ingestion of ascorbic acid
    D. Ingestion of certain medications

43. Urobilinogen is formed from the
    A. conjugation of bilirubin in the liver.
    B. reduction of conjugated bilirubin in bile.
    C. reduction of bilirubin by intestinal bacteria.
    D. oxidation of urobilin by anaerobic intestinal bacteria.

44. Which of the following statements about urobilinogen is true?
    A. Urobilinogen is not normally present in urine.
    B. Urobilinogen excretion usually is decreased following a meal.
    C. Urobilinogen excretion is an indicator of renal function.
    D. Urobilinogen is labile and readily photo-oxidizes to urobilin.

45. The classic Ehrlich's reaction is based on the reaction of urobilinogen with
    A. diazotized dichloroaniline.
    B. *p*-aminobenzoic acid.
    C. *p*-dichlorobenzene diazonium salt.
    D. *p*-dimethylaminobenzaldehyde.

46. Which of the following chemical principles is most specific for the detection of urobilinogen?
    A. Azocoupling reaction
    B. Ehrlich's reaction
    C. Hoesch test
    D. Watson-Schwartz test

47. Which of the following statements about porphobilinogen is true?
    A. Porphobilinogen is red and fluoresces.
    B. Normally, only trace amounts of porphobilinogen are formed.
    C. Porphobilinogen is an intermediate product in bilirubin formation.
    D. Porphobilinogen production is the rate-limiting step in heme synthesis.

48. A Watson-Schwartz test is performed on a urine specimen. The following results are seen: chloroform tube—red color in the bottom layer; butanol tube: red color in the top layer. These results indicate the presence of
    A. urobilinogen
    B. porphobilinogen
    C. urobilinogen and other Ehrlich's reactive substances
    D. porphobilinogen and other Ehrlich's reactive substances

49. Which of the following features is/are different when the Hoesch and Watson-Schwartz tests are compared?
    1. The pH of the reaction mixture
    2. The concentration of the Ehrlich's reagent used
    3. The volume ratio of urine to Ehrlich's reagent in the reaction mixture
    4. The sensitivity and specificity for porphobilinogen and urobilinogen
    A. 1, 2, and 3 are correct.
    B. 1 and 3 are correct.
    C. 4 is correct.
    D. All are correct.

50. Which of the following reagent strip tests can be affected by ascorbic acid, resulting in falsely low or false-negative results?
    1. Blood
    2. Bilirubin
    3. Glucose
    4. Nitrite
    A. 1, 2, and 3 are correct.
    B. 1 and 3 are correct.
    C. 4 is correct.
    D. All are correct.

51. Which of the following best describes the mechanism of ascorbic acid interference?
    A. Ascorbic acid inhibits oxidation of the chromogen.
    B. Ascorbic acid inactivates a reactant, promoting color development.
    C. Ascorbic acid removes a reactant from the intended reaction sequence.
    D. Ascorbic acid interacts with the reactants, producing a color that masks the results.

CASE 7-1

A 45-year-old woman with type 1 diabetes mellitus is admitted to the hospital and has been given a preliminary diagnosis of the nephrotic syndrome. She has not been feeling well for the past week and has bilateral pitting edema in her lower limbs. Her admission urinalysis results follow.

Results

Physical Examination	Chemical Examination	Confirmatory Tests
Color: colorless	SG: 1.010	
Clarity: clear	pH: 5	
Odor: —	Blood: small	
Large amount of white foam noted	Protein: 500 mg/dL	SSA: 4+
	LE: negative	
	Nitrite: negative	
	Glucose: 250 mg/dL	
	Ketones: negative	
	Bilirubin: negative	
	Urobilinogen: normal	

LE, Leukocyte esterase.

1. Circle any abnormal or discrepant urinalysis findings.
2. Which substance most likely accounts for the large amount of white foam observed?
    A. Fat
    B. Protein
    C. Glucose
    D. Blood/hemoglobin
3. Explain the most likely reason for the presence of increased red blood cells in this patient's urine.
4. Is the hemoglobin present (blood reaction: small) contributing to the protein test result? Explain.
5. If this patient has the nephrotic syndrome, the proteinuria in this patient should be classified as
    A. glomerular proteinuria.
    B. tubular proteinuria.
    C. overflow proteinuria.
    D. postrenal proteinuria.
6. In progressive renal disease, when solute discrimination by the glomerular filtration barrier is lost, monitoring which protein is most useful in identifying these glomerular changes?
7. Why is glucose present in the urine of this patient? Explain briefly.

CASE 7-2

An 82-year-old woman was admitted to the hospital with back and left rib pain. Radiographic examination revealed lytic lesions of the lumbar vertebrae and ribs, and sheets of plasma cells were present on bone marrow biopsy. A diagnosis of multiple myeloma is made. Her admission urinalysis results follow.

Results

Physical Examination	Chemical Examination	Confirmatory Tests
Color: yellow	SG: 1.020	
Clarity: slightly cloudy	pH: 5.5	
Odor: —	Blood: negative	
	Protein: trace	SSA: 3+
	LE: negative	
	Nitrite: negative	
	Glucose: negative	
	Ketone: negative	
	Bilirubin: negative	
	Urobilinogen: normal	

1. Circle any abnormal or discrepant urinalysis findings.
2. Explain the most probable cause for the discrepancy between the reagent pad test for protein and the SSA test results.
3. A 24-hour urine collection reveals an increase in urine total protein. Which protein(s) is most likely responsible for the proteinuria in this patient?
   A. Albumin
   B. Globulins
   C. Hemoglobin
   D. Uromodulin
4. The proteinuria in this patient would be classified as
   A. glomerular proteinuria.
   B. tubular proteinuria.
   C. overflow proteinuria.
   D. postrenal proteinuria.

LE, Leukocyte esterase.

CASE 7-3

A 23-year-old woman is seen in the emergency room with acute abdominal pain, nausea, and hypertension. She had a previous admission 1 year ago for intestinal problems and neurologic symptoms (depression). At that time, gastrointestinal and neurologic examinations were negative. She recently started taking oral contraceptives and states that she is taking no other medications. In addition, she has a family history of acute intermittent porphyria. Routine hematologic and chemistry tests are ordered, and all results are normal. A routine urinalysis is performed.

Results

Physical Examination	Chemical Examination	Confirmatory Tests
Color: yellow	SG: 1.015	
Clarity: clear	pH: 5.0	
Odor: —	Blood: negative	
	Protein: negative	
	LE: negative	
	Nitrite: negative	
	Glucose: negative	
	Ketones: negative	
	Bilirubin: negative	
	Urobilinogen: normal	
		Hoesch test: positive

1. Circle any abnormal or discrepant urinalysis findings.
2. For academic reasons, the urine specimen was refrigerated and was examined the next day for any change in color. The yellow urine now had a pink hue; however, it was not prominent. What substance most likely is causing the pink hue now observed in the urine?
3. If the results of the Hoesch test were questionable or if reagents were not available, what test could be performed to confirm the presence of this substance?
4. Explain the physiologic process that results in the appearance of this substance in the urine.
5. What is this patient's most likely diagnosis?
6. In addition to the substance observed, this patient would most likely have increased levels of
   A. blood porphyrins.
   B. fecal porphyrins.
   C. urinary coproporphyrin.
   D. urinary δ-aminolevulinic acid.
7. Are any reagent strip tests capable of detecting the substance identified in Question 2 in urine?

LE, Leukocyte esterase.

CASE 7-4

A 51-year-old woman is admitted to the hospital for a vaginal hysterectomy. During surgery, she is placed in Simon's position (exaggerated lithotomy position) for 6 hours because of surgical complications. She receives 2 units of packed red blood cells following surgery. Twenty-four hours after surgery, a routine urinalysis, hemoglobin, hematocrit, and various chemistry tests are performed. The chemistry and urinalysis results follow.

Serum Chemistry Results

Test Result	Reference Range
Creatine kinase: 5800 U/L	10-130 U/L
Myoglobin: 400 U/L	<120 U/L
Haptoglobin: 175 mg/dL	83-267 mg/dL

Urine Results

Physical Examination	Chemical Examination	Confirmatory Tests
Color: brown	SG: 1.015	
Clarity: clear	pH: 5.5	
Odor: —	Blood: large	
	Protein: trace	SSA: trace
	LE: negative	
	Nitrite: negative	
	Glucose: negative	
	Ketones: negative	
	Bilirubin: negative	
	Urobilinogen: normal	

1. Circle any abnormal or discrepant urinalysis findings.
2. In this specimen, which substance most likely is causing the urine to appear brown?
   A. Bilirubin
   B. Hemoglobin
   C. Myoglobin
   D. A drug the patient is taking
3. Which of the following substances is causing the blood reaction to be large?
   A. Ascorbic acid
   B. Bilirubin
   C. Hemoglobin
   D. Myoglobin
4. What protein is responsible for the trace strip result? Explain.
5. Suggest a cause for the myoglobinuria.

LE, Leukocyte esterase.

CASE 7-5

A 26-year-old man is seen by his physician and reports sudden weight loss, polydipsia, and polyuria. A routine urinalysis and plasma glucose level are obtained. The patient was fasting before blood collection.

Chemistry Results

Plasma glucose: 230 mg/dL (reference ranges: fasting ≤110 mg/dL; diabetic ≥126 mg/dL)

Results

Physical Examination	Chemical Examination	Confirmatory Tests
Color: colorless	SG: 1.010	Refractometer: 1.029
Clarity: clear	pH: 5.5	
Odor:	Blood: negative	
	Protein: negative	
	LE: negative	
	Nitrite: negative	
	Glucose: >2000	Clinitest (2-drop): ≥5000
	Ketones: small	Clinitest (5-drop): >2000*
	Bilirubin: negative	
	Urobilinogen: normal	

1. List any abnormal or discrepant urinalysis findings.
2. Explain the pass-through effect exhibited by the Clinitest method in this patient.
3. What is the concern about observing the pass-through effect?
4. Is this patient showing any signs of renal damage or dysfunction? Yes No
5. Select the diagnosis that best accounts for the glucosuria observed in this patient.
   A. Normal; glucose renal threshold exceeded
   B. Type 1 diabetes mellitus
   C. Type 2 diabetes mellitus
   D. Impaired glucose tolerance
6. Explain why the reagent strip ketone test is positive.
7. Explain the two different specific gravity results obtained. Which result most accurately reflects the ability of the kidneys to concentrate renal solutes (i.e., renal concentrating ability)?

LE, Leukocyte esterase.
*The pass-through effect was noted during performance of this test.

CASE 7-6

A 36-year-old man sees his doctor and reports fatigue, nausea, and concern about a yellowish discoloration in the sclera of his eyes. Physical examination reveals a tender liver. The following urinalysis results are obtained.

Results

Physical Examination	Chemical Examination	Confirmatory Tests
Color: amber	SG: 1.015	
Clarity: slightly cloudy	pH: 6.5	
Odor: —	Blood: negative	
Yellow coloration of foam noted	Protein: trace	
	LE: negative	
	Nitrite: negative	
	Glucose: negative	
	Ketones: negative	
	Bilirubin: negative	Ictotest: positive
	Urobilinogen: normal	

1. List any abnormal or discrepant urinalysis findings.
2. What substance most likely accounts for the urine color and foam color observations?
3. Why is the reagent strip bilirubin test negative, whereas the Ictotest is positive?
4. Should the bilirubin on this urine be reported as negative or positive?
5. Explain the physiologic process that accounts for the bilirubin in this urine.
6. What form of bilirubin is present in this urine: unconjugated or conjugated?
7. Why is the urobilinogen normal and not increased?

LE, Leukocyte esterase.

REFERENCES

1. Clinical and Laboratory Standards Institute: Urinalysis: approved guideline, ed 3, CLSI Document GP16-A3, Wayne, PA, 2009, CLSI.
2. Shihabi ZK, Hamilton RW, Hopkins MB: Myoglobinuria, hemoglobinuria, and acute renal failure. Clin Chem 35:1713-1720, 1989.
3. McPherson RA, Ben-Ezra J, Zhao S: Basic examination of urine. In Henry JB, editor: Henry's clinical diagnosis and management by laboratory methods, ed 21, Philadelphia, 2007, WB Saunders.
4. Waller KV, Ward MW, Mahan JD, Wismatt DK: Current concepts in proteinuria. Clin Chem 35:755-765, 1989.
5. Robinson RR, Glover SN, Phillippi PJ, et al: Fixed and reproducible orthostatic proteinuria. Am J Pathol 39:405-417, 1961.
6. Gyure WL: Comparison of several methods for semiquantitative determinations of urinary protein. Clin Chem 23:876-879, 1977.
7. American Diabetes Association: Position statement: diabetic nephropathy. Diabetes Care 21:S50-S53, 1998.
8. Alzaid AA: Microalbuminuria in patients with NIDDM: an overview. Diabetes Care 19:79-89, 1996.
9. Peterson JC, Adler S, Burkart JM, et al: Blood pressure control, proteinuria, and the progression of renal disease. Ann Intern Med 123:754-762, 1995.
10. Fredrickson RA, MacKay D, Boudreau M, MacCabe R; Diagnostics Chemicals Limited: Rapid, semi-quantitative urinary albumin ImmunoDip stick assay for microalbuminuria. Paper presented at Oak Ridge Conference, April 1998, Raleigh, NC.
11. Mogensen CE, Viberti GC, Peheim E, et al: Multicenter evaluation of the Micral-Test II test strip, an immunologic rapid test for the detection of microalbuminuria. Diabetes Care 20:1642-1646, 1997.
12. Chemstrip Micral product insert, Indianapolis, IN, 2001, Roche Diagnostics Corporation.
13. Clinitek Microalbumin Reagent Strips product insert, Elkhart, IN, May 1999, Bayer Corporation.
14. Multistix PRO Reagent Strips product insert, Elkhart, IN, October 2001, Bayer Corporation.
15. Pugia MJ, Lott JA, Wallace JF, et al: Assay of creatinine using the peroxidase activity of copper-creatinine complexes. Clin Biochem 33:63-73, 2000.
16. Pugia MJ, Lott JA, Profitt JA, et al: High-sensitivity dye binding assay for albumin in urine. J Clin Lab Anal 13:180-187, 1999.
17. Wallace JF, Pugia MJ, Lott JA, et al: Multisite evaluation of a new dipstick for albumin, protein, and creatinine. J Clin Lab Anal 15:231-235, 2001.
18. Brigden ML, Edgell D, McPherson M, et al: High incidence of significant urinary ascorbic acid concentrations in a West Coast population: implications for routine urinalysis. Clin Chem 38:426-431, 1992.
19. Benedict SR: A reagent for the detection of reducing sugars. J Biol Chem 5:485, 1909.
20. Montgomery R, Conway TW, Spector AA: Lipid metabolism. In Biochemistry: a case-oriented approach, St Louis, 1990, Mosby.
21. Cotran RS, Kumar V, Robbins SL: Robbins' pathologic basis of disease, ed 4, Philadelphia, 1989, WB Saunders.
22. Caraway WT, Watts NB: Carbohydrates. In Tietz NW, editor: Fundamentals of clinical chemistry, ed 3, Philadelphia, 1987, WB Saunders.
23. Csako G: Causes, consequences, and recognition of false-positive reactions for ketones. Clin Chem 36:1388-1389, 1990.
24. Sherwin JE: Liver function. In Kaplan LA, Pesce AJ, editors: *Clinical chemistry, theory, analysis, and correlation*, ed 2, St Louis, 1989, Mosby.
25. Kanis JA: Detection of urinary porphobilinogen. Lancet 1:1511, 1973.
26. Pierach CA, Cardinal R, Bossenmaier I, Watson CJ: Comparison of the Hoesch and Watson-Schwartz tests for urinary porphobilinogen. Clin Chem 23:1666-1668, 1977.
27. Csako G: Mesna and other free-sulfhydryl compounds produce false-positive results in a urine test strip method for ascorbic acid. Clin Chem 45:2295-2296, 1999.

BIBLIOGRAPHY

Agrawal B, Berger A, Wolf K, Luft F: Microalbuminuria screening by reagent strip predicts cardiovascular risk in hypertension. J Hypertens 14:223-228, 1996.

American Diabetes Association: Nephropathy in Diabetes. Diabetes Care 27:S79-S83, 2004.

Brunzel NA: Renal function: nonprotein nitrogen compounds, function tests, and renal disease. In Clinical chemistry: concepts and applications, New York, 2003, McGraw-Hill.

de la Sierra A, Bragulat E, Sierra C, et al: Microalbuminuria in essential hypertension: clinical and biochemical profile. Br J Biomed Sci 57:287-291, 2000.

Ehrmeyer S: Using a creatinine ratio in urinalysis to improve the reliability of protein and albumin results. Medical Laboratory Observer 35:26-28, 2003.

Finnegan K: Routine urinalysis. In Saunders manual of clinical laboratory science, Philadelphia, 1998, WB Saunders.

Ben-Ezra J, Zhao S, McPherson RA: Basic examination of urine. In McPherson RA and Pincus MR, editors: Clinical diagnosis and management by laboratory methods, ed 21, Philadelphia, 2007, Saunders.

Giampietro O, Penno G, Clerico A, et al: Which method for quantifying microalbuminuria in diabetics? Acta Diabetol 28:239-245, 1992.

Kaplan LA, Pesce AJ, Kazmierczak SC, editors: Clinical chemistry: theory, analysis, correlation, ed 4, St Louis, 2003, Mosby.

Labbe RF, Lamon JM: Porphyrins and disorders of porphyrin metabolism. In Tietz NW, editor: Fundamentals of clinical chemistry, ed 3, Philadelphia, 1987, WB Saunders.

Marshall SM, Shearing PA, Alberti KG: Micral-Test strips evaluated for screening for albuminuria. Clin Chem 38:588-591, 1992.

Mogensen CE, Keane WF, Bennett PH, et al: Prevention of diabetic renal disease with special reference to microalbuminuria. Lancet 346:1080-1084, 1995.

Mundt LA, Shanahan K: Graff's textbook of urinalysis and body fluids, ed 2, Philadelphia, 2011, Lippincott Williams & Wilkins.

Strasinger SK, Di Lorenzo MS: Urinalysis and body fluids, ed 5, Philadelphia, 2008, FA Davis.

Tiu SC, Lee SS, Cheng MW: Comparison of six commercial techniques in the measurement of microalbuminuria in diabetic patients. Diabetes Care 16:616-620, 1993.

Warram JH, Gearin G, Laffel L, et al: Effect of duration of type I diabetes on the prevalence of stages of diabetic nephropathy defined by urinary albumin/creatinine ratio. J Am Soc Nephrol 7:930-937, 1996.

Yudkin JS, Forrest RD, Jackson CA: Microalbuminuria as predictor of vascular disease in nondiabetic subjects. Lancet 2:531-534, 1988.

Zelmanovitz T, Gross JL, Oliveira JR, et al: The receiver operating characteristics curve in the evaluation of a random urine specimen as a screening test for diabetic nephropathy. Diabetes Care 20:516-519, 1997.

Microscopic Examination of Urine Sediment

KEY TERMS

casts Cylindrical bodies that form in the lumen of the renal tubule. Their core matrix is principally made up of uromodulin (formerly known as Tamm-Horsfall glycoprotein), although other plasma proteins can be incorporated. Because casts are formed in the tubular lumen, any chemical or formed element present—such as cells, fat, and bacteria—can be incorporated into its matrix. Casts are enumerated and classified by the types of inclusions present.

clue cells Squamous epithelial cells with large numbers of bacteria adhering to them. Clue cells appear soft and finely granular with indistinct or "shaggy" cell borders. To be considered a clue cell, the bacteria do not need to cover the entire cell, but the bacterial organisms must extend beyond the cytoplasmic borders of the cell. Clue cells are characteristic of bacterial vaginosis, a synergistic infection involving *Gardnerella vaginalis* and anaerobic bacteria.

collecting duct cells Cuboidal or polygonal cells approximately 12 to 20 mm in diameter with a large, centrally located dense nucleus. These cells form the lining of the collecting tubules and become larger and more columnar as they approach the renal calyces.

crystals Entities formed by the solidification of urinary solutes. These urinary solutes can be made of a single element, a compound, or a mixture and are arranged in a regular, repeating pattern throughout the crystalline structure.

cytocentrifugation A specialized centrifuge procedure used to produce a monolayer of the cellular constituents in various body fluids on a microscope slide. The slides are fixed and stained, providing a permanent preparation for cytologic studies.

distal convoluted tubular cells Oval to round cells approximately 14 to 25 mm in diameter with a small, central to slightly eccentric nucleus and a dense chromatin pattern. These cells form the lining of the distal convoluted tubules.

KOH preparation A preparation technique used to enhance the

viewing of fungal elements. Secretions obtained using a sterile swab are suspended in saline. A drop of this suspension is placed on a microscope slide, followed by a drop of 10% KOH. The slide is warmed and is viewed microscopically. KOH destroys most formed elements, with the exception of bacteria and fungal elements.

lipiduria The presence of lipids in the urine.

Maltese cross pattern A design that appears as an orb divided into four quadrants by a bright Maltese-style cross. When the microscopist uses polarizing microscopy, cholesterol droplets exhibit this characteristic pattern, which aids in their identification. Other substances, such as starch granules, can show a similar pattern.

oval fat bodies Renal tubular epithelial cells or macrophages with inclusions of fat or lipids. Often these cells are engorged such that specific cellular identification is impossible.

proximal convoluted tubular cells Large (approximately 20 to 60 mm in diameter) oblong or cigar-shaped cells with a small, often eccentric, nucleus (or they can be multinucleated) and a dense chromatin pattern; these cells form the lining of the proximal tubules.

Prussian blue reaction (also called the Rous test) A chemical reaction used to identify the presence of iron. Iron-containing granules such as hemosiderin stain a characteristic blue color when mixed with a

freshly prepared solution of potassium ferricyanide–HCl.

squamous epithelial cells Large (approximately 40 to 60 mm in diameter), thin, flagstone-shaped cells with a small, condensed, centrally located nucleus (or they can be anucleated) that form the lining of the urethra in the female and the distal urethra in the male.

Tamm-Horsfall protein See *uromodulin.*

transitional (urothelial) epithelial cells Round or pear-shaped cells with an oval to round nucleus and abundant cytoplasm. These cells form the lining of the renal calyces, renal pelves, ureters, and bladder. They vary considerably in size, ranging from 20 to 40 mm in diameter, depending on their location in the three principal layers of this epithelium, that is, the superficial layer, the intermediate layers, and the basal layer.

uromodulin A glycoprotein (formerly known as Tamm-Horsfall protein)[1] that is produced and secreted only by renal tubular cells, particularly those of the thick ascending limbs of the loop of Henle and the distal convoluted tubules.[2] Studies have demonstrated that uromodulin plays a role in the following functions in the kidney: water impermeability of the tubules where it is expressed, defense against infectious agents (e.g., bacteria), and inhibition of calcium salt aggregation.[3]

The standardized quantitative microscopic examination of urine sediment made its clinical laboratory debut in 1926. At that time, Thomas Addis developed a procedure to quantitate formed elements in a 12-hour overnight urine collection. The purpose of this test, the Addis count, was to follow the progress of renal diseases, particularly acute glomerulonephritis. Increased numbers of red blood cells, white blood cells, or **casts** in the urine indicated disease progression. A disease process was indicated when one or more of the following cell changes occurred: The number of red blood cells exceeded 500,000; the number of white blood cells exceeded 2 million; or the number of casts exceeded 5000. Because other, primarily chemical, methods are currently available to monitor the progression of renal disease, the

Addis count is no longer routinely performed, despite its ability to accurately detect changes in the excretion of urinary formed elements. However, microscopic examination of urine sediment continues to play an important role in the initial diagnosis and monitoring of renal disease.

STANDARDIZATION OF SEDIMENT PREPARATION

Ensuring the accuracy and precision of the urine microscopic examination requires standardization. This demands that established laboratory protocols for manually preparing the urine sediment, including using the same supplies, step sequences, timing intervals, and

TABLE 8-1	Factors That Require Standardization in the Microscopic Examination

Urine volume used (e.g., 10 mL, 12 mL, 15 mL)
Speed of centrifugation (400 or 450 × g)
Time of centrifugation (5 minutes)
Concentration of sediment prepared (e.g., 10:1, 12:1, 15:1, 30:1)
Volume of sediment examined—determined by commercial slides used and microscope optical properties (i.e., ocular field number)
Result reporting—format, terminology, reference intervals, magnification used for assessment

TABLE 8-2	Comparison of Selected Standardized Urinalysis Systems

Features	Count-10 System (V-Tech, Inc.)	Kova System (Hycor Scientific)	UriSystem Features (Fisher HealthCare)
Initial volume of urine used	12 mL	12 mL	12 mL
Final urine volume with sediment	0.8 mL	1.0 mL	0.4 mL
Sediment concentration	15:1	12:1	30:1
Volume of sediment used	6 mL	6 mL	16 mL
Area for viewing	36 mm²	32 mm²	90 mm²
Number of 100× fields*	11	10	28
Number of 400× fields*	183	163	459
Coverslip type	Acrylic	Acrylic	Acrylic
Number of specimens per slide	10	4, 10	10

*Calculated using a "field of view" diameter for high power (400×) of 0.5 mm and for low power (100×) of 2 mm. The number of fields possible is equal to the area for viewing divided by the area per low- or high-power field. Note that the field of view diameter is determined by the lens systems of the microscope.

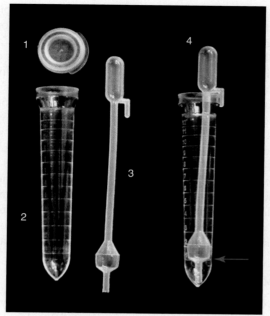

FIGURE 8-1 A commercial urine sediment preparation system. The KOVA System consists of a KOVA tube (2), a KOVA Pettor (3), and a KOVA cap (1). The clear plastic centrifuge tube is filled to the appropriate graduation mark with well-mixed urine and is capped. After centrifugation, the specially designed KOVA Pettor is gently slid into the tube, and the end is firmly seated into the base (4). The bulblike end fits snuggly, such that all but 1 mL of urine can be easily decanted *(red arrow)*. The retained supernatant urine is used to resuspend the sediment for the microscopic examination.

equipment, are adhered to by all personnel. Table 8-1 lists various factors that must be established and followed to obtain standardization in the microscopic examination. Note that all personnel must follow all testing aspects consistently to ensure comparable urinalysis results.

Commercial Systems

To achieve consistency, several commercial urinalysis systems are available (Table 8-2). Each system seeks to consistently (1) produce the same concentration of urine or sediment volume; (2) present the same volume of sediment for microscopic examination; and (3) control microscopic variables such as the volume of sediment viewed and the optical properties of the slides. All of these systems surpass the outdated practice of using a drop of urine on a glass slide and covering it with a coverslip. In addition, commercial slides are cost competitive, easy to adapt to, and necessary to ensure reproducible and accurate results.

Commercial systems feature disposable plastic centrifuge tubes with gradations for consistent urine volume measurement (Figure 8-1). The tubes are clear, allowing for assessment of urine color and clarity, and conical, which facilitates sediment concentration during centrifugation. The centrifuge tubes of each commercial system are unique. The UriSystem tube (Fisher HealthCare, Houston, TX) is designed such that after centrifugation, it can be decanted with a quick smooth motion and consistently retains 0.4 mL of urine for sediment resuspension. The KOVA System (Hycor Biomedical, Garden Grove, CA) uses a specially designed pipette (KovaPettor) that snuggly fits the diameter and shape of the tube to retain 1 mL of urine during decanting. The Count-10 System (V-Tech, Inc., Lake Mary, FL) offers several options to retain 0.8 mL for sediment resuspension.

Each commercial system provides tight-fitting plastic caps for the tubes to prevent spillage and aerosol formation during centrifugation.

A laboratory need not purchase all aspects of a commercial system to obtain a standardized urine sediment for microscopic analysis. In fact, laboratories have considerable flexibility and can blend the systems. For example, a laboratory could choose to use KOVA System tubes to prepare the urine sediment but UriSystem slides or the RS2005 Urine Sediment Workstation (DiaSys Ltd., New York, NY), a semiautomated slide system, to view the sediment. Regardless of the system or combination of products used when preparing and performing the microscopic examination of urine sediment, the imperative is that all personnel adhere to established protocols to ensure that accurate and reproducible results are obtained.

Specimen Volume

The volume of urine recommended for a urinalysis is 12 mL; however, volumes ranging from 10 to 15 mL can be used. This volume from a well-mixed specimen will contain a representative sampling of urine formed elements. However, this amount of urine is not always available, especially from pediatric patients. In these instances, the volume of urine can be reduced to 6 mL, and all numeric counts from the sediment examination must be doubled. In some laboratories, when less than 3 mL of urine is available for testing, the urine is examined microscopically, without concentration of the sediment. Whenever the actual volume used to prepare the sediment for the microscopic examination is less than that routinely required, a notation must accompany the specimen report. The decision to accept specimens with volumes less than 12 mL for urinalysis, as well as the protocol used for testing, is determined by each individual laboratory.

Centrifugation

After well-mixed urine is poured into a centrifuge tube, it is covered and centrifuged at 400 to 450 g for 5 minutes. This centrifugation speed allows for optimal sediment concentration without damaging fragile formed elements such as cellular casts. All personnel must adhere to this 5-minute centrifugation time with all specimens to ensure uniformity. Note that the speed is given in relative centrifugal force (RCF, g) because this term is not dependent on the centrifuge used. In contrast, the speed in revolutions per minute (RPM) required to obtain 400 to 450 g varies with each centrifuge and is directly dependent on the rotor size. For example, one centrifuge may obtain $450 \times g$ at 1200 RPM, whereas another may require 1500 RPM to obtain this same g-force. The RPM necessary to achieve 400 to 450 g can be determined from a nomogram or by using Equation 8-1.

Equation 8-1

$$RCF\,(g) = 1.118 \times 10^{-5} \times radius\,(cm) \times RPM^2$$

In this equation, the radius in centimeters refers to the distance from the center of the rotor to the outermost point of the cup, tube, or trunnion when the rotor is in motion (Figure 8-2).

It is important that the centrifuge brake is not used because this will cause the sediment to resuspend, resulting in erroneously decreased numbers of formed

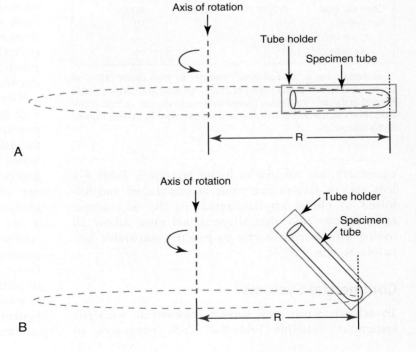

FIGURE 8-2 The rotor radius (R) is the distance measured from the rotor's axis of rotation to the bottom of the specimen tube at its greatest horizontal distance from the rotor axis. **A,** The radius when a horizontal rotor is used. **B,** The radius when a fixed-angle rotor is used.

elements in the concentrated sediment. In many laboratories, multiple personnel use centrifuges to perform numerous and varied procedures. If all centrifuge settings, including the brake, are not checked before use, the resultant urine sediments can show dramatic variations in their formed elements because of processing differences in speed, time, or braking. Using control materials for the microscopic examination or performing interlaboratory duplicate testing is valuable in its ability to detect these important changes in sediment preparation.

Sediment Concentration

Following centrifugation, the covered urine specimens should be carefully removed and the sediments concentrated using the established protocol. Standardized commercial systems accomplish this task through consistent retention of a specific volume of urine. Note that different brands of centrifuge tubes and pipettes should not be intermixed. This can cause variation in the volume of urine retained, which will change the concentration of the sediment. Table 8-2 shows how commercial systems vary in the sediment concentration produced, ranging from a 12:1 to a 30:1 concentration. Manual techniques traditionally strive toward a 12:1 concentration. Supernatant urine is removed by decanting or using a disposable pipette until 1 mL of urine is retained. Then, a pipette is used to gently resuspend the sediment. Too vigorous agitation of the sediment can cause fragile and brittle formed elements, such as red blood cell (RBC) casts and waxy casts, to break into pieces.

Volume of Sediment Viewed

A standardized slide should be used for the microscopic examination of urine sediment to ensure that the same volume of sediment is presented for viewing each time. Commercial standardized slides are made of molded plastic and have a built-in coverslip or provide a glass coverslip for use (Figure 8-3). With a disposable transfer pipette, urine sediment is presented to a chamber, which fills by capillary action. This technique facilitates uniform distribution of the formed elements throughout the viewing area of the slide.

Another option for standardizing the volume of sediment viewed is the RS2005 Urine Sediment Workstation. The RS2005 is a semiautomated microscopic analysis system, which includes an optical slide assembly (approximately 3 inches × 1 inch) that is placed on the microscope stage. The slide assembly resembles a hemocytometer chamber with a fixed glass coverslip and is connected to the RS2005 unit by a single piece of tubing. The RS2005 unit houses a peristaltic pump responsible for liquid flow into and out of the slide assembly. Concentrated urine sediment is aspirated into the viewing chamber with the use of a stainless steel sampling probe that extends from

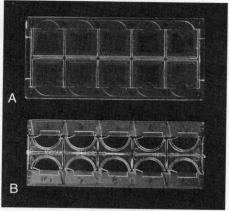

FIGURE 8-3 Commercial microscope slides. **A,** A 10-position Uri-System slide with integrated coverslips. **B,** A plastic 10-chamber KOVA Glasstic slide.

one end of the slide assembly. This probe is placed into the well-mixed urine sediment suspension at the bottom of a centrifuge tube, and the "Sample" button on the RS2005 unit is pressed. Within 3 seconds, the suspension is aspirated from the centrifuge tube and is transferred into the assembly for microscopic viewing. When the microscopic examination is complete, the "Purge" button causes the pump to start and reverse the flow of liquid. The urine sediment is flushed from the viewing chamber back through the sample probe; this is followed by purging with a solution that decontaminates the viewing chamber and prepares it for the next sample.

Glass microscope slides and coverslips are not recommended because they do not yield standardized, reproducible results.[4] If glass slides are used, the laboratorian should always pipette an exact amount (e.g., 15 mL) of the resuspended sediment onto the glass slide using a calibrated pipette. The volume of sediment dispensed is determined by each laboratory and depends on the size of the coverslip used. The urine sediment volume must fill the entire area beneath the coverslip without excess. Bubbles and uneven distribution of the sediment components can result when the coverslip is applied (e.g., heavier components such as casts are pushed or concentrate near the coverslip edges). If the microscopic examination reveals that the distribution of formed elements is uneven, a new suspension of the sediment should be prepared for viewing. Because all commercial systems have proved superior to the "drop on a slide" method, this technique should not be used for the microscopic examination of urine.[5]

Reporting Formats

In a manual microscopic examination, urine components are assessed or enumerated using at least 10 low-power (lpf) or 10 high-power fields (hpf). The quantity of some

TABLE 8-3	Qualitative Terms and Descriptions for Fields of View (FOVs)	
Term		**Description**
Rare	1+	Present, but hard to find
Few	1+	One (or more) present in *almost* every field of view (FOV)
Moderate	2+	Easy to find; number present in FOV varies; "more than few, less than many"
Many	3+	Prominent; large number present in all FOVs
Packed	4+	FOV is crowded by or overwhelmed with the elements

components (e.g., mucus, **crystals,** bacteria) is *qualitatively* assessed per field of view (FOV) in descriptive or numeric terms. Table 8-3 lists commonly used terms and typical descriptions. Each laboratory determines which terms are used, as well as the definition for each term. Other sediment components (RBCs, white blood cells [WBCs], casts) are *enumerated* as a range of formed elements present (e.g., 0 to 2, 2 to 5, 5 to 10). Note that although a component may be reported using low-power magnification, high-power magnification may be needed to specifically identify or categorize it, for example, to identify the cell type in a cellular cast. In this case, the cells were determined to be RBCs, and the quantity of cellular casts present is reported as the average number viewed using low power (e.g., 2 to 5 RBC casts/lpf).

When a microscopic examination is performed, the volume of sediment viewed in each microscopic FOV is determined by two factors: the optical lenses of the microscope and the standardized slide system used. The ocular field number of the microscope and the objective lens determine the area of the FOV (see Chapter 1). The larger the FOV, the greater is the number of components that may be visible. To obtain reproducible results when manual microscopic examinations are performed, the same microscope must be used, or when multiple microscopes are available, the diameters of their FOVs (i.e., ocular field numbers) must be identical.

These viewing factors and sediment preparation protocols account for the differences observed in reference ranges for microscopic formed elements. They also prevent comparison of the microscopic results obtained in laboratories using different microscopes and commercial slides. However, if each laboratory would relate sediment elements as the "number present per volume of urine" instead of per low- or high-power field, interlaboratory result comparisons would be possible and comparisons between manual and automated microscopy systems (e.g., iQ200 [Iris Diagnostics, Chatsworth, CA]; UF-1000i [bioMerieux Inc., Durham, NC]) would be facilitated.

To convert the number of formed elements observed per low- or high-power field to the number present per milliliter of urine tested, a few calculations are necessary (Box 8-1). First, the area of the field of view for the

BOX 8-1	Conversion of the Number of Formed Elements Present in a Microscopic Field to the Number of Formed Elements Present in a Volume of Urine

1. Calculate the areas of the low-power and high-power fields of view for your microscope using the formula: Area $= \pi r^2$.
   For example:
   Diameter of high-power field view $= 0.5$ mm (ocular field number 20)
   Radius of high-power field view $= 0.25$ mm
   Area of high-power field view $= 0.196$ mm^2

2. Calculate the maximum number of low-power and high-power fields possible using your microscope and the standardized microscope slides (see manufacturer's information or Table 8-1) in use as follows:

$$\frac{\text{Total coverslip area for viewing}}{\text{Area per high-power field (or low-power field)}} = \text{Number of view fields possible}$$

For example, using a KOVA slide and the microscopic lenses given in step 1,

$$\frac{32 \, mm^2}{0.196 \, mm^2} = 163 \text{ fields of view possible using high power}$$

3. Calculate the field conversion factor, which is the number of microscope fields per milliliter of urine tested, as follows:

$$\frac{\text{Number of view fields possible}}{\text{Volume of sediment viewed (mL)} \times \text{Concentration factor}} = \frac{\text{Number of view fields}}{1 \, mL \text{ of urine tested}}$$

For example, using the KOVA system specimen preparation and a KOVA slide,

$$\frac{163 \text{ high-power fields of view possible}}{0.006 \, mL \text{ sediment} \times 12} = \frac{\approx 2200 \text{ high-power fields}}{mL \text{ urine}}$$

$$= \text{Field Conversion Factor}$$

4. Convert the number of formed elements observed per high-power field (or low-power field) to the number present per milliliter of urine by multiplying the number observed per view field by the appropriate field conversion factor.
   For example, 2 red blood cells (RBCs) are observed per high-power field. Therefore,

$$\frac{2 \, RBCs}{\text{High-power field}} \times \frac{2200 \text{ high-power fields}}{mL \text{ urine}} = \frac{4400 \, RBCs}{mL \text{ urine}}$$

low- and high-power fields must be determined. This calculation uses the diameter for the field of view, which is determined by the ocular field number of the microscope and the formula for the area of a circle (Area $= \pi r^2$). Because a standardized commercial microscope slide provides the same volume of sediment in a known viewing area (see Table 8-2), and the area viewed in each

TABLE 8-4	Visualization Techniques to Aid in the Microscopic Examination of Urine Sediment
Technique	**Features**
Staining Techniques	
Sternheimer-Malbin	• A supravital stain that characteristically stains cellular structures and other formed elements • Enables detailed viewing and differentiation of cells, cast inclusions, and low refractile elements (e.g., hyaline casts, mucus)
0.5% toluidine blue	• A metachromatic stain that enhances the nuclear detail of cells • Aids in differentiating WBCs and renal tubular epithelial cells
2% acetic acid	• Accentuates the nuclei of leukocytes and epithelial cells • Lyses RBCs
Fat stains: Sudan III, Oil Red O	• Stains triglyceride (neutral fat) globules a characteristic orange (Sudan III) or red (Oil Red O) color • Used to confirm the presence of fat in urine
Gram stain	• Identifies and classifies bacteria as gram-negative or gram-positive • Aids in the identification of bacterial and fungal casts
Prussian blue reaction	• Identifies hemosiderin, which can be free-floating, in epithelial cells, or in casts
Hansel stain	• Aids in the identification of eosinophils
Microscopic Techniques	
Phase-contrast microscopy	• Enhances the imaging of translucent or low-refractile formed elements
Interference contrast microscopy	• Enhances the imaging of formed elements by producing three-dimensional images
Polarizing microscopy	• Used to confirm the presence of cholesterol globules by their characteristic *Maltese cross* pattern • Aids in the identification of crystals • Assists in differentiating "look-alike" components *Do NOT polarize light:* *DO polarize light:* RBCs Monohydrate calcium oxalate crystals Casts, mucus Fibers (clothing, diapers), plastic fragments Bacteria Amorphous crystals (urates: strongly; phosphates: very weakly) Cells, cellular debris (membrane phospholipids) Cholesterol globules, starch granules

microscopic field is known, the "field conversion factors" remain constant. Once the field conversion factors for a particular microscope and the standardized microscope slide system used have been established, determining the number of formed elements per milliliter of urine requires a single multiplication step. Box 8-1 outlines these calculations and includes an example.

ENHANCING URINE SEDIMENT VISUALIZATION

Visualization of urine sediment components can be difficult when brightfield microscopy is used because the refractive index of urine and some sediment components are similar, lacking sufficient contrast for optimal viewing. Staining changes the refractive index of formed elements and increases their visibility. Another approach is to change the type of microscopy, which can also facilitate visualization of low-refractility components or can be used to confirm the identity of suspected substances such as fat. Hyaline casts, mucous threads, and bacteria are difficult to see under brightfield microscopy; the use of stains or phase microscopy enhances their visualization. These techniques facilitate observation of the fine detail necessary for specific identification (e.g., distinguishing a white blood cell from a renal tubular cell). They also help to differentiate look-alike entities,

such as monohydrate calcium oxalate crystals, which can resemble red blood cells, and can be used to distinguish between mucous threads and hyaline casts. Table 8-4 summarizes the visualization techniques discussed in this chapter.

Staining Techniques

Supravital Stains. Numerous stains have been used to enhance the visualization of urine sediment. Each laboratory should have a stain available because stains are inexpensive and can significantly assist in the identification of some urine sediment components. The most commonly used stain is a supravital stain consisting of crystal-violet and safranin, also known as the Sternheimer-Malbin stain (Figure 8-4). This stain enhances formed element identification by enabling more detailed viewing of internal structures, particularly of white blood cells, epithelial cells, and casts. Other formed elements (e.g., red blood cells, mucus) stain characteristically, and their descriptions are noted on the package inserts provided with commercially prepared stains. Although the Sternheimer-Malbin stain is available commercially, it can also be readily prepared in the laboratory if desired.[6] One disadvantage of its use is that in strongly alkaline urines, this stain can precipitate, which obstructs the visualization of sediment components.

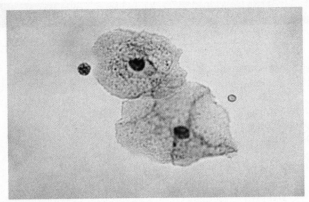

FIGURE 8-4 Two squamous epithelial cells stained with Sternheimer-Malbin stain. Brightfield, 100×.

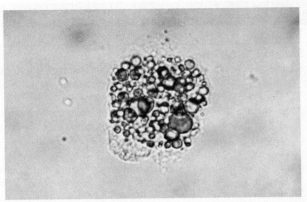

FIGURE 8-7 Oval fat body stained with Sudan III stain. Note the characteristic orange-red coloration of neutral fat globules. Brightfield, 400×.

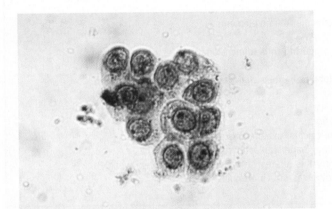

FIGURE 8-5 Fragment of renal collecting duct epithelial cells stained with 0.5% toluidine blue. Brightfield, 400×.

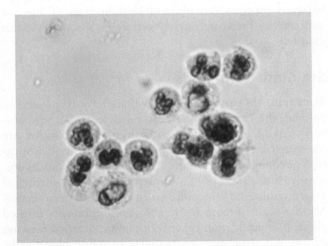

FIGURE 8-6 Leukocytes stained with 0.5% toluidine blue. Brightfield, 400×.

Another good supravital stain for urine sediment is a 0.5% solution of toluidine blue (Figures 8-5 and 8-6). The stain is a metachromatic dye that stains various cell components differently, hence the differentiation between the nucleus and the cytoplasm becomes more apparent. The toluidine blue stain enhances the specific identification of cells and aids in distinguishing cells of similar size, such as leukocytes from renal **collecting duct cells.**

Acetic Acid. Although acetic acid is not actually a stain, it can be helpful in identifying white blood cells. White blood cells can appear small, especially in hypertonic urine, with their nuclei and granulation not readily apparent. By adding 1 to 2 drops of a 2% solution of acetic acid to a few drops of urine sediment, the nuclear pattern of white blood cells and epithelial cells is accentuated, whereas red blood cells are lysed.

Fat or Lipid Stains. Sudan III or Oil Red O is often used to confirm the presence of neutral fat or triglyceride suspected during the microscopic examination (Figure 8-7). These lipids stain orange or red and may be found (1) free floating as droplets or globules; (2) within renal cells or macrophages, aptly termed *oval fat bodies;* or (3) within the matrix of casts as globules or oval fat bodies. An important note is that only neutral fats (e.g., triglycerides) stain. In contrast, cholesterol and cholesterol esters do not stain and must be confirmed by polarizing microscopy. The distinction between triglyceride and cholesterol is primarily academic because the implications for renal disease are the same regardless of the identity of the fat. In other words, changes have occurred in the glomeruli such that triglycerides and cholesterol from the bloodstream are now passing the glomerular filtration barriers with the plasma ultrafiltrate. The urinalysis laboratory can use a fat stain or polarizing microscopy to confirm the presence of fat; the confirmation method selected is usually determined by cost, personnel preference, and convenience.

Gram Stain. Although Gram stain is used primarily in the microbiology laboratory, it may at times be used in the urinalysis laboratory. Gram stain provides a means of positively identifying bacteria in the urine and differentiating them as gram-negative or gram-positive (Figure 8-8). To perform a Gram stain, a dry preparation of the urine sediment is made on a microscope slide by

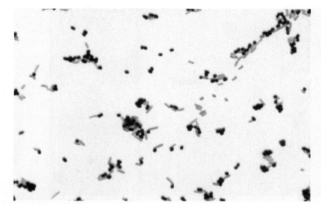

FIGURE 8-8 Bacteria. Gram stain of gram-negative rods and gram-positive cocci. Brightfield, 1000×.

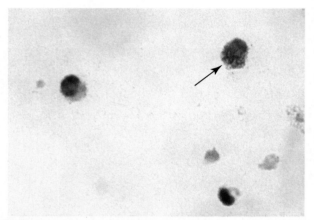

FIGURE 8-9 Eosinophil *(arrow)* in urine stained with Hansel stain. Cytospin, 400×.

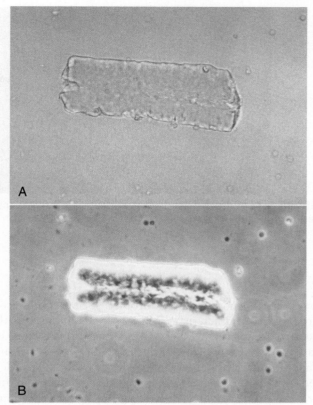

FIGURE 8-10 Waxy cast. **A,** Brightfield, 100×. **B,** Phase contrast, 100×. Note the central fissure and increased detail revealed using phase-contrast microscopy.

smearing and air drying or by cytocentrifugation. As in the microbiology laboratory, the slide is heat-fixed then stained. Gram-negative bacteria appear pink, whereas gram-positive bacteria appear dark purple. Because these slides can be viewed using a high-power oil immersion (100×) objective, additional characterization of the bacteria (e.g., cocci, rods) could be made, but this is rarely done by the urinalysis laboratory.

Prussian Blue Reaction. To facilitate the visualization of hemosiderin, free floating or in epithelial cells and casts, the **Prussian blue reaction** is used. First described by Rous in 1918 to identify urinary siderosis, the Prussian blue reaction stains the iron of hemosiderin granules a characteristic blue.[7] See "Hemosiderin" later in this chapter for more discussion of this reaction and its use.

Hansel Stain. Hansel stain (methylene blue and eosin-Y in methanol) is used in the urinalysis laboratory specifically to identify eosinophils in the urine (Figure 8-9). Whereas Wright's stain or Giemsa stain also distinguishes eosinophils, Hansel stain is preferred.[8] Patients with acute interstitial nephritis caused by hypersensitivity to a medication such as a penicillin derivative can have increased numbers of eosinophils in the urine sediment.

Identification of this renal disease is important because it is one of the few renal diseases for which quick and effective treatment is available: cessation of drug administration. Failure to do so can result in permanent renal damage.

Microscopy Techniques

Phase-Contrast Microscopy. As described in Chapter 1, phase-contrast microscopy converts variations in refractive index into variations in contrast and is ideally suited for viewing urine sediment (Figure 8-10). Phase-contrast microscopy permits more detailed visualization of translucent or low-refractile components and living cells than is possible with brightfield microscopy. This technique enables identification of traditionally difficult-to-view formed elements: hyaline casts and mucous threads. In addition, microscopic examinations are generally faster to perform; this is a direct reflection of the increased visualization afforded by phase-contrast microscopy.

Polarizing Microscopy. In the urinalysis laboratory, polarizing microscopy is most often used to confirm the presence of fat, specifically cholesterol. Cholesterol is birefringent, and, similar to its counterpart triglyceride, it can be found as free-floating droplets or in cells (oval

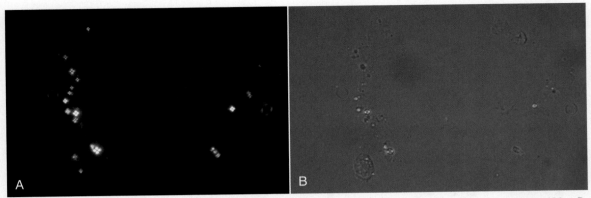

FIGURE 8-11 A, Cholesterol droplets displaying their characteristic Maltese cross pattern using polarizing microscopy, 400×. **B,** Polarizing microscopy with a first-order red compensator plate, 400×.

fat bodies) and casts. In droplet form, cholesterol produces a characteristic **Maltese cross pattern** with polarized light (Figure 8-11, *A*). These droplets appear as orbs against a black background divided into four quadrants by a bright Maltese-style cross. If a first-order red compensator plate is used, opposing quadrants in the orb are yellow or blue depending on their orientation, and the background is red to violet (Figure 8-11, *B*). Starch granules also show a similar Maltese cross pattern; however, when brightfield microscopy is used, starch granules are readily distinguishable from cholesterol by their refractility, characteristic dimple, and variations in size and shape. Because fatty acids and triglycerides are not anisotropic, they are not identified by polarizing microscopy.

Polarizing microscopy can also assist in differentiating urine sediment components that may "look alike" (see Table 8-4). Red blood cells can be distinguished from monohydrate calcium oxalate crystals; casts or mucus from fibers; and amorphous material from coccoid bacteria.

Interference Contrast Microscopy. Chapter 1 discusses two types of interference microscopy. Differential interference contrast (Nomarski) microscopy and modulation contrast (Hoffman) microscopy provide detailed three-dimensional images of high contrast and resolution (Figure 8-12). Although their use is suited ideally for microscopic examination of the formed elements found in urine sediment, the increased cost often cannot be justified by the traditional urinalysis laboratory. With experience, however, these microscopic techniques are easy to use and less time-consuming than brightfield microscopy because of the enhanced imaging. In addition, once a brightfield microscope has been modified for modulation contrast microscopy, it can easily be used for brightfield, polarizing, and other techniques by simply removing the specialized slit aperture from the light path.

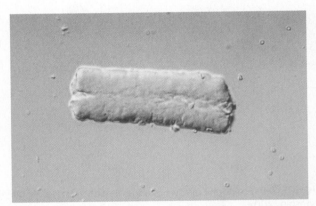

FIGURE 8-12 Three-dimensional image of the waxy cast in Figure 8-7 using differential interference contrast (Nomarski) microscopy, 100×. Compare images obtained in these two figures.

CYTOCENTRIFUGATION AND CYTODIAGNOSTIC URINALYSIS

Cytocentrifugation

Cytocentrifugation is a technique used to produce permanent microscope slides of urine sediment and body fluids (see Chapter 18). Because a monolayer of sediment components is desired, an initial microscopic examination is required to determine the amount or volume of urine sediment to use when preparing the slide. After which, the appropriate amount of concentrated urine sediment is added to a specially designed cartridge fitted with a microscope slide that is placed in a cytocentrifuge (e.g., Shandon Cytospin, Thermo Shandon, Pittsburgh, PA). After cytocentrifugation, a dry circular monolayer of sediment components remains on the slide. The slide is fixed permanently using an appropriate fixative and is stained. For cytologic studies, Papanicolaou's stain is preferred; however, if Papanicolaou's stain is not available, or if time is a factor, Wright's stain can be used. The end result is a monolayer of the urine sediment components with their structural details greatly enhanced by staining. This enables the quantitation and differentiation of white blood cells and epithelial cells in the urine sediment. If desired, these slides can also be viewed using high-power oil immersion objectives and can be retained permanently in the laboratory for later reference or review.

Cytodiagnostic Urinalysis

In 1926, Thomas Addis established the value of identifying increased numbers of urine cellular elements as evidence of disease progression. Today, the ability to perform urine differential cell counts enables identification of and discrimination between renal disease and urinary tract disorders. Although a cytodiagnostic urinalysis should not be performed on all urine specimens, it can play an important role in the early detection of renal allograft rejection and in the differential diagnosis of renal disease. Cytodiagnostic urinalysis involves making a 10:1 concentration of a first morning urine specimen, followed by cytocentrifugation of the urine sediment and Papanicolaou's staining.[9] Although cytodiagnostic urinalysis requires more time to perform, it is uniquely valuable in identification of blood cell types, cellular fragments, epithelial cells (atypical and neoplastic), cellular inclusions (viral and nonviral), and cellular casts.

FORMED ELEMENTS IN URINE SEDIMENT

A wide range of formed elements can be encountered in the microscopic examination of urine sediment. These formed components can originate from throughout the urinary tract—from the glomerulus to the urethra—or can result from contamination (e.g., menstrual blood, spermatozoa, fibers, starch granules). Many components, such as blood cells and epithelial cells, are cellular; others are chemical precipitates, such as the variety of crystalline and amorphous material that can be present in the sediment. **Casts**—cylindrical bodies with a glycoprotein matrix—form in the lumen of the renal tubules and are flushed out with the urine. Opportunistic microorganisms such as bacteria, yeast, and trichomonads can also be encountered in urine sediment. Not all of these formed elements indicate an abnormal or pathologic process. However, the presence of large numbers of "abnormal" components is diagnostically significant.

Identifying and enumerating the components found in urine sediment provide a means of monitoring disease progression or resolution. Determining at what point the amount of each element present indicates a pathologic process requires familiarity with the expected normal or

TABLE 8-5	Reference Intervals for Microscopic Examination*	
Component	**Number**	**Magnification**
Red blood cells	0-3	Per HPF
White blood cells	0-8	Per HPF
Casts	0-2 hyaline (or finely granular[†])	Per LPF
Epithelial cells		
Squamous	Few	Per LPF
Transitional	Few	Per HPF
Renal	Few	Per HPF
Bacteria and yeast	Negative	Per HPF
Abnormal crystals	None	Per LPF

HPF, High-power field (400×); *LPF,* low-power field (100×).
*Using the UriSystem. Values vary with concentration of urine sediment, microscope slide technique, and microscope optical properties. See Appendix B for reference intervals for a "complete" urinalysis.
[†]Following physical exercise, cast numbers increase and include finely granular casts (1991, Haber).

reference interval for each component (Table 8-5). (See Appendix B for reference intervals of all parameters in a complete urinalysis.) Normally, a few red blood cells, white blood cells, epithelial cells, and hyaline casts are observed in the urine sediment from normal, healthy individuals. Their actual number varies depending on the sediment preparation protocol and the standardized slide system used for the microscopic examination.[10] Because changes occur in unpreserved urine, factors such as the type of urine collection and how the specimen has been stored also affect the formed elements observed during microscopic examination.

This section discusses in detail the variety of formed elements possible in urine sediment and presents the origin of each component and its clinical significance, possible variations in shape and composition, and techniques used to facilitate differential identification. A wide range of additional images of urine sediment components can be found in the Urine Sediment Image Gallery, which is arranged alphabetically at the end of this chapter.

Blood Cells

Red Blood Cells (Erythrocytes). The name *erythrocyte* is derived from the Greek word "erythros," meaning "red" and the suffix element "-cyte," meaning "cell." Hence, these cells are more frequently called red blood cells (RBCs), and this term will be used predominantly throughout this text. RBCs were one of the first cells recognized and described after the discovery of the microscope.

Microscopic Appearance. Because of their small size—approximately 8 μm in diameter and 3 μm in

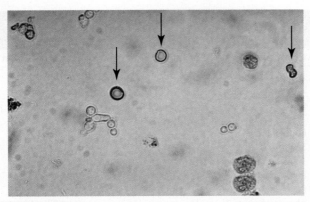

FIGURE 8-13 Three red blood cells: Two viewed from above appear as biconcave disks, and one viewed from the side appears hourglass-shaped *(arrows)*. Also present are budding yeast and several white blood cells. Brightfield, Sedi-Stain, 400×.

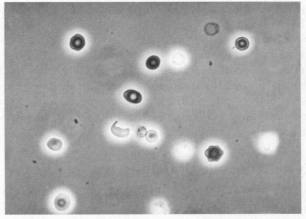

FIGURE 8-14 Dysmorphic and crenated red blood cells. A single ghost red blood cell is located at top of view. Phase contrast, 400×.

depth—RBCs in urine are viewed and enumerated using high-power magnification. RBCs have no nucleus, they normally appear as smooth biconcave disks, and they are moderately refractile. RBCs may be viewed from any angle in urine sediment. When viewed from the side, they have an hourglass shape; when viewed from above, they appear as disks with a central pallor (Figure 8-13). When present in *hypertonic urine,* RBCs become smaller as intracellular water is lost from the cell by osmosis, which causes them to become crenated. As they crenate, erythrocytes lose their biconcave disk shape and become spheres covered with spicules or crenations. Because of these membrane changes, these crenated cells appear rough microscopically compared with normal erythrocytes. In *hypotonic urine,* erythrocytes swell and release their hemoglobin to become "ghost" cells, which are cells with intact cell membranes but no hemoglobin. These empty cells, outlined by their membranes, appear as colorless, empty circles. Because their hemoglobin has been lost, ghost cells are difficult to see using brightfield microscopy; however, they are readily visible with phase-contrast or interference contrast microscopy (Figure 8-14). Alkaline urine promotes red blood cell lysis and disintegration, resulting in ghost cells and erythrocyte remnants. All of the red blood cell shapes described—normal biconcave disks, crenated cells, and ghost cells—can be found in the same urine sediment.

Dysmorphic or distorted erythrocytes can also be observed (see Figure 8-14). Occasionally these cells are present with normal erythrocytes in the urine of healthy individuals. However, increased numbers of particularly acanthocytes are associated with glomerular disorders.[11,12,13] Sickle cells have also been observed in the urine sediment of patients suffering from sickle cell disease.

Normally, RBCs are found in the urine of healthy individuals and do not exceed 0 to 3 per high-power field or 3 to 12 per microliter of urine sediment.[14]

Semiquantitation is made by observing 10 representative high-power fields and averaging the number of erythrocytes seen in each. Although RBCs are nonmotile, they are capable of passing through pores only 0.5 mm (500 nm) in diameter as foot processes.[15] In addition, during inflammation, RBCs can be transported out of capillaries by the same mechanism as inert, insoluble substances.[13] All RBCs in urine originate from the vascular system. The integrity of the normal vascular barrier in the kidneys or the urinary tract can be damaged by injury or disease, causing leakage of RBCs into any part of the urinary tract. Increased numbers of RBCs along with red blood cell casts indicate renal bleeding, either glomerular or tubular. These urines also have significant proteinuria. When an increased number of RBCs is present without casts or proteinuria, the bleed is occurring below the kidney or may be caused by contamination (e.g., menstrual, hemorrhoidal).

Correlation With Physical and Chemical Examinations. RBCs observed during the microscopic examination should be correlated with the physical and chemical examinations (Table 8-6). Macroscopically, the urine sediment may indicate the presence of RBCs when the sediment button is characteristically red in color. Sometimes specimens have a positive chemical test for blood, but the microscopic examination reveals no RBCs. This can be explained by the fact that RBCs readily lyse and disintegrate in hypotonic or alkaline urine; such lysis can also occur within the urinary tract before urine collection. As a result, urine specimens can be encountered that contain only hemoglobin from RBCs that are no longer intact or microscopically visible. However, it is important to note that other substances, such as myoglobin, microbial peroxidases, and strong oxidizing agents, can cause a positive blood chemical test (see Chapter 7). Note that these reactions are considered "false-positive" reactions because RBCs or blood is not present.

TABLE 8-6	Red Blood Cells: Microscopic Features and Correlations
Microscopic features	• Typical form—smooth, biconcave disks, 6-8 μm in diameter; no nucleus • Crenated forms—in concentrated urine (high SG) • Ghost cells—in dilute urine (low SG) • Dysmorphic forms and cell fragments
Look-alike elements	• Monohydrate calcium oxalate crystals • Yeast cells
Correlation with physical and chemical examinations	• Urine color—note that a normal appearing urine can still have increased RBCs present • Blood reaction—can be negative owing to ascorbic acid interference; degree of interference varies with reagent strip brand

In specimens in which RBCs are present microscopically but the chemical screen for blood is negative, ascorbic acid interference should be suspected. If ascorbic acid is ruled out, it is possible that the formed elements observed are not RBCs but a "look-alike" component such as yeast or monohydrate calcium oxalate crystals. In these cases, their identity should be confirmed by an alternative technique such as staining or using polarizing microscopy.

Even though hemoglobin is a protein, in most cases of hematuria, it does not contribute to the protein result obtained by the chemical reagent strip. Hemoglobin must be present in the urine in an amount exceeding 10 mg/dL before it is detected by routine protein reagent strip tests. In other words, when the chemical reagent strip test for blood reads less than large (3+), hemoglobin is not causing or contributing to the protein result; when the blood result is greater than or equal to large (3+), hemoglobin may be contributing to the protein reagent strip test result.

Look-Alikes. Other components in urine sediment such as yeast, monohydrate calcium oxalate crystals, small oil droplets, or air bubbles can resemble RBCs. Even white blood cells can be difficult to distinguish from crenated RBCs in a hypertonic urine specimen. In the latter case, using acetic acid or toluidine blue stain can be advantageous because these solutions make it easier to see the nuclei of white blood cells. The techniques described earlier in this chapter are useful for differentiation of these formed elements. A Sternheimer-Malbin stain characteristically colors RBCs, whereas neither yeast nor calcium oxalate crystals stain. Polarizing microscopy can identify calcium oxalate crystals, or 2% acetic acid can be added, which lyses RBCs but does not eliminate yeast or calcium oxalate crystals.

Yeast varies in size, tends to be spherical or ovoid rather than biconcave, and often exhibits budding. Each of these characteristics helps to differentiate yeast from RBCs.

Small bubbles or droplets of oil contaminating the urine sediment can be distinguished from RBCs by their variation in size, uniformity in appearance, and high refractility. Although these characteristics are usually evident to an experienced microscopist, they may not be obvious to a novice.

Clinical Significance. Numerous conditions can result in hematuria. Box 7-3 categorizes them into kidney and urinary tract disorders (e.g., glomerulonephritis, pyelonephritis, cystitis, calculi), non-renal disorders such as hypertension, appendicitis, tumors, trauma, strenuous exercise, and drugs. However, it is interesting to note that smoking as well as normal exercise has also been associated with hematuria.[16] Anticoagulant drugs and drugs that induce a toxic reaction, such as sulfonamides, can also cause increased numbers of RBCs in the urine sediment. Therefore any condition that results in inflammation or that compromises the integrity of the vascular system throughout the urinary tract can result in hematuria. Keep in mind that specimens contaminated with blood from vaginal secretions or hemorrhoidal blood can falsely imply hematuria. Table 8-6 summarizes the microscopic features of RBCs and the expected correlation between physical and chemical examinations when RBCs are present.

White Blood Cells (Leukocytes). *Leukocyte* is a collective term that refers to any type of white blood cell. In health, the distribution of white blood cells (WBCs) in the urine essentially mirrors that of peripheral blood. The five types of cells that can be present are neutrophils, lymphocytes, eosinophils, basophils, and monocytes (macrophages). Because neutrophils predominate in the peripheral blood, they are the white blood cell most often observed in urine; however, with some renal conditions, other leukocytes predominate in the urine. For example, in acute interstitial nephritis caused by drug hypersensitivity, the predominant leukocytes observed are eosinophils, whereas in renal allograft rejection, lymphocytes predominate.

Neutrophils

Microscopic Appearance. Neutrophils are the most common granulocytic leukocytes present in urine. They measure approximately 14 μm in diameter but can range from 10 to 20 μm, depending on the tonicity of the urine. They are larger than erythrocytes and can be similar in size to the small epithelial cells that line the collecting ducts of nephrons. Neutrophils are spherical cells with characteristic cytoplasmic granules and lobed or segmented nuclei (Figure 8-15). Unstained, neutrophils have a grayish hue and appear grainy. Neutrophils may occur singly or aggregated in clumps; clumping, which often occurs in acute inflammatory conditions, makes their enumeration difficult (Figure 8-16).

In fresh urine specimens, the characteristic features of neutrophils are often readily apparent by brightfield microscopy; however, as neutrophils age and begin to disintegrate, their lobed nuclei fuse, and they can

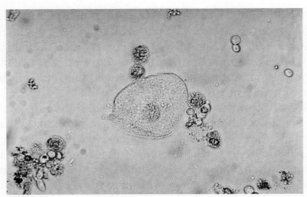

FIGURE 8-15 Several white blood cells with characteristic cytoplasmic granules and lobed nuclei surrounding a squamous epithelial cell. Budding yeast cells are also present. Brightfield, Sedi-Stain, 400×.

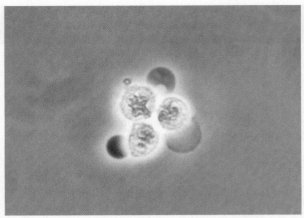

FIGURE 8-17 Disintegrating white blood cells with the formation of blebs. Phase contrast, 400×.

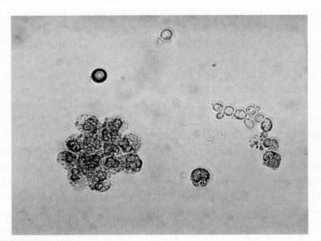

FIGURE 8-16 A clump of white blood cells. One red blood cell and budding yeast are also present. Brightfield, Sedi-Stain, 400×.

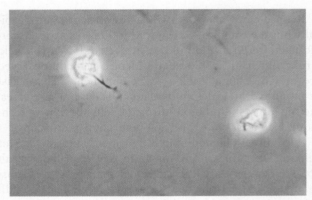

FIGURE 8-18 Formation of myelin filaments in disintegrating white blood cells. Phase contrast, 400×.

resemble a mononuclear cell. These changes can make neutrophils difficult to distinguish from renal tubular collecting duct cells. *Hypotonic* urine causes white blood cells to swell and become spherical balls that lyse as rapidly as 50% in 2 to 3 hours at room temperature. In these large swollen cells, brownian movement of the refractile cytoplasmic granules is often evident, giving the descriptive name "glitter cells" to these edemic leukocytes. In *hypertonic* urine, leukocytes become smaller as water is lost osmotically from the cells, but they do not crenate.

In addition to fusion of lobed nuclei (neutrophils), further evidence of cellular disintegration is seen in the formation of blebs (Figure 8-17). These vacuoles develop within the cell periphery or on their outer membranes; they appear to be empty or may contain a few small granules. As these changes continue, the blebs or vacuoles can detach and become free floating in the urine. They may also develop and remain within the cell, pushing the cytoplasm to one side and giving rise to large

pale areas intracellularly. Another degenerative change is the development of numerous finger-like or wormlike projections protruding from their surfaces (Figure 8-18). These long filaments, termed *myelin forms*, result from the breakdown of the cell membrane. As these cells die, additional vacuolization, rupturing, or pseudopod formation may be observed.

Normally, leukocytes are present in the urine of healthy individuals. When manual microscopic examinations are conducted, semiquantitation is performed by observing 10 representative high-power fields and determining the average number of WBCs present in each field. Note that values depend on the protocol used. Typically in health, 0 to 8 WBCs are present per high-power field, or approximately 10 WBCs per microliter of urine sediment using a standardized microscope slide. Any clumping of WBCs evident during the microscopic examination should be reported because leukocyte enumeration is directly affected. The presence of WBCs in urine is not surprising because they are a normal component in secretions of the male and female genital tracts. Because WBCs are motile, they are capable of entering the urinary tract at any point. In response to an inflammatory process, WBCs move through the tissues in an ameboid fashion (chemotaxis). Although they are spherical within the bloodstream or in the urine, the cytoplasm and the nucleus of leukocytes readily deform; this enables them to leave the peritubular capillaries and migrate through renal tissue (interstitium).

When microscopic examination reveals WBC casts, this finding provides diagnostic evidence of an upper urinary tract infection. Similarly, cellular casts (i.e., cell identity cannot be determined) and coarsely granular casts (which result from cell degradation) may also support a diagnosis of an upper urinary tract infection. In these cases, the protein reagent strip test should be positive. In contrast, with lower urinary tract infections (those localized below the kidney, such as in the bladder), microscopic examination would reveal increased WBCs but without cellular casts; if protein is present, it is usually at a low level.

Correlation With Physical and Microscopic Examinations.

When WBCs are present in the urine in increased numbers, the urine may be cloudy. Depending on the extent of the infection, the urine may have a strong, foul odor. A macroscopic examination of the sediment button may show a large amount of gray-white material: the concentrated leukocytes. Because leukocytes readily lyse in urine, discrepancies can occur between the number of cells seen microscopically and the leukocyte esterase (LE) screening test. A positive LE test, despite few or no white blood cells present microscopically, can occur because of WBC lysis and disintegration. Also, different populations of WBCs have varying quantities of cytoplasmic granules and therefore differing amounts of leukocyte esterase. In fact, lymphocytes have no leukocyte esterase. When increased numbers of WBCs are present in urine, but the LE test is negative, the microscopist must ensure that the cells are granulocytic leukocytes, and that the reagent strips are functioning properly. Although the LE screening test usually detects 10 to 25 white blood cells per microliter, the amount of esterase present may be insufficient to produce a positive response. Note that owing to hydration, hypotonic urine could cause the leukocyte esterase to be diluted such that it is below the detection limit of the LE reaction. Table 8-7 summarizes the microscopic features of WBCs and the expected correlation between physical and chemical examinations when WBCs are present.

Look-Alikes.

As was mentioned earlier, some renal tubular epithelial cells and at times even RBCs can be difficult to distinguish from leukocytes. A 2% acetic acid solution or, better yet, a 0.5% toluidine blue stain helps reveal the nuclear details of the cells present, which in turn enables proper cell identification. The large, dense nuclei of collecting duct cells and their polygonal shape help to distinguish collecting duct cells from spherical

TABLE 8-7	White Blood Cells (WBCs): Microscopic Features and Correlations
Microscopic features	*Neutrophils* • Spherical cells, 12-14 μm in diameter • Granular cytoplasm • Lobed nuclei • Glitter cells—dilute urine (low SG) *Lymphocytes* • Spherical cells, 6-9 μm in diameter • Mononuclear *Monocytes and macrophages* • Spherical cells, 20-25 μm in diameter • Granular cytoplasm • Mononuclear • Cytoplasm often vacuolated with ingested debris
Look-alike elements	• Renal tubular epithelial cells (collecting duct cells) • Dead trichomonads • Crenated red blood cells (RBCs)
Correlation with physical and chemical examinations	• Leukocyte esterase reaction—can be negative despite increased WBCs owing to excess hydration or when the WBCs are lymphocytes • Negative nitrite reaction: suggestive of inflammation or nonbacterial infection • Positive nitrite reaction: suggests bacterial infection

white blood cells that have characteristic cytoplasmic granulation (Figure 8-19). Staining with Sternheimer-Malbin stain or toluidine blue can produce more detailed cellular images for specific identification.

Clinical Significance.

An increased number of WBCs in urine is termed *leukocyturia*. Inflammatory conditions of the urinary tract and almost all renal diseases show increased numbers of WBCs, particularly neutrophils, in the urine. Note that both bacterial and nonbacterial causes of inflammation can result in leukocyturia. Bacterial infections include pyelonephritis, cystitis, urethritis, and prostatitis; nonbacterial infections include nephritis, glomerulonephritis, chlamydia, mycoplasmosis, tuberculosis, trichomonads, and mycoses. The latter two organisms, trichomonads and mycoses, often appear in urine from women as contaminants from vaginal secretions. Although they can infect the urinary tract, infection is rare. In contrast, when these organisms are present in the urine from a male, a urinary tract infection is implied.

Eosinophils. In a routine microscopic examination of unstained urine sediment, the discrimination of eosinophils from neutrophils is often impossible despite their

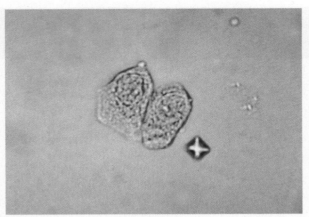

FIGURE 8-19 Two renal collecting duct cells stained with 0.5% toluidine blue. Their polygonal shape and nuclear detail distinguish them from leukocytes. Brightfield, 400×.

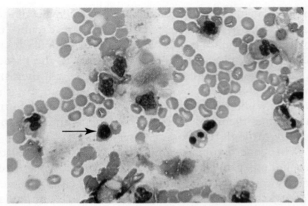

FIGURE 8-21 Lymphocyte *(arrow)* in a cytospin of urine sediment. Brightfield, 400×.

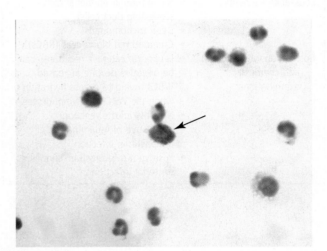

FIGURE 8-20 Eosinophil *(arrow)* in a cytospin of urine stained with Hansel stain. Brightfield, 400×.

Lymphocytes. Although lymphocytes are normally present in the urine, these leukocytes are usually not recognized because of their small numbers. When supravital stains are used or a cytodiagnostic urinalysis using Wright's or Papanicolaou's stain is performed, lymphocytes are more readily apparent and identifiable (Figure 8-21). Most prevalent in the urine are small lymphocytes, approximately 6 to 9 μm in diameter. They have a single, round to slightly oval nucleus and scant clear cytoplasm that usually extends out from one side of the cell. Lymphocytes are present in inflammatory conditions such as acute pyelonephritis; however, because neutrophils predominate, lymphocytes often are not recognized. In contrast, lymphocytes predominate in urine from patients experiencing renal transplant rejection. Because lymphocytes do not contain leukocyte esterases, they will not produce a positive LE test, regardless of the number of lymphocytes present.

Monocytes and Macrophages (Histiocytes). Monocytes and macrophages can be observed in urine sediment. They are actively phagocytic cells that are capable of phagocytizing bacteria, viruses, antigen-antibody complexes, RBCs, and organic and inorganic substances (e.g., fat, hemosiderin). The primary functions of these cells are (1) to defend against microorganisms, (2) to remove dead or dying cells and cellular debris, and (3) to interact immunologically with lymphoid cells. Renal tubulointerstitial diseases resulting from infections or immune reactions draw monocytes and macrophages to the site of inflammation by chemotaxis, that is, their movement from the bloodstream into renal tissue occurs in response to a chemoattractant stimulus.

Monocytes range in diameter from 20 to 40 μm. They have a single, large nucleus that is round to oval and often indented. The cytoplasm can be abundant and contains azurophilic granules. Because monocytes are actively phagocytic cells, large vacuoles often containing debris or organisms within them can be observed (Figure 8-22).

bilobed nuclei and slightly larger size. When specifically requested, urine specimens for eosinophil detection should be cytocentrifuged and stained using Hansel stain. This stain is considered superior to Wright's stain in detecting eosinophils in urine[17] (Figure 8-20). Acute interstitial nephritis (AIN) and, occasionally, chronic urinary tract infections (UTIs) occur with eosinophiluria. The presence of eosinophil casts is diagnostic of AIN. Overall, eosinophiluria is a good predictor of AIN associated with drug hypersensitivity, particularly hypersensitivity to penicillin and its derivatives. Untreated AIN can lead to permanent renal damage; however, if AIN is detected early, simply ceasing administration of the drug can result in the return of normal renal function. In cases of acute allograft rejection, the presence of large numbers of eosinophils in a kidney biopsy specimen is considered a poor prognostic indicator.[18]

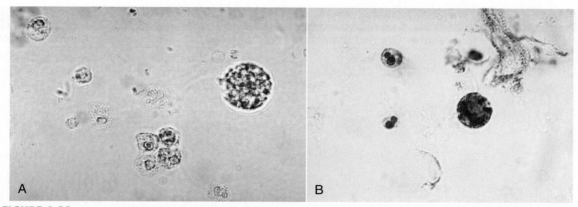

FIGURE 8-22 Macrophages and several other white blood cells. **A,** Brightfield, 400×. **B,** Brightfield, Sedi-Stain, 400×.

Macrophages are derived from monocytes; when they reside in interstitial tissues, they are often called *histiocytes*. Although macrophages average 30 to 40 μm in diameter, they can be as small as 10 μm or as large as 100 μm in diameter. When they are small, their oval nuclei and azurophilic granules make them difficult to distinguish from neutrophils. Because macrophages are transformed from monocytes, they usually have irregular, kidney-shaped nuclei and abundant cytoplasm. They are actively phagocytic, so their cytoplasm is often vacuolated. Because of their variable size and appearance, macrophages can be difficult to identify in an unstained urine sediment.

Monocytes and macrophages are identified more easily by using supravital stains on the urine sediment or by making a cytocentrifuged preparation followed by Wright's or Papanicolaou's stain. In addition, because monocytes and macrophages contain azurophilic granules, they can be detected by the chemical screening test for leukocyte esterase if they are present in sufficient numbers.

During microscopic examination of an unstained urine sediment, monocytes can be misidentified as renal tubular cells. They are of similar size, and both are mononucleated. However, monocytes or macrophages are spherical in urine, whereas renal tubular epithelial cells have dense nuclei and tend to be polygonal with one or more flat edges.

When monocytes or macrophages have ingested lipoproteins and fat, these globular inclusions are distinctly refractile (Figure 8-23). Called *oval fat bodies*, these cells are impossible to distinguish from renal tubular cells that can also absorb fat. The microscopist can use polarizing microscopy or fat stains to confirm the identity of the lipid inclusions.

Epithelial Cells

Various types of epithelial cells are seen in urine sediment. Some epithelial cells result from normal cell

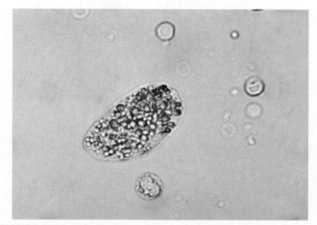

FIGURE 8-23 Oval fat body. A cell with numerous highly refractile fat globules and other inclusions. Brightfield, 400×.

turnover of aging cells, whereas others represent epithelial damage and sloughing caused by inflammatory processes or renal disease. Familiarity with the type of epithelium present in each portion of a nephron and in the urinary tract (e.g., urethra, bladder, ureters) facilitates identification of cells in urine sediment. In addition, the presence of large numbers of some cell types can indicate an improperly collected specimen, whereas increased numbers of others indicate a severe pathologic process. Whenever epithelial cells with abnormal characteristics are observed, such as unusual size, shape, inclusions, or nuclear chromatin pattern, additional cytologic studies are necessary. These cells may indicate neoplasia in the genitourinary tract or can result from treatments, such as chemotherapy or radiation.

Basically three types of epithelial cells are observed in urine sediment: squamous, transitional (urothelial), and renal tubular epithelial cells (Table 8-8). By far the most common epithelial cells encountered are **squamous epithelial cells.** Renal epithelial cells are those from the nephrons of the kidney. They consist of several

TABLE 8-8	Epithelial Cells: Microscopic Features and Clinical Significance			
Cell Type	**Site**	**Relative Size and Diameter**	**Morphology**	**Clinical Significance**
Squamous	Females: line entire urethra Males: distal portion of urethra only	40-60 μm	• Shape: thin, flagstone-shaped with distinct cell borders • Abundant cytoplasm; cytoplasmic granulation increases as cell ages • Nucleus: ≈8-14 μm,* centrally located; can be anucleated or multinucleated	• Increased numbers due to poor collection technique (i.e., not a "clean catch")

Transitional	Bladder
	Ureters
	Renal pelves
	Males: majority of urethra
		20-40 μm	• Shape varies with site:
			  Superficial cells: round or pear-shaped
			  Intermediate layer: smaller and round
			  Basal layer: small, elongated (or columnar-like)
			• Moderate amount of cytoplasm
			• Distinct cell borders that appear "firm"
			• Nucleus: ≈8-14 μm,* round or oval, centrally located
				• Increased numbers with infection or inflammation of bladder, ureters, renal pelves, or male urethra
				• Cell clusters or sheets can occur after catheterization or instrumentation of urinary tract (e.g., cystoscopy)

Renal	Collecting duct cells	Small ducts: 12-20 μm	*Small duct cells*
			• Shape: polygonal or cuboidal (*Hint:* Look for a flat edge†)
			• Nucleus: large, covers 60%-70% of cell
				• Increased numbers with ischemic events:
				  Shock
				  Anoxia
				  Sepsis

		Large ducts: 6-10 μm	*Large duct cells* • Shape: columnar • Nucleus: ≈6-8 μm, eccentric	• Trauma

	Convoluted tubular cells	Distal tubular cells: 14-25 μm	*Distal tubular cells*
			• Shape: oval to round
			• Cytoplasm: grainy
			• Nucleus: small, round, central, or eccentric
				• Increased numbers with toxic events:
				  Heavy metals
				  Hemoglobinuria, myoglobinuria
				• Poisons

		Proximal tubular cells: 20-60 μm	*Proximal tubular cells* • Shape: large, oblong or cigar-shaped with indistinct cell membrane (*Note:* Resemble granular casts with single inclusion) • Cytoplasm: grainy • Nucleus: usually eccentric; can be multinucleated	• Drugs

*Approximately the size of a red blood cell or a white blood cell.
†Over time, cells in urine absorb water to become swollen, and the flat edge may not be as noticeable.

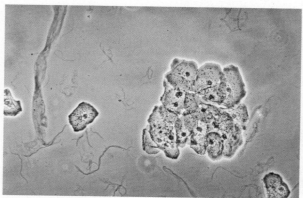

FIGURE 8-24 Squamous epithelial cells: one large clump and several individual cells. Note their large, thin, flagstone-shaped appearance, centrally located nuclei, and stippled cytoplasm (stippling increases with cellular degeneration). A few ribbon-like mucous threads are also present. Phase contrast, 100×.

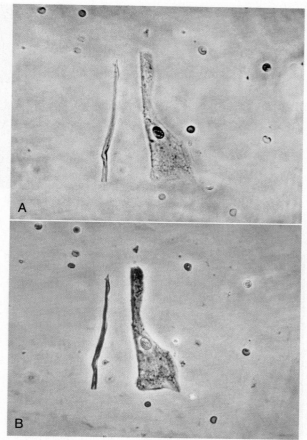

FIGURE 8-25 Two squamous epithelial cells. The cell on the left is presenting a side view, demonstrating how flat these cells are. The upper edge of the cell on the right is curled, producing an unusual form. **A,** Brightfield, Sedi-Stain, 200×. **B,** Phase contrast, 200×.

distinctively different cell types, with each originating from a specific part of the nephron (i.e., collecting duct cells, **proximal convoluted tubular cells, distal convoluted tubular cells**). The type of cell encountered depends on the location of the disease process that is causing the epithelium to be injured and sloughed. Although identification of some epithelial cells can be difficult in wet preparations, techniques are available to facilitate proper cell identification. Each laboratory should have a policy that addresses urine sediments with unusual or abnormal cellularity, such as atypical cells or cellular fragments. This policy may simply involve forwarding the specimen to the cytology department for analysis or performing a cytodiagnostic urinalysis. Because both the presence of certain types of epithelial cells and the number of epithelial cells present can be clinically significant, it is important that the microscopist use any techniques available to ensure the proper identification and reporting of epithelial cells.

During the microscopic examination, squamous epithelial cells are easily observed using low-power magnification because of their large size. In contrast, transitional and renal epithelial cells are better assessed using high-power magnification. After epithelial cells are observed in 10 representative fields of view at the appropriate magnification, the report should indicate each type of epithelial cell encountered. The report format may use descriptive terms such as *few, moderate,* or *many* per field of view or may be numeric such as 5 to 10 cells per field of view.

Squamous Epithelial Cells. Squamous epithelial cells are the most common and the largest epithelial cells found in the urine (Figure 8-24). These cells line the entire urethra in the female but only the distal portion of the urethra in the male. Routinely, the superficial layers of the squamous epithelium are desquamated and replaced by new, underlying epithelium. In women, large

numbers of squamous epithelial cells in the urine sediment often indicate vaginal or perineal contamination; similarly in uncircumcised men, large numbers suggest specimen contamination. Squamous epithelial cells are large (40 to 60 μm), thin, flagstone-shaped cells with distinct edges that may be present in clumps. They have a small, condensed, centrally located nucleus about the size of an erythrocyte, or they can be anucleated. Their large amount of cytoplasm is often stippled with fine granulation (keratohyalin granules), which increases as the cells degenerate. Squamous epithelial cells can be observed in unusual conformations because their edges can fold over or curl while they are suspended in urine (Figure 8-25).

Squamous cells, which are easily identified using low-power magnification, are the only epithelial cells evaluated using this magnification. Squamous epithelial cells in urine specimens rarely have diagnostic significance and usually indicate specimen contamination.

Transitional (Urothelial) Epithelial Cells. The renal calyces, renal pelves, ureters, and bladder are lined with

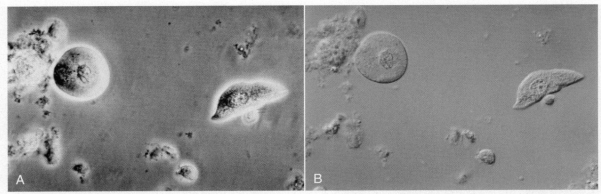

FIGURE 8-26 Two transitional (urothelial) epithelial cells. **A,** Phase contrast, 400×. **B,** Interference contrast, 400×.

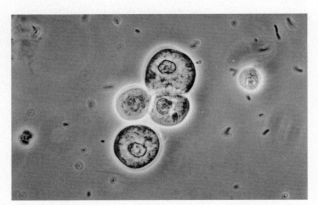

FIGURE 8-27 Four transitional (urothelial) epithelial cells. Phase contrast, 400×.

several layers of transitional epithelium (Figure 8-26). In the male, this type of epithelium also lines the urethra except for the distal portion, whereas in the female, transitional epithelium ceases at the base of the bladder. **Transitional (urothelial) epithelial cells** vary considerably in size. This size variation relates primarily to the three principal layers of transitional epithelium in the bladder. The cells in the uppermost or superficial layer are large (30 to 40 μm) and round or pear-shaped. Cells from the intermediate layers are smaller and rounder (20 to 30 μm), whereas those from the single basal layer tend to be elongated or columnar.

A few transitional epithelial cells are present in the urine sediment from normal, healthy individuals and represent routine sloughing of old epithelium. In urine sediments, the most prevalent form of transitional cells is the superficial type: round or pear-shaped, with a dense oval to round nucleus and abundant cytoplasm (Figure 8-27). The nucleus is about the size of a red or white blood cell, and the peripheral borders of the nucleus and cell membrane are distinctly outlined.

With urinary tract infection, increased numbers of transitional epithelial cells are often present in the urine.

At times, clusters or sheets of transitional epithelium are observed following urinary catheterization or other types of instrumentation procedures. However, when sheets of cells appear without these procedures, they indicate a pathologic process that requires further investigation, such as transitional cell carcinoma.

Renal Tubular Epithelial Cells. As described in Chapter 4, each portion of a nephron or renal tubule is lined with a single layer of a characteristic epithelium. A few renal tubular cells appear in urine from normal healthy individuals and represent routine replacement of aging or old epithelium. Newborn infants have more renal tubular cells in their urine than do older children or adults.

In routine microscopic examinations of urine, two types of renal epithelial cells are enumerated and reported: convoluted tubular cells and collecting duct cells.

Convoluted Renal Tubular Cells. Because the cytoplasm of convoluted tubular cells is coarsely granular, their nuclei are not readily visible when phase-contrast microscopy is used, and these cells can resemble granular casts. Using brightfield microscopy and staining the urine sediment greatly enhance visualization of the nuclei and correct identification of these cells. Cytocentrifugation followed by Papanicolaou's staining of the urine sediment can be used to specifically identify these cells.

Differentiating between proximal convoluted tubular cells and distal convoluted tubular cells is difficult and is based primarily on size and shape. Usually differentiation between proximal and distal convoluted tubular cells is not necessary, and these cells are collectively reported as "convoluted" renal tubular cells.

Proximal Convoluted Tubular Cells. These are large cells (20 to 60 μm in diameter) with granular cytoplasm. They are oblong or cigar-shaped (Figure 8-28)—a characteristic that makes them resemble granular casts. They have a nucleus with a dense chromatin pattern that is usually eccentric, and they can be multinucleated.

Distal Convoluted Tubular Cells. These round to oval cells measuring approximately 14 to 25 μm in diameter are smaller than cells of the proximal tubule

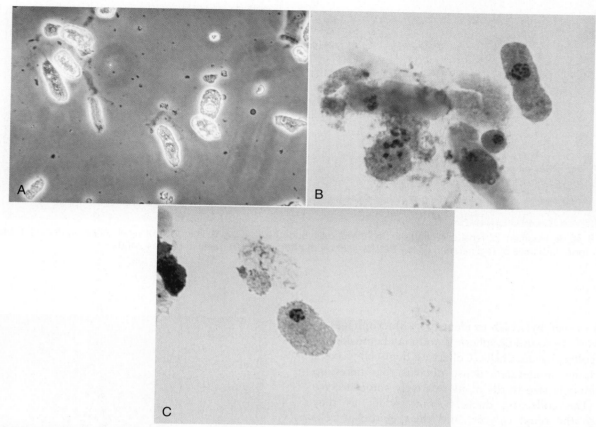

FIGURE 8-28 Convoluted tubular epithelial cells. **A,** Numerous proximal convoluted tubular cells. Note the similarity in shape to granular casts and that their nuclei are not readily apparent in many cells. Phase contrast, 200×. **B,** Sediment stained with 0.5% toluidine blue. A large, castlike proximal tubular cell and a smaller, round distal tubular cell are present with two hyaline casts and other debris. Brightfield, 400×. **C,** A single proximal tubular cell stained with 0.5% toluidine blue. Note the indistinct cell margins, granular cytoplasm, and small eccentric nucleus. Brightfield, 400×.

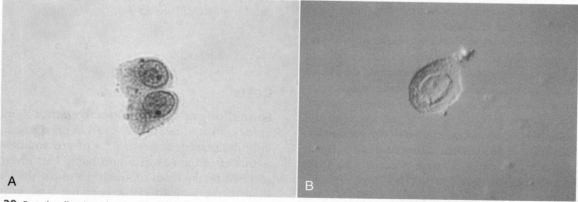

FIGURE 8-29 Renal collecting duct epithelial cells. **A,** Two cells with an intact edge. Brightfield, toluidine blue stain, 400×. **B,** A single cell. Interference contrast, 400×.

(Figure 8-28, *B*). They have a small, dense nucleus that is usually eccentric, and they have a granular cytoplasm, much like that of proximal tubular cells.

Proximal and distal convoluted tubular cells are found in the urine as a result of acute ischemic or toxic renal tubular disease (e.g., acute tubular necrosis) from heavy metals or drug (aminoglycosides) toxicity (see Chapter 9, "Acute Tubular Necrosis").

Collecting Duct Cells. Collecting duct cells range from 12 to 20 μm in diameter and are cuboidal, polygonal, or columnar (Figure 8-29). They are rarely round or spherical. Therefore, always look for a corner or a flat

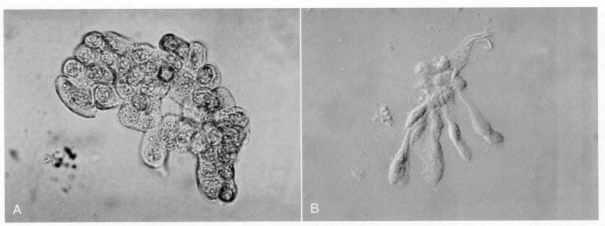

FIGURE 8-30 A, Fragment of renal collecting duct epithelial cells. Brightfield, 400×. **B,** Fragment of renal collecting duct epithelial cells in "spindle" form, indicative of regeneration of the tubular epithelium after injury. Interference contrast, 400×.

edge on the cell by which to identify it. Macrophages or monocytes are round or spherical and may be misidentified as collecting duct cells. Collecting duct cells have a single, large, moderately dense nucleus that takes up approximately two-thirds of its relatively smooth cytoplasm. The collecting ducts become wider as they approach the renal calyces, and their epithelial cells become larger and more columnar. Increased numbers of collecting duct cells accompany all types of renal diseases, including nephritis, acute tubular necrosis, kidney transplant rejection, and salicylate poisoning.

In contrast to proximal and distal convoluted tubular cells, collecting duct cells can be observed as fragments of undisrupted tubular epithelium (Figure 8-30; see Figure 8-5). To be identified as a fragment, at least three cells must be sloughed together with a bordering edge intact. Their presence reveals severe tubular injury and damage to the epithelial basement membrane. Collecting duct fragments are found following trauma, shock, or sepsis, and indicate ischemic necrosis of the tubular epithelium. In addition to these renal cell fragments, pathologic casts (e.g., granular, waxy, renal tubular cell) and increased numbers of blood cells are usually present.

Renal Tubular Cells With Absorbed Fat. Renal tubular cells that are engorged with absorbed fat from the tubular lumen or are degenerating their own intracellular lipids are called *oval fat bodies* (Figure 8-31). These cells may have many large, highly refractile droplets, or they can have only a small number of apparently glistening granules. Because oval fat bodies often indicate glomerular dysfunction and renal tubular cell death, they are always accompanied by an increased amount of urine protein and cast formation. Oval fat bodies are positively identified using polarizing microscopy or fat stains such as Sudan III or Oil Red O (see Figure 8-7). (For continued discussion on fat identification in urine, see the section "Fat," later in this chapter.)

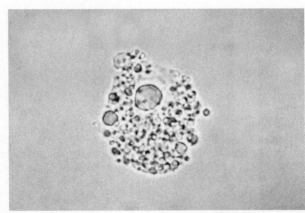

FIGURE 8-31 Oval fat body. Note the size variation of the fat globules. Brightfield, 400×.

Casts

Formation and General Characteristics. Unique to the kidney, urinary casts are formed in the distal and collecting tubules with a core matrix of **uromodulin** (formerly known as **Tamm-Horsfall protein**). This glycoprotein is secreted by the renal tubular cells of the thick ascending limb of the loop of Henle (i.e., the straight portion of the distal tubules) and by the distal convoluted tubules.[2,19] As the contents of the tubular lumen become concentrated, uromodulin forms fibrils that attach it to the lumen cells, holding it temporarily in place while it enmeshes into its matrix many substances that are present. Any urinary component, whether chemical or a formed element, can be found incorporated into a cast. Eventually, the formed cast detaches from the tubular epithelial cells and is flushed through the remaining portions of the nephron with the lumen fluid.

Because casts are formed within the tubules, they are cylindrical and microscopically always appear thicker in the middle than along their edges (Figure 8-32). They have essentially parallel sides with ends that can be rounded or straight (abrupt). The shape and size of urinary casts can vary greatly depending on the diameter and shape of the tubule in which they form. The narrower the tubular lumen, the narrower is the resulting cast. Sometimes casts are well formed at one end but are tapered or have a tail at the other end (Figure 8-33). These casts, often called *cylindroids,* result from (1)

incomplete cast formation, (2) formation of a cast in a tubule where the lumen width differs (naturally or from disease), or (3) cast disintegration. Because they have the same clinical significance as completely formed casts, cylindroids are not enumerated separately. When wide or broad casts are observed, they indicate cast formation in extremely dilated tubules or in a wide collecting duct (Figure 8-34). Because a single collecting duct serves numerous nephrons, cast formation within them indicates pronounced urine stasis and renal disease.

Casts can be short and stubby, long and thin, or any combination. They may be straight, curved, or convoluted. A cast becomes convoluted when after formation and release from a tubule, it encounters a tubular obstruction, such as another cast being formed. The first (narrower) cast becomes compressed to form a cast that appears convoluted (Figure 8-35). Because casts can be retained in the tubule for varying lengths of time, the substances enmeshed in their matrices can disintegrate. In addition, the cast matrix itself can undergo changes that become apparent microscopically, for example, transition from a granular to a waxy cast (see Figures 8-34 and 8-36). Some casts are fragile and are easily broken into chunks if the urine sediment is mixed too vigorously during resuspension (Figure 8-37). Also note

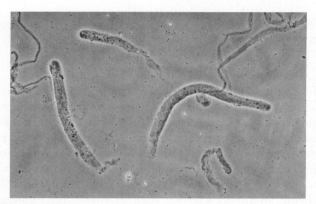

FIGURE 8-32 Three hyaline casts and several mucous threads. Phase contrast, 100×.

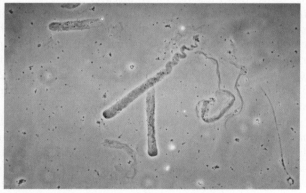

FIGURE 8-33 Three hyaline casts. The cast with a tapered end is frequently called a *cylindroid.* Phase contrast, 100×.

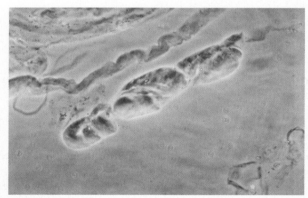

FIGURE 8-35 Convoluted hyaline cast, initially formed in a tubule and later compressed in a tubule of larger diameter. Phase contrast, 200×.

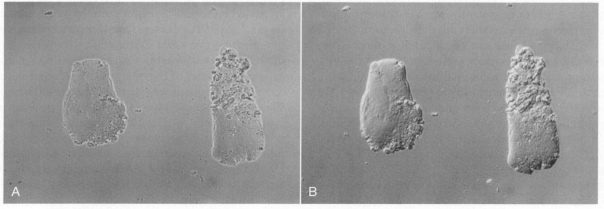

FIGURE 8-34 Two broad, granular to waxy casts. **A,** Brightfield, 100×. **B,** Interference contrast, 100×.

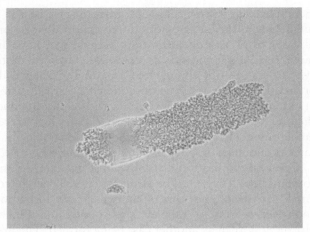

FIGURE 8-36 Coarsely granular going to waxy cast. Brightfield, 100×.

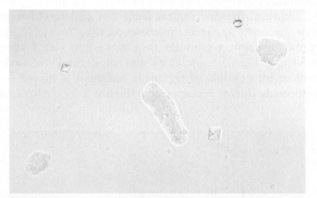

FIGURE 8-37 One intact finely granular/waxy cast and two broken pieces of a cast. Brightfield, 100×.

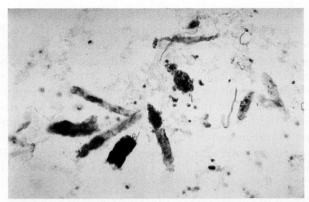

FIGURE 8-38 A low-power field of view revealing casts of various types: cellular, granular, and mixed. Brightfield, Sedi-Stain, 100×.

that hypotonic and alkaline urine promotes the disintegration of casts in the urine sediment.

Numerous factors such as an acid pH, increased solute concentration, urine stasis, and increased plasma proteins (particularly albumin) enhance cast formation.[2] In an acidic environment, gelation of protein and the precipitation of solutes are enhanced. Because acidification and concentration of urine occur in the distal and collecting tubules, these tubules are the sites of most cast formation. Urinary stasis can occur because of obstruction from disease processes or congenital abnormalities. This stasis promotes the accumulation and concentration of ultrafiltrate components, hence cast formation. In conditions that cause increased quantities of plasma proteins (e.g., albumin, globulins, hemoglobin, myoglobin) in the lumen ultrafiltrate, cast formation is enhanced greatly. These proteins become incorporated into the uromodulin protein matrix, along with any cells and cellular or granular debris that happen to be present.

Clinical Significance. A few hyaline or finely granular casts may be present in the urine sediment from normal, healthy individuals. Casts reflect the status of the renal tubules; therefore with renal disease, increased numbers of casts are found in urine sediment (Figure 8-38). The number of casts reflects the extent of tubular involvement and the severity of disease. Both the types of casts and their numbers provide valuable information to health care providers. Two exceptions are notable. Following strenuous exercise such as marathon running, increased numbers of casts can be found in the urine of normal individuals (athletic pseudonephritis); their presence does not indicate renal disease. These casts are linked to the increased albuminuria resulting from exercise-induced glomerular permeability changes. The urine sediment may show as many as 30 to 50 hyaline or finely granular casts per low-power field but returns to normal (showing no proteinuria or casts) within 24 to 48 hours. Increased numbers of casts have also been associated with some diuretic therapies.[2]

The importance of a patient history including the diagnosis and a list of medications cannot be overemphasized. A patient history provides information that can support or account for the numbers and types of formed elements observed. Note that physical exercise and emotional stress can affect the number of formed elements observed in the urine sediment. Increased excretion of casts is thought to be caused at least in part by increased secretion of uromodulin by renal tubular cells. A careful patient history can prevent misdiagnosis or overdiagnosis of renal dysfunction.

Classification of Casts. Casts are classified microscopically on the basis of the composition of their matrix and the types of substances or cells enmeshed within them (Box 8-2). Because any substance can be incorporated into a cast, Box 8-2 could be expanded to include all possible inclusions; those that are listed represent the most commonly encountered casts. One should keep in mind that casts can contain more than one formed element or can be of two matrix types. Mixed cellular casts often are reported as such with a description of the entities involved, for example, cellular cast—leukocytes

BOX 8-2 | Classification of Urinary Casts

Homogeneous matrix
- Hyaline
- Waxy

Cellular inclusions
- Red blood cells
- Leukocytes
- Renal tubular epithelial cells
- Mixed cells
- Bacteria

Other inclusions
- Granular
- Fat globules—cholesterol, triglycerides
- Hemosiderin granules
- Crystals

Pigmented
- Bilirubin
- Hemoglobin
- Myoglobin

Size
- Broad

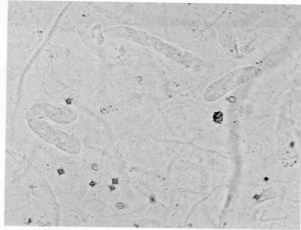

FIGURE 8-39 Hyaline casts. Three hyaline casts and mucous threads. Brightfield, 200×.

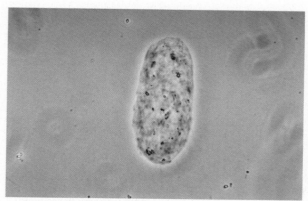

FIGURE 8-40 Hyaline cast. Note the appearance of the fibrillar protein matrix and the presence of fine granulation. Phase contrast, 400×.

and renal tubular cells. When a cast of two matrix types (half granular and half waxy) is encountered, the cast is identified using the term that has the greatest clinical significance. In this example, the cast should be enumerated and reported as a waxy cast. Table 8-9 lists the characteristic features, chemical examination, and other correlations that are associated with each cast type.

Homogeneous Matrix Composition. Hyaline Casts. Hyaline casts, composed primarily of a homogeneous uromodulin protein matrix, are the most commonly observed casts in the urine sediment (Figure 8-39). This protein matrix gives hyaline casts a low refractive index that is similar to that of urine and makes them difficult to see using brightfield microscopy. These casts appear colorless in unstained urine sediment, with rounded ends and in various shapes and sizes. When phase-contrast or interference contrast microscopy is used, their fibrillar protein matrix is more apparent and often includes some fine granulation (Figure 8-40).

In healthy individuals, two or fewer hyaline casts per low-power field is considered normal. Increased numbers of hyaline casts can be found following extreme physiologic conditions such as strenuous exercise, dehydration, fever, or emotional stress. They also accompany pathologic casts in renal disease and in cases of congestive heart failure.

If brightfield microscopy is used, staining the sediment greatly enhances the visualization of hyaline casts and helps differentiate them from mucous threads that may also be present. Hyaline casts become pink with Sternheimer-Malbin stain, and their edges are more clearly defined. With phase-contrast or interference contrast microscopy, hyaline casts are readily identified by

the homogeneity of their matrix and by their characteristic shape. Occasionally, a hyaline cast may have a single epithelial or blood cell within its matrix. These casts, as well as cylindroids, are enumerated as hyaline casts and have no diagnostic significance.

Waxy Casts. Named as such because of their waxy appearance, these casts have a high refractive index and are readily visible using brightfield microscopy. Waxy casts appear homogeneous, with their edges well defined, and often have sharp, blunt, or uneven ends. Cracks or fissures from their lateral margins or along their axes are often present and are characteristic of these casts (Figure 8-41). In unstained urine sediment, they are colorless, gray, or yellow; with Sternheimer-Malbin stain, they become darker pink than hyaline casts and have a diffuse, ground-glass appearance.

Waxy casts indicate prolonged stasis and tubular obstruction. They are believed to represent an advanced stage of other casts (e.g., hyaline, granular, cellular) that

TABLE 8-9	Casts: Microscopic Features and Correlations		

Cast Type	Microscopic Features	Chemical Examination Correlation	Correlations
Hyaline	• Colorless, fibrillar matrix • Low refractive index		• Most commonly observed • Increased numbers with strenuous exercise, stress, dehydration, fever • Accompany other pathologic casts in urine sediment
Granular	*Finely granular casts* • Small granules dispersed throughout matrix, giving it a sandpaper appearance • Granules from renal cell metabolic by-products	• Protein +/– • Blood +/–	• Accompany strenuous exercise, stress, dehydration, fever
	Coarsely granular casts • Large, coarse granules within matrix • Granules primarily from degenerating cells, trapped cellular debris, and metabolic by-products	• Protein positive • Blood +/–	• Not associated with any specific disease • Accompany other pathologic casts in urine sediment
Cellular	*Red blood cell (RBC) casts* • Intact RBCs within matrix	• Blood positive • Protein positive	• Associated with glomerular diseases (e.g., glomerulonephritis, nephritis) • A rare cast may be observed following contact sports (i.e., athletic pseudonephritis)
	White blood cell (WBC) casts • Intact WBCs within matrix	• Protein positive • Leukocyte esterase (LE) positive • Blood +/– • Nitrite +/–	• Associated with infectious diseases (e.g., bacterial or viral pyelonephritis) and inflammatory disorders (e.g., interstitial nephritis, lupus erythematosus, glomerulonephritis)
	Renal tubular epithelial cell (RTE) casts • RTE cells within matrix	• Protein positive • Blood +/–	• Most often associated with acute tubular necrosis but present in all types of renal disease
Waxy	• Ground glass appearance • High refractive index (i.e., easy to see using brightfield microscopy) • Homogeneous matrix • Cracks or fissures from margins or along length of cast often present	• Protein positive • Blood +/–	• Associated with nephrotic syndrome and chronic renal disease (glomerulonephritis, pyelonephritis), transplant rejection, and malignant hypertension
Fatty	• Fat globules or oval fat bodies (OFBs) within matrix • Highly refractile fat globules have yellowish to green sheen (brightfield microscopy) • Cholesterol globules form Maltese cross under polarizing microscopy; triglycerides stain orange or red using Sudan III or Oil Red O, respectively	• Protein positive • Blood +/–	• Associated with nephrotic syndrome, diabetic nephropathy (acute tubular necrosis and crush injuries) • May be present with acute tubular necrosis and crush injuries
Other	*Bacterial casts* • Bacteria within matrix	• Protein positive • LE positive • Blood +/– • Nitrite +/–	• Associated with bacterial pyelonephritis
	Crystal casts • Crystals within matrix	• Protein positive • Blood +/–	• Associated with renal calculi (kidney stone) formation or drug precipitation due to insufficient hydration
	Fungal casts • Yeast within matrix	• Protein positive • LE positive • Blood +/–	• Associated with fungal pyelonephritis
Cast look-alikes	*Mucous threads* • Ribbon-like with twists and folds • Ends are serrated or irregular • Low refractive index		• Increased with infection or inflammation of urinary tract

are transformed during urinary stasis, taking as long as 48 hours or more to form (Figure 8-42). They are often broad, indicating their formation in dilated tubules or collecting ducts. Waxy casts are found most frequently in patients with chronic renal failure, hence they are frequently referred to as *renal failure casts*. They are also encountered in patients with acute renal disease (e.g., acute glomerulonephritis, nephrotic syndrome) or malignant hypertension and during renal allograft rejection.

Cellular Inclusion Casts

Red Blood Cell Casts. The microscopic appearance of red blood cell casts varies. Some casts are packed with RBCs; others may present principally as a hyaline cast with several clearly defined RBCs embedded within its matrix (Figures 8-43 and 8-44). In either case, the RBCs must be unmistakably identified in at least a portion of the cast before it can be called a red blood cell cast. In unstained urine sediments, erythrocytes within the cast matrix cause them to be characteristically yellow or red-brown. The latter color indicates degeneration of the erythrocytes with hemoglobin oxidation. In Sternheimer-Malbin–stained sediments, intact RBCs may appear colorless or lavender in a pink homogeneous matrix.

If urine stasis is sufficient, erythrocyte casts degenerate into pigmented, granular casts called *blood casts* or *muddy brown casts* (Figure 8-45). These red to golden-brown granular casts contain no distinct RBCs in their matrix because the cells have lysed and undergone degeneration. This process can also occur in vitro when the

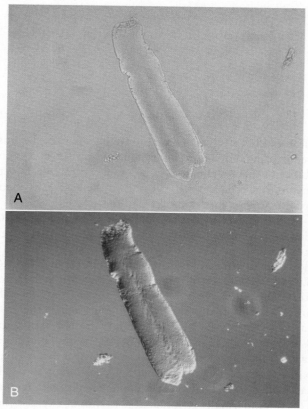

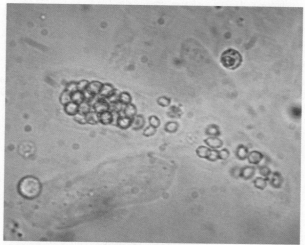

FIGURE 8-41 Waxy cast. **A,** Brightfield, 100×. **B,** Interference contrast, 100×.

FIGURE 8-43 Red blood cell cast. Red blood cells are embedded in the cast matrix. Brightfield, 400×.

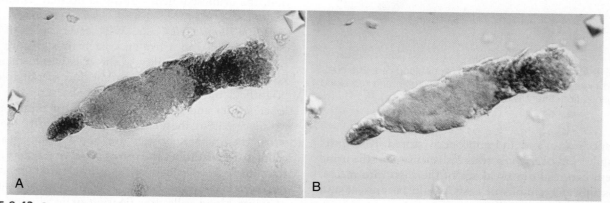

FIGURE 8-42 Cast, part granular and part waxy. Note the difference in cast diameter at one end compared with the other. This indicates initial cast formation in a narrow tubular lumen followed by stasis in a tubule with a wider lumen and further cast formation. **A,** Brightfield, Sedi-Stain, 200×. **B,** Interference contrast, 200×.

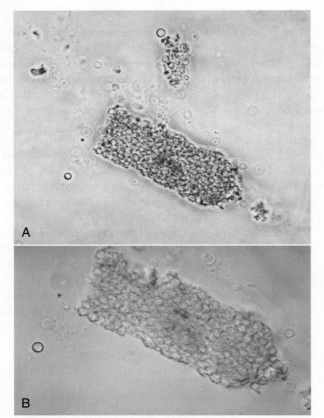

A

B

FIGURE 8-44 Red blood cell cast. This cast is packed with intact red blood cells. **A,** Brightfield, 200×. **B,** Interference contrast, 400×.

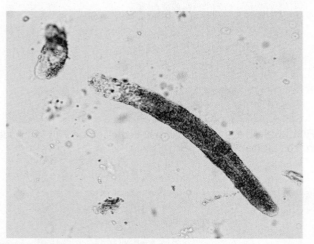

FIGURE 8-45 A pigmented granular cast or blood cast. The granules and pigmentation originate from hemoglobin and red blood cell degeneration. Brightfield, 200×.

urine specimen is old and improperly stored. RBC casts are fragile, and overly vigorous resuspension of the urine sediment can result in breakage of the casts into pieces. Microscopically, chunks of casts would be present and may be difficult to identify.

Phase-contrast and interference contrast microscopy aid in identification of red blood cell casts by enhancing

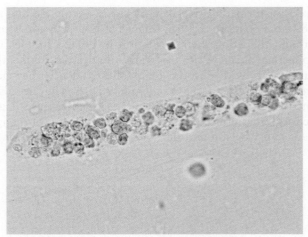

FIGURE 8-46 White blood cell cast. Brightfield, 400×.

the detail of cells trapped within the cast matrix. Because free-floating RBCs are also present, the optical sectioning ability of these techniques enables better visualization to ensure that cells are actually within the cast matrix and are not simply superimposed on its surface.

Red blood cell casts are diagnostic of intrinsic renal disease. The RBCs are most often of glomerular origin (i.e., passage across glomerular filtration barriers as in glomerulonephritis) but can result from tubular damage (i.e., blood leakage into the tubules, as with acute interstitial nephritis). When RBCs are able to pass into the tubular ultrafiltrate, so are plasma proteins; therefore varying degrees of proteinuria are present (see Table 8-9). The detection and monitoring of red blood cell casts in urine sediment provide a means of evaluating a patient's response to treatment. Occasionally, an RBC cast may be observed in the urine of a healthy individual. This finding usually is noted after strenuous exercise (i.e., athletic pseudonephritis), particularly after participation in contact sports such as football, basketball, or boxing. As with other urine findings associated with this condition, the urine sediment returns to normal within 24 to 48 hours.

White Blood Cell Casts. WBC casts consist of leukocytes embedded in a hyaline cast matrix (Figure 8-46). Because of the refractility of the cells within them, leukocyte casts are readily apparent and identifiable with brightfield microscopy. When the characteristic multilobed nuclei and granular cytoplasm of these cells are readily apparent, these casts are easy to identify. However, when these characteristics are not evident because of cellular degeneration, the use of supravital stains or contrast microscopy is necessary to differentiate them from renal epithelial cells. The presence of increased numbers of white blood cells, free-floating or in clumps, would suggest strongly that the cells within these casts are leukocytes.

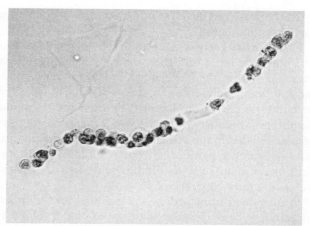

FIGURE 8-47 Renal tubular cell cast. Brightfield, 200×.

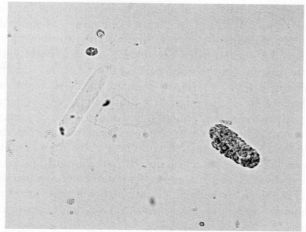

FIGURE 8-48 Two casts, one hyaline, the other with coarsely granular inclusions. Brightfield, 200×.

The presence of WBC casts indicates renal inflammation or infection and requires further clinical investigation. The origin of the white blood cells, glomerular or tubular, can be difficult to determine. If glomerular (e.g., glomerulonephritis), red blood cell casts will also be present and in greater numbers than white blood cell casts. With tubular diseases (e.g., pyelonephritis), leukocytes migrating into the tubular lumen from the interstitium are enmeshed in the cast matrix. In these cases, bacteriuria and varying degrees of proteinuria and hematuria usually accompany the white blood cell casts (see Table 8-9). Renal infections from agents other than bacteria (e.g., cytomegalovirus) are possible and must be considered when bacteriuria is not present and negative bacterial cultures are obtained.

Renal Tubular Cell Casts. Renal tubular cells can become enmeshed in the uromodulin matrix of casts; these casts are nonspecific markers of tubular injury. They have a high refractive index and are readily visible on brightfield microscopy. When the characteristic large central nuclei and shape of these cells are apparent, these casts are easily identified (Figure 8-47). However, as renal tubular cells become damaged, they undergo degenerative changes that can make specific identification of these casts difficult. Individual renal tubular cells may be found randomly arranged within a cast, or they may appear aligned as fragments of the tubular lining removed intact from the tubule. These latter casts indicate that a portion of a nephron has been severely damaged, with the tubular basement membrane stripped of its epithelium.

Because the size of some renal tubular cells is similar to that of leukocytes, degenerating renal tubular cells in casts may need enhanced visualization to be differentiated and specifically identified. Supravital stains or microscopy techniques such as phase-contrast or interference contrast microscopy can be used. The presence of degenerating tubular cell casts in urine sediment indicates intrinsic renal tubular disease. Proteinuria and often granular casts accompany renal tubular cell casts.

Mixed Cell Casts. It is common to find casts that have incorporated within their matrix multiple cell types, such as renal epithelial cells and leukocytes or erythrocytes and leukocytes. Any combination is possible. These casts are often enumerated and reported as cellular casts, with their composition provided in the report.

Bacterial Casts. Because visualizing these small organisms within the cast matrix is difficult, bacterial casts are rarely identified as such. Bacterial casts are diagnostic of pyelonephritis. Because these casts usually include leukocytes, they are often reported as leukocyte casts. They are actually mixed casts. With the use of brightfield microscopy and a stain (supravital or Gram), careful scrutiny of the cast matrix between leukocytes can often reveal embedded bacteria. Contrast interference microscopy allows even better visualization of bacteria within casts because of its optical sectioning ability. Occasionally, casts that consist of bacteria without leukocytes incorporated in the protein matrix have been observed.

Casts With Inclusions

Granular Casts. Granular casts come in a variety of granular textures. They range from small, fine granules dispersed throughout the cast matrix to large, coarse granules (Figures 8-48 and 8-49). They are composed primarily of uromodulin protein and cast granulation is not clinically significant. Easily viewed with brightfield microscopy because of their high refractive index, granular casts often appear colorless to shades of yellow. Granular casts can appear in all shapes and sizes, and broad granular casts are considered to be an indicator of a poor prognosis.

Several mechanisms account for the granular casts observed in the urine sediment. The granules in finely granular casts have been identified as by-products of protein metabolism, in part lysosomal, that are excreted by renal tubular epithelial cells[20]—this accounts for the appearance of granular casts in the urine of normal, healthy individuals. A variation of this mechanism is believed to account for the finding of some casts with large, coarse granulation, particularly when no accompanying cellular casts are present. In these cases, as tubular cells degenerate, their intracellular components are released into the tubular lumen and become enmeshed in a cast. Other coarsely granular casts result from the degeneration of cellular casts. These casts often contain identifiable cellular remnants. In patients with intrinsic renal disease, these coarsely granular casts are usually accompanied by cellular casts. Further degeneration of granular casts into waxy casts can occur during urine stasis (see Figure 8-36, 8-42).

Urine sediment from normal healthy individuals may have an occasional finely granular cast. These casts are not as common as hyaline casts, but their numbers can increase following exercise. Patients with various types of renal disease can have varying quantities of coarse and finely granular casts.

Fatty Casts. Fatty casts contain free fat globules, oval fat bodies, or both, and their matrix can be hyaline or granular. Within the cast, fat globules can vary in size and are highly refractile (Figures 8-50 and 8-51). Oval fat bodies in casts are identified by their intact cellular membranes. Because oval fat bodies often indicate renal tubular cell death, the presence of oval fat bodies in fatty casts indicates a significant renal pathologic condition. Cells other than oval fat bodies may also be present within the fatty cast matrix.

In unstained urine sediment examined by brightfield microscopy, lipid globules may appear light yellow or darker, depending on microscope adjustments. If fat stains such as Sudan III or Oil Red O are used, triglyceride (neutral fat) globules within casts stain characteristically orange or red (see Figure 8-7), whereas cholesterol and cholesterol esters do not. In contrast,

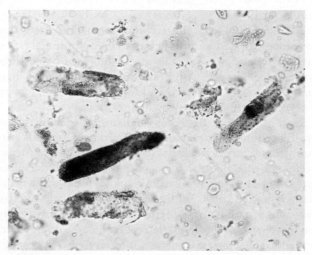

FIGURE 8-49 Finely granular and coarsely granular casts. Pigmentation from hemoglobin degradation. Brightfield, 200×.

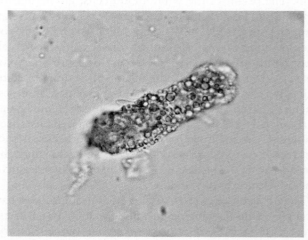

FIGURE 8-50 A fatty cast. Note the globules and their characteristic refractility. Brightfield, 400×.

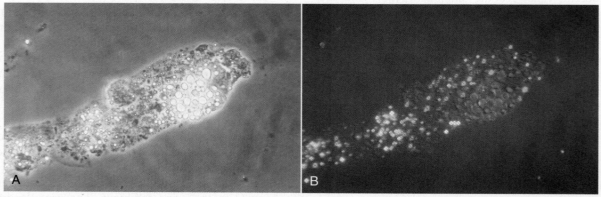

FIGURE 8-51 Fatty cast. Note the high refractility of the fat globule inclusions in the matrix of the cast. **A,** Phase contrast, 400×. **B,** Polarizing microscopy, 400×. The highly refractile fat globules apparent in **A** do not exhibit a Maltese cross pattern, identifying them as neutral fat; those with a Maltese cross pattern are cholesterol.

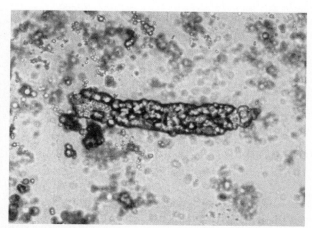

FIGURE 8-52 Cast with sulfamethoxazole crystal inclusions. Brightfield, 200×.

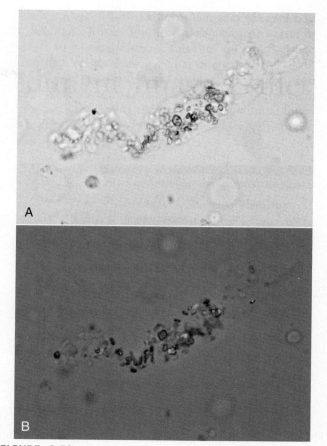

FIGURE 8-53 Cast with monohydrate calcium oxalate crystal inclusions. **A,** Brightfield, 400×. **B,** Polarizing microscopy with first-order red compensator, 400×.

polarized microscopy can identify cholesterol and cholesterol esters by their characteristic birefringence; these globules form a Maltese cross pattern (see Figure 8-51, *B,* and Figure 8-11). Note that lipids do not take up Sternheimer-Malbin stain, although the protein matrix of the cast does.

Fatty casts are accompanied by significant proteinuria and may be found in numerous renal diseases, particularly nephrotic syndrome (see Table 8-9). In addition, a severe crush injury with disruption of body fat can result in the presence of fatty casts in the urine sediment.

Other Inclusion Casts. Because during cast formation any substance present in the tubular lumen can be incorporated into the uromodulin matrix, hemosiderin granules and crystals have been found in casts. Because crystals can aggregate along mucous threads to simulate a cast, it is important that the hyaline matrix is observed and that it actually encases the crystals. Crystal casts are not common; those encountered are usually composed of calcium oxalate or sulfonamide crystals (Figures 8-52 and 8-53). The presence of crystal casts indicates crystal precipitation within the tubules, which can damage tubular epithelium as well as cause tubular obstruction. As a result, varying amounts of hematuria usually accompany crystalline casts in the urine sediment.

Pigmented Casts. Pigmented casts, usually of a hyaline matrix with distinct coloration, are characterized by incorporation of the pigment within the casts (Figure 8-54). Hemoglobin, myoglobin, or bilirubin (bile) casts can be encountered in the urine sediment. Hemoglobin casts appear yellow to brown and are accompanied by hematuria. Because myoglobin casts are similar in appearance to hemoglobin casts, differentiation requires a patient history with a possible diagnosis of rhabdomyolysis or confirmation that myoglobin is present. Bilirubin characteristically colors all urine sediment constituents, including casts, yellow- or golden-brown (Figure 8-55). In contrast, urobilin, a pigment that can impart an orange-brown color to urine, does not color

the formed elements of the sediment. Highly pigmented drugs, such as phenazopyridine, can also characteristically color sediment elements.

Size. Broad casts indicate cast formation in dilated tubules or in the large collecting ducts (Figure 8-56). Because several nephrons empty into a single collecting duct, cast formation here indicates significant urinary stasis due to obstruction or disease. The presence of many broad casts in urine sediment indicates a poor prognosis. Broad casts may be of any type; however, when a significant amount of urinary stasis is involved, they principally present as granular or waxy casts (see Figure 8-34). In chronic renal diseases in which nephrons have sustained previous damage, broad hyaline casts may be encountered. These casts form as a result of continued proteinuria and other factors that enhance their formation.

Correlation With Physical and Chemical Examinations. When significant numbers of casts, particularly pathologic casts, are identified in urine sediment, correlation with the physical and chemical examinations must be made. Increased numbers of casts or abnormal casts must be accompanied by proteinuria, although the degree of proteinuria can vary. In contrast, proteinuria can

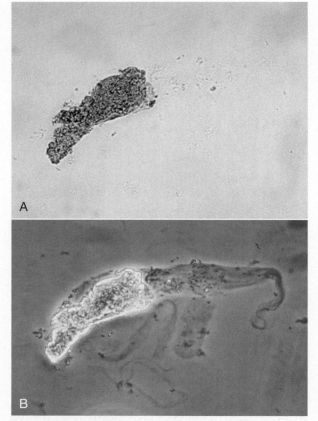

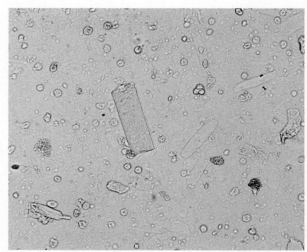

FIGURE 8-56 Broad waxy cast and numerous hyaline casts. Bright-field, 200×.

FIGURE 8-54 Pigmented granular cast. **A,** Brightfield, 200×. **B,** Phase contrast, 200×. Note the enhanced visualization of low-refractile components such as the hyaline matrix and mucus using phase-contrast microscopy.

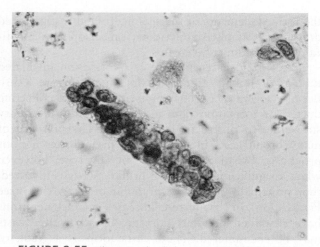

FIGURE 8-55 Bile-stained cellular cast. Brightfield, 200×.

occur without cast formation. If red blood cell casts are identified, the chemical test for blood should be positive, or its negativity accounted for before these casts are reported. Leukocyte casts may or may not be associated with a positive leukocyte esterase test, depending on the types and numbers of leukocytes present. Leukocyte

casts often are accompanied by bacteriuria, the most common causative agent of UTI. In these cases, the nitrite test may also be positive. Bile-pigmented casts should be accompanied by a positive chemical test for bilirubin; similarly, hemoglobin- or myoglobin-pigmented casts should be accompanied by a positive chemical test for blood.

Look-Alikes. For the novice microscopist, several formed elements in urine sediment can be confused with casts. Mucous threads can be misidentified as hyaline casts (see Figure 8-32). Although mucous threads have a similar low refractive index, they are ribbon-like, and their ends are not rounded but are serrated. They are irregular, whereas hyaline casts are more formed.

Various fibers, such as cotton threads or diaper fibers, can resemble waxy casts (Figure 8-57). Several distinguishing characteristics allow for their differentiation. Fibers tend to be flatter in the middle and thicker at their margins, whereas casts are cylindrical and thicker in the center. In addition, fibers are more refractile than casts. Under polarizing microscopy, fibers polarize light, whereas casts do not (see Figure 8-53, *B* and note the appearance of the "cast matrix"). Finally, fibers may contaminate the urine at any time, whereas casts, particularly waxy casts, must be accompanied by protein-uria. Other entities, such as squamous epithelial cells folded into a tubular shape or scratches on the coverslip surface, may be misidentified as casts. With practice, proper identification of these components is not difficult.

Crystals such as amorphous urates and phosphates can aggregate together or along a mucous thread to simulate a cast. With polarizing microscopy, their bire-fringence identifies them as crystalline entities, and the lack of a distinct matrix differentiates them from a true cast.

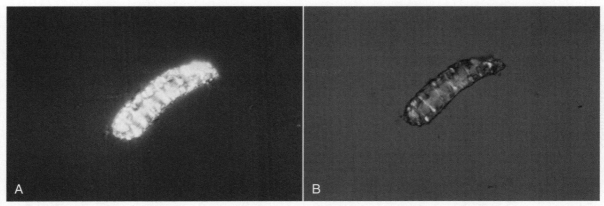

FIGURE 8-57 A, Diaper fiber demonstrating anisotropism (strong birefringence) with polarizing microscopy, 200×. **B,** Polarizing microscopy with first-order red compensator, 200×.

Crystals

Crystals result from the precipitation of urine solutes out of solution. They are not normally present in freshly voided urine but form as urine cools to room or refrigerator temperature (depending on storage). When crystals are present in freshly voided urine, they indicate formation in vivo and are always clinically significant. Regardless of the crystal type, crystal formation within the nephrons can cause significant tubular damage. Most crystals are not clinically significant and can be distracting when the laboratorian is performing the microscopic examination. In addition, they can make visualization of important formed elements difficult, especially when they are present in large numbers. Some crystals indicate a pathologic process; therefore it is important that they are correctly identified and reported. Crystals are identified on the basis of their microscopic appearance and the pH at which they are present. The urine pH provides the information necessary to positively identify several look-alike crystals (e.g., amorphous urates from phosphates, ammonium biurate from sulfonamides).

Contributing Factors. Several factors influence crystal formation, including (1) the concentration of the solute in the urine, (2) the urine pH, and (3) the flow of urine through the tubules. As the glomerular ultrafiltrate passes through the tubules, solutes within the lumen fluid are concentrated. If an increased amount of a solute is present because of dehydration, dietary excess, or medications, the ultrafiltrate can become supersaturated. This can result in precipitation of the solute into its characteristic crystalline form. Because solutes differ in their solubility, this characteristic provides a means of identifying and differentiating them. For example, inorganic salts such as oxalate, phosphate, calcium, ammonium, and magnesium are less soluble in neutral or alkaline urine. As a result, when the urine pH becomes neutral or alkaline, these solutes can precipitate out in their crystalline form. In contrast, organic solutes such as uric acid, bilirubin, and cystine are less soluble in acidic conditions and can form crystals in acidic urine. Most

clinically significant crystals (e.g., cystine, tyrosine, leucine) are found in acidic urine, including those of iatrogenic origin (e.g., sulfonamides, ampicillin).

Crystal formation, similar to cast formation, is enhanced by slow urine flow through the renal tubules. This flow reduction allows time for maximum concentration of solutes in the ultrafiltrate. At the same time, the tubules are effecting pH changes in the ultrafiltrate. When the pH becomes optimal for a supersaturated solute, crystals form.

Although these factors account for crystal formation within the renal tubules, they are also involved in the development of crystals during urine storage. The solute concentration, the pH, the time allowed for formation, and the temperature play a role in crystal formation. When these conditions are optimized, the chemicals in urine can exceed their solubility and precipitate in their uniquely characteristic crystalline or amorphous forms.

The following section discusses normal and abnormal crystals and loosely categorizes them according to the pH at which they typically form. Crystals are routinely reported as few, moderate, or many under high-power magnification. The characteristics and clinical significance of crystals formed from normal urine solutes are provided in Table 8-10; those from, abnormal and iatrogenic solutes are provided in Table 8-11.

Acidic Urine

Amorphous Urates. When the urine pH is acid (between pH 5.7 and 7.0), uric acid exists in its ionized form as a urate salt. Some of these urate salts (sodium, potassium, magnesium, and calcium) can precipitate in amorphous or noncrystalline forms. Microscopically, these precipitates appear as small, yellow-brown granules (Figure 8-58), much like sand, and they can interfere with the visualization of other formed elements present in the urine sediment. Because refrigeration enhances precipitation, performance of the microscopic examination on fresh urine specimens often avoids the formation of amorphous urates. The urinary pigment uroerythrin readily deposits on the surfaces of urate crystals,

TABLE 8-10 Crystals of Normal Urine Solutes Arranged According to pH

Solute	pH			Color	Microscopic Appearance	Solubility Characteristics	Comments and Clinical Significance
	Acid	Neutral	Alkaline				
Uric acid (pH <5.7)	+	—	—	Colorless to yellow to golden brown	Pleomorphic; often flat, diamond,, or rhombic; cubic and barrels forms; can layer or form rosettes; color varies with thickness; strong birefringence	Soluble with alkali	Increased excretion following chemotherapy and gout
Amorphous urates (Ca, Mg, Na, K)	+	+	—	Colorless to yellow-brown	Amorphous, granular; strong birefringence	Soluble with alkali; soluble at ≈60° C; convert to uric acid with concentrated HCl	Common; macroscopic appearance—orange-pink precipitate ("brick dust")
Monosodium urates	+	+	—	Colorless to light yellow	Slender, pencil-like prisms with blunt ends; often in small clusters of 2-3 crystals	Soluble with alkali; soluble at ≈60° C	Uncommon
Acid urates (Na, K, NH4)	(+)	+	—	Yellow-brown	Balls or spheres; resemble biurates; strong birefringence	Soluble at ≈60° C; convert to uric acid with glacial acetic acid	Common in old urine
Calcium oxalate	+	+	(+)	Colorless	Dihydrate; octahedral or envelope form; weak to moderate birefringence Monohydrate; ovoid or dumbbell form; strong birefringence	Soluble in dilute HCl	Common; often accompanies ethylene glycol ingestion
Calcium phosphate	(+)	+	+	Colorless	Dibasic (Ca [HPO4]): thin prisms in rosette or stellar form; prisms have one tapered end; rarely, as long, thin needles, weak birefringence	Soluble in dilute acid	Common
					Monobasic (Ca[H2PO4]2): irregular, granular-appearing sheets or plates		Rare
Magnesium phosphate	(+)	+	+	Colorless	Elongated rectangular or rhomboid plates; end or corner may be notched; edges can be irregular or eroded; weak birefringence	Soluble in acetic acid; insoluble in potassium hydroxide	Rare
Amorphous phosphate (Ca, Mg)	—	+	+	Colorless	Amorphous, granular	Soluble with acid; insoluble at ≈60° C	Common; macroscopic appearance—white to beige precipitate
Calcium carbonate	—	+	+	Colorless	Tiny granular spheres; often in pairs (dumbbells) or tetrads; strong birefringence	With acetic acid produces CO_2 gas (effervescence)	Rare
Triple phosphate (NH4, Mg, PO4)	—	+	+	Colorless	Prism with three to six sides ("coffin lids") or less common flat, fern-like form (associated with rapid formation or prisms dissolving); moderate birefringence	Soluble in acetic acid; fern-like form can be induced by addition of ammonia	Common
Ammonium biurate	—	+	+	Dark yellow-brown	Spheres with striations or spicules; "thorny apple", strong birefringence	Soluble with acetic acid; soluble at ≈60° C; convert to uric acid with concentrated HCl or acetic acid	Rare in fresh urine; iatrogenic alkalinization can induce; common in old urine; can resemble sulfonamides

TABLE 8-11   Abnormal Crystals of Metabolic and Iatrogenic* Origin Arranged According to pH

Solute	pH Acid	pH Neutral	pH Alkaline	Color	Microscopic Appearance	Solubility Characteristics	Comments and Clinical Significance
Crystals of Metabolic Origin							
Bilirubin	+	—	—	Yellow-brown highly pigmented	Fine needles or granules that form clusters	Soluble in alkali; soluble in strong acid	Rare; crystals induced by storage at 2-8° C; bilirubinuria associated with liver disease or obstruction
Leucine	+	—	—	Dark yellow to brown	Spheres with concentric circles or striations; strong birefringence	Soluble in alkali	Rare; liver disease, aminoaciduria; accompanies tyrosine; crystals induced by storage at 2° C to 8° C
Tyrosine	+	—	—	Colorless to yellow	Fine, delicate needles in clusters or sheaves	Soluble in alkali	Rare; liver disease, aminoaciduria; crystals induced by storage at 2° C to 8° C
Cholesterol	+	+	—	Colorless	Flat, rectangular plates with notched corners; weak birefringence	Soluble in chloroform and ether	Rare; crystals induced by storage at 2° C to 8° C; indicates lipiduria; found with proteinuria and other forms of urinary fat
Hemosiderin	+	+	—	Golden brown	Granules; free floating, in clumps, or in cells and casts		Rare; present 2-3 days after hemolytic event; confirm with Prussian blue test
Cystine	+	+	(+)	Colorless	Hexagonal plates, often layered; weak to moderate birefringence that varies with thickness	Soluble in alkali; pKa 8.3, solubility increases with pH	Rare; cystinosis or cystinuria; confirm with nitroprusside test
Crystals of Iatrogenic Origin							
Ampicillin	+	—	—	Colorless	Long, thin needles or prisms; strong birefringence		Rare; high-dose antibiotic therapy
Radiographic contrast media (meglumine diatrizoate)	+	—	—	Colorless	Form varies with administration; strong birefringence: *Intravenous administration:* flat, elongated rectangular plates; *Retrograde administration:* long, slat-like prisms		Radiographic procedures; causes high specific gravity (>1.040); can resemble cholesterol crystals
Sulfonamides	+	—	—	Yellow-brown	Form varies with drug; strong birefringence: *Sulfamethoxazole, sulfadiazine*—spheres with striations or dense globules. *Acetylsulfadiazine*—sheaves of wheat with eccentric binding; fan forms		Rare; accompany antibiotic therapy; confirm with diazo reaction test; some forms resemble acid urates and ammonium biurate
Indinavir sulfate	(+)	+	+	Colorless; gray to brown when aggregated	Slender, feather-like crystals that aggregate into wing-like bundles; moderate to strong birefringence		Antiretroviral therapy

*Solutes that originate from medications, imaging procedures, or treatments (e.g., drugs, radiographic contrast media).

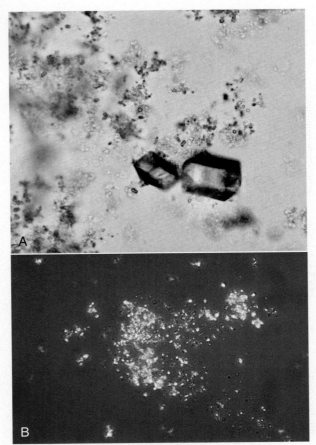

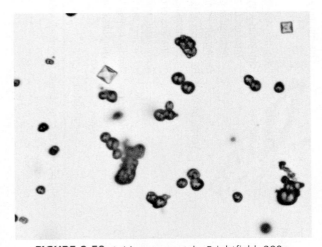

FIGURE 8-58 Amorphous urates. **A,** Two uric acid crystals are also present. Brightfield, 400×. **B,** Polarizing microscopy, 400×.

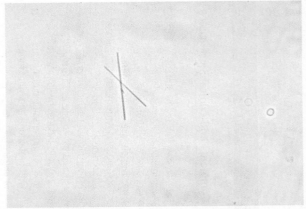

FIGURE 8-60 Monosodium urate crystals. Brightfield, 200×.

approximately 60° C. If concentrated acetic acid is added and time allowed, amorphous urates will convert to uric acid crystals. Amorphous urates have no clinical significance and are distinguished from amorphous phosphates on the basis of urine pH, their macroscopic appearance, and their solubility characteristics.

Acid Urates. Acid urate crystals are sodium, potassium, and ammonium salts of uric acid that appear as small, yellow-brown balls or spheres (Figure 8-59). Their color is distinctive and is similar to that of their alkaline counterpart, ammonium biurate crystals. Acid urate crystals can be present when the urine pH is neutral to slightly acidic but frequently are not observed in fresh urine. Because of their small, spherical shape and color, they may be misidentified as leucine crystals. Similar to other urate crystals, acid urates dissolve at 60° C and can be converted to uric acid crystals by the addition of glacial acetic acid. They have no clinical significance and are reported as "urate crystals."

Monosodium Urate. Monosodium urate crystals, a distinct form of a uric acid salt, appear as colorless to light-yellow slender, pencil-like prisms (Figure 8-60). They may be present singly or in small clusters, and their ends are not pointed. Monosodium urate crystals can be present when the urine pH is acid and dissolve at 60° C. They have no clinical significance and usually are reported as "urate crystals."

Uric Acid. Uric acid crystals occur in many forms; the most common form is the rhombic or diamond shape (Figures 8-61 and 8-62). However, the crystals may be appear as cubes, barrels or bands and may cluster together to form rosettes (Figures 8-63 and 8-64); they often show layers or laminations on their surfaces (Figure 8-65). Although they present most often in various forms with four sides, they occasionally have six sides and may require differentiation from colorless cystine crystals. Uric acid crystals are yellow to golden brown, and the intensity of their color varies directly with the thickness of the crystal. As a result, crystals may appear colorless when they are thin or when the urine is low in uroerythrin (a urine pigment). With the use of polarizing

FIGURE 8-59 Acid urate crystals. Brightfield, 200×.

imparting to them a characteristic pink-orange color. This coloration is apparent macroscopically during the physical examination. Often referred to as "brick dust," urate crystals indicate that the urine is acidic.

Amorphous urates are present in acidic (or neutral) urine specimens. They can be identified by their solubility in alkali or their dissolution when heated to

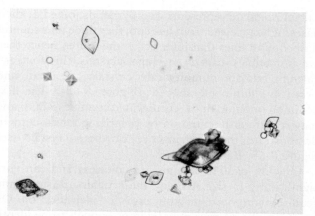

FIGURE 8-61 Uric acid crystals (diamond-shaped) and a few calcium oxalate crystals. Note the darker coloration as the crystals layer and thicken. Brightfield, 200×.

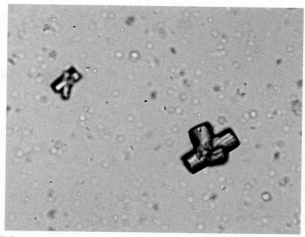

FIGURE 8-64 Uric acid crystals. Barrel form. Brightfield, 200×.

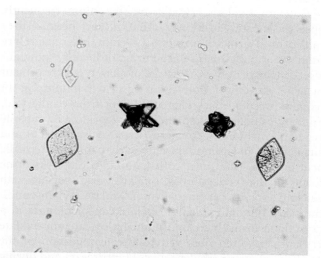

FIGURE 8-62 Uric acid crystals. Single and cluster forms. Brightfield, 200×.

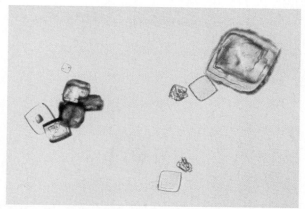

FIGURE 8-65 Uric acid crystals. These crystals can layer or laminate on top of one another. Brightfield, 100×.

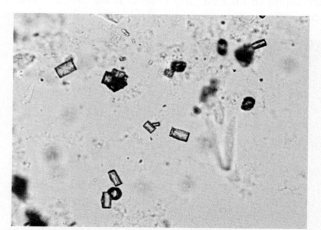

FIGURE 8-63 Uric acid crystals. Less common barrel forms. Brightfield, 200×.

microscopy, uric acid crystals exhibit strong birefringence and produce a variety of interference colors.

Uric acid crystals can be present only if the urine pH is less than 5.7. At a pH greater than 5.7, uric acid is in its ionized form as urate and forms urate salts (e.g., amorphous urates, sodium urate). Uric acid crystals are 17 times less soluble than urate salt crystals. If urine with uric acid crystals is adjusted to an alkaline pH, the crystals readily dissolve. Similarly, if urine with urate salt crystals is acidified adequately, uric acid crystals form.

Uric acid is a normal urine solute that originates from the catabolism of purine nucleosides (adenosine and guanosine from RNA and DNA). Hence, uric acid crystals can appear in urine from healthy individuals. Increased amounts of urinary uric acid can be present following the administration of cytotoxic drugs (e.g., chemotherapeutic agents) and with gout. With these conditions, if the urine pH is appropriately acid, large numbers of uric acid crystals can be present.

Calcium Oxalate. The most common shape of calcium oxalate crystals is their octahedral or pyramid form (Figures 8-66 and 8-67). This dihydrate form of

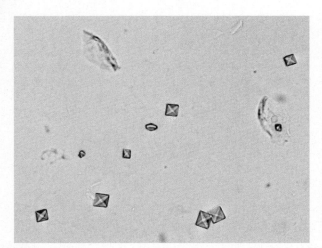

FIGURE 8-66 Calcium oxalate crystals. Octahedral (envelope) form of dihydrate crystals. Brightfield, 200×.

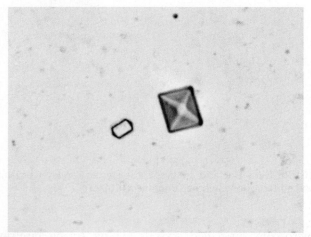

FIGURE 8-67 Calcium oxalate crystals. An unusual barrel form and a typical dehydrate form. Brightfield, 400×.

calcium oxalate represents two pyramids joined at their bases. When viewed from one end, they appear as squares scribed with lines that intersect in the center, hence they are sometimes called envelope crystals. In contrast, calcium oxalate monohydrate crystals are small and ovoid or dumbbell shaped (Figure 8-68). The less common monohydrate form can resemble RBCs and may require differentiation by polarizing microscopy to demonstrate the birefringence of these crystals (see Figure 8-68, *B*).

Calcium oxalate crystals are colorless and can vary significantly in size. Usually the crystals are small and require high-power magnification for identification. On occasion, the crystals may be large enough to be identified under low-power magnification. Calcium oxalate crystals may cluster together and can stick to mucous threads. When this occurs, they may be mistaken for crystal casts.

Calcium oxalate crystals are the most frequently observed crystals in human urine, in part because they can form in urine of any pH. Calcium and oxalate are solutes normally found in the urine of healthy individuals. Approximately 50% of the oxalate typically present in urine is derived from ascorbic acid (vitamin C), an oxalate precursor (see Figure 7-13) or from oxalic acid. Foodstuffs high in oxalic acid or ascorbic acid include vegetables (rhubarb, tomatoes, asparagus, spinach) and citrus fruits. In addition, beverages that are high in oxalic acid include cocoa, tea, coffee, and chocolate. As urine forms in the renal tubules, oxalate ions associate with calcium ions to become calcium oxalate. When conditions are optimal, calcium oxalate can precipitate in a crystalline form. Increased numbers of calcium oxalate crystals are often observed following ingestion of the oxalate precursor ethylene glycol (antifreeze) and during severe chronic renal disease.

Alkaline Urine

Amorphous Phosphate. Amorphous phosphates are found in alkaline and neutral urine and are microscopically indistinguishable from amorphous urates.

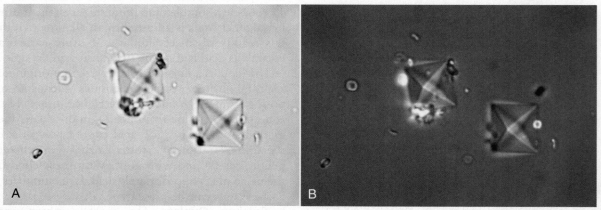

FIGURE 8-68 Calcium oxalate crystals. Small ovoid monohydrate crystals that resemble erythrocytes, and two large typical envelope forms of dihydrate crystals. **A,** Brightfield, 400×. **B,** Polarizing microscopy, 400×. The birefringence of these small ovoid crystals helps distinguish them from erythrocytes.

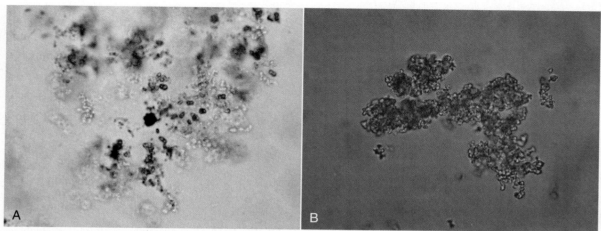

FIGURE 8-69 Amorphous phosphates. Note the lack of birefringence under polarizing microscopy. **A,** Brightfield microscopy, 400×. **B,** Polarizing microscopy with first-order red compensator, 400×.

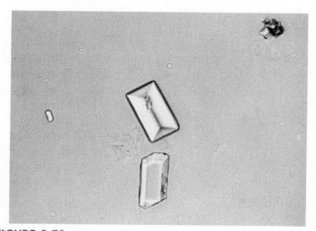

FIGURE 8-70 Triple phosphate crystals. Typical "coffin lid" form. Brightfield, 100×.

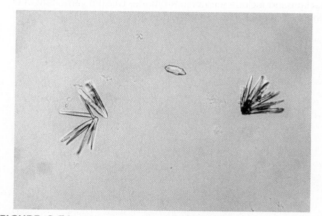

FIGURE 8-71 Calcium phosphate crystals. Prisms are arranged singly and in rosette forms. Brightfield, 100×.

This noncrystalline form of phosphates resembles fine, colorless grains of sand in the sediment (Figure 8-69). Amorphous phosphates are differentiated from amorphous urates on the basis of urine pH, their solubility characteristics, and, to a lesser degree, their macroscopic appearance. Large quantities of amorphous phosphates cause a urine specimen to appear cloudy; the precipitate is white or gray, in contrast to the pink-orange color of amorphous urates. Unlike urates, amorphous phosphates are soluble in acid and do not dissolve when heated to approximately 60° C.

Similar to amorphous urates, amorphous phosphates have no clinical significance and can make the microscopic examination difficult when a large quantity is present. Because refrigeration enhances their deposition, specimens maintained at room temperature and analyzed within 2 hours of collection minimize amorphous phosphate formation.

Triple Phosphate. Triple phosphate (NH_4MgPO_4, ammonium magnesium phosphate) crystals are colorless and appear in several different forms. The most common and characteristic forms are three- to six-sided prisms with oblique terminal surfaces, the latter described as

"coffin lids" (Figure 8-70). Not all crystals are perfectly formed, and their size can vary greatly. With prolonged storage, these crystals can dissolve, taking on a feathery form that resembles a fern leaf.

Among the crystals observed in alkaline urine, triple phosphate crystals are common. They can also be present in neutral urine specimens. Ammonium magnesium phosphate is a normal urine solute, hence triple phosphate crystals can be present in urine from healthy individuals. Triple phosphate crystals have little clinical significance but have been associated with UTIs characterized by an alkaline pH and have been implicated in the formation of renal calculi.

Calcium Phosphate. Calcium phosphate is present in urine as dibasic calcium phosphate (i.e., $CaHPO_4$, calcium monohydrogen phosphate) and as monobasic calcium phosphate (i.e., $Ca[H_2PO_4]_2$, calcium biphosphate). These similar yet different compounds precipitate out of solution in distinctly different crystalline shapes. Dibasic calcium phosphate crystals, sometimes called *stellar phosphates,* appear as colorless, thin, wedgelike prisms arranged in small groupings or in a rosette pattern (Figure 8-71). Each prism has one tapered or pointed

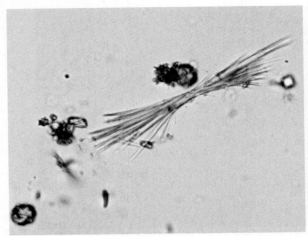

FIGURE 8-72 Calcium phosphate crystals. Uncommon slender needles arranged in bundles or sheaves. Other crystals present in background include ammonium biurate, calcium carbonate, and a single calcium oxalate. Brightfield, 400×.

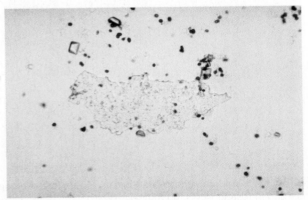

FIGURE 8-73 Calcium phosphate sheet or plate. Brightfield, 100×.

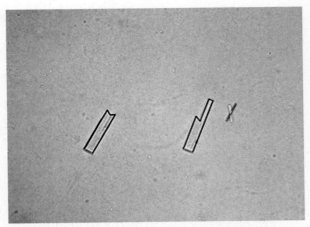

FIGURE 8-74 Magnesium phosphate crystals. Brightfield, 400×.

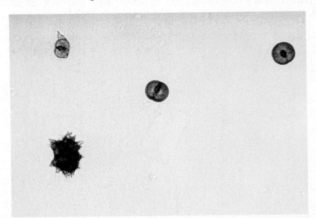

FIGURE 8-75 Ammonium biurate crystals. Spheres and a "thorny apple" form. Brightfield, 200×.

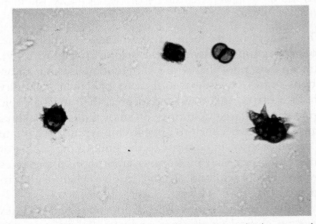

FIGURE 8-76 Ammonium biurate crystals. Several "thorny apple" forms. Brightfield, 200×.

end, with the other end squared off. Another, less commonly observed form of dibasic calcium phosphate is seen in those crystals shaped as thin, long needles arranged in bundles or sheaves (Figure 8-72). In contrast, monobasic calcium phosphate crystals usually appear microscopically as irregular, granular sheets (Figure 8-73) or flat plates that can be large and may be noticed floating on the top of a urine specimen. These colorless crystalline sheets can resemble large degenerating squamous epithelial cells.

Classified as alkaline crystals because they are usually present in neutral or slightly alkaline urine specimens, calcium phosphate crystals can also form in slightly acidic urine. They are weakly birefringent with polarizing microscopy. Calcium phosphate crystals are common and have no clinical significance.

Magnesium Phosphate. Magnesium phosphate crystals are large, colorless crystals that appear as elongated rectangular or rhomboid plates. These flattened prisms can be notched and their edges can be irregular or eroded (Figure 8-74).[21] They are weakly birefringent under polarizing microscopy. Although magnesium

phosphate crystals form from normal urine solutes in neutral or alkaline urine, they are rarely seen.

Ammonium Biurate. Ammonium biurate crystals appear as yellow-brown spheres with striations on the surface (Figure 8-75). Irregular projections or spicules can also be present, giving these crystals a "thorny apple" appearance (Figure 8-76). They can form in alkaline or neutral urine.

Ammonium biurate is a normal urine solute. These crystals occur most frequently in urine specimens that have undergone prolonged storage. However, when they precipitate out of solution in fresh urine specimens (e.g., following iatrogenically induced alkalinization), they are clinically significant, because in vivo precipitation can cause renal tubular damage. Their presence most often indicates inadequate hydration of the patient. Therefore when ammonium biurate crystals are encountered in a urine specimen, investigation is required to determine whether (1) the integrity of the urine specimen has been compromised (improper storage), or (2) in vivo formation is taking place.

Ammonium biurate crystals are strongly birefringent and dissolve in acetic acid or on heating to approximately 60° C. Similar to other urate salts (amorphous urates, acid urates), ammonium biurate crystals can be converted to uric acid crystals with the addition of concentrated hydrochloric or acetic acid.

An important note is that ammonium biurate crystals can resemble some forms of sulfonamide crystals. One differentiates between them on the basis of urine pH, a sulfonamide confirmatory test, and the solubility characteristics of the crystals.

Calcium Carbonate. Calcium carbonate crystals appear as tiny, colorless granular crystals (Figure 8-77, *A*). Slightly larger than amorphous material, these crystals sometimes are misidentified as bacteria because of their size and occasional rod shape. Under polarizing microscopy, they are strongly birefringent, which aids in differentiating them from bacteria. Calcium carbonate crystals are usually found in pairs, giving them a dumbbell shape, or as tetrads. They may also be encountered as aggregate masses that are difficult to distinguish from amorphous material (Figure 8-77, *B*).

Present primarily in alkaline urine, calcium carbonate crystals are not found frequently in the urine sediment. Although they have no clinical significance, one can identify calcium carbonate crystals positively through the production of carbon dioxide gas (effervescence) with the addition of acetic acid to the sediment.

Crystals of Metabolic Origin

Bilirubin. The amount of bilirubin in urine can be so great that on refrigeration, its solubility is exceeded and bilirubin crystals precipitate out of solution (Figure 8-78). Bilirubin crystals usually appear as small clusters of fine needles (20 to 30 μm in diameter), but granules and plates have been observed. Always characteristically yellow-brown, these crystals indicate the presence of large amounts of bilirubin in the urine. Bilirubin crystals are confirmed by correlation with the chemical examination, that is, the crystals can be present only if the chemical screen for bilirubin is positive.

Bilirubin crystals only form in an acidic urine. They dissolve when alkali or strong acids are added. They are classified as abnormal crystals because bilirubinuria indicates a metabolic disease process. However, because these crystals form in the urine after excretion and cooling (i.e., storage), they are not frequently observed and they are not usually reported.

Cystine. Cystine crystals appear as colorless, hexagonal plates with sides that are not always even (Figure 8-79). These clear, refractile crystals are often laminated or layered and tend to clump.

Present primarily in acidic urine, cystine crystals are clinically significant and indicate disease, that is,

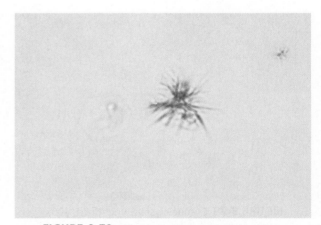

FIGURE 8-78 Bilirubin crystal. Brightfield, 400×.

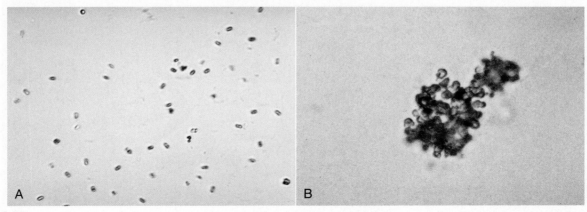

FIGURE 8-77 Calcium carbonate. **A,** Numerous single crystals. Brightfield, 400×. **B,** Aggregate of calcium carbonate crystals. Brightfield, 400×.

congenital cystinosis or cystinuria. These crystals tend to deposit within the tubules as calculi, resulting in renal damage; therefore proper identification is important. Thin, hexagonal uric acid crystals can resemble cystine; therefore a confirmatory test should be performed before cystine crystals are reported. The chemical confirmatory test for cystine is based on the cyanide-nitroprusside reaction. Sodium cyanide reduces cystine to cysteine, and the free sulfhydryl groups subsequently react with nitroprusside to form a characteristic purple color.

Cystine crystals can be present in urine with a pH of less than 8.3 (pK_a of cystine). They dissolve in alkali and hydrochloric acid (pH <2). In vivo, the solubility of cystine rises exponentially with urine pH (i.e., it is almost four times more soluble at pH 8 than at pH 5).[22] The excessive excretion of cystine and the formation of cystine crystals is abnormal and indicates a disease process.

Tyrosine and Leucine. Tyrosine crystals appear as fine, delicate needles that are colorless or yellow (Figure 8-80). They frequently aggregate to form clusters or sheaves but also may appear singly or in small groups.

Leucine crystals are highly refractile, yellow to brown spheres. They have concentric circles or radial striations on their surface and can resemble fat globules. Unlike fat, leucine crystals do not stain with fat stains. They are birefringent under polarized microscopy but the light pattern produced is not a true Maltese cross pattern.

Tyrosine and leucine crystals can form in acidic urine and dissolve in alkaline solution. They are rarely seen today because of the rapid turnaround time for a urinalysis, and because they require refrigeration to force them out of solution. Of the two, tyrosine is found more often in urine because it is less soluble than leucine. Sometimes leucine crystals can be forced out of solution by the addition of alcohol to tyrosine-containing urines.

These amino acid crystals are abnormal and are present in the urine of patients with overflow aminoacidurias—rare inherited metabolic disorders. In these disorders, the concentrations of these amino acids in the blood are high (aminoacidemia), resulting in increased renal excretion. Although rare, these crystals have been observed in the urine of patients with severe liver disease. These abnormal crystals are confirmed, preferably by chromatographic methods, before they are reported.

Cholesterol. Cholesterol crystals appear as clear, flat, rectangular plates with notched corners (Figure 8-81). These crystals can be present in acidic urine and, because of their organic composition, are soluble in chloroform and ether.

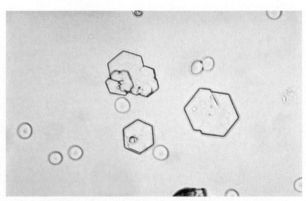

FIGURE 8-79 Cystine crystals. Brightfield, 400×.

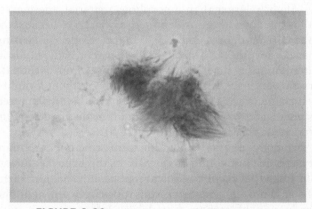

FIGURE 8-80 Tyrosine crystals. Brightfield, 400×.

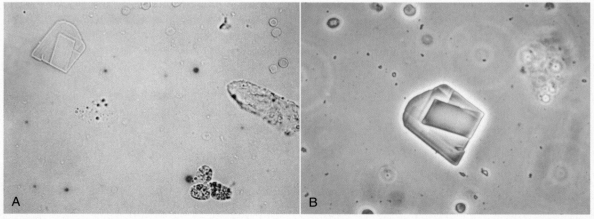

FIGURE 8-81 A, View of urine sediment with a cholesterol crystal, free-floating fat, and oval fat bodies. Brightfield, 200×. **B,** Cholesterol crystal. Phase contrast, 400×.

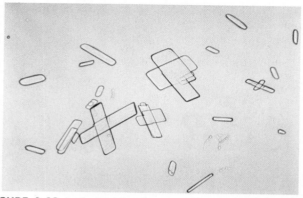

FIGURE 8-82 Radiographic contrast medium, meglumine diatri-zoate (Renografin). The crystals appear as plates. Brightfield, 100×. Compare with cholesterol crystals (intravenous administration), Figure 8-71.

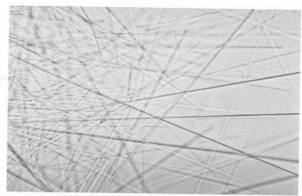

FIGURE 8-83 Ampicillin crystals. Brightfield, 400×. *(Courtesy Patrick C. Ward.)*

Rarely observed in urine sediment, cholesterol crystals indicate large amounts of urine cholesterol and ideal conditions that have promoted supersaturation and pre-cipitation. Other evidence of lipids, such as free-floating fat droplets, fatty casts, or oval fat bodies and large amounts of protein, accompany these crystals.

Cholesterol crystals can be seen with the nephrotic syndrome and in conditions resulting in chyluria: the rupture of lymphatic vessels into the renal tubules as a result of tumors, filariasis, and so on.

Intravenous radiopaque contrast media (x-ray dye) such as meglumine diatrizoate and diatrizoate sodium form flat and layered rectangular crystals that are mor-phologically similar to and need to be differentiated from cholesterol crystals (Figure 8-82). Differentiation is achieved by correlating microscopic findings with chemi-cal examination results. For example, radiopaque con-trast media produces an abnormally high urine specific gravity (i.e., greater than 1.040), and they are not associ-ated with proteinuria or **lipiduria;** in contrast, cholesterol crystals are seen in urine with a normal specific gravity and must be accompanied by proteinuria and lipiduria.

Cholesterol crystal formation occurs in vitro, that is, the crystals are induced out of solution by the cooling of urine after collection and storage. Therefore in some institutions, these crystals are not reported. Instead, lipi-duria or chyluria is documented in the urinalysis report by the enumeration and reporting of oval fat bodies, free-floating fat, and fatty casts.

Crystals of Iatrogenic Origin

Medications. Most medications (drugs) and their metabolites are eliminated from the body by the kidneys. As urine forms within the nephrons, high concentrations of these agents can cause their precipitation out of solu-tion. These crystals are termed *iatrogenic,* which means that they are induced in the patient as the result of a treatment (e.g., the prescribed drug). Proper identifica-tion and reporting of drug crystals are important because if the crystals are forming in vivo (i.e., in the renal tubules), they can cause kidney damage. When unusual

crystals are encountered in urine sediment, the health care provider should be contacted to obtain a list of the patient's medications and to determine whether any recent diagnostic procedures involving infusion of medi-cations or dyes have been performed (e.g., intravenous pyelogram). When in vivo crystalline formation is sus-pected, treatments such as increased hydration or the infusion of pH-adjusting agents can be initiated to prevent adverse effects. Two common antibiotics, sulfon-amides and ampicillin, are known for their propensity to form crystals in urine.

Ampicillin. Ampicillin crystals appear as long, color-less, thin prisms or needles (Figure 8-83). The individual needles may aggregate into small groupings or, with refrigeration, into large clusters. Present in acidic urine, ampicillin crystals indicate large doses of ampicillin and are rarely observed with adequate hydration.

Indinavir. Indinavir sulfate crystals are slender feather-like crystals that aggregate into wing-like bundles, which can also associate into a rosette-like or cross form (Figure 8-84). The crystals are strongly birefringent when observed under polarizing microscopy. In contrast to most drug crystals that are only present in acid urine, indinavir and other antiviral drugs (e.g., acyclovir) can be present in acid urine but are more often observed in neutral and alkaline urines.

Sulfonamides. Sulfonamides appear in various forms that differ depending on the particular form of the drug prescribed. When initially manufactured, sul-fonamide preparations were relatively insoluble and resulted in kidney damage caused by crystal formation within the renal tubules. Currently, these drugs have been modified, and their solubility is no longer a problem. As a result, sulfonamide crystals are not found as often in urine sediment, and renal damage caused by them is uncommon.

Sulfadiazine drug crystals usually appear yellow to brown and as bundles of needles that resemble sheaves of wheat (Figure 8-85). The constriction of the bundle may be located centrally or extremely eccentric, resulting

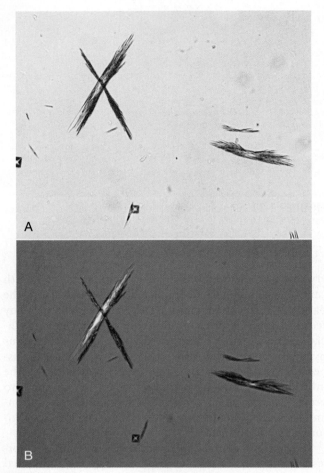

FIGURE 8-84 Indinavir sulfate crystals. **A,** Brightfield, 200×. **B,** Polarizing microscopy with first-order red compensator, 200×.

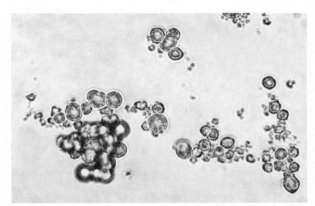

FIGURE 8-86 Sulfamethoxazole (Bactrim) crystals. Brightfield, 400×.

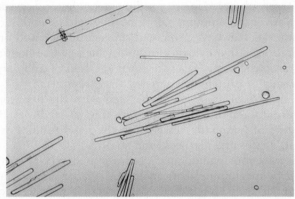

FIGURE 8-87 Radiographic contrast medium following retrograde administration; meglumine diatrizoate (Renografin). The crystals appear in needle forms. Brightfield, 100×.

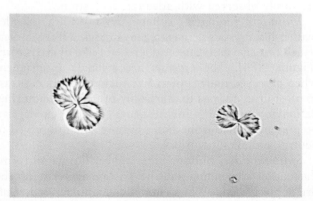

FIGURE 8-85 Sulfadiazine crystals. Brightfield, 400×. *(Courtesy Patrick C. Ward.)*

in a fan formation. Sulfamethoxazole (e.g., Bactrim, Septra) is more commonly encountered and appears as brown rosettes or spheres with irregular radial striations (Figure 8-86). All sulfonamide crystals are highly refractile and birefringent.

Sulfonamide crystals can be present in acid urine and should be confirmed chemically before they are reported.

The diazotization of sulfanilamide followed by an azo-coupling reaction is the preferred method to confirm their presence. In shape and color, these crystals closely resemble ammonium biurate crystals but can be differentiated from them on the basis of their pH, their solubility, and the chemical confirmatory test. A list of the patient's current and past medications can be of value in confirming the identity of these urine crystals.

Radiographic Contrast Media. Diatrizoate salts are used as an intravenous radiographic contrast medium in x-ray procedures. They are water-soluble derivatives of triiodobenzene and are available in many preparations of meglumine or sodium salts or in mixtures of the two. Diatrizoate salts are known by numerous product names such as Hypaque, Renografin, Cystografin, and Renovist. Because of their water solubility, they are readily excreted in the urine.

Crystals of radiographic contrast media following retrograde administration appear as colorless, long, rectangular needles that occur singly or clustered in sheaves (Figure 8-87); when administered intravenously, they appear as flat, elongated rectangular plates (see Figures 8-82 and 8-88). One distinguishes the latter crystalline form from cholesterol crystals by (1) the large number of crystals usually present, (2) the high urine specific gravity (greater than 1.040) that accompanies them, and (3) the lack of significant proteinuria and lipiduria.

Diatrizoate crystals appear in acidic urine. Clearance of radiographic contrast media is highly variable, with the greatest excretion noted during the first 24 hours, but excretion can persist as late as 3 days.[23] Besides significantly elevating urine specific gravity, diatrizoate crystals can cause a false-positive sulfosalicylic acid precipitation test for protein. A microscopic examination of the precipitate formed in this test identifies it as a crystalline substance and not amorphous material like protein. With interference contrast and polarizing microscopy, diatrizoate crystals are strongly birefringent producing a variety of interference colors (Figure 8-88).

Microorganisms in Urine Sediment

In health, the urinary tract is sterile, i.e., no microorganisms are present. Consequently, the presence of bacteria, yeast, trichomonads, or parasites in urine indicates an infection or that contamination occurred during the collection process. Table 8-12 lists characteristic microscopic features and urinalysis findings associated with commonly observed microorganisms as well as some less common.

Bacteria. Observing bacteria in the urine sediment requires high-power magnification (Figure 8-89). The most commonly encountered bacteria in urine are rod-shaped (bacilli), but coccoid forms can also be present. These microorganisms can vary in size from long, thin rods to short, plump rods. They may appear singly or in chains, depending on the species present. In wet preparations, their motility often distinguishes bacteria from amorphous substances that may be present. Because the skin, vagina, and gastrointestinal tract normally contain bacteria, the presence of bacteria in urine often reflects contamination from these sources.

Bacteria are reported as few, moderate, or many per high-power field. Because urine from normal healthy individuals is sterile, the presence of bacteria in the urine sediment implies a UTI or urine contamination. Bacteria most often ascend the urethra to cause a UTI. They can also be present because of a fistula—a narrow pathway—between the urinary tract and the bowel. In addition, contaminating bacteria multiply rapidly in improperly stored urine. Therefore the presence of bacteria has clinical significance only if the urine specimen has been properly collected and stored.

For urine sediment in which identification of bacteria is difficult, a cytospin preparation followed by Gram staining could be performed. During UTI, bacteriuria usually is accompanied by leukocytes in the urine sediment. When significant bacteriuria is present without leukocytes, the specimen collection and handling should be investigated.

Yeast. Yeasts are ovoid, colorless cells that can closely resemble RBCs (Figure 8-90). More refractile than erythrocytes, yeasts often have characteristic budding forms and pseudohyphae (Figure 8-91). Yeasts can vary in size, and some species are very large (10 to 12 μm). Yeasts do not dissolve in acid and usually do not stain with

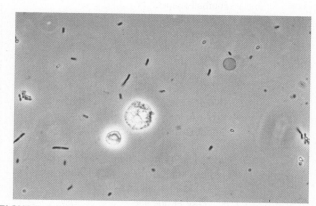

FIGURE 8-89 Urine sediment with bacteria (rods), two erythrocytes, and a leukocyte. Phase contrast, 400×.

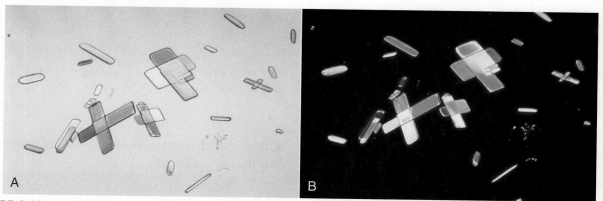

FIGURE 8-88 Intravenous radiographic contrast medium. **A,** Interference contrast microscopy, 100×. **B,** Polarizing microscopy, 100×.

Organism	Characteristic Features	UA Correlations
TABLE 8-12	**Microorganisms in Urine Sediment**	
Bacteria	Bacilli (rods) or cocci (spheres) Single organisms, in chains, or in groups (e.g., diplococci, tetrads)	WBCs increased; WBC clumps and macrophages with severe infection LE +/− Nitrite +/−
Yeast	Ovoid, colorless, refractile cells No nucleus Characteristic budding forms Pseudohyphae may be present	WBCs increased LE +/−
Trichomonads	Pear-shaped organisms Average length ≈15 μm 4 anterior flagella, 1 posterior axostyle, undulating membrane Identify based on characteristic flitting or jerky motion	WBCs increased, WBC clumps present LE +/−
Other parasites	*Enterobius vermicularis* (pinworm) Football-shaped* or ovoid eggs 50-60 μm long by 20-30 μm wide Transparent cell wall, larva visible inside	None; fecal contaminant
	Giardia lamblia Ovoid eggs 8-12 μm long Smooth, well-defined cell wall	None; fecal contaminant
	Schistosoma haematobium Football-shaped* or ovoid eggs with a spike at one end Thick, transparent cell wall; larva visible inside	Blood positive RBCs increased

*Shape of the American football.

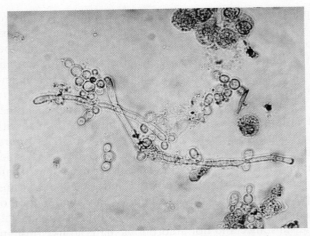

FIGURE 8-90 Budding yeast and pseudohyphae. Leukocytes are also present singly and as a clump. Brightfield, Sedi-Stain, 400×.

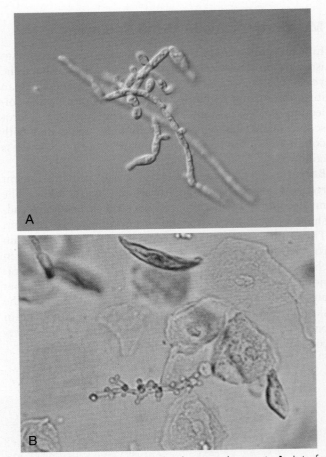

FIGURE 8-91 Pseudohyphae development by yeast. **A,** Interference contrast, 400×. **B,** Brightfield, 400×.

supravital stains; these two characteristics can aid in differentiating them from erythrocytes.

In women, yeast in the urine sediment most often indicates contamination of the urine with vaginal secretions. However, because yeasts are ubiquitous—present in the air and on skin—their presence could indicate contamination from these sources. Although infrequent, primary UTIs resulting from yeasts are possible, hence health care providers must correlate the finding of yeast with the patient's clinical picture to determine whether an actual infection, vaginal or urethral, is present. Certain situations such as pregnancy, use of oral contraceptives, and diabetes mellitus promote the development of vaginal yeast infection.

The most commonly encountered yeast in urine sediment is *Candida albicans*. The characteristic budding and the development of pseudohyphae make C. *albicans*

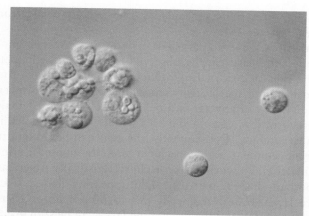

FIGURE 8-92 Leukocytes with intracellular yeast. Interference contrast, 400×.

readily identifiable as yeast. Another species found less frequently is *C. glabrata,* formerly called *Torulopsis glabrata.* This species does not form pseudohyphae, and these yeast cells may be found phagocytized within white blood cells (Figure 8-92). In immunosuppressed patients, systemic *Candida* infections are common; for some unknown reason, yeasts have a predilection for the kidneys. During the microscopic examination, only the presence of yeast can be determined; identification of the species present requires fungal culture.

A **KOH preparation** is often used to detect yeast, hyphae, and other fungal cells in vaginal secretions. See Chapter 16, "Analysis of Vaginal Secretions."

Trichomonas Vaginalis. Trichomonads, protozoan flagellates, can be observed in the urine sediment. Trichomonads appear as turnip-shaped flagellates whose unicellular bodies average 15 μm in length, although organisms as small as 5 μm and as large as 30 μm are possible. They have four anterior flagella, a single posterior axostyle, and an undulating membrane that extends halfway down the body of the organism (Figure 8-93). The beating flagella propel the organism while the undulating membrane rotates it. The result is a characteristic flitting or jerky motility in wet preparations. Because of their similarity in size to both leukocytes and renal tubular cells, this motility is critical for their identification (Figure 8-94).

Trichomonas vaginalis is the most common cause of parasitic gynecologic infection in female patients (see Chapter 16, "Analysis of Vaginal Secretions"). Transmitted sexually, trichomonads most frequently represent an infection of the vagina and/or urethra, and their presence in the urine often indicates contamination with vaginal secretions. In male patients, trichomonad infections of the urethra are usually asymptomatic. In either case, when observed in urine sediment, trichomonads are not quantitated but are simply reported as present.

Urine is not an optimal medium for trichomonads. Because their characteristic motility provides the best

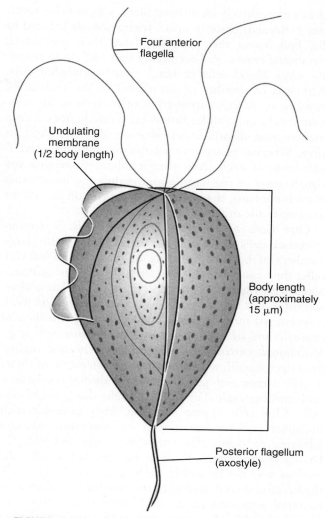

FIGURE 8-93 Schematic diagram of *Trichomonas vaginalis.*

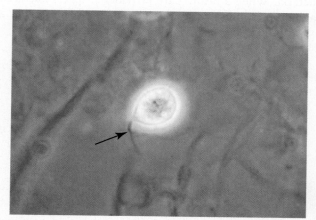

FIGURE 8-94 A trichomonad in urine sediment. Because of their rapid flitting motion, only one of the flagella is visible in this view *(arrow).* Mucus, white blood cells, and other trichomonads are present but are not in focus at this focal plane. Phase contrast, 400×.

means of positively identifying them, a fresh urine specimen is needed. Once in urine, trichomonads proceed to die, first losing their motility; later, their undulating membrane ceases, and eventually they ball up to resemble white blood cells or renal tubular epithelial cells. With loss of motility or movement of the undulating membrane, differentiation from other cells in the sediment can be impossible. Supravital stains do not enhance trichomonad identification, whether they are dead or alive. Whereas phase-contrast microscopy and interference contrast microscopy permit enhanced imaging and visualization of the flagella and undulating membranes of trichomonads, these techniques depend on movement to identify the organisms specifically.

Clue Cells and Gardnerella Vaginalis. Squamous epithelial cells from the vaginal mucosa with large numbers of bacteria adhering to them are called **clue cells;** they can be present in urine specimens contaminated with vaginal secretions (Figure 8-95). These characteristic cells are indicative of bacterial vaginosis (BV), a synergistic infection most often involving *Gardnerella vaginalis* and an anaerobe, usually *Mobiluncus* spp. (e.g., *Mobiluncus curtisii*). A disruption in the normal vaginal flora (lactobacilli) with subsequent proliferation of these, usually minor, endogenous bacterial species results in a foul-smelling vaginal discharge and the sloughing of clue cells. Clue cells appear soft and finely granular with indistinct cell borders caused by numerous bacteria adhering to them, hence they are often described as having shaggy edges. In these bacteria-laden cells, the nucleus may not be visible. To be considered a clue cell, the bacteria do not need to cover the entire cell; however, bacterial organisms must extend beyond the cell's cytoplasmic borders. Be aware that with an inexperienced microscopist, normal intracellular keratohyalin granulation can be misidentified as bacteria adhering to squamous epithelial cells. However, these granules are variable in size and are usually larger and more refractile than bacteria. When a health care provider suspects bacterial vaginosis, a pelvic examination is performed and a

vaginal secretions specimen is collected for evaluation (see Chapter 16).

Parasites. Several parasites, in addition to trichomonads and yeast, can be observed in the urine sediment. The eggs or ova of *Enterobius vermicularis* (pinworm) can be found in urine from school-aged children; however, individuals of any age can be infected. The adult female pinworm lays eggs in the area around the rectum; this causes itching. Consequently, the eggs can be present in urine sediment if the specimen is contaminated during collection. Pinworm eggs are characteristically American football–shaped, with one side appearing flatter. They are large, transparent cells (50 to 60 μm long; 20 to 30 μm wide), and the developing larva can be seen inside (Figure 8-96).

Cysts of *Giardia lamblia* may be observed in urine sediment as the result of fecal contamination of infected individuals. Giardiasis is most often acquired by drinking contaminated water. It can occur from inadequate sanitation of city water supplies or from contamination of fresh water lakes and streams. *Giardia* organisms have contaminated recreational water sources such as swimming pools and water parks. The cysts are small, ovoid

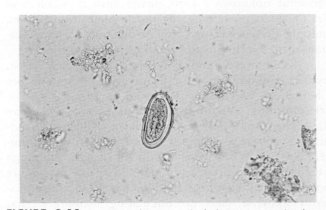

FIGURE 8-96 An *Enterobius vermicularis* egg, unstained wet mount. Note its oval shape with a slightly flattened side and the developing larva within.

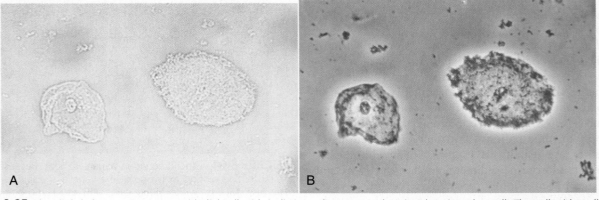

FIGURE 8-95 The slightly larger squamous epithelial cell with indistinct, shaggy cytoplasmic edges is a clue cell. The cell with well-defined cytoplasmic edges is a normal squamous epithelial cell. **A,** Brightfield, 200×. **B,** Phase contrast, 200×.

cells about 8 to 12 μm in length, with smooth, well-defined cell walls (Figure 8-97). When viewing using brightfield microscopy and high power (400×) magnification, the cytoplasm appears to be filled with nuclear material, but distinct nuclei (up to four) usually are not apparent without specific staining.

Finally, the eggs of the blood fluke *Schistosoma haematobium* can be present in urine sediment. Schistosomiasis is endemic in Africa and the Middle East and is acquired upon exposure to water where infected snails live (e.g., fishermen, swimmers, workers in irrigation canals). Infections are most often diagnosed when the eggs are found in urine sediment or in biopsies of the bladder, rectum, or vaginal wall. *Schistosoma* eggs are distinctively large (100 to 170 μm long and 40 to 70 μm wide) and shaped like an American football with a spike at one end (Figure 8-98). Their cell walls are thick but transparent, revealing the larva that fills its interior. Hematuria is often present as well.

Miscellaneous Formed Elements

Mucus. Mucus, a fibrillar protein, commonly appears in urine sediment and has no clinical significance. In unstained urine sediment with brightfield microscopy, mucus can be difficult to observe because of its low refractive index. However, when phase-contrast or interference contrast microscopy is used, mucous threads are readily identifiable by their delicate, ribbon-like strands and irregular or serrated ends. Muous strands appear wavy and can take various forms as they surround other sediment elements. They can be present as distinct strands or as a clumped mass (Figure 8-99).

Because some mucus has been shown immunohistochemically to contain uromodulin (formerly Tamm-Horsfall protein), and because this protein is produced solely by the renal tubular epithelium, some mucus found in urine is derived at least partially from the renal tubules.[15] The genitourinary tract, particularly the vaginal epithelium, is also a source of the mucus frequently observed in urine sediments from women.

Muous threads can be misidentified as hyaline casts because of their similar low refractive index and fibrillar protein structure. The cylindrical composition of casts and their rounded ends aid in their differentiation from mucus.

Fat. Fats or lipids are found in urine sediment in three forms: as free-floating fat globules, within oval fat bodies (cells with fat globules), or within a cast matrix as fat globules or entrapped oval fat bodies. During the microscopic examination, a distinguishing feature of lipids is their high refractility. With the use of brightfield microscopy, these highly refractive globules are spherical; they vary in size, and, depending on the optics used, they can appear colorless to yellow-green or even brownish (see Figure 8-31).

The type of fat present can vary; often both triglyceride and cholesterol can be demonstrated (Figure 8-100). Triglyceride, also called *neutral fat*, is composed of a glycerol backbone with three fatty acids esterified to it.

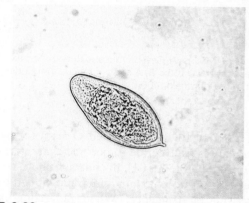

FIGURE 8-98 A *Schistosoma haematobium* egg, unstained wet mount Note the terminal spine on this large, American football shaped egg.

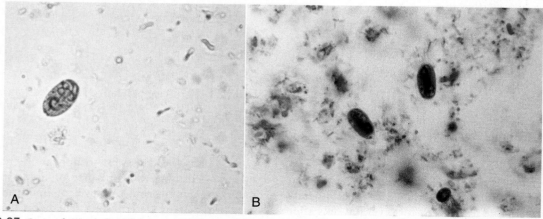

FIGURE 8-97 Cysts of *Giarda lamblia*. **A,** A single *Giardia lamblia* cyst, unstained. **B,** Two *Giardia lamblia* cysts, trichrome stained.

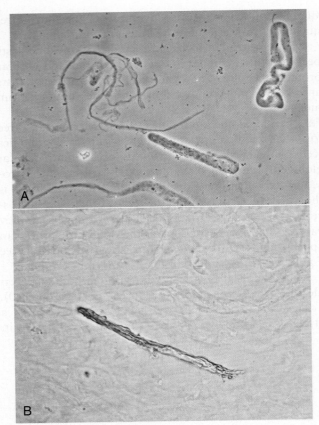

FIGURE 8-99 Mucus. **A,** Several mucous threads and two hyaline casts. Phase contrast, 100×. **B,** A mass of mucus surrounding a fiber (contaminant). Brightfield, 400×.

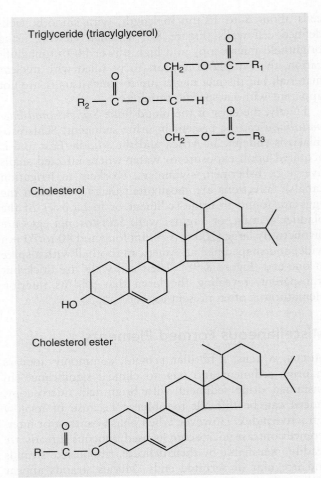

FIGURE 8-100 Chemical structures of triglyceride (triacylglycerol or neutral fat), cholesterol, and cholesterol esters.

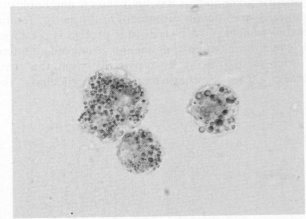

FIGURE 8-101 Three oval fat bodies stained with Sudan III stain. Note the characteristic orange-red staining of neutral fat globules. Brightfield, 400×.

Adding a Sudan III or an Oil Red O stain to the urine sediment causes triglyceride to become characteristically orange or red (Figure 8-101). In contrast, cholesterol and cholesterol esters do not stain and are identified by their characteristic birefringence. When polarizing microscopy is used, cholesterol globules produce a distinctive Maltese cross pattern, that is, an orb that appears divided into four quadrants by a bright Maltese-style cross (Figure 8-102). In urine specimens that contain significant amounts of fat, cholesterol crystals may form on storage at refrigerator temperature. The section "Crystals" contains more discussion of these unique cholesterol crystals.

Lipiduria is always clinically significant, although its presence does not pinpoint a specific diagnosis. Lipiduria is present with a variety of renal diseases and may occur following severe crush injuries. It is a characteristic feature of the nephrotic syndrome, along with severe proteinuria, hypoproteinemia, hyperlipidemia, and edema. Because the nephrotic syndrome can occur with other kidney diseases, as well as with metabolic diseases such as diabetes mellitus, lipids are often encountered in the urine sediment from these patients. In preeclampsia, fat is often present and can persist for several weeks after delivery. Extreme physical exercise (e.g., marathon racing) can also cause fat to appear in the urine sediment.[2] Identifying the presence of lipids in urine sediment and monitoring the level of lipiduria aids health care providers in determining whether a disease process is progressing or resolving.

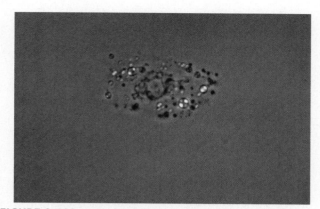

FIGURE 8-102 Cholesterol droplets demonstrating the characteristic Maltese cross pattern. Polarizing microscopy with first-order red compensator, 400×.

Lipids most often enter the urine because of adverse changes in the glomerular filtration barriers, which allow the plasma lipids to pass. If large lipid molecules are able to cross into Bowman's space, so can plasma proteins, most notably albumin. Therefore lipiduria is always accompanied by some degree of proteinuria. Note however that the level of proteinuria in a random urine specimen can be disguised by hydration. In other words, a low reagent strip protein test can be caused by the large amount of water excreted (dilute urine). When protein excretion is 300 mg/dL or greater, the urine sediment should be specifically screened for fat with the use of polarizing microscopy or fat stains such as Sudan III or Oil Red O.

It is also important to note that urine from men with prostatitis, could be contaminated with prostatic fluid. During prostatitis, prostatic fluid contains many WBCs, macrophages, as well as oval-fat bodies (fat-laden macrophages) and free-floating fat globules.[24] Note that urine contaminated with this type of prostatic fluid could resemble the nephrotic syndrome—lipiduria and proteinuria—and may require investigation. Contamination of urine with normal prostatic fluid may be suspected when numerous fine secretory granules are present, giving the urine a grainy appearance microscopically. These secretory granules vary in size, from fine granules to about half the size of an RBC. In elderly men, prostatic fluid may contain free-floating fat globules. Therefore, when the finding of urinary fat is unexpected in the urine from a male, it could be the result of prostatic fluid contamination.

Because other entities in urine sediment can resemble fat, it is important to distinguish these look-alike substances. Starch granules form a similar Maltese pattern with polarizing microscopy; however, they are easily distinguished from fat globules with the use of brightfield microscopy. Starch granules are highly refractile, tend to have a central dimple, and are not spherical. The variation in size demonstrated by fat globules aids in

differentiating them from RBCs. In addition, RBCs do not stain with fat dyes and are not birefringent. When a Sternheimer-Malbin stain is used, lipids retain their high refractility and yellow-green to gold color, whether free floating, held intracellularly (oval fat bodies), or enmeshed within a cast matrix.

Oils and fats from lubricants, ointments, creams, and lotions can also contaminate urine. They may be introduced during specimen collection from vaginal creams, topical ointments, or catheter lubricants. In the laboratory, immersion oil left on an objective lens can contaminate urine sediment during the microscopic examination. Regardless of the source, these contaminating lipids are often indicated by the lack of associated abnormalities (proteinuria, fatty casts, oval fat bodies) and are identified by (1) their presence only as free-floating globules, (2) homogeneity, (3) lack of structure, and (4) size (often droplets coalesce to become unusually large).

Hemosiderin. Hemosiderin is a form of iron that results from ferritin denaturation. These insoluble granules can become large enough to be observed microscopically in the urine sediment, especially after they have been stained to a Prussian blue color. Unstained hemosiderin granules appear as coarse yellow-brown granules and are difficult to distinguish from amorphous crystalline material in the sediment (Figure 8-103, *A*).

Hemosiderin granules are found in the urine sediment 2 to 3 days after a severe hemolytic episode (e.g., transfusion reaction, paroxysmal nocturnal hemoglobinuria). In these cases, plasma haptoglobin is saturated with hemoglobin, and any remaining free hemoglobin is able to pass through the glomerular filtration barrier to be absorbed by the renal tubular epithelium. The tubular cells metabolize the hemoglobin to ferritin and subsequently denature it to form hemosiderin. Hemoglobin is toxic to cells, and as these cells degenerate, hemosiderin granules appear in the urine. Hemosiderin granules may be found free floating or within macrophages, casts, or tubular epithelial cells.

The **Prussian blue reaction,** also known as the *Rous test,* is used to identify hemosiderin in the urine sediment and in tissues. A concentrated urine sediment is examined for the presence of coarse yellow-brown hemosiderin granules, free floating or within casts or tubular epithelial cells. The urine sediment is suspended in a freshly prepared solution of potassium ferricyanide–HCl and is allowed to stand at room temperature for 10 minutes. After centrifugation and discarding of the supernatant, the sediment is reexamined for the presence of coarse blue granules. In this preparation, hemosiderin iron causes the granules to stain Prussian blue (Figure 8-100, *B*). Because the reaction can be delayed, negative sediments are examined a second time after 30 minutes.[12]

Sperm. Sperm cells or spermatozoa may be present in urine sediment from males and females. They have oval heads approximately 3.0 to 5.0 µm long and thin, thread-like tails about 40 to 60 µm long (Figure 8-104). A variety

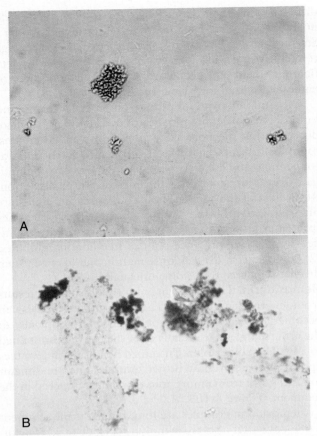

FIGURE 8-103 **A,** Hemosiderin granules floating free in urine sediment. Brightfield, 400×. **B,** Hemosiderin granules after staining with Prussian blue. Brightfield, 400×.

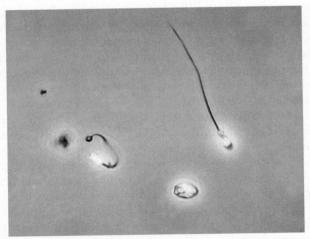

FIGURE 8-104 Spermatozoa in urine sediment. One typical and two atypical forms. Phase contrast, 400×.

of forms may be encountered, and at times sperm may be found in clumps of mucus in the sediment. See Chapter 11 for additional discussion of sperm morphology.

Because urine is not a viable medium for sperm, the presence of motile sperm indicates recent intercourse or ejaculation. In urine from women, sperm are usually

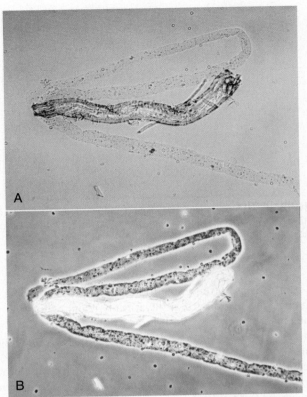

FIGURE 8-105 Hyaline cast and a fiber. Note the difference in form and refractility. **A,** Brightfield, 100×. **B,** Phase contrast, 100×.

considered a vaginal contaminant. It is important to report the presence of sperm in urine from females because it could potentially identify sexual abuse in underage and other vulnerable females. This information enables the health care provider to appropriately intervene, if necessary.

In urine from men, sperm can be present owing to nocturnal emissions, from normal or retrograde ejaculation. Sperm in urine sediment have no clinical significance and are simply reported as present.

Contaminants

Fibers. Numerous types of fibers, such as hair, cotton, and other fabric threads, often appear in the urine sediment. They are considered contaminants and are disregarded during the microscopic examination. It is important to ensure their proper identification by the novice microscopist. Fibers can be large with distinct edges and are often moderately to highly refractile. Fibers may resemble urinary casts; several features aid in their differentiation. Fibers tend to be flat and thicker at their margins, in contrast to casts, which are thicker in the middle (Figure 8-105). Fibers are anisotropic, and polarizing microscopy demonstrates their birefringence; casts are not anisotropic (see Figure 8-57 (fiber), 8-53, *B* [cast]).
Starch. Starch granules originating from body powders or those found in protective gloves worn by health care

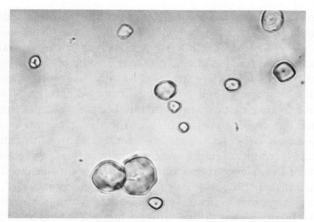

FIGURE 8-106 Starch granules. Brightfield, 400×.

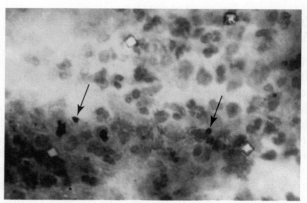

FIGURE 8-108 Charcoal granules (arrows) in urine sediment. Numerous leukocytes are present. Cytospin preparation, Wright's stain, brightfield microscopy, 400×.

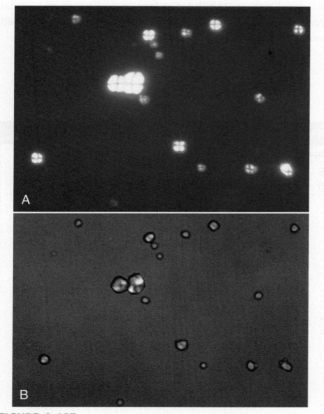

FIGURE 8-107 Starch granules. **A,** Demonstration of a Maltese cross pattern using polarizing microscopy, 400×. **B,** Polarizing microscopy with first-order red compensator, 400×.

visual differences on brightfield microscopy, starch granules and cholesterol droplets are usually readily differentiated.

Because starch granules are a urine contaminant, they are not reported. Excessive quantities could interfere with the examination, however, and may necessitate specimen re-collection.

Fecal Matter. Fecal material contaminates urine primarily by two modes: through improper collection technique and through an abnormal connection or fistula between the urinary tract and the bowel. Specimens received from infants and from patients who are extremely ill or physically compromised are most likely to be contaminated with fecal material because of the difficulty involved in performing the urine collection. With the assistance of a health care worker for ill or physically compromised patients or the use of collection bags for infants, these specimens can be obtained without contamination. In contrast, when a fistula that continually channels fecal material into the urinary tract is present, optimizing the collection technique will not eliminate the contamination. In the latter condition, the patient has a persistent UTI from the constant influx of normal bacterial flora from the intestine into the urinary tract; food remnants may also be present in the urine sediment.

Fecal contamination of urine specimens often is not grossly apparent. Microscopic examination of the urine sediment reveals the abnormal presence of partially digested vegetable cells and muscle fibers from ingested foods. One method that can be used to confirm a suspected fistular connection is to have the patient ingest charcoal particles. After ingestion, the patient's urine is collected for 24 hours or longer, and the entire collection is concentrated by centrifugation. The resultant urine sediment is thoroughly screened microscopically for the presence of charcoal particles. If charcoal particles are found, they confirm the diagnosis of a fistula between the bowel and the urinary tract (Figure 8-108).

workers are frequently encountered microscopically in the urine sediment. Starch has unique characteristics that make it easy to identify. Starch granules can vary greatly in size and usually have a centrally located dimple (Figure 8-106). They are not perfectly round; rather they have scalloped or faceted edges. Under polarizing microscopy, starch granules exhibit a Maltese cross pattern similar to that of cholesterol (Figure 8-107). Because they are not round like cholesterol droplets, however, the edges of the Maltese pattern are less defined. Because of their

Correlation of Urine Sediment Findings With Disease

Most urine sediment findings are not unique for a specific disorder; rather they indicate a process (e.g., infection, inflammation) or functional change (e.g., glomerular changes, tubular dysfunction, obstruction) that is occurring in the kidneys or urinary tract. An exception is the presence of cystine crystals that points to the hereditary diseases of cystinuria or cystinosis. A challenge for health care providers can be determining the cause of the disorder and its location within the urinary tract. Consequently, it is the entire urinalysis—the physical, chemical, and microscopic examinations—that best enables healthcare providers to detect and monitor disease in the urinary tract. When serial specimens (daily or weekly) are obtained from a patient, the urinalysis test provides an economical means to monitor the progression or resolution of a disorder.

Table 8-13 links the urine sediment findings discussed in this chapter to selected disorders of the urinary tract to be discussed in Chapter 9. In health, the urine sediment may have a few epithelial cells, a rare RBC and few WBCs (see Table 8-5). A few hyaline casts or an occasional finely granular cast may also be observed but because the urinary tract is sterile, microorganisms such as bacteria and yeast should not be present. Note that hyaline casts are not listed in this table because they are not considered pathologic casts (i.e., indicative of disease). However, increased numbers of hyaline casts may be observed in the urine sediment with each of these disorders. Some urine sediment findings point specifically to a disease process (e.g., presence of bacteria and WBCs indicate an infection), whereas other findings identify the location of a disease process (e.g., WBC casts, RBC casts indicate process occurring in the kidneys where casts are formed). See Chapter 9 for further discussion of renal and metabolic diseases including their clinical features, pathogenesis, and urinalysis results associated with each.

TABLE 8-13	Urine Sediment Findings With Selected Diseases										
	Blood Cells		Epithelial Cells		Pathologic Casts*							
Disease	RBC	WBC	TE	RTE	RBC[†]	WBC	RTE Cell	Coarsely Granular	Waxy	Fat[‡]	Bacteria[§]	Other
Infection or Inflammation												
Lower UTI Cystitis or urethritis (bacterial)	++	+++	++								+	
Upper UTI Acute pyelonephritis (bacterial)	+	+++	+			++	+	++	+/−		+/−	Macrophages with severe infection
Acute interstitial nephritis (drug-induced)	++	+++	++			+	++	++	+/−			Eosinophils predominate
Glomerular Disease												
Acute glomerulonephritis (AGN)	+++	+	+		+++	+	+	++				Dysmorphic RBCs
Chronic glomerulonephritis	+	+	+		+/−		++	++	++			Broad casts
Nephrotic syndrome	+		+				+/−	+	+	+++		
Tubular Disease												
Acute tubular necrosis (ATN)	++	++	+++		+/−	++	++	++	(+/−)			Proximal RTE cells with toxic ATN Collecting duct RTE cells with ischemic ATN Epithelial fragments

*Note that hyaline casts, which are not considered pathological, are often present in increased numbers in the listed conditions.
[†]Includes blood and hemoglobin casts.
[‡]Includes fatty casts, oval fat bodies (OFB), and free-floating fat globules.
[§]Quantity of bacteria observed can vary from few to many; does not reflect severity of bacterial infection.

STUDY QUESTIONS

1. Which of the following are not standardized when commercial systems are used for the processing and microscopic examination of urine sediment?
   A. Microscopic variables, such as the number of focal planes
   B. The concentration and volume of the urine sediment prepared
   C. The volume of the urine sediment dispensed for microscopic viewing
   D. Identification and enumeration of formed elements in the urine sediment

2. When urine sediment is viewed, stains and various microscopic techniques are used to
   1. enhance the observation of fine detail.
   2. confirm the identity of suspected components.
   3. differentiate formed elements that look alike.
   4. facilitate the visualization of low-refractile components.
   A. 1, 2, and 3 are correct.
   B. 1 and 3 are correct.
   C. 4 is correct.
   D. All are correct.

3. The microscopic identification of hemosiderin is enhanced when the urine sediment is stained with
   A. Gram stain.
   B. Hansel stain.
   C. Prussian blue stain.
   D. Sudan III stain.

4. When the laboratorian performs the microscopic examination of urine sediment, which of the following are enumerated using low-power magnification?
   A. Bacteria
   B. Casts
   C. Red blood cells
   D. Renal tubular cells

5. A urine sediment could have which of the following formed elements and still be considered "normal"?
   A. Two or fewer hyaline casts
   B. Five to 10 red blood cells
   C. A few bacteria
   D. A few yeast cells

6. Which of the following statements about red blood cells in urine is true?
   A. Red blood cells crenate in hypotonic urine.
   B. Red blood cell remnants are called "ghost cells."
   C. Alkaline and hypotonic urine promotes red blood cell disintegration.
   D. Dysmorphic red blood cells often are associated with renal tubular disease.

7. Hemoglobin is a protein and will
   A. not react in the protein reagent strip test.
   B. interfere with the protein reagent strip test, producing erroneous results.
   C. always contribute to the protein reagent strip result, regardless of the amount of hemoglobin present.
   D. contribute to the protein reagent strip result only when large concentrations of hemoglobin are present.

8. Which urinary sediment component(s) when observed microscopically can resemble red blood cells?
   1. Yeasts
   2. Air bubbles
   3. Oil droplets
   4. Calcium oxalate crystals
   A. 1, 2, and 3 are correct.
   B. 1 and 3 are correct.
   C. 4 is correct.
   D. All are correct.

9. Which of the following is not a characteristic of neutrophils found in the urine sediment?
   A. They are approximately 10 to 14 μm in diameter.
   B. They form "ghost cells" in hypotonic urine.
   C. They shrink in hypertonic urine but do not crenate.
   D. As they disintegrate, vacuoles and blebs form and their nuclei fuse.

10. How do increased numbers of leukocytes usually get into the urine?
    A. Through a renal bleed
    B. By passive movement through pores in the vascular epithelium
    C. By active ameboid movement through tissues and epithelium
    D. Through damage to the integrity of the normal vascular barrier

11. Which statement regarding lymphocytes found in urine sediment is correct?
    A. They are not normally present in the urine.
    B. They produce a positive leukocyte esterase test.
    C. Their number is increased in patients with drug hypersensitivity.
    D. Their number is increased in patients experiencing kidney transplant rejection.

12. Which of the following urinary tract structures is not lined with transitional epithelium?
    A. Bladder
    B. Nephrons
    C. Renal pelves
    D. Ureters

13. Match the number of the epithelial cell type with its characteristic feature. Only one type is correct for each feature.

Characteristic Feature	Epithelial Cell Type
__ A. Large and flagstone; can be anucleated	1. Collecting tubular cell
__ B. Oblong or cigar shaped; small eccentric nucleus	2. Distal tubular cell
__ C. Polygonal; large nucleus	3. Proximal tubular cell
__ D. Oval to round; small nucleus that is	4. Squamous epithelial cell centered or slightly eccentric
__ E. Round, pear-shaped, or columnar with a small oval to round nucleus	5. Transitional epithelial cell

14. Which of the following can be observed in the urine sediment as an intact fragment or sheet of cells?
    1. Collecting tubular epithelium
    2. Distal tubular epithelium
    3. Transitional epithelium
    4. Proximal tubular epithelium
A. 1, 2, and 3 are correct.
B. 1 and 3 are correct.
C. 4 is correct.
D. All are correct.

15. Urinary casts are formed in
A. the distal and collecting tubules.
B. the distal tubules and the loops of Henle.
C. the proximal and distal tubules.
D. the proximal tubules and the loops of Henle.

16. Urinary casts are formed with a core matrix of
A. albumin.
B. Bence Jones protein.
C. transferrin.
D. uromodulin.

17. Which of the following does not contribute to the size, shape, or length of a urinary cast?
A. The concentration of protein in the core matrix of the cast
B. The configuration of the tubule in which the cast is formed
C. The diameter of the tubular lumen in which the cast is formed
D. The duration of time the cast is allowed to form in the tubule

18. All of the following enhance urinary cast formation except
A. an alkaline pH.
B. urinary stasis.
C. an increase in the solute concentration of the ultrafiltrate.
D. an increase in the quantity of plasma proteins in the ultrafiltrate.

19. When the laboratorian is using brightfield microscopy, a urinary cast that appears homogeneous with well-defined edges, blunt ends, and cracks is most likely a
A. fatty cast.
B. granular cast.
C. hyaline cast.
D. waxy cast.

20. All of the following can be found incorporated into a cast matrix except
A. bacteria.
B. crystals.
C. transitional epithelial cells.
D. white blood cells.

21. Which of the following urinary casts are diagnostic of glomerular or renal tubular damage?
A. Bacterial casts
B. Red blood cell casts
C. Renal tubular cell casts
D. White blood cell casts

22. Which of the following characteristics best differentiates waxy casts from fibers that may contaminate urine sediment?
A. Waxy casts do not polarize light; fibers do.
B. Waxy casts are more refractile than fibers.
C. Waxy casts have rounded ends; fibers do not.
D. Waxy casts are thicker at their margins; fibers are thicker in the middle.

23. Which of the following does not affect the formation of urinary crystals within nephrons?
A. The pH of the ultrafiltrate
B. The diameter of the tubular lumen
C. The flow of urine through the tubules
D. The concentration of solutes in the ultrafiltrate

24. The formation of urinary crystals is associated with a specific urine pH. Match the urine pH that facilitates crystalline formation with the appropriate crystal type. More than one number (pH) can be used.

Crystal Type	Urine pH
__ A. Ammonium biurate	1. Acid
__ B. Amorphous urates	2. Neutral
__ C. Amorphous phosphates	3. Alkaline
__ D. Calcium oxalate	
__ E. Cholesterol	
__ F. Cystine	
__ G. Radiographic contrast media	
__ H. Sulfonamides	
__ I. Triple phosphate	
__ J. Tyrosine	
__ K. Uric acid	

25. Match the crystal composition with the microscopic description that best characterizes it.

Microscopic Description	Crystal Composition
__ A. Colorless "coffin lid" form	1. Ammonium biurate
__ B. Colorless hexagonal plates	2. Amorphous urates
__ C. Colorless "envelope" form	3. Amorphous phosphates
__ D. Colorless rectangular plates with notched corners	4. Calcium oxalate
__ E. Yellow-brown "thorny apple" form	5. Cholesterol
	6. Cystine
__ F. Colorless to yellow; diamond-shaped or rhombic-; can form layers	7. Sulfonamides
	8. Triple phosphate
__ G. Yellow-brown sheaves of wheat	9. Uric acid

26. Which of the following crystals, when found in the urine sediment, most likely indicates an abnormal metabolic condition?
    A. Bilirubin
    B. Sulfonamides
    C. Triple phosphate
    D. Uric acid

27. During the microscopic examination of a urine sediment, cystine crystals are found. The laboratorian should perform which of the following before reporting the presence of these crystals?
    1. Perform a confirmatory chemical test
    2. Ensure that the urine specimen has an acid pH
    3. Assess the number of crystals per high-power field
    4. Check the current medications that the patient is taking
    A. 1, 2, and 3 are correct.
    B. 1 and 3 are correct.
    C. 4 is correct.
    D. All are correct.

28. Mucous threads can be difficult to differentiate from
    A. fibers.
    B. hyaline casts.
    C. pigmented casts.
    D. waxy casts.

29. Which of the following is not a distinguishing characteristic of yeast in the urine sediment?
    A. Motility
    B. Budding forms
    C. Hyphae formation
    D. Colorless ovoid forms

30. Fat can be found in the urine sediment in all of the following forms except
    A. within casts.
    B. within cells.
    C. as free-floating globules.
    D. within hemosiderin granules.

31. Which of the following statements regarding the characteristics of urinary fat is true?
    A. Cholesterol droplets stain with Sudan III stain.
    B. Triglyceride or neutral fat stains with Oil Red O stain.
    C. Cholesterol droplets do not form a Maltese cross pattern under polarized light.
    D. Triglycerides and neutral fat are anisotropic and form a Maltese cross pattern under polarized light.

32. Which of the following statements regarding the microscopic examination of urine sediment is false?
    A. If large numbers of leukocytes are present microscopically, then bacteria are present.
    B. If urinary fat is present microscopically, then the chemical test for protein should be positive.
    C. If large numbers of casts are present microscopically, then the chemical test for protein should be positive.
    D. If large numbers of red blood cells are present microscopically, then the chemical test for blood should be positive.

33. The following are initial results obtained during a routine urinalysis. Which results should be investigated further?
    A. Negative protein; 2 to 5 waxy casts
    B. Cloudy, brown urine; 2 to 5 red blood cells
    C. Urine pH 7.5; ammonium biurate crystals
    D. Clear, colorless urine; specific gravity 1.010

34. The following are initial results obtained during a routine urinalysis. Which results should be investigated further?
    A. Negative protein; 0 to 2 hyaline casts
    B. Urine pH 6.0; calcium oxalate crystals
    C. Cloudy, yellow urine; specific gravity 1.050
    D. Amber urine with yellow foam; negative bilirubin by reagent strip; positive Ictotest

35. Which of the following when found in the urine sediment from a female patient is not considered a vaginal contaminant?
    A. Fat
    B. Clue cells
    C. Spermatozoa
    D. Trichomonads

CASE 8-1

A routine urinalysis specimen is sent to the laboratory from a patient suspected of having renal calculi. When the microscopic examination is performed, unusual crystals that resemble cholesterol plates are observed. The technologist is suspicious and performs a sulfosalicylic acid precipitation test (SSA test for protein) and checks the specific gravity by refractometry. The patient care unit is contacted for a list of current medications. The list reveals that the patient had an intravenous pyelogram 6 hours earlier. The patient is taking no other medications except those given during the intravenous pyelogram procedure (Demerol and Xylocaine).

Results

Physical Examination	Chemical Examination	Microscopic Examination
Color: yellow	SG: 1.020	RBC/hpf: 0-2
Clarity: cloudy	Refractometry: >1.035	WBC/hpf: 0-2
Odor: —	pH: 5.0	Casts: negative
	Blood: negative	Epithelials: few TE cells/hpf
	Protein: negative	
	SSA: 4+ (crystalline precipitate)	Crystals: moderate; type unknown per hpf
	LE: negative	
	Nitrite: negative	
	Glucose: negative	
	Ketones: negative	
	Bilirubin: negative	
	Urobilinogen: normal	

1. List any abnormal or discrepant urinalysis findings.
2. What is the most likely identity of this crystal?
   A. Cystine
   B. Cholesterol
   C. Triple phosphate
   D. Uric acid, rare form
   E. X-ray contrast media
3. State two results that support the crystal selection made in question 2.
4. Which chemical examination result does not support the presence of lipids in the urine? Explain.
5. Which specific gravity result best indicates this patient's renal ability to concentrate urine?
   A. Reagent strip result: 1.020
   B. Refractometer result: >1.035

hpf, High-power field; *LE,* leukocyte esterase; *RBC,* red blood cell; *TE,* transitional epithelial; *WBC,* white blood cell.

CASE 8-2

A 22-year-old woman is seen in the emergency department. She complains of a painful burning sensation (dysuria) when urinating. She also states that she feels as if she has "to go" all the time. A midstream clean catch urine specimen is collected for a routine urinalysis and culture.

Results

Physical Examination	Chemical Examination	Microscopic Examination
Color: yellow	SG: 1.015	RBC/hpf: 0-2
Clarity: cloudy	pH: 6.0	WBC/hpf: 10-25
Odor: —	Blood: trace	Casts/hpf: 2-5 hyaline
	Protein: trace	Epithelials: few SE cells/lpf; moderate TE cells/hpf
	LE: negative	
	Nitrite: negative	
	Glucose: negative	Bacteria: moderate/hpf
	Ketones: negative	
	Bilirubin: negative	
	Urobilinogen: normal	

1. List any abnormal or discrepant urinalysis findings.
2. Based on the patient's symptoms and the urinalysis results, select the most probable diagnosis.
   A. Normal urinalysis
   B. Urinary tract infection
   C. Acute glomerulonephritis
   D. Nephrotic syndrome
3. Assume that no patient information is available, and that the number of squamous epithelial cells observed microscopically was "many." Would your suspected diagnosis change?
4. State three reasons why the nitrite test can be negative despite bacteriuria.
5. State two reasons why the leukocyte esterase test can be negative despite increased numbers of white blood cells in the urine sediment.
6. Suggest a cause for the increased number of transitional epithelial cells observed in the urine sediment.

hpf, High-power field; *LE,* leukocyte esterase; *lpf,* low-power field; *RBC,* red blood cell; *SE,* squamous epithelial; *TE,* transitional epithelial; *WBC,* white blood cell.

CASE 8-3

A 36-year-old man with a history of diabetes mellitus is admitted to the hospital with the following complaints: decreased frequency of urination, constant "bloated" feeling, weight gain, puffy eyes in the morning, and scrotal swelling. Mild edema of the ankles, abdomen, and eyes is also noted. Routine chemistry tests reveal hypoalbuminemia and hyperlipidemia ($\uparrow$ triglycerides and $\uparrow$ cholesterol). Urinalysis results follow:

Results

Physical Examination	Chemical Examination	Microscopic Examination
Color: yellow	SG: 1.015	RBC/hpf: 2-5
Clarity: slightly cloudy	pH: 5.0	WBC/hpf: 0-2
	Blood: small	Casts/lpf: 2-5 hyaline;
Odor: —	Protein: 2000 mg/dL	0-2 fatty;
Large amount of white foam noted.	SSA: 4+	0-2 waxy
	LE: negative	Epithelials: few TE cells/
	Nitrite: negative	hpf; few
	Glucose: 100 mg/dL	OFBs/hpf
	Ketones: negative	
	Bilirubin: negative	
	Urobilinogen: normal	

1. List any abnormal or discrepant urinalysis findings.
2. Based on the patient's symptoms and urinalysis results, select the most probable diagnosis:
   A. Acute pyelonephritis
   B. Nephrotic syndrome
   C. Acute glomerulonephritis
   D. Lipiduria of unknown cause
3. The proteinuria in this patient should be classified as
   A. glomerular proteinuria.
   B. tubular proteinuria.
   C. overflow proteinuria.
   D. postrenal proteinuria.
4. What substance is responsible for the large amount of white foam observed?
   A. Fat
   B. Protein
   C. Glucose
   D. Casts
5. Explain the physiologic processes responsible for the edema exhibited in this patient.
6. In progressive renal disease with loss of glomerular filtering ability, which plasma protein is usually lost first? Explain why.
7. Explain the physiologic process responsible for the glucose present in this patient's urine.
8. Why is the ketone test not positive?

hpf, High-power field; *LE,* leukocyte esterase; *lpf,* low-power field; *OFBs,* oval fat bodies; *RBC,* red blood cell; *TE,* transitional epithelial; *WBC,* white blood cell.

CASE 8-4

A 30-year-old man is admitted to the hospital with headache, anorexia, and passing red-colored urine. Examination reveals mild edema of the eyes and mild hypertension. Medical history reveals that the patient's daughter had strep throat about a month ago and was treated successfully. Subsequently, he developed a sore throat that lasted a few days but did not seek treatment. Urinalysis results follow.

Results

Physical Examination	Chemical Examination	Microscopic Examination
Color: red	SG: 1.010	RBC/hpf: 25-50
Clarity: cloudy	pH: 5.5	WBC/hpf: 0-2
Odor: —	Blood: moderate	Casts/lpf: 2-5 hyaline;
	Protein: 300 mg/dL	0-2 RBCs;
	SSA: 3+	0-2 granular
	LE: negative	Epithelials: few TE
	Nitrite: negative	cells/hpf
	Glucose: negative	Bacteria: negative
	Ketones: negative	
	Bilirubin: negative	
	Urobilinogen: normal	

1. List any abnormal or discrepant urinalysis findings.
2. What is the most likely process by which red blood cells are getting into this patient's urine?
3. At this level of hematuria, is the blood that is present most likely contributing to the reagent strip protein result?
   A. Yes
   B. No
4. This patient is determined to have acute glomerulonephritis. Based on this diagnosis, the proteinuria in this patient would be classified as
   A. glomerular proteinuria.
   B. tubular proteinuria.
   C. overflow proteinuria.
   D. postrenal proteinuria.
5. Of the microscopic findings, which sediment entity specifically indicates adverse glomerular changes and the presence of a renal disorder?

hpf, High-power field; *lpf,* low-power field; *RBC,* red blood cell; *TE,* transitional epithelial; *WBC,* white blood cell.

CASE 8-5

An obese 58-year-old woman is seen by her physician. Her chief complaint is perineal itching and soreness. When giving her health history, she also complains of being thirsty "all the time" and of urinating more frequently. On pelvic examination, a white discharge is noted. A urine specimen is collected for a routine urinalysis.

Results

Physical Examination	Chemical Examination	Microscopic Examination
Color: yellow	SG: 1.015	RBC/hpf: 0-2
Clarity: cloudy	pH: 6.0	WBC/hpf: 10-25;
Odor: —	Blood: moderate	clumps
	Protein: trace	Casts/lpf: 0-2
	LE: positive	hyaline
	Nitrite: negative	Epithelials: many SE
	Glucose: 500 mg/dL	cells/lpf
	Ketones: trace	Bacteria: negative
	Bilirubin: negative	Yeast/hpf: moderate
	Urobilinogen: normal	Crystals/hpf: few urates

1. List any abnormal or discrepant urinalysis findings.
2. What is the most likely cause of this patient's vaginitis?
3. What is the most likely origin or source of the white blood cells in this urine?
4. Which two microscopic findings suggest that this urine is not a midstream clean catch specimen?
5. Is this patient showing signs/symptoms of any urinary tract disorder or dysfunction? Yes No
6. Explain the physiologic processes responsible for ketonuria.

hpf, High-power field; *LE,* leukocyte esterase; *lpf,* low-power field; *RBC,* red blood cell; *SE,* squamous epithelial; *WBC,* white blood cell.

CASE 8-6

A 48-year-old woman is admitted to a hospital for an emergency appendectomy. Because of bleeding complications, she receives a unit of packed red blood cells after surgery. Two hours later, she develops fever, chills, and nausea. Two days following surgery, a routine urinalysis and hemosiderin test (Rous test) are performed, and the following results are obtained.

Results

Physical Examination	Chemical Examination	Microscopic Examination
Color: brown	SG: 1.015	RBC/hpf: 0-2
Clarity: slightly	pH: 5.0	WBC/hpf: 0-2
cloudy	Blood: large	Casts/lpf: 5-10 granular
Odor: —	Protein: trace	Epithelials: few TE cells/
	SSA: trace	hpf; few RTE
	LE: negative	cells/hpf; few
	Nitrite: negative	SE cells/hpf
	Glucose: negative	Crystals/hpf: few
	Ketones: negative	amorphous
	Bilirubin: negative	urates
	Urobilinogen: 4 mg/dL	Hemosiderin
		test: positive

1. List any abnormal or discrepant urinalysis findings.
2. What is hemosiderin?
3. Explain how hemosiderin gets into the urine sediment.
4. What substance most likely is causing the brown color observed in this urine?
5. Explain the physiologic mechanism that leads to increased urobilinogen in this patient's urine.
6. Because of the intravascular hemolytic episode experienced by this patient, her serum bilirubin is significantly increased. Why is her urine bilirubin still normal?

hpf, High-power field; *LE,* leukocyte esterase; *lpf,* low-power field; *RBC,* red blood cell; *RTE,* renal tubular epithelial; *SE,* squamous epithelial; *TE,* transitional epithelial; *WBC,* white blood cell.

CASE 8-7

A 19-year-old female college athlete visits the campus health clinic for a mandatory sports physical. She claims no health problems and is taking no medications. A clean catch urine specimen is collected for a routine urinalysis, and the following results are obtained.

Results

Physical Examination	Chemical Examination	Microscopic Examination
Color: yellow	SG: 1.020	RBC/hpf: 50-100
Clarity: clear	pH: 7.0	WBC/hpf: 25-50;
Odor: —	Blood: trace	clumps
	Protein: trace	Casts/lpf: 5-10 cellular
	LE: negative	Epithelials: few RTE
	Nitrite: negative	cells/hpf;
	Glucose: negative	few SE cells/
	Ketones: negative	lpf
	Bilirubin: negative	Crystals/hpf: few uric acid
	Urobilinogen: normal	
	Ascorbic acid: negative	

The technologist performing the microscopic examination checks the pH of the urine sediment and rechecks that of the specimen in the urine cup. The following results are obtained:

Urine sediment: pH 5.0

Urine in specimen cup: pH 7.0

1. List any abnormal or discrepant urinalysis findings.
2. Suggest a cause for the discrepancies observed.

hpf, High-power field; *lpf,* low-power field; *RBC,* red blood cell; *RTE,* renal tubular epithelial; *SE,* squamous epithelial; *WBC,* white blood cell.

REFERENCES

1. Pennica D, Kohr WJ, Juang WJ, et al: Identification of human uromodulin as the Tamm-Horsfall urinary glycoprotein. Science 236:83–88, 1998.
2. Carlson JA, Harrington JT: Laboratory evaluation of renal function. In Diseases of the kidney, ed 5, Boston, 1993, Little, Brown & Company.
3. Kumar S, Muchmore A: Tamm-Horsfall protein—uromodulin (1950-1990). Kidney Int 37:1395–1401, 1990.
4. National Committee for Clinical Laboratory Standards: Routine urinalysis: tentative guideline, NCCLS Document GP16-T, vol 12, No 26, Wayne, PA, 1992, NCCLS.
5. Schumann GB, Tebbs RD: Comparison of slides used for standardized routine microscopic urinalysis. J Med Technol 3:54–58, 1986.
6. Sternheimer R, Malbin B: Clinical recognition of pyelonephritis with a new stain for urinary sediments. Am J Med 11:312–323, 1951.
7. Rous P: Urinary siderosis. J Exp Med 28:645–658, 1918.
8. Nolan CR, Anger MS, Kelleher SP: Eosinophiluria: a new method of detection and definition of the clinical spectrum. N Engl J Med 315:1516–1519, 1986.
9. Schumann GB: Cytodiagnostic urinalysis for the nephrology practice. Semin Nephrol 6:308–345, 1986.
10. Mahon CS, Smith LA: Standardization of the urine microscopic examination. Clin Lab Sci 3:328–332, 1990.
11. Fairley KF, Birch DF: Hematuria: a simple method for identifying glomerular bleeding. Kidney Int 21:105–108, 1982.
12. Kohler H, Wandel E, Brunck B: Acanthocyturia—a characteristic marker for glomerular bleeding. Kidney Int 40:115–120, 1991.
13. Crop MJ, de Rijke YB, Verhaugen PC, et al: Diagnostic value of urinary dysmorphic erythrocytes in clinical practice. Nephron Clin Pract 115:c203–c212, 2010.
14. Schumann GB, Schweitzer SC: Examination of urine. In Henry JB, editor: Clinical diagnosis and management by laboratory methods, ed 18, Philadelphia, 1991, WB Saunders.
15. Bessis M: Living blood cells and their ultrastructure, New York, 1973, Springer-Verlag.
16. Freni SC, Dalderup LM, Oudegeest JJ, Wensveen N: Erythrocyturia, smoking and occupation. J Clin Pathol 30:341–344, 1977.
17. Corwin HL, Bray RA, Haber MH: The detection and interpretation of urinary eosinophils. Arch Pathol Lab Med 113:1256–1258, 1989.
18. Weir MR, Hall-Craggs M, Shen SY, et al: The prognostic value of the eosinophil in acute allograft rejection. Transplantation 41:709–712, 1986.
19. Orskov I, Ferencz A, Orskov F: Tamm-Horsfall protein or uromucoid is the normal urinary slime that traps type 1 fimbriated Escherichia coli. Lancet 1:887, 1980.
20. Haber MH: Composition of the normal urinary sediment. In A primer of microscopic urinalysis, ed 2, Garden Grove, CA, 1991, Hycor Biomedical.
21. Dukes CE: Urinary crystals and amorphous deposits. In Urine—Examination and clinical interpretation, London, 1939, Oxford University Press.
22. Resnick MI, Schaeffer AJ: Patient 68. In Urology Pearls, Philadelphia, 2000, Hanley & Belfus, Inc.
23. Henry RJ: Proteins. In Clinical chemistry principles and technics, New York, 1968, Harper & Row.
24. Stamey TA, Kindrachuk RW: Examination of Expressed Prostatic Secretions. In Urinary Sediment and Urinalysis, Philadelphia, 1985, WB Saunders Company.

BIBLIOGRAPHY

Clinical and Laboratory Standards Institute (CLSI): Urinalysis: approved guideline, ed 3, CLSI Document GP16-A3, Wayne, PA, 2009, CLSI.

Finnegan K: Routine urinalysis. In Saunders manual of clinical laboratory science, Philadelphia, 1998, WB Saunders.

Kaplan LA, Pesce AJ, Kazmierczak SC, editors: Clinical chemistry: theory, analysis, correlation, ed 4, St Louis, 2003, Mosby.

McPherson RA, Ben-Ezra J: Basic examination of urine. In McPherson RA, Pincus MR, editors: Henry's Clinical diagnosis and management by laboratory methods, ed 22, Philadelphia, 2011, WB Saunders.

Ringsrud KM, Linne JJ: Urinalysis and body fluids: a color text and atlas, St Louis, 1995, Mosby-Year Book.

Strasinger SK, Di Lorenzo MS: Urinalysis and body fluids, ed 5, Philadelphia, 2008, FA Davis.

Urine Sediment Image Gallery

ARTIFACTS/CONTAMINANTS

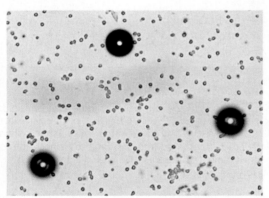

FIGURE 1 Three air bubbles trapped beneath a coverslip observed using low-power (100×) magnification. Numerous white blood cells (WBCs) are also present.

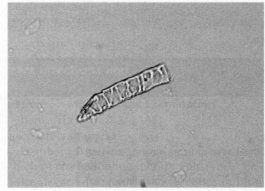

FIGURE 2 A diaper fiber. Note its flat, wrinkled appearance and strong refractility. For an inexperienced microscopist, these fibers may be misidentified as waxy casts.

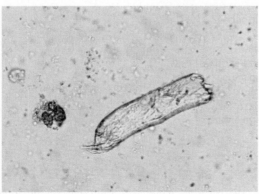

FIGURE 3 A clothing fiber. Its refractility, frayed ends, and flatness aid in its proper identification.

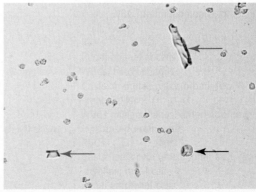

FIGURE 4 A starch granule *(black arrow)* demonstrating a characteristic dimple. When glass slides and coverslips are used, glass fragments *(red arrows)* can be present. Numerous white blood cells are also present.

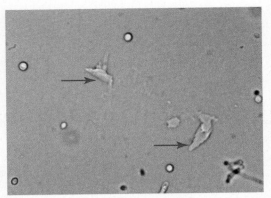

FIGURE 5 When plastic commercial standardized slides are used, fragments of plastic *(red arrows)* can be present in the sediment. Red blood cells, yeasts, and pseudohyphae are also present.

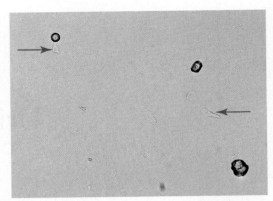

FIGURE 6 Three starch granules, all highly refractile, with slightly differing appearances, yet each has a centrally located dimple. Fragments of plastic *(red arrows)* are also present.

BLOOD CELLS

Red Blood Cells

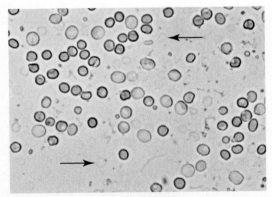

FIGURE 7 Numerous intact and ghost red blood cells *(black arrows)*. In this image, intact cells have a characteristic appearance caused by the hemoglobin within them. In contrast, ghost red blood cells (RBCs) have intact cell membranes but have lost their hemoglobin. This urine was hypotonic (dilute; low specific gravity), and many of the RBCs appear swollen and rounded because of the diffusion of fluid into the cells.

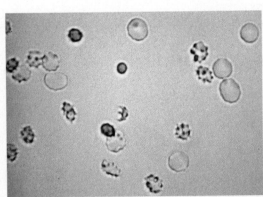

FIGURE 8 Red blood cells in hypertonic urine (concentrated; high specific gravity). Many of the cells in this field of view have lost their typical biconcave shape and are crenated. This happens when fluid within the cell is transferred into the urine to balance the tonicity of the environment. Consequently, the cell membrane shrinks, forming folds or projections.

White Blood Cells

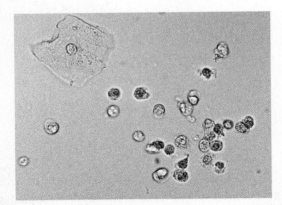

FIGURE 9 White blood cells and a single squamous epithelial cell.

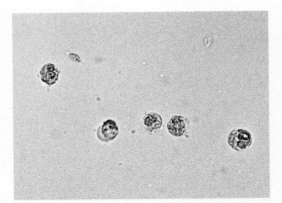

FIGURE 10 Five white blood cells. Note that the lobed nuclei in several of these neutrophils are readily apparent, whereas in those that are degenerating, the nucleus has become mononuclear.

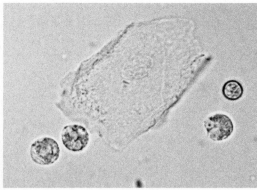

FIGURE 11 Three white blood cells, a single red blood cell, and a squamous epithelial cell.

CASTS

Cellular Casts

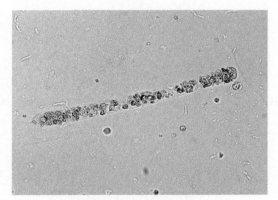

FIGURE 12 A mixed cellular cast.

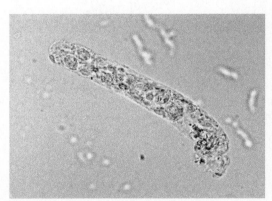

FIGURE 13 Renal tubular epithelial cell cast with one end broken or incompletely formed.

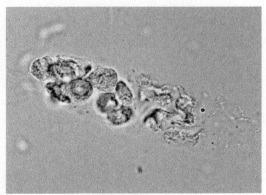

FIGURE 14 Renal tubular epithelial cell cast. Note the cuboidal shape of the entrapped cells. The nuclei were also apparent when focusing up and down during the microscopic examination.

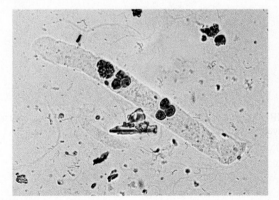

FIGURE 15 A renal tubular cell cast and several free-floating renal tubular cells in a Sternheimer-Malbin stained sediment. A highly refractile glass fragment is present in the center of this field of view.

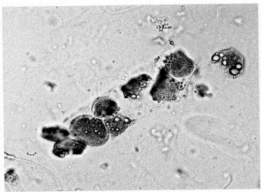

FIGURE 16 A cast with oval fat bodies (i.e., renal tubular cells that contain fat). In this Sternheimer-Malbin stained sediment, the fat globules take on a yellow or greenish appearance.

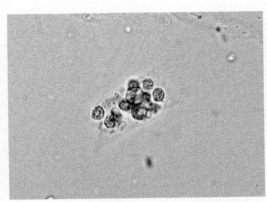

FIGURE 17 A white blood cell cast. Note the spherical or round shape of entrapped cells.

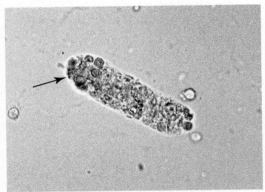

FIGURE 18 A mixed cell cast. This cast contains both white blood cells and red blood cells *(arrow)*.

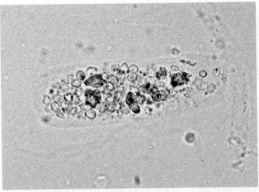

FIGURE 19 A mixed cell cast, predominantly red blood cells.

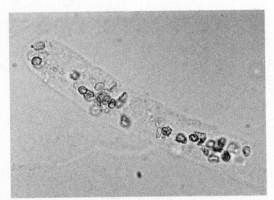

FIGURE 20 A red blood cell cast. Red blood cells are dispersed in the hyaline matrix of this cast.

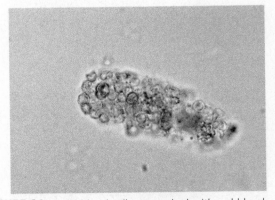

FIGURE 21 A red blood cell cast packed with red blood cells.

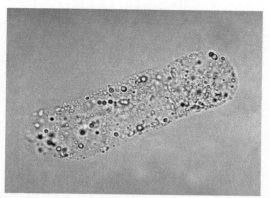

FIGURE 22 A fatty cast. Note the refractility, color, and size variation of fat globules in this cast.

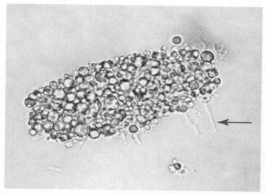

FIGURE 23 A fatty cast loaded with fat. With the passage of time and cooling (this urine specimen was stored in a refrigerator), a cholesterol crystal *(arrow)* has started to form from the fat (cholesterol) in this cast.

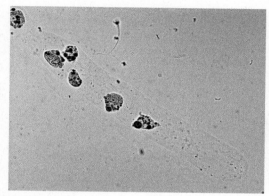

FIGURE 24 Oval fat bodies in a hyaline matrix (i.e., a fatty cast). In this sediment stained using Sudan III, the fat in the oval fat bodies has taken on the characteristic terra-cotta or red-orange color, indicating that the fat present is neutral fats (triglycerides).

Granular Casts

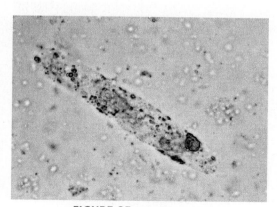

FIGURE 25 Granular cast.

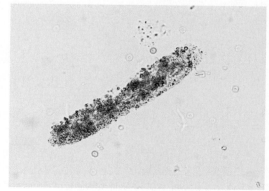

FIGURE 26 Granular cast.

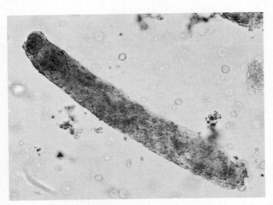

FIGURE 27 Coarsely granular cast.

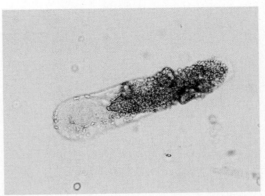

FIGURE 28 Cast transitioning from cellular to granular to waxy. The intense brown color suggests that pigmentation is derived from hemoglobin. This sediment also contained numerous red blood cells and red blood cell casts.

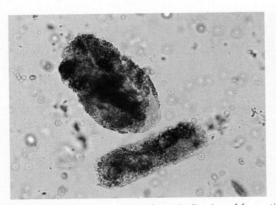

FIGURE 29 Granular casts. A broad cast indicative of formation in a large collecting duct or in dilated tubules indicates significant renal pathology. The granules in these casts most likely originated from red blood cells/hemoglobin.

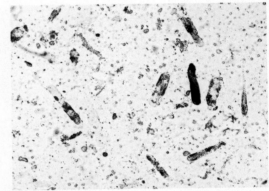

FIGURE 30 A low-power (100×) field of view of urine sediment containing numerous casts: hyaline, granular, red blood cell, and cellular.

Hyaline Casts

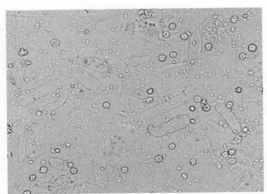

FIGURE 31 A low-power (100×) field of view of urine sediment containing numerous hyaline casts. Because their refractive index is similar to that of urine, they can be difficult to observe on bright-field microscopy. Focusing up and down during the microscopic examination aids in the detection of hyaline casts because they are often more apparent when slightly out of focus.

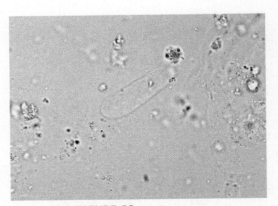

FIGURE 32 Hyaline cast.

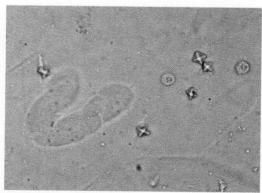

FIGURE 33 A U-shaped hyaline cast, two white blood cells, and several dihydrate calcium oxalate crystals.

Waxy Casts

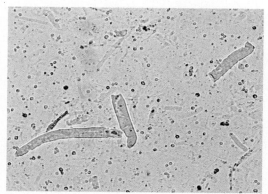

FIGURE 34 A low-power (100×) field of view of a urine sediment containing numerous casts, particularly hyaline and waxy (three predominate).

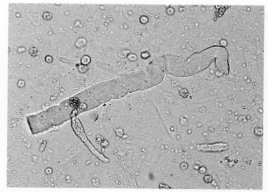

FIGURE 35 A long, broad waxy cast predominates in this field of view. Also present are other waxy and hyaline casts, as well as renal tubular cells and oval fat bodies.

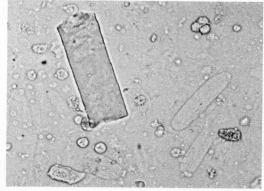

FIGURE 36 A single waxy cast and two hyaline casts. Note the difference in refractility between these two types of casts. In this image, the hyaline casts are actually out of focus, which makes them easier to see.

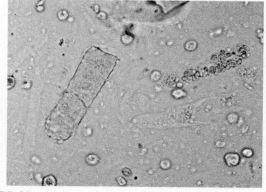

FIGURE 37 A waxy cast (left) lying almost vertical and two red blood cell casts (right) lying horizontally.

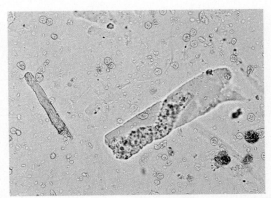

FIGURE 38 Two waxy casts. One typical in size and one broad cast that is transitioning from granular to waxy. Note ground-glass appearance and blunt end, which are characteristics of waxy casts.

CRYSTALS

Ammonium Biurate Crystals

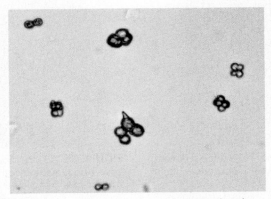

FIGURE 39 Ammonium biurate crystals. Note the characteristic yellow to brown color. With the passage of time (urine storage), these crystals will grow to form spicules or thorns.

Bilirubin Crystals

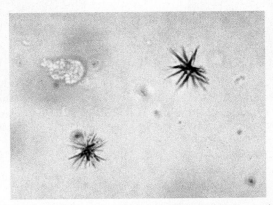

FIGURE 40 Bilirubin crystals. Small, finely spiculated crystals with the characteristic golden yellow color indicative of bilirubin. These crystals may form when urine with large amounts of bilirubin is refrigerated and stored.

Calcium Carbonate Crystals

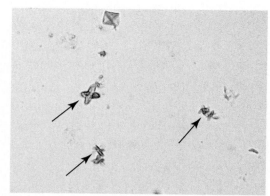

FIGURE 41 Calcium carbonate crystals *(arrows)* and single dihydrate calcium oxalate crystal.

Calcium Oxalate Crystals

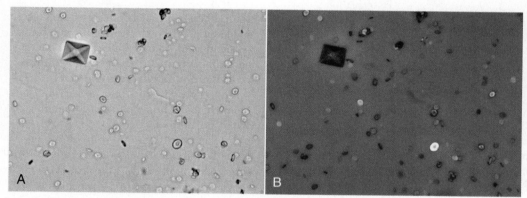

FIGURE 42 A, A single dihydrate calcium oxalate crystal and numerous monohydrate calcium oxalate crystals that look similar to red blood cells. **B,** Same field of view using polarizing microscopy. Rule of thumb: Crystals can polarize light; red blood cells do not.

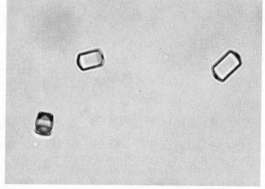

FIGURE 43 Calcium oxalate crystals, atypical barrel form.

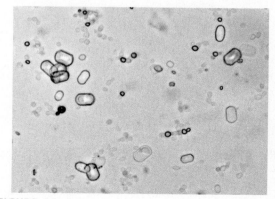

FIGURE 44 Calcium oxalate crystals, atypical ovoid form.

Cholesterol Crystal

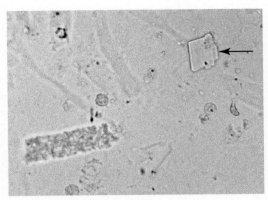

FIGURE 45 Cholesterol crystal *(arrow).*

Cystine Crystal

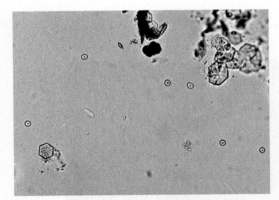

FIGURE 46 Cystine crystals. A single cystine crystal appears in the lower left corner, and several cystine crystals are layered and clustered together at the upper right corner. Several red blood cells are also present.

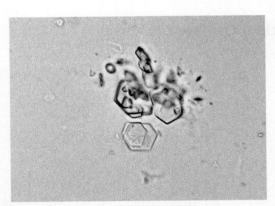

FIGURE 47 Several cystine crystals layered and clustered together.

Drug Crystals

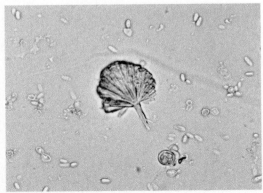

FIGURE 48 Acetylsulfadiazine crystal surrounded by numerous yeasts.

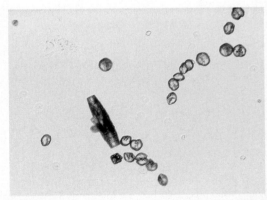

FIGURE 49 Numerous sulfamethoxazole (Bactrim) crystals surrounding a single barrel-shaped uric acid crystal. Note the yellow-brown color and the similar shape of sulfamethoxazole crystals to those of ammonium biurate. Urine pH aids in differentiating these two crystals.

Phosphate Crystals

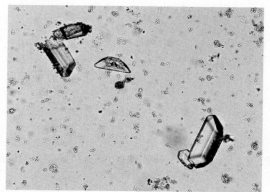

FIGURE 50 Triple phosphate crystals and numerous amorphous phosphates.

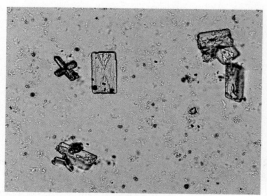

FIGURE 51 Dissolving triple phosphate crystals and numerous amorphous phosphates.

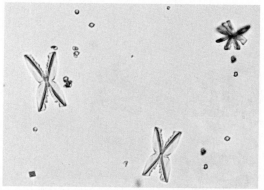

FIGURE 52 Two atypical triple phosphate crystals and a single stellate calcium phosphate crystal *(upper right)*.

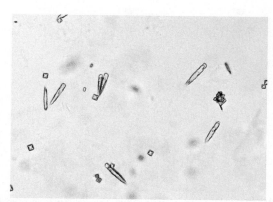

FIGURE 53 Wedge-shaped calcium phosphate crystals and dihydrate calcium oxalate crystals.

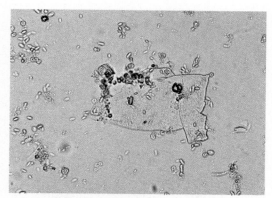

FIGURE 54 A calcium phosphate sheet.

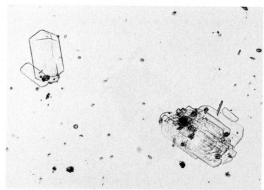

FIGURE 55 Calcium phosphate crystals. Unusual flat, plate-like form that layers.

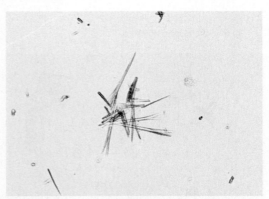

FIGURE 56 Calcium phosphate crystals. Uncommon slender wedges or needles.

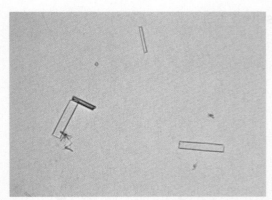

FIGURE 57 Magnesium phosphate crystals. Elongated rhomboid plates; rare.

Urate Crystals

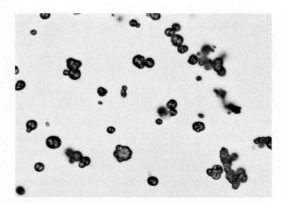

FIGURE 58 Acid urate crystals. Note the yellow to brown color characteristic of thick urate crystals.

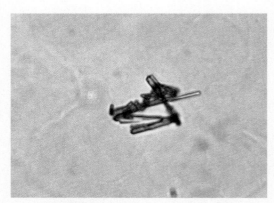

FIGURE 59 Monosodium urate crystals.

Uric Acid Crystals

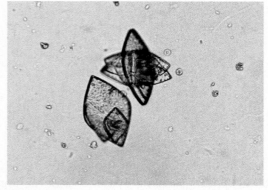

FIGURE 60 Uric acid crystals in the common diamond shape.

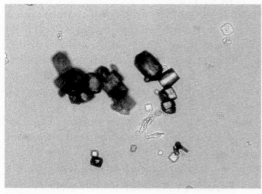

FIGURE 61 Uric acid crystals, barrel or cube forms.

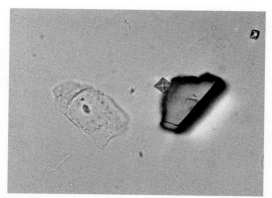

FIGURE 62 A chunk of a uric acid crystal. Note the characteristic color.

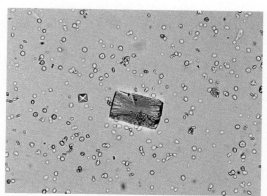

FIGURE 63 A single uric acid crystal in an unusual band form and numerous calcium oxalate crystals (mono- and dihydrate forms).

X-Ray Contrast Media Crystals

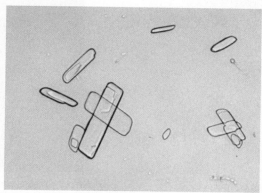

FIGURE 64 X-ray contrast media following intravenous (IV) administration (i.e., meglumine diatrizoate [Renografin]) crystals.

EPITHELIAL CELLS

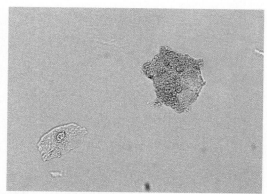

FIGURE 65 Two squamous epithelial cells covered with bacteria, known as *clue cells* and a single typical or "normal" squamous epithelial cell. In urine that has been contaminated with vaginal secretions, clue cells may be observed. This is not a common occurrence.

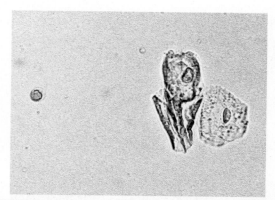

FIGURE 66 Three squamous epithelial cells and a single white blood cell. Note the similarity in size between the white blood cells and the nuclei of these epithelial cells.

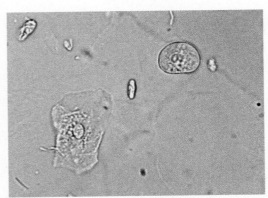

FIGURE 67 A squamous epithelial cell *(lower left cell)* and a transitional epithelial cell *(upper right cell)*. Note the similarity in sizes of their nuclei, yet the difference in the amount of cytoplasm (i.e., different nucleus-to-cytoplasm ratios). Several large rod-shaped bacteria are also present.

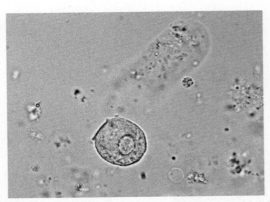

FIGURE 68 A typical transitional epithelial cell and a hyaline cast.

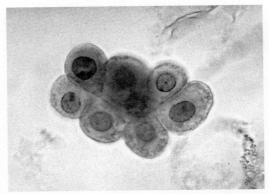

FIGURE 69 A fragment of transitional epithelial cells.

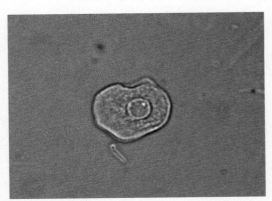

FIGURE 70 Transitional epithelial cell or squamous epithelial cell? Reasoning could be used to justify classification into either category. Cells lining the urinary system convert from squamous to transitional (urothelial) epithelium. This cell most likely originated from this area of transition.

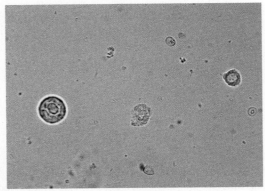

FIGURE 71 A transitional epithelial cell *(left)* and two typical cuboidal renal tubular (collecting duct) cells.

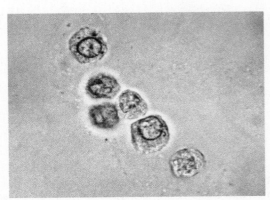

FIGURE 72 Renal tubular epithelial cells. These cells came from a small collecting duct based on their cuboidal shape and their nucleus-to-cytoplasm ratio.

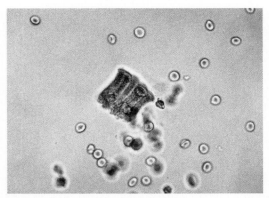

FIGURE 73 Renal tubular epithelial cells. This fragment of columnar epithelial cells with their eccentric nuclei derived from a large collecting duct. Numerous red blood cells are also present.

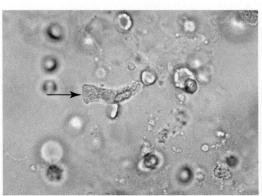

FIGURE 74 A single renal tubular cell *(arrow)* from a large collecting duct. Note the similarity in size of the nucleus of this cell to that of the red blood cells that are present.

FAT GLOBULES AND OVAL FAT BODIES

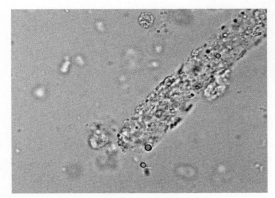

FIGURE 75 Several free fat globules and a fatty cast. Note refractility, variation in size, and greenish hue of the fat globules.

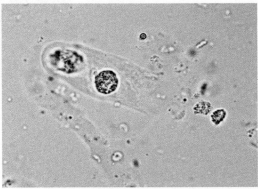

FIGURE 76 An oval fat body in the hyaline matrix of a cast. Also present in this field of view are another free-floating oval fat body, a fat globule, and a hyaline cast. Note the similarity in size and shape of the fat globule to a red blood cell.

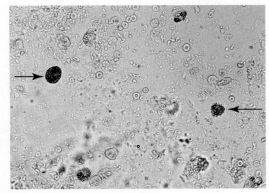

FIGURE 77 Two oval fat bodies *(arrows)* loaded with fat, hence their intense refractility. Numerous red blood cells, amorphous materials, and debris are also present.

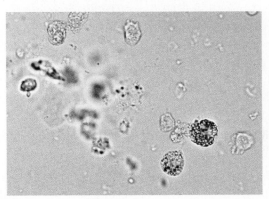

FIGURE 78 Two oval fat bodies and several renal tubular cells.

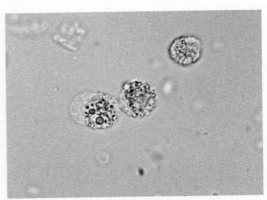

FIGURE 79 Three oval fat bodies. As with free-floating fat, the globules within cells often vary in size, are highly refractile, and have a greenish sheen.

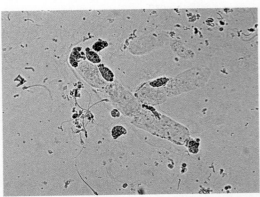

FIGURE 80 Several oval fat bodies enmeshed within casts and free in the urine sediment. Bacteria and spermatozoa are also present.

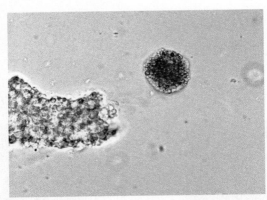

FIGURE 81 An oval fat body engorged with fat (triglycerides or neutral fat) stained using Sudan III.

MICROORGANISMS

Bacteria

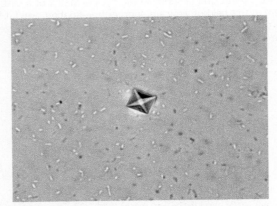

FIGURE 82 Numerous rod-shaped bacteria and a single dihydrate calcium oxalate crystal.

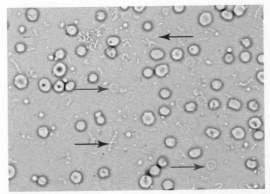

FIGURE 83 Numerous bacteria, singly and in chains, with several indicated by *blue arrows*. Many red blood cells (RBCs) and intact and ghost cells *(red arrows)* are present.

Trichomonads

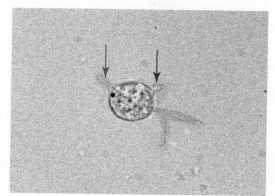

FIGURE 84 A trichomonad. Their characteristic rapid flitting motion results from their undulating membrane *(blue arrow),* anterior flagella *(two indicated by yellow arrows),* and axostyle *(red arrow).* Because of their size and granular appearance, nonmotile (or dead) trichomonads may be misidentified as white blood cells.

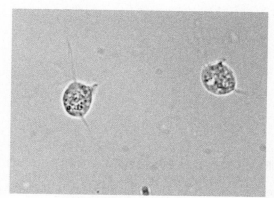

FIGURE 85 Two trichomonads.

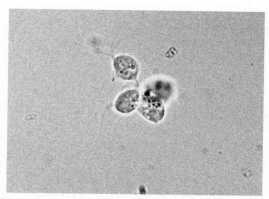

FIGURE 86 A cluster of four trichomonads. It is common to observe trichomonads clustered together along with white blood cell (WBC) clumps in urine sediment.

Yeast

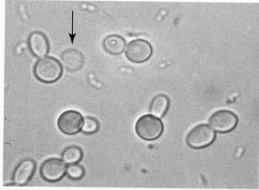

FIGURE 87 Several budding yeast (blastoconidia), bacteria, and a single ghost red blood cell. Note the refractility and sheen of the yeast, which is made most evident by focusing up and down during the microscopic examination.

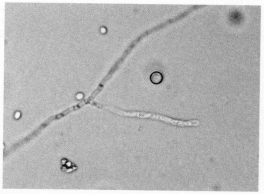

FIGURE 88 A branch of pseudohyphae (*Candida* spp.) and two red blood cells demonstrating typical pink-red coloration. Several ovoid yeasts are present in a different focal plane.

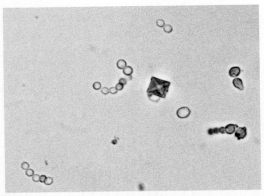

FIGURE 89 Yeast cells and blastoconidia (budding yeast). These yeast cells appear more round than oval, highlighting the fact that different species of yeast will appear differently. A single dihydrate calcium oxalate crystal is also present.

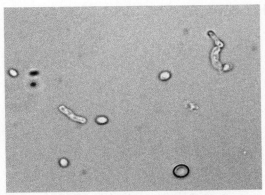

FIGURE 90 Early germ tube formation and several yeast cells. A single red blood cell is also present.

MISCELLANEOUS FORMED ELEMENTS

Hemosiderin

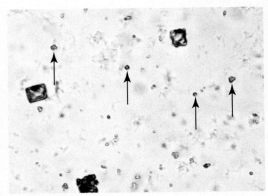

FIGURE 91 Hemosiderin granules in urine sediment appear yellow-brown. Numerous granules as well as a clump are present in this field of view. Four granules are identified by the *arrows.* Two dissolving dihydrate calcium oxalate crystals are also present.

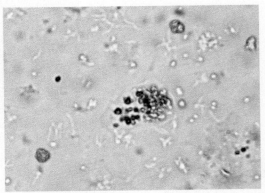

FIGURE 92 Hemosiderin granules in the hyaline matrix of a cast (i.e., a hemosiderin cast).

Mucus

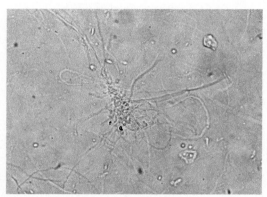

FIGURE 93 A cluster of mucous threads. Because the refractive index of muous is similar to that of urine, it can be difficult to observe using brightfield microscopy. Focusing up and down during the microscopic examination aids in the detection of mucus because it is often more apparent when slightly out of focus. A couple of squamous epithelial cells and other elements, on a different focal plane, are also present.

Sperm

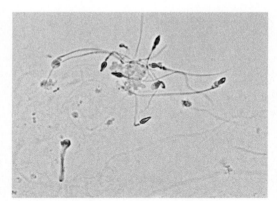

FIGURE 94 A cluster of sperm trapped in mucus.

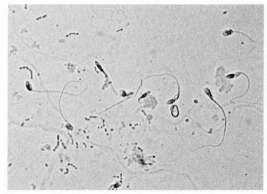

FIGURE 95 Sperm and bacteria in urine sediment. Note that several abnormal spermatozoa forms are present.

Renal and Metabolic Disease

LEARNING OBJECTIVES

After studying this chapter, the student should be able to:

1. Discuss the pathogenesis of glomerular damage and describe four morphologic changes that occur in glomeruli.
2. Describe the clinical features associated with glomerular disease and discuss factors that affect the degree to which they are present.
3. Describe briefly the morphologic appearances of the glomeruli, the mechanisms of glomerular damage, and the clinical presentations of the following glomerular diseases:
   • Acute glomerulonephritis
   • Chronic glomerulonephritis
   • Rapidly progressive glomerulonephritis
   • Focal proliferative glomerulonephritis
   • Focal segmental glomerulosclerosis
   • IgA nephropathy
   • Membranoproliferative glomerulonephritis
   • Membranous glomerulonephritis
   • Minimal change disease
4. Describe the pathologic mechanisms of glomerular damage in the following systemic diseases:
   • Systemic lupus erythematosus
   • Diabetes mellitus
   • Amyloidosis
5. State at least five clinical features that characterize the nephrotic syndrome and identify diseases that are associated with this syndrome.
6. Differentiate between ischemic and toxic acute tubular necrosis and discuss the clinical presentation and urinalysis findings associated with this disease.
7. Describe the renal dysfunction and clinical features of the following renal tubular disorders:
   • Cystinosis
   • Cystinuria
   • Fanconi's syndrome
   • Renal glucosuria

   • Renal phosphaturia
   • Renal tubular acidosis
8. Compare and contrast the causes, clinical features, and typical urinalysis findings in the following tubulointerstitial diseases and urinary tract infections:
   • Acute and chronic pyelonephritis
   • Acute interstitial nephritis
   • Lower urinary tract infections
   • Yeast infections
9. Describe briefly the effects of vascular disease on renal function.
10. Compare and contrast the causes and clinical features of acute and chronic renal failure.
11. Summarize the pathogenesis of calculus formation; discuss four factors that influence the formation of urinary tract calculi and briefly review current treatment options.
12. Describe briefly the physiologic mechanisms, clinical features, and roles of the urinalysis laboratory in the diagnosis of the following amino acid disorders:
    • Cystinuria and cystinosis
    • Homogentisic acid (alkaptonuria)
    • Maple syrup urine disease
    • Phenylketonuria
    • Tyrosinuria and melanuria
13. Describe briefly the physiologic mechanisms, clinical features, and typical urinalysis findings in the following carbohydrate disorders:
    • Glucosuria
    • Diabetes mellitus
    • Galactosuria
14. Describe briefly the physiologic mechanisms, clinical features, and typical urinalysis findings in the following metabolic disorders:
    • Diabetes insipidus
    • Porphyrin disorders

CHAPTER OUTLINE

Renal Diseases
  Glomerular Disease
  Tubular Disease
  Tubulointerstitial Disease and
  Urinary Tract Infections

Vascular Disease
Acute and Chronic Renal Failure
Calculi
Metabolic Diseases
  Amino Acid Disorders

Carbohydrate Disorders
Diabetes Insipidus
Porphyrias

KEY TERMS

acute interstitial nephritis An acute inflammatory process that develops 3 to 21 days following exposure to an immunogenic drug (e.g., sulfonamides, penicillins) and results in injury to the renal tubules and interstitium. The condition is characterized by fever, skin rash, leukocyturia (particularly eosinophiluria), and acute renal failure. Discontinuation of the offending agent can result in full recovery of renal function.

acute poststreptococcal glomerulonephritis A type of glomerular inflammation that occurs 1 to 2 weeks after a group A β-hemolytic streptococcal infection. Onset is sudden, and the glomerular damage is immune mediated.

acute pyelonephritis An inflammatory process involving the renal tubules, interstitium, and renal pelvis. The condition is caused most often by a bacterial infection and is characterized by the sudden onset of symptoms (i.e., flank pain, dysuria, frequency of micturition, and urinary urgency).

acute renal failure (ARF) A renal disorder characterized by a sudden decrease in the glomerular filtration rate that results in azotemia and oliguria. It is a consequence of numerous conditions that can be categorized as prerenal (e.g., decrease in renal blood flow), renal (e.g., acute tubular necrosis), or postrenal (e.g., urinary tract obstruction). The disease course varies greatly, and survivors usually regain normal renal function.

acute tubular necrosis (ATN) A group of renal diseases characterized by destruction of renal tubular epithelium. Acute tubular necrosis is classified into two types based on initiating event and the epithelium predominantly involved. Ischemic ATN is caused by decreased renal perfusion and results in increased sloughing of primarily renal collecting duct cells. Toxic ATN results from nephrotoxic substances (drugs, chemicals) and is characterized by increased sloughing of primarily convoluted tubular cells.

alkaptonuria A rare recessively inherited disease caused by a deficiency of the enzyme homogentisic acid oxidase. This disorder is characterized by the excretion of large amounts of homogentisic acid (i.e., alcapton bodies).

aminoaciduria The presence of increased quantities of amino acids in the urine.

amyloidosis A group of systemic diseases characterized by deposition of amyloid, a proteinaceous substance, between cells in numerous tissues and organs.

calculi (also called *stones*) Solid aggregates or concretions of chemicals, usually mineral salts, that form in secreting glands of the body.

chronic glomerulonephritis A slowly progressive glomerular disease that develops years after other forms of glomerulonephritis. The condition usually leads to irreversible renal failure, requiring renal dialysis or kidney transplantation.

chronic pyelonephritis A renal inflammatory process involving the tubules, interstitium, renal calyces, and renal pelves, most often caused by reflux nephropathies that lead to chronic bacterial infections of the upper urinary tract. This chronic inflammation results in fibrosis and scarring of the kidney and eventually in loss of renal function.

chronic renal failure A renal disorder characterized by progressive loss of renal function caused by an irreversible, intrinsic renal disease. The glomerular filtration rate decreases progressively. Chronic renal failure concludes with end-stage renal disease, characterized by isosthenuria, significant proteinuria, variable hematuria, and numerous casts of all types, particularly waxy and broad casts.

cystinosis An autosomal recessive inherited disorder characterized by intracellular deposition of the amino acid cystine in all cells throughout the body. Cystine deposition within renal tubular cells results in renal dysfunction (Fanconi's syndrome) and eventually in renal failure.

cystinuria An autosomal recessive inherited disorder characterized by an inability to reabsorb the amino acids cystine, arginine, lysine, and ornithine in the renal tubules and in the intestine. This results in the loss of cystine and the other dibasic amino acids in the urine, despite normal cellular metabolism of cystine. Because cystine is insoluble at an acid pH, it can precipitate in the renal tubules to cause calculi formation, or the crystals can be observed in urine sediment. Note that all other dibasic amino acids are soluble in an acid pH, and their presence in urine goes undetected unless sensitive amino acid methods are used.

diabetes insipidus A metabolic disease caused by defective antidiuretic hormone production (neurogenic) or lack of renal tubular response to antidiuretic hormone (nephrogenic). It is characterized by polyuria and polydipsia.

diabetes mellitus A metabolic disease characterized by an inability to metabolize glucose, resulting in hyperglycemia, glucosuria, and alterations in fat and protein metabolism. Diabetes mellitus develops when (1) insulin production, (2) insulin action, or (3) both are defective. The disease is classified as type 1 or type 2, depending on age of onset, initial presentation, insulin requirements, and other factors.

Fanconi syndrome A renal disorder characterized by generalized proximal tubular dysfunction resulting in aminoaciduria, proteinuria, glucosuria, and phosphaturia. It is a complication of inherited and acquired diseases.

focal proliferative glomerulonephritis A type of glomerular inflammation characterized by cellular proliferation in a specific part of the glomeruli (segmental) and limited to a specific number of glomeruli (focal).

focal segmental glomerulosclerosis A type of glomerular disease characterized by sclerosis of the glomeruli. Not all glomeruli are affected, hence the term *focal*, and of those that are, only certain portions become diseased, hence the term *segmental*.

galactosuria The presence of galactose in urine.

glomerulonephritides (plural) or glomerulonephritis (singular) Nephritic conditions characterized by damage to and inflammation of the glomeruli. Causes are varied and include immunologic, metabolic, and hereditary disorders.

IgA nephropathy A type of glomerular inflammation characterized by the deposition of immunoglobulin A in the glomerular mesangium. The condition often occurs 1 to 2 days following a mucosal infection of the respiratory, gastrointestinal, or urinary tract.

maple syrup urine disease (MSUD) A rare autosomal recessive inherited defect or deficiency in the enzyme responsible for the oxidation of the branched-chain amino acids leucine, isoleucine, and valine. As a result, these amino acids along with their corresponding α-keto acids accumulate in the blood, cerebrospinal fluid, and urine. The name derives from the subtle maple syrup odor of the urine from these patients.

melanuria Increased excretion of melanin in urine.

membranoproliferative glomerulonephritis A type of glomerular inflammation characterized by cellular proliferation of the mesangium, with leukocyte infiltration and thickening of the glomerular basement membrane. Immunologically based, the disease is slowly progressive.

membranous glomerulonephritis A type of glomerular inflammation characterized by deposition of immunoglobulins and complement along the epithelial side (podocytes) of the basement membrane. The condition is associated with numerous immune-mediated diseases and is the major cause of nephrotic syndrome in adults.

minimal change disease A type of glomerular inflammation characterized by loss of the podocyte foot processes. An immune-mediated condition that is the major cause of nephrotic syndrome in children.

nephritic syndrome A group of clinical findings indicative of glomerular damage that include hematuria, proteinuria, azotemia, edema, hypertension, and oliguria. Severity and combinations of features vary with the glomerular disease.

nephrotic syndrome A collection of clinical findings indicating adverse glomerular changes. It is characterized by proteinuria, hypoalbuminemia, hyperlipidemia, lipiduria, and generalized edema. A nonspecific disorder associated with renal as well as systemic diseases.

phenylketonuria An autosomal recessive inherited enzyme defect or deficiency characterized by an inability to convert phenylalanine to tyrosine. Consequently, phenylalanine is converted to phenylketones, which are excreted in the urine.

porphyria Increased production of porphyrin precursors or porphyrins.

rapidly progressive glomerulonephritis (RPGN; also called *crescentic glomerulonephritis*) A type of glomerular inflammation characterized by cellular proliferation into Bowman's space to form "crescents." Numerous disease processes, including systemic lupus erythematosus, vasculitis, and infection, can lead to its development.

renal phosphaturia A rare hereditary disease characterized by an inability of the distal tubules to reabsorb inorganic phosphorus.

renal tubular acidosis A renal disorder characterized by an inability of renal tubules to secrete adequate hydrogen ions. Four types are recognized, and they can be inherited or acquired. Patients are unable to produce an acidic urine, regardless of their acid-base status.

rhabdomyolysis The breakdown or destruction of skeletal muscle cells.

systemic lupus erythematosus An autoimmune disorder that affects numerous organ systems and is characterized by autoantibodies. The disease is chronic and frequently insidious, often causes fever, and involves varied neurologic, hematologic, and immunologic abnormalities. Renal involvement, as well as pleuritis and pericarditis, is common. The clinical presentation varies greatly and is associated with a constellation of symptoms such as joint pain, skin lesions, leukopenia, hypergammaglobulinemia, antinuclear antibodies, and LE cells.

tyrosinuria The presence of the amino acid tyrosine in urine.

yeast infection An inflammatory condition that results from the proliferation of a fungus, most commonly *Candida* species.

For centuries, the study of urine has been used to obtain information about the health status of the body. From the time of Hippocrates (5th century BCE) to the present, the diagnosis of renal diseases and many metabolic diseases has been aided by the performance of a routine urinalysis. Because the onset of disease can be asymptomatic, a urinalysis may often detect abnormalities before a patient exhibits any clinical manifestations. In addition, urinalysis provides a means of monitoring disease progression and the effectiveness of treatments. This chapter discusses the clinical features of renal and metabolic diseases and the typical urinalysis results associated with them. Because extensive coverage of these diseases is beyond the scope of this text, the reader should see the bibliography for additional resources.

RENAL DISEASES

Diseases of the kidney are often classified into four types based on the morphologic component initially affected: glomerular, tubular, interstitial, or vascular. Initially, renal disease may affect only one morphologic component; however, with disease progression, other components are involved because of their close structural and functional interdependence. Susceptibility to disease varies with each structural component. Glomerular diseases most often are immune-mediated, whereas tubular and interstitial diseases result from infectious or toxic substances. In contrast, vascular diseases cause a reduction in renal perfusion that subsequently induces both morphologic and functional changes in the kidney.

Glomerular Disease

Diseases that damage glomeruli are varied and include immunologic, metabolic, and hereditary disorders (Box 9-1). Systemic disorders are technically *secondary* glomerular diseases because they initially and principally involve other organs; the glomeruli become involved as a consequence as the systemic disease progresses. In contrast, primary glomerular diseases specifically affect the kidney, which is often the only organ involved. *Primary* glomerular disorders, collectively called **glomerulonephritides**, consist of several different types of **glomerulonephritis**.

Morphologic Changes in the Glomerulus. Four distinct morphologic changes of glomeruli are recognized: cellular proliferation, leukocytic infiltration, glomerular basement membrane thickening, and hyalinization with sclerosis. One or more of these changes accompany each type of glomerulonephritis and form the basis for characterizing glomerular diseases.

In the glomerular tuft, cellular proliferation is characterized by increased numbers of endothelial cells (capillary endothelium), mesangial cells, and epithelial cells (podocytes). This proliferation may be segmental, involving only a part of each glomerulus. At the same time, proliferation can be focal, involving only a certain number of glomeruli, or diffuse, involving all glomeruli.

Drawn by a local chemotactic response, leukocytes, particularly neutrophils and macrophages, can readily infiltrate glomeruli. Present in some types of acute glomerulonephritis, leukocyte infiltration may also be accompanied by cellular proliferation.

Glomerular basement membrane thickening includes any process that results in enlargement of the basement membrane. Most commonly, thickening results from the deposition of precipitated proteins (e.g., immune complexes, fibrin) on either side of or within the basement membrane. However, in diabetic glomerulosclerosis, the basement membrane thickens without evidence of deposition of any material.

Hyalinization of glomeruli is characterized by the accumulation of a homogeneous, eosinophilic extracellular material in the glomeruli. As this amorphous substance accumulates, glomeruli lose their structural detail and become sclerotic. Various glomerular diseases lead to these irreversible changes.

Pathogenesis of Glomerular Damage. The primary mode of glomerular injury results from immune-mediated processes. Circulating antigen-antibody complexes and complexes that result from antigen-antibody reactions that occur within the glomerulus (i.e., in situ) play a role in glomerular damage.

Circulating immune complexes are created in response to endogenous (e.g., tumor antigens, thyroglobulin) or exogenous (e.g., viruses, parasites) antigens. These circulating immune complexes become trapped within the glomeruli. The antibodies associated with them have no specificity for the glomeruli; rather they are present in the glomeruli because of glomerular hemodynamic characteristics and physicochemical factors (e.g., molecular charge, shape, size). The result is that the immune complexes become entrapped in the glomeruli and bind complement, which subsequently causes glomerular injury.

A second immune mechanism involves antibodies that react directly with glomerular tissue antigens (e.g., anti–glomerular basement membrane disease) or with

---

BOX 9-1 | Glomerular Diseases

Primary Glomerular Diseases
- Acute glomerulonephritis
  - Poststreptococcal
  - Non-poststreptococcal
- Crescentic glomerulonephritis
- Membranous glomerulonephritis
- Minimal change disease (lipoid nephrosis)
- Focal glomerulosclerosis
- Membranoproliferative glomerulonephritis
- IgA nephropathy
- Focal glomerulonephritis
- Chronic glomerulonephritis

Secondary Glomerular Diseases
Systemic Diseases
- Diabetes mellitus
- Systemic lupus erythematosus
- Amyloidosis
- Vasculitis, such as polyarteritis nodosa
- Bacterial endocarditis

Hereditary Disorders
- Alport's syndrome
- Fabry's disease

nonglomerular antigens that currently reside in the glomeruli. These latter nonglomerular antigens can originate from a variety of sources such as drugs and infectious agents (i.e., viral, bacterial, parasitic). Because immune complexes, immunoglobulins, and complement retain reactive sites even after their deposition, their presence in the glomeruli actually induces further immune complexation.

Glomerular injury does not result from the immune complexes but rather from the chemical mediators and toxic substances that they induce. Complement, neutrophils, monocytes, platelets, and other factors at the site produce proteases, oxygen-derived free radicals, and arachidonic acid metabolites. These substances, along with others, stimulate a local inflammatory response that further induces glomerular tissue damage. The coagulation system also plays a role, with fibrin frequently present in these diseased glomeruli. Fibrinogen that has leaked into Bowman's space also induces cellular proliferation.

Clinical Features of Glomerular Diseases. Glomerular damage produces characteristic clinical features or a syndrome—a group of symptoms or findings that occur together. These nephritic syndromes occur with primary glomerular diseases, as well as in patients with glomerular injury due to a systemic disease (Box 9-1). It becomes the clinician's task to differentiate between these conditions, identify the specific disease processes, and determine appropriate treatment.

The features that characterize glomerular damage (i.e., nephritic syndrome) include hematuria, proteinuria, oliguria, azotemia, edema, and hypertension (see Table 9-1). The severity of each feature and the combination present vary depending on the number of glomeruli involved, the mechanism of injury, and the rapidity of disease onset. A classic example of a condition characterized by all the features of a **nephritic syndrome** is acute poststreptococcal glomerulonephritis. In contrast, some forms of glomerulonephritis are asymptomatic and are detected only when routine screening reveals microscopic hematuria or subnephrotic proteinuria (e.g., membranoproliferative glomerulonephritis, **focal proliferative glomerulonephritis**). Another syndrome that is a frequent manifestation of glomerular diseases is the *nephrotic syndrome* (see next section). Glomerular diseases that manifest the nephritic or nephrotic syndrome have the potential to ultimately develop into chronic renal failure. When this occurs, 80% to 85% of the functioning ability of the kidney is gone. Table 9-2 presents selected glomerular diseases along with a summary of their typical urinalysis results.

Nephrotic Syndrome. The **nephrotic syndrome** is a group of clinical features that occur simultaneously. Representing increased permeability of the glomeruli to the passage of plasma proteins, most notably albumin, nephrotic syndrome is characterized by heavy proteinuria (3.5 g/day or more). Additional features include hypoproteinemia, hyperlipidemia, lipiduria, and edema. Plasma albumin levels are usually less than 3 g/dL because liver synthesis is unable to compensate for the large amounts of protein being excreted in the urine. Albumin is the predominant protein lost because of its high plasma concentration. However, proteins of equal or smaller size, such as immunoglobulins,

TABLE 9-1	Syndromes That Indicate Glomerular Injury	
Syndrome	**Clinical Features**	
Asymptomatic hematuria or proteinuria	Variable hematuria, subnephrotic proteinuria	
Acute nephritic syndrome	Hematuria, proteinuria, oliguria, azotemia, edema, hypertension	
Nephrotic syndrome	Proteinuria (>3 g/day), lipiduria, hypoproteinemia, hyperlipidemia, edema	

TABLE 9-2	Typical Urinalysis Findings With Selected Glomerular Diseases	
Disease	**Physical and Chemical Examination**	**Microscopic Examination**
Acute glomerulonephritis	Protein: mild (<1.0 g/day), can reach nephrotic level (>3-3.5 g/day) Blood: positive (degree variable)	↑ RBCs, often dysmorphic ↑ WBCs ↑ Renal tubular epithelial cells ↑ Casts: RBC, hemoglobin casts (pathognomonic), granular; occasional WBC and renal cell casts
Chronic glomerulonephritis	Protein: heavy (>2.5 g/day) Blood: positive (usually small) Specific gravity: low and fixed	↑ RBCs ↑ WBCs ↑ Casts: all types, particularly granular, waxy, broad ↑ Renal epithelial cells
Nephrotic syndrome	Protein: severe (>3.5 g/day) Blood: positive (usually small)	Lipiduria: oval fat bodies, free fat globules ↑ Casts: all types, particularly fatty, waxy, renal cell casts ↑ Renal epithelial cells ↑ RBCs

↑, Increased; *RBC,* red blood cell; *WBC,* white blood cell.

low-molecular-weight complement components, and anticoagulant cofactors, are also excreted in increased amounts. As a result, patients with the nephrotic syndrome are more susceptible to infections and thrombotic complications.

Hyperlipidemia in the nephrotic syndrome is caused by increased plasma levels of triglycerides, cholesterol, phospholipids, and very-low-density lipoproteins. Whereas the exact mechanisms causing hyperlipidemia are still unknown, it is caused at least in part by increased synthesis of these lipids by the liver and is compounded by a decrease in their catabolism. Because of increased glomerular permeability, these lipids are able to cross the glomerular filtration barrier and appear in the urine. They may be present as free-floating fat globules, found within renal epithelial cells or macrophages (i.e., oval fat bodies), or encased in casts.

The generalized edema present with the nephrotic syndrome is characteristically soft and pitting (i.e., when the flesh is depressed, an indentation remains). Development of edema is due primarily to decreased excretion of sodium.[1] Whereas the exact mechanism is not clearly understood, it is due in part to increased reabsorption of sodium and water by the distal tubules. Loss of protein and its associated oncotic pressure from the blood plasma also results in the movement of fluid into interstitial tissues; however, its role is minor compared with that of sodium in the development of edema in these patients. Edema is usually apparent around the eyes (periorbital) and in the legs, but in severe cases, patients also develop pleural effusions and ascites.

Along with heavy proteinuria and lipiduria in these patients, urine microscopic examination often shows a mild microscopic hematuria. In addition, pathologic casts such as fatty, waxy, and renal tubular casts are often present (see Table 9-2).

Nephrotic syndrome occurs in patients with minimal change disease (lipoid nephrosis), membranous glomerulonephritis, focal segmental glomerulosclerosis, and membranoproliferative glomerulonephritis. These glomerular diseases account for about 90% of all nephrotic syndrome cases in children and about 75% of those in adults. Systemic diseases that can present with the nephrotic syndrome include diabetes mellitus, systemic lupus erythematosus, amyloidosis, malignant neoplasms, and infection, as well as renal responses to nephrotoxic agents (e.g., drugs, poisons).

Types of Glomerulonephritis. Each glomerulonephritis can be classified on the basis of its characteristic anatomic alterations to the glomeruli. These morphologic and immunologic changes are apparent in renal biopsy specimens by light microscopy or with the use of special stains (e.g., immunofluorescent stain) and other microscopy techniques (e.g., fluorescent microscopy, electron microscopy). The different types of glomerulonephritis are not disease specific. For example, a patient recovering from an infection can have glomerulonephritis of the crescentic type, typical acute glomerulonephritis, or minimal change disease. In addition, although initial presentation may be of one type, the disease can progress into that of another. A classic example is the eventual development of chronic glomerulonephritis in 90% of patients with crescentic or rapidly progressive glomerulonephritis. Table 9-3 summarizes the predominant forms of primary glomerulonephritides discussed in this section.

Acute Glomerulonephritis. One cause of acute glomerulonephritis (AGN) is a streptococcal infection, and it is specifically known as **acute poststreptococcal glomerulonephritis.** It is a common glomerular disease that occurs 1 to 2 weeks after a streptococcal infection of the throat or skin. Although the disease appears most often in children, AGN can affect individuals at any age. Only certain strains of group A β-hemolytic streptococci—those with M protein in their cell walls—induce this nephritis. The time delay between streptococcal infection and the clinical presentation of AGN actually correlates with the time required for antibody formation.

Morphologically, all glomeruli show cellular proliferation of the mesangium and endothelium, as well as leukocytic infiltration. Swelling of the interstitium caused by edema and inflammation obstructs capillaries and tubules. As a result, fibrin forms in the capillary lumina, and red blood cell casts form in the tubules. In addition, deposits of immune complexes, complement, and fibrin can be shown in the mesangium and along the basement membrane with the use of special staining and microscopy techniques.

Typically, the onset of AGN is sudden and includes fever, malaise, nausea, oliguria, hematuria, and proteinuria. Edema may be present, often around the eyes (periorbital), knees, or ankles, and hypertension is usually mild to moderate. Because this disease is immune mediated, any blood or urine cultures for infectious agents are negative. Blood tests reveal an elevated antistreptolysin O titer, a decrease in serum complement, and the presence of cryoglobulins. In addition, the creatinine clearance is decreased, and the ratio of blood urea nitrogen to creatinine is increased. Serum albumin levels can be normal; however, if large amounts of protein are lost in the urine, these levels are decreased.

More than 95% of children who develop acute poststreptococcal glomerulonephritis recover spontaneously or with minimal therapy. In contrast, only about 60% of adults recover rapidly; the remaining affected adults recover more slowly with a subset ultimately developing chronic glomerulonephritis.

Although rare, AGN caused by nonstreptococcal agents has been reported. It has been associated with other bacteria (e.g., pneumococci), viruses (e.g., mumps, hepatitis B), and parasitic infection (e.g., malaria). Note that the clinical features of AGN are the same, regardless of which agent is causing the immune complex formation that induces the disorder.

TABLE 9-3	Summary of Predominant Forms of Primary Glomerulonephritis		
Disease	**Typical Outlook Solution**	**Pathogenesis**	**Glomerular Changes**
Acute glomerulonephritis (AGN), poststreptococcal	Acute nephritic syndrome	Antibody mediated	Cellular proliferation (diffuse); leukocytic infiltration; interstitial swelling
Rapidly progressive glomerulonephritis (RPGN)	Acute nephritic syndrome	Antibody mediated; often anti-GBM	Cellular proliferation to form characteristic "crescents"; leukocytic infiltration; fibrin deposition; GBM disruptions
Membranous glomerulonephritis (MGN)	Nephrotic syndrome	Antibody mediated	Basement membrane thickening because of immunoglobulin (Ig) and complement (C) deposits; loss of foot processes (diffuse)
Minimal change disease (MCD)	Nephrotic syndrome	T cell immunity dysfunction; loss of glomerular polyanions	Loss of foot processes
Focal segmental glomerulosclerosis (FSGS)	Proteinuria variable; subnephrotic to nephrotic	Unknown; possibly a circulating systemic factor; can reoccur after kidney transplant	Sclerotic glomeruli with hyaline and lipid deposits (focal and segmental); diffuse loss of foot processes; focal IgM and C3 deposits
Membranoproliferative glomerulonephritis (MPGN)	Depends on type: nephrotic syndrome or hematuria or proteinuria	Immune complex or complement activation	Cellular proliferation (mesangium); leukocytic infiltration; IgG and complement deposits
IgA nephropathy	Recurrent hematuria and proteinuria	IgA mediated; complement activation	Deposition of IgA in mesangium; variable cellular proliferation
Chronic glomerulonephritis	Chronic renal failure	Variable	Hyalinized glomeruli

GBM, Glomerular basement membrane; *Ig,* immunoglobulin.

Rapidly Progressive Glomerulonephritis. **Rapidly progressive glomerulonephritis** (RPGN) is also termed *crescentic glomerulonephritis.* It is characterized by cellular proliferation in Bowman's space to form crescents, from which its initial name was derived. These cellular crescents within the glomerular tuft cause pressure changes and can even occlude the entrance to the proximal tubule. Infiltration with leukocytes and fibrin deposition within these crescents are also characteristic of this type of glomerulonephritis. As a result of these degenerative glomerular changes, characteristic wrinkling and disruptions in the glomerular basement membrane are evident by electron microscopy.

RPGN develops (1) following an infection, (2) as a result of a systemic disease, such as systemic lupus erythematosus or vasculitis, or (3) idiopathically (usually following a flulike episode). Hematuria is present, and the level of proteinuria varies. Edema or hypertension may or may not be present. Although an antibody to the basement membrane can be demonstrated in most patients, others may show few or no immune deposits in the glomeruli. This fact supports the theory of multiple pathways leading to severe glomerular damage. Regardless of therapy, 90% of patients with RPGN eventually develop chronic glomerulonephritis and require long-term renal dialysis or kidney transplantation.

Membranous Glomerulonephritis. The deposition of immunoglobulins and complement along the epithelial (podocytes) side of the basement membrane characterizes **membranous glomerulonephritis** (MGN). With time, the basement membrane thickens, enclosing the embedded immune deposits and causing loss of the foot processes. Eventually, thickening of the basement membrane severely reduces the capillary lumen, causing glomerular hyalinization and sclerosis. No cellular proliferation or leukocytic infiltration is evident.

MGN is the major cause of the nephrotic syndrome in adults. Complement activation (specifically the action of C5b-9, the membrane attack complex of complement) is responsible for the glomerular damage that results in leakage of large amounts of protein into the renal tubules.

In approximately 85% of patients, MGN is idiopathic. In remaining patients, MGN is associated with immune-mediated disease. The antigens implicated can be exogenous *(Treponema)* or endogenous (thyroglobulin, DNA), and many antigens remain unknown. MGN frequently occurs secondary to other conditions, such as systemic lupus erythematosus, diabetes mellitus, or thyroiditis, or following exposure to metals (e.g., gold, mercury) or drugs (e.g., penicillamine).

The typical clinical presentation of MGN is sudden onset of the nephrotic syndrome. Hematuria and mild hypertension may be present. The clinical course varies, with no resolution of proteinuria in up to 90% of patients. Although this may take many years, eventually 50% of patients with MGN progress to chronic glomerulonephritis. Only 10% to 30% of patients with MGN show complete or partial recovery.

Minimal Change Disease. **Minimal change disease** (MCD) is characterized by glomeruli that look normal by light microscopy; however, electron microscopy reveals the loss of podocyte foot processes. These foot processes are replaced by a simplified structure, and their cytoplasm shows vacuolization. No leukocyte infiltration or cellular proliferation is present.

Despite the absence of any immunoglobulin or complement deposits, MCD is believed to be immunologically based, involving a dysfunction of T cell immunity. Various factors support this theory; the most notable factor is the onset of MCD following infection or immunization and its rapid response to corticosteroid therapy. T cell dysfunction causes loss of the glomerular "shield of negativity" or polyanions (e.g., heparan sulfate proteoglycan). Remember, albumin can pass readily through the glomerular filtration barrier if the negative charge is removed; hence MCD is characterized by the nephrotic syndrome (i.e., massive proteinuria).

In children, MCD is responsible for most cases of the nephrotic syndrome. Usually, no hypertension or hematuria is associated with it. Clinically, differentiation of MCD from MGN is based on the dramatic response of MCD to corticosteroid therapy. Although patients may become steroid dependent to keep the disease in check, the prognosis for recovery is excellent for children and adults.

Focal Segmental Glomerulosclerosis.
Focal segmental glomerulosclerosis (FSGS) is characterized by *sclerosis* of glomeruli. The process is both focal (occurring in some glomeruli) and segmental (affecting a specific area of the glomerulus). Morphologically, sclerotic glomeruli show hyaline and lipid deposition, collapsed basement membranes, and proliferation of the mesangium. FSGS is characterized most by diffuse damage to the glomerular epithelium (podocytes). Although not readily apparent by light microscopy, electron microscopy reveals the diffuse loss of foot processes in both sclerotic and nonsclerotic glomeruli. Glomerular hyalinization and sclerosis result from the mesangial response to the accumulation of plasma proteins and fibrin deposits. In addition, immunoglobulin (Ig)M and C3 are evident by immunofluorescence in these sclerotic areas.

FSGS can occur (1) as a primary glomerular disease, (2) in association with another glomerular disease, such as IgA nephropathy, or (3) secondary to other disorders. Heroin abuse, acquired immunodeficiency syndrome (AIDS), reflux nephropathy, and analgesic abuse nephropathy are some conditions that can precede FSGS.

Proteinuria is a predominant feature of FSGS. In 10% to 15% of patients, it initially presents as the nephrotic syndrome. The remaining patients exhibit moderate to heavy proteinuria. Hematuria, reduced glomerular filtration rate (GFR), and hypertension can also be present. Patients with FSGS usually have little or no response to corticosteroid therapy, which helps to differentiate this disorder from MCD. Many patients develop chronic

glomerulonephritis at variable rates. An interesting note is that FSGS can recur following renal transplantation (25% to 50%), sometimes within days, suggesting a circulating systemic factor as the causative agent.

Membranoproliferative Glomerulonephritis.
Membranoproliferative glomerulonephritis (MPGN) is characterized by cellular proliferation, particularly of the mesangium, along with leukocyte infiltration and thickening of the glomerular basement membrane. As a result of the increased numbers of mesangial cells, the glomeruli take on a microscopically visible lobular appearance. Ultrastructural characteristics subdivide MPGN into two types, types I and II.

Most cases of MPGN are immune mediated with the formation of immune complexes in the glomeruli or the deposition of complement in the glomeruli followed by its activation.

MPGN is a slow, progressive disease, with 50% of patients eventually developing chronic renal failure. MPGN has a varied presentation pattern with some patients showing only hematuria or subnephrotic proteinuria (less than 3 to 3.5 g/day), whereas it accounts for 5% to 10% of patients who present with the nephrotic syndrome. MPGN is similar to FSGS in that it also has an unusually high incidence of recurrence following renal transplant.

IgA Nephropathy.
The deposition of IgA in the glomerular mesangium characterizes **IgA nephropathy,** one of the most prevalent types of glomerulonephritis worldwide. However, IgA deposits are detectable only with the use of special stains and microscopy techniques (e.g., immunofluorescence). Apparently, circulating IgA complexes or aggregates become trapped and engulfed by mesangial cells. Aggregated IgA is known to be capable of activating the alternative complement pathway, resulting in glomerular damage. Morphologically, the glomerular lesions are varied. Some may appear normal, whereas others may show evidence of focal or diffuse cellular proliferation.

A common finding is recurrent hematuria in a range from gross to microscopic amounts. Proteinuria is usually present, varying in degree from mild to severe. IgA nephropathy often occurs 1 to 2 days following a mucosal infection of the respiratory, gastrointestinal, or urinary tract from infectious agents (e.g., bacteria, viruses) that stimulate mucosal IgA synthesis. As a result, serum IgA levels are frequently elevated, and circulating IgA immune complexes are present in these patients.

IgA nephropathy primarily affects children and young adults. The disease is slow and progressive, eventually causing chronic renal failure in 50% of patients. When disease onset occurs in old age or is associated with severe proteinuria and hypertension, renal failure develops more quickly.

Chronic Glomerulonephritis.
In time, numerous glomerular diseases result in the development of **chronic glomerulonephritis.** Morphologically, the glomeruli

TABLE 9-4	Percentage of Glomerular Diseases Resulting in Chronic Glomerulonephritis	
Disease		**Approximate Percentage**
Rapidly progressive glomerulonephritis (RPGN)		90%
Focal glomerulosclerosis (FSGS)		50%–80%
Membranous glomerulonephritis (MGN)		50%
Membranoproliferative glomerulonephritis (MPGN)		50%
IgA nephropathy		30%–50%
Poststreptococcal glomerulonephritis		1%–2%

Ig, Immunoglobulin.

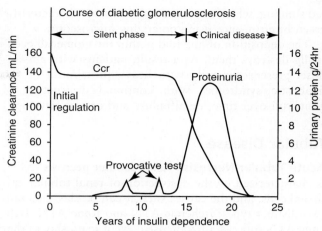

FIGURE 9-1 A composite drawing showing the course of diabetic nephropathy. Exercise and other stress cause intermittent proteinuria before a sustained protein leak, which may lead to nephrotic syndrome. Initial regulation indicates initiation of insulin therapy. *(From Friedman EA, Shieh SD: Clinical management of diabetic nephropathy. In Friedman EA, L'Esperance FA, editors: Diabetic renal-retinal syndrome, New York, 1980, Grune-Stratton. [Used with permission.])*

become hyalinized, appearing as acellular eosinophilic masses. In addition, the renal tubules are atrophied, fibrosis is evident in the renal interstitium, and lymphocytic infiltration may be present.

About 80% of patients who develop chronic glomerulonephritis have previously had some form of glomerulonephritis (Table 9-4). The remaining 20% of cases represent forms of glomerulonephritis that were unrecognized or subclinical in their presentation.

The development of chronic glomerulonephritis is slow and silent, taking many years to progress. Some patients may present only with edema, which leads to the discovery of an underlying renal disease. Occasionally, hypertension and cerebral or cardiovascular conditions manifest first clinically. Other clinical findings associated with chronic glomerulonephritis include proteinuria, hypertension, and azotemia. Death resulting from uremia and pathologic changes in other organs (e.g., uremic pericarditis, uremic gastroenteritis) occurs if patients are not maintained on dialysis or do not undergo renal transplantation.

Systemic Diseases and Glomerular Damage. Systemic lupus erythematosus (SLE), a systemic autoimmune disorder, presents with a constellation of lesions and clinical manifestations. Almost all patients with SLE show some type of kidney involvement. The pathogenesis of glomerular damage involves the deposition of immune complexes (specifically anti-DNA complexes) and complement activation. Five morphologic patterns of lupus nephritis are recognized; however, none of them is diagnostic or unique to SLE. In other words, patients with SLE may exhibit any of the clinical glomerular syndromes (see Table 9-1): recurrent hematuria, acute nephritic syndrome, or the nephrotic syndrome. An important note is that chronic renal failure is a leading cause of death in these patients.

Diabetes mellitus is another systemic disorder that frequently results in kidney disease. The most common renal conditions in diabetic patients present as a glomerular syndrome. However, other renal diseases occur and include vascular lesions of the renal arterioles, which

are associated with hypertension, as well as enhanced susceptibility to pyelonephritis and papillary necrosis. Consequently, renal disease is a major cause of death in the diabetic population.

Thickening of the glomerular basement membrane is evident by electron microscopy in all diabetic patients. Proteinuria eventually develops in up to 55% of diabetic patients and can range from subnephrotic to nephrotic levels. Within 10 to 20 years of disease onset, pronounced cellular proliferation of the glomerular mesangium eventually results in glomerulosclerosis (Figure 9-1). Chronic renal failure usually develops within 4 to 5 years following the onset of persistent proteinuria and requires long-term renal dialysis or transplantation.

The development of diabetic glomerulosclerosis occurs more often with type 1 diabetes mellitus than with type 2. The Diabetes Control and Complications Trial demonstrated that blood glucose control significantly influences the development of microvascular complications in subjects with type 1 diabetes.[2] A similar correlation was demonstrated in individuals with type 2 diabetes during the United Kingdom Prospective Diabetes Study.[3] Therefore the same or similar underlying mechanisms of disease likely apply, and any improvement in blood glucose control can prevent the development and progression of diabetic nephropathy.

Amyloidosis is a group of systemic diseases that involve many organs and is characterized by the deposition of amyloid, a pathologic proteinaceous substance, between cells in numerous tissues and organs. Amyloid is made up of about 90% fibril protein and 10% glycoprotein. Microscopically in tissue, amyloid initially appears as an eosinophilic hyaline substance. It is differentiated from hyaline (e.g., collagen, fibrin) by Congo red staining, which imparts amyloid with a characteristic green birefringence using polarizing microscopy.

The deposition of amyloid within the glomeruli eventually destroys them. As a result, patients with amyloidosis present clinically with heavy proteinuria or the nephrotic syndrome. With continual destruction of glomeruli over time, renal failure and uremia develop.

Tubular Disease

Acute Tubular Necrosis.
Acute tubular necrosis (ATN) is characterized by the destruction of renal tubular epithelial cells, and the causes vary. It can be classified into two distinct types: ischemic ATN and toxic ATN. Ischemic ATN follows a hypotensive event (e.g., shock) that results in decreased perfusion of the kidneys followed by renal tissue ischemia. In contrast, toxic ATN results from exposure to nephrotoxic agents that have been ingested, injected, absorbed, or inhaled. The tubular damage that results from either type of ATN can be reversed once the initiating event or agent has been identified and addressed. An interesting note is that approximately 50% of all cases of ATN result from surgical procedures.[4]

The three principal causes of *ischemic ATN* are sepsis, shock, and trauma. However, any obstruction to renal blood flow or occlusion of renal arteries or arterioles can result in the hypoperfusion of renal tissue and ischemia. Examples of sepsis and shock include extensive bacterial infections and severe burns; examples of trauma include crush injuries and numerous surgical procedures.

Toxic ATN is caused by a variety of agents that can be separated into two categories: endogenous and exogenous nephrotoxins. The tubular necrosis induced by these nephrotoxins can cause oliguria and acute renal failure. Endogenous nephrotoxins are normal solutes or substances that become toxic when their concentration in the bloodstream is excessive. They are primarily hemoglobin and myoglobin and to a lesser degree uric acid and immunoglobulin light chains. Renal injury is due to a combination of factors, including volume depletion, renal vasoconstriction (ischemia), direct heme-protein–mediated cytotoxicity, and cast formation.[5,6] Myoglobin and hemoglobin are two heme-containing proteins that are known to be toxic to renal tubules. Myoglobinuria results from **rhabdomyolysis**—the breakdown or destruction of skeletal muscle cells. It can occur as the result of traumatic muscle injury (e.g., crush injuries, surgery) or following nontraumatic muscle damage that occurs with excessive immobilization (due to intoxication or seizure), ischemia, inflammatory myopathies, heat stroke, or drugs. In contrast, hemoglobinuria follows severe hemolytic events in which haptoglobin—the plasma protein that normally binds free hemoglobin to prevent its loss in the urine—has been depleted, and free hemoglobin readily passes the glomerular filtration barrier into the tubules.

Exogenous nephrotoxins—substances ingested or absorbed—include numerous therapeutic agents (aminoglycosides, cephalosporins, amphotericin B, indinavir, acyclovir, foscarnet), anesthetics (enflurane, methoxyflurane), radiographic contrast media, chemotherapeutic drugs (cyclosporine), recreational drugs (heroin, cocaine), and industrial chemicals such as heavy metals (mercury, lead), organic solvents (carbon tetrachloride, ethylene glycol), and other poisons (mushrooms, pesticides).

Morphologically, ischemic ATN affects short segments (i.e., focal) of the tubules in random areas throughout the nephron, from the medullary segments of the proximal tubules and ascending loops of Henle to the collecting tubules. The tubular basement membrane is often disrupted (i.e., tubulorrhexis) as a result of complete necrosis of the tubular cells; consequently, the renal interstitium is exposed to the tubular lumen. As a result, renal cell fragments are sloughed into the urine. These cell fragments consist of three or more tubular cells shed intact and usually originate in the collecting duct (see Figure 8-30). In contrast, toxic ATN causes tubular necrosis primarily in the proximal tubules and usually does not involve their basement membranes. Convoluted renal tubular epithelial cells are found in the urine sediment; the presence of these distinctively large proximal tubular epithelial cells indicates toxic ATN (see Figure 8-28). In addition to tubular cell death, nephrotoxins in high concentrations often cause renal vasoconstriction. Because of this, patients may have characteristics associated with ischemic ATN. Both types of ATN show cast formation within the distal convoluted and collecting tubules. Compared with toxic ATN, however, ischemic ATN shows an increased number and variety of casts in the urine sediment, including granular, renal tubular cell, waxy, and broad casts.

The clinical presentation of ATN often is divided into three phases: onset, renal failure, and recovery. The onset of ATN may be abrupt following a hypotensive episode or deceptively subtle in a previously healthy individual following exposure to a toxin or administration of a nephrotoxic drug. This variable presentation develops into a renal failure phase with azotemia, hyperkalemia, and metabolic acidosis. At this time, approximately 50% of patients have a reduction in urine output to less than 400 mL/day (oliguria). The recovery phase is indicated by a steady increase in urine output; levels may reach 3 L/day. This diuretic state is exhibited by oliguric and nonoliguric patients and is explained best by the return to normal GFR before full recovery of the damaged tubular epithelium. This increased diuresis results in the loss of large amounts of water, sodium, and potassium until tubular function returns and the azotemia resolves. It takes about 6 months for full renal tubular function and concentrating ability to return.

Tubular Dysfunction.
Renal tubular dysfunction may result from a primary renal disease or may be induced secondarily. The dysfunction may involve a single

TABLE 9-5	Proximal Tubular Dysfunctions
Dysfunction	**Disease**
Single Defect in Proximal Tubular Function	
Impaired ability to reabsorb glucose	Renal glucosuria
Impaired ability to reabsorb specific amino acids	Cystinuria (cystine and dibasic amino acids)
	Hartnup disease (monoamino-monocarboxylic amino acids)
Impaired ability to reabsorb sodium	Bartter's syndrome
Impaired ability to reabsorb bicarbonate	Renal tubular acidosis type II
Impaired ability to reabsorb calcium	Idiopathic hypercalciuria
Excessive reabsorption of calcium	Hypocalciuric familial hypercalcemia
Excessive reabsorption of sodium	Gordon's syndrome
Excessive reabsorption of phosphate	Pseudohypoparathyroidism
Multiple Defects in Proximal Tubular Function	
Inherited Diseases	Cystinosis
	Tyrosinemia
	Wilson's disease
	Galactosemia
	Hereditary fructose intolerance
	Glycogen storage disease
Metabolic Diseases	Bone diseases, such as osteomalacia, primary hyperparathyroidism, vitamin D–dependent rickets
Renal Diseases	Amyloidosis
	Nephrotic syndrome
	Transplant rejection
	Renal vascular injury
Toxin Induced	Heavy metals, such as lead, mercury, cadmium
	Drugs, such as aminoglycosides, cephalosporins, mercaptopurine, expired tetracycline

pathway with only one solute type affected or may involve multiple pathways, thereby affecting a variety of tubular functions. Tables 9-5 and 9-6 summarize proximal and distal tubular dysfunctions and associated disorders. Isolated areas of the nephrons (e.g., proximal tubule) can be affected, while the other regions retain essentially normal function. Because renal tubular disorders do not affect glomerular function, the GFR is usually normal. This section discusses commonly encountered tubular dysfunctions, and Table 9-7 outlines the typical urinalysis findings associated with them.

Fanconi Syndrome. The term **Fanconi syndrome** is used to characterize any condition that presents with a generalized loss of proximal tubular function. As a consequence of this dysfunction, amino acids, glucose, water, phosphorus, potassium, and calcium are not reabsorbed from the ultrafiltrate and are excreted in the urine. A spectrum of disorders, including inherited diseases (e.g., cystinosis), toxin exposure (e.g., lead), metabolic bone diseases (e.g., rickets), and renal diseases (e.g., amyloidosis), can present with this syndrome.

TABLE 9-6	Distal Tubular Dysfunctions
Dysfunction	**Disease**
Impaired ability to reabsorb phosphate	Familial hypophosphatemia (vitamin D–resistant rickets)
Impaired ability to reabsorb calcium	Idiopathic hypercalciuria
Impaired ability to acidify	Renal tubular acidosis types, urine I and IV
Impaired ability to retain	Renal salt-losing disorders, sodium
Impaired ability to concentrate urine	Nephrogenic diabetes
Excessive reabsorption of sodium	Liddle's syndrome

Cystinosis and Cystinuria. Both cystinosis and cystinuria are inherited autosomal recessive disorders that cause renal tubular dysfunction and urinary excretion of the amino acid cystine. These disorders are distinctively different in the gene involved, their clinical

TABLE 9-7	Typical Urinalysis Findings With Selected Tubular Diseases	
Disease	**Physical and Chemical Examination**	**Microscopic Examination**
Acute tubular necrosis	Protein: mild (<1 g/day) Blood: positive Specific gravity: low	↑ RBCs ↑ WBCs ↑ Renal epithelial cells, including renal cell fragments; proximal tubular cells in toxic ATN; collecting tubular cells in ischemic ATN ↑ Casts: renal cell, granular, waxy, and broad
Cystinuria and cystinosis	Blood: positive (usually small) Cystinosis: Protein: mild (<1 g/day)	↑ RBCs Cystine crystals
Renal tubular acidosis*	pH >5.5	Unremarkable
Fanconi syndrome	Protein: moderate (<2.5 g/day) Glucose: positive; amount variable	Unremarkable

↑, Increased; *ATN,* acute tubular necrosis; *RBCs,* red blood cells; *WBCs,* white blood cells.
*Patients with renal tubular acidosis can develop Fanconi syndrome.

presentations, and the physiologic mechanisms responsible for cystine in the urine. For additional discussion, see "Amino Acid Disorders" later in this chapter.

Renal Glucosuria. Glucosuria can result from a lowered maximal tubular reabsorptive capacity (T_m) for glucose. Normally, the T_m for glucose is approximately 350 mg/min by the proximal tubules. Renal glucosuria is a benign inherited condition that results in excretion of glucose in the urine despite normal blood glucose levels. In these patients, glucosuria is caused by a reduction in the glucose T_m.

As discussed in Chapter 7, glucosuria also occurs with prerenal conditions (e.g., diabetes mellitus) and intrinsic renal disease (i.e., defective tubular absorption) (see Box 7-8).

Renal Phosphaturia. Renal phosphaturia is an uncommon hereditary disorder characterized by an inability of the distal tubules to reabsorb inorganic phosphorus. The tubular defect appears to be twofold: a hypersensitivity of the distal tubules to the parathyroid hormone that causes increased phosphate excretion, and a decreased proximal tubular response to lowered plasma phosphate levels. Because of low plasma phosphate levels, bone growth and mineralization are decreased.

Patients with renal phosphaturia may be asymptomatic or can exhibit signs of severe deficiency such as osteomalacia or rickets and growth retardation. Inherited as a dominant sex-linked characteristic, this disorder is often termed *familial hypophosphatemia* or *vitamin D–resistant rickets.*

Renal Tubular Acidosis. Renal tubular acidosis (RTA) is characterized by the inability of the tubules to secrete adequate hydrogen ions despite a normal GFR. Consequently, despite being in acidosis, these patients are unable to produce an acid urine (i.e., urine pH <5.3). Renal tubular acidosis can be inherited as an autosomal dominant trait, with partial or complete expression, or it can occur secondary to a variety of diseases.

Several forms of RTA (types I, II, III, and IV) are identified based on their renal tubular defect(s). In type

I RTA, the tubular dysfunction appears to be twofold: an inability to maintain the normal hydrogen ion gradient and an inability to increase tubular ammonia secretion to compensate. The defect in maintaining the hydrogen ion gradient results from a tubular secretory defect or from increased back-diffusion of hydrogen ions into the distal tubular cells. Regardless, patients with RTA become acidotic, and their bodies compensate by removing calcium carbonate from bone to buffer the retained acids. Consequently, these patients develop osteomalacia and hypercalcemia. The resultant hypercalciuria can cause the precipitation of calcium salts in the tubules and renal parenchyma (nephrocalcinosis).

Type II RTA is characterized by decreased proximal tubular reabsorption of bicarbonate. As a result, an increased amount of bicarbonate remains for distal tubular reabsorption. To compensate, most of the hydrogen ions that the distal tubule secretes are used to retain bicarbonate and are not eliminated in the urine. Consequently, hydrogen ion excretion decreases and urine pH increases. This type of RTA rarely occurs without additional abnormalities of the proximal tubule (e.g., Fanconi's syndrome).

Patients with type III RTA express characteristics of type I and type II RTA. Type IV RTA is characterized by an impaired ability to exchange sodium for potassium and hydrogen in the distal tubule.

Numerous conditions can give rise to acquired RTA. Approximately 30% of patients with acquired RTA type I have an autoimmune disorder that has an associated hypergammaglobulinemia such as biliary cirrhosis or thyroid disease. Drugs, nephrotoxins, and kidney transplant rejection can result in the development of RTA, as can inborn errors of metabolism such as Wilson's disease or cystinosis.

Individualized treatment for RTA consists of reducing acidemia by oral administration of alkaline salts (e.g., sodium bicarbonate) and potassium. This serves to raise the plasma pH toward normal and to replace lost potassium (primarily in RTA types I and II). Other clinical problems such as the development of renal calculi (stones) and upper urinary tract infection may require additional treatment regimens.

Tubulointerstitial Disease and Urinary Tract Infections

Because of their close structural and functional relationships, a disease process affecting the renal interstitium inevitably involves the tubules, leading to tubulointerstitial disease. Numerous conditions or factors are capable of causing a tubulointerstitial disease process, and the pathogenic mechanism for each can differ (Box 9-2). Tubulointerstitial disease and lower urinary tract infection can be intimately involved because the latter represents the principal mechanism leading to the development of acute pyelonephritis. Table 9-8 outlines typical routine urinalysis findings in selected urinary tract infections and tubulointerstitial diseases.

Urinary Tract Infections. Urinary tract infections (UTIs) can involve the upper or lower urinary tract. A lower UTI can involve the urethra (urethritis), the bladder (cystitis), or both, whereas an upper UTI can involve the renal pelvis alone (pyelitis) or can include the interstitium (pyelonephritis). Urinary tract infections are common and affect females approximately 10 times more often than males. This predisposition in females is due to several factors: short urethra with close proximity to the vagina and rectum; hormones that enhance bacterial adherence to mucosa; the absence of prostatic fluid and its antibacterial action; and the "milking" of bacteria up the urethra during sexual intercourse.

Normally, urine and the urinary tract are sterile, except for the normal bacterial flora at the extreme outermost (distal) portion of the urethra. Continual flushing of the urethra during voiding of urine normally prevents

---

BOX 9-2 | Causes of Tubulointerstitial Diseases

- Infection
  - Acute pyelonephritis
  - Chronic pyelonephritis
- Toxins
  - Drugs
    - Acute interstitial nephritis
    - Analgesic nephritis
    - Heavy metal poisonings, such as lead
- Metabolic disease
  - Urate nephropathy
  - Nephrocalcinosis
- Vascular diseases
- Irradiation
  - Radiation nephritis
- Neoplasms
- Multiple myeloma
- Transplant rejection

TABLE 9-8 | Typical Urinalysis Findings in Selected Urinary Tract Infections and Tubulointerstitial Diseases

Disease	Physical and Chemical Examination	Microscopic Examination
Lower Urinary Tract Infection		
Cystitis	Protein: small (<0.5 g/day) Blood: + (usually small) Leukocyte esterase: ±; usually + Nitrite: ±; usually +	↑ WBCs ↑ Bacteria: variable, small to large numbers ↑ RBCs ↑ Transitional epithelial cells
Tubulointerstitial Disease (Upper Urinary Tract Infection)		
Acute pyelonephritis	Protein: mild (<1 g/day) Blood: + (usually small) Leukocyte esterase: ±; usually + Nitrite: ±; usually + Specific gravity: normal to low	↑ WBCs, often in clumps; macrophages ↑ Bacteria: variable, small to large numbers ↑ Casts: WBC (pathognomonic), granular, renal cell, waxy ↑ RBCs ↑ Renal epithelial cells
Chronic pyelonephritis	Protein: moderate (<2.5 g/day) Leukocyte esterase: ± Specific gravity: low	↑ WBCs, macrophages ↑ Casts: granular, waxy, broad; few WBC and renal cells
Acute interstitial nephritis	Protein: mild (≈1 g/day) Blood: + (degree variable) Leukocyte esterase: ±; usually +	↑ WBCs, macrophages; differential reveals increased eosinophils ↑ RBCs ↑ Casts: leukocyte (eosinophil) cast, granular, hyaline, renal cell ↑ Renal epithelial cells (Crystals—drug crystals possible, if drug is inducing the disease)

±, Either positive or negative; +, positive; ↑, increased; *RBC,* red blood cell; *WBC,* white blood cell.

the movement of bacteria into sterile portions of the urinary tract. In spite of this, UTIs are caused most often by bacteria from the GI tract (fecal flora) and are considered endogenous infections (i.e., infecting agent originates from within the organism). In other words, because of various factors, intestinal bacteria get introduced into the urinary tract, where they proliferate and cause an infection. Approximately 85% of all UTIs are caused by the gram-negative rods present in normal feces. The most common pathogen is *Escherichia coli*; however, *Proteus, Klebsiella, Enterobacter,* and *Pseudomonas* are other gram-negative rods that are often encountered. *Streptococcus faecalis* (enterococci) and *Staphylococcus aureus* are gram-positive organisms that have also been implicated in UTIs. It is worth noting, however, that essentially any bacterial or fungal agent can cause a UTI.

Lower UTIs are often characterized by pain or burning on urination (dysuria) and the frequent urge to urinate even when the bladder has just been emptied (urgency). Other symptoms that may or may not be present include low-grade fever and pressure or cramping in the lower abdomen. It is important to note that in the elderly, a common initial and only sign of a UTI is mental confusion or distress.

With a lower UTI, routine urinalysis reveals leukocyturia and bacteriuria. Of particular note is the absence of pathologic casts; this differentiates a lower UTI from one of the upper urinary tract in which casts are present. A quantitative urine culture can be used to establish the diagnosis and to identify the causative agent, with a finding of 1×10^5 bacterial colonies per milliliter indicating infection. Minimal hematuria and proteinuria can also be present. Owing to irritation and inflammation of the bladder epithelium, increased numbers of transitional epithelial cells may also be sloughed and noted microscopically (see Table 9-8).

Symptoms of a UTI usually disappear within 2 days after initiation of antibiotic treatment. The urinary analgesic phenazopyridine (Pyridium) may also be prescribed to relieve dysuria and urgency; note that this drug is not an antibiotic. Phenazopyridine will distinctly change the color of the urine to a characteristically bright orange.

The clinical presentation and findings in an upper urinary tract infection (e.g., acute pyelonephritis) are discussed in the next section.

Acute Pyelonephritis. Acute pyelonephritis is a bacterial infection that involves the renal tubules, interstitium, and renal pelvis. Two different mechanisms can lead to a kidney infection: (1) movement of bacteria from the lower urinary tract to the kidneys, or (2) localization of bacteria from the bloodstream in the kidneys (hematogenous infection). The most common cause is an ascending urinary tract infection from gram-negative organisms that are normal intestinal flora. Usually if bacteria reach the bladder, they are prevented from ascending the ureters to the kidneys by the continual flow of urine into the bladder and by other antibacterial mechanisms.

However, when bladder emptying is incomplete (e.g., obstruction, dysfunction), a few bacteria can exponentially proliferate in the residual urine in the bladder. When these bacteria move up the ureters to the kidneys, an upper UTI or pyelonephritis can be established.

Acute pyelonephritis is associated with predisposing conditions that enhance the proliferation and movement of bacteria to the kidneys. One of these conditions is vesicoureteral reflux (VUR), which causes the abnormal flow of urine up into the ureters. VUR is most commonly diagnosed in infancy or childhood and is associated with a congenital, inherited anatomic variation at the junction of the ureter and bladder (e.g., the valve), which allows the backward flow of urine up the ureters. VUR can also occur following bladder or other abdominal surgery. Other conditions that lead to upper UTIs include catheterization, urinary tract obstruction, sepsis (blood infection), pregnancy, diabetes mellitus, and immunosuppressive conditions. After bacteria reach the kidney, they multiply predominantly in the interstitium, causing an acute inflammation. The inflammation eventually involves the tubules, which become necrotic, and bacterial toxins along with leukocytic enzymes cause abscesses to form. Large numbers of neutrophils accumulate in these tubules in an attempt to prevent further spread of the infection. Note that the glomeruli are rarely involved in these infections.

Clinically, acute pyelonephritis has a sudden onset characterized by flank (side), back, or groin pain, dysuria, and a frequent urge to urinate (urgency), which includes nocturia. Patients may also present with a high fever, chills, nausea, headache, and generalized malaise. As with a lower UTI, elderly individuals frequently have mental confusion or distress, and this may be the only symptom noted.

Urinalysis will reveal bacteria and large numbers of leukocytes (leukocyturia) and other inflammatory cells (e.g., macrophages) that derive from the inflammatory infiltrate in the kidney. The presence of leukocyte casts, as well as other casts (e.g., granular, renal tubular cell, broad), is pathognomonic of renal involvement (i.e., an upper UTI). Minimal to mild proteinuria and hematuria are present, and the urine specific gravity is usually low (see Table 9-8).

Acute pyelonephritis lasts 1 to 2 weeks and is most often benign. With appropriate antibiotic therapy, symptoms may take a week or longer to disappear. If predisposing conditions are not resolved, ongoing or chronic infection can eventually lead to permanent renal damage.

Chronic Pyelonephritis. Chronic pyelonephritis develops when persistent inflammation of renal tissue causes permanent scarring that involves the renal calyces and pelvis. Many diseases can cause chronic tubulointerstitial disease; however, most do not involve the renal calyces and pelvis. The most common causes of chronic pyelonephritis are reflux nephropathies, such as VUR and intrarenal reflux, and chronic urinary tract obstruction. VUR was discussed previously (see "Acute Pyelonephritis"). Intrarenal reflux occurs within the renal pelvis owing to anatomic variations of the renal papillae; these structural abnormalities cause urine to move backward (up the collecting ducts) and into the renal cortex instead of down the ureters into the bladder.

When bacteria-laden urine is sent to the renal interstitium by reflux nephropathies or obstruction, an upper UTI develops. If infection and inflammation are ongoing or *chronic,* fibrosis and scarring of the renal tissue occur. Over time, the renal calyces become dilated and deformed; this is a characteristic feature of chronic pyelonephritis.

The onset of reflux nephropathies is usually subtle and is often detected by routine urinalysis or after a patient develops hypertension and renal failure. Urinalysis reveals increased leukocytes and proteinuria; bacteria may or may not be present. Whereas casts are present in early stages, they are usually absent in later chronic stages. Polyuria and nocturia develop as tubular function is lost; hence the urine specific gravity is low. With disease progression and the development of hypertension, renal blood flow and the glomerular filtration rate are affected. Approximately 10% to 15% of patients with chronic pyelonephritis develop chronic renal failure (end-stage renal disease) and require dialysis.

Acute Interstitial Nephritis. Any allergic response in the interstitium of the kidney can cause **acute interstitial nephritis** (AIN). Although various drugs and conditions can be involved, the most common cause is acute allograft rejection of a transplanted kidney.[6] Among medications, antibiotics, particularly methicillin, cephalosporins, sulfonamides, rifampin, and ciprofloxacin, are most notably associated with AIN. Other medications associated with AIN include nonsteroidal anti-inflammatory drugs (NSAIDs), such as ibuprofen, antiepileptic agents (phenytoin, carbamazepine), and allopurinol. Conditions such as leukemia, lymphoma, sarcoidosis, bacterial infection (e.g., *Escherichia coli, Staphylococcus, Streptococcus,* tuberculosis), and viral infection (e.g., cytomegalovirus, Epstein-Barr virus) can also cause AIN.

Whether a medication, a microorganism, or tissue, these agents induce a cell-mediated immune response that causes damage to the interstitium and the renal tubular epithelium. The renal interstitium becomes edemic and infiltrated with white blood cells (WBCs), particularly lymphocytes, macrophages, eosinophils, and neutrophils. Although varying degrees of renal tubular necrosis may occur, it is interesting to note that the glomeruli and the renal blood vessels usually are not involved and retain normal functioning ability.

With AIN, routine urinalysis will reveal hematuria, mild proteinuria, and leukocyturia without bacteria (i.e., sterile leukocyturia). A differential analysis of the urine WBCs will reveal increased numbers of eosinophils (eosinophiluria). WBC or eosinophil casts may also be present in the urine sediment.

With antibiotic-related AIN, typical symptoms include fever, skin rash (25% of individuals), and eosinophilia. Other cases of AIN (e.g., NSAIDs, systemic conditions) do not present with these symptoms. The development of AIN usually begins 3 to 21 days following exposure to the offending agent. With medications, discontinuation of the offending drug can result in full recovery of renal function; however, irreversible damage can occur, especially in elderly individuals.

Yeast Infections. The urinary tracts of men and women are susceptible to **yeast infection,** although such infections occur more commonly in the vagina. *Candida* species (e.g., *Candida albicans*) are normal flora in the gastrointestinal tract and vagina, and their proliferation is kept in check by the normal bacterial flora in these areas. When the bacterial flora is adversely disrupted by antibiotics or pH changes, yeasts proliferate. Urine and blood catheters provide a mode of inoculating yeasts into the urinary tract or bloodstream. *Candida* has a predilection for renal tissue and can cause an upper or lower UTI. Yeast infections can be particularly severe and difficult to manage in immunocompromised patients.

Vascular Disease

Because kidney function is directly dependent on receiving 25% of the cardiac output, any disruption in the blood supply will affect renal function. Likewise, any changes in the vasculature of the kidney directly affect the close interrelationship and interdependence of the blood vessels with the renal interstitium and tubules. Therefore, disorders that alter the blood vessels or the blood supply to the kidney can cause renal disease. Atherosclerosis of intrarenal arteries causes a reduction in renal blood flow, whereas hypertension, polyarteritis nodosa, eclampsia, diabetes, and amyloidosis often cause significant changes in the renal arterioles and glomerular capillaries such that severe and fatal renal ischemia can result. Hypertension is a frequent finding in many kidney disorders when the role of the kidneys in blood pressure control is compromised by disease.

Acute and Chronic Renal Failure

Acute Renal Failure. Acute renal failure (ARF) is characterized clinically by a sudden decrease in the GFR, azotemia, and oliguria (i.e., urine output less than 400 mL). Although the nephrons are "functionally" abnormal, no histologic abnormality is usually present. Often the initial oliguria leads to anuria, and, despite the fact that ARF is usually reversible, it has a high mortality rate.

The mechanisms that cause ARF can be classified as prerenal, renal, and postrenal. Approximately 25% of

ARF cases are prerenal and result from a decrease in renal blood flow. Any event that reduces the mean arterial blood pressure in the afferent arterioles to below 80 mm Hg causes a reduction in the GFR. The most common initiator is a decreased cardiac output, which causes a decrease in renal perfusion. If this condition lasts long enough, tissue ischemia results. In fact, ischemic ATN is the most common cause of ARF. Other conditions that cause a sudden reduction in blood volume and are associated with this type of ARF include hemorrhages, burns, and surgical procedures, as well as acute diarrhea and vomiting. In response to decreased blood pressure, the kidneys increase sodium and water reabsorption in an attempt to restore normal blood volume and perfusion. If this process is unsuccessful, ischemic renal injury can occur, and the development of a renal-type ARF is superimposed on the initiating prerenal cause.

The urine sediment in prerenal ARF is not distinctive. In contrast, urine electrolytes provide information that aids in identifying this disease process. The urine sodium concentration is low because an increased amount of sodium is being reabsorbed. Despite this, the urine osmolality is usually greater than the serum osmolality, and the ratio of blood urea nitrogen to creatinine is significantly increased.

Renal causes of ARF account for approximately 65% of cases. Characterized by renal damage, ARF can result from any glomerular, tubular, or vascular disease process. Most patients (99%) present clinically with ATN. As ATN progresses, renal tubular destruction leads to loss of water and electrolytes (e.g., sodium, potassium). The increased urinary excretion of sodium in renal ARF contrasts with the decreased urine sodium excretion from prerenal causes of ARF and aids in their differentiation.

Postrenal causes of ARF include obstructions in urine flow and account for approximately 10% of patients with ARF. Mechanical obstruction within the kidney can result from various sources such as crystalline deposition (e.g., drugs, amino acids, solutes) and neoplasms. The obstruction causes an increase in hydrostatic pressure within the tubules and Bowman's space. As a result, normal filtration pressures across the glomerular filtration barrier are disrupted and the GFR is decreased. Eventually, the tubules become damaged and renal function is lost.

Regardless of the cause of ARF, the urinalysis findings are not characteristically diagnostic. However, careful examination is important to aid in diagnosing the underlying cause (e.g., ATN, obstruction, myoglobinuria, nephrotoxin). The clinical course of ARF varies greatly; patients who survive usually regain normal renal function. Monitoring of the patient's fluids and electrolytes is crucial during the course of ARF, with dialysis often needed to control the azotemia. If a patient becomes overhydrated, edema and heart failure can result. The high mortality of ARF is due principally to concomitant infection or potassium intoxication.

Chronic Renal Failure. Progressive loss of renal function caused by an irreversible and intrinsic renal disease characterizes **chronic renal failure** (CRF). With CRF, the GFR slowly but continuously decreases. Note that the decreasing GFR becomes clinically recognizable only after 80% to 85% of normal renal function has been lost (i.e., GFR ≈15 to 20 mL/min). Hence the course of CRF is often described as "slow and silent." Early in the course of CRF, the remaining healthy nephrons hypertrophy to compensate for those destroyed and in doing so are able to maintain the "appearance" of normal renal function.

Numerous diseases result in CRF, with the glomerulonephropathies accounting for 50% to 60% of cases. Diabetic nephropathy, chronic pyelonephritis, hypertension, collagen vascular diseases (e.g., systemic lupus erythematosus), and congenital abnormalities are some other causes.

Clinically, CRF presents with azotemia, acid-base imbalance, water and electrolyte imbalance, and abnormal calcium and phosphorus metabolism. Periodic measurement of the GFR or estimated GFR (eGFR) assists the clinician in monitoring CRF. Other clinical features include anemia, bleeding tendencies, hypertension, weight loss, nausea, and vomiting. Eventually, CRF progresses to an advanced renal disease often termed *end-stage renal disease* or *end-stage kidneys*. When patients reach this stage, they require dialysis or renal transplantation to survive.

Urinalysis findings associated with end-stage renal disease include a fixed specific gravity (isosthenuria, at 1.010), significant proteinuria, minimal to moderate hematuria, and the presence of all types of casts, particularly waxy and broad casts.

Calculi

Pathogenesis. Calculi are aggregates of solid chemicals (mineral salts) interlaid with a matrix of proteins and lipids. They form within the body and may be found in any secreting gland, including the pancreas, gallbladder, salivary gland, lacrimal gland, and urinary tract. This discussion focuses on calculi or "stones" of the urinary tract. They are found primarily in the renal calyces, pelvis, ureter, or bladder.

Only about 0.1% of the population develops renal calculi, and approximately 75% of these calculi contain calcium (Table 9-9). Calculi are rarely composed of a single chemical component; rather they are mixtures that most often include calcium, oxalate, or both. Magnesium ammonium phosphate (triple phosphate), phosphate, uric acid, and cystine are also frequently involved. The organic matrix of calculi incorporates a variety of proteins such as Tamm-Horsfall protein (uromodulin), albumin, prothrombin fragments, and other urine

TABLE 9-9	Renal Calculi Composition	
Chemical Component		**Approximate Frequency**
Calcium		75%
with oxalate		35%
with phosphate		15%
with others		25%
Magnesium ammonium phosphate		15%
Uric acid		6%
Cystine		2%
All others		<1%

proteins. Similarly, lipids of the matrix include cholesterol, triglycerides, phospholipids, and gangliosides.[7]

Underlying metabolic or endocrine disorders, as well as infections and isohydria (fixed urinary pH), can cause or enhance calculi formation. When the urine becomes supersaturated with chemical salts and the pH is optimal, renal calculi begin to form. Stone formation may or may not be associated with a concomitant increase of these solutes in the blood. For example, about 25% of individuals who develop calcium stones do not have hypercalcemia or hypercalciuria; similarly, more than 50% of patients with uric acid stones do not have hyperuricemia or hyperuricosuria. However, patients with hypercalciuria, hyperoxaluria, and hyperuricemia have an increased risk of developing renal calculi. These conditions occur when renal tubular reabsorption mechanisms are dysfunctional, allowing increased urinary excretion of a chemical salt, or when intestinal absorption is increased.

It is postulated that calculi formation is affected by the absence of natural inhibitors. The molecules identified have demonstrated inhibition to one or more of the steps that lead to stone formation: crystal aggregation, crystal growth, nucleation, or adherence to renal epithelium.[8] Together, as a mixture, these molecules may be responsible for preventing calculi formation; however, their definitive roles have yet to be elucidated. Inhibitors identified and studied include nephrocalcin, osteopontin (uropontin), citrate, Tamm-Horsfall protein (uromodulin), chondroitin sulfate, calgranulin, bikunin, prothrombin F1 fragment, heparan sulfate, pyrophosphate, and CD59.[8,9]

Factors Influencing Calculi Formation. Essentially four factors influence renal calculi formation:

1. Supersaturation of chemical salts in urine
2. Optimal urinary pH
3. Urinary stasis
4. Nucleation or initial crystal formation

Increases in the concentration of urinary solutes can result from external causes, endocrine disorders, or metabolic conditions. External causes include dehydration, in which the urinary solutes are excreted in as small an amount of water as possible to conserve body water. Increased urine concentrations of particular solutes can occur owing to dietary excesses or increased intestinal absorption, as in patients with inflammatory bowel disease. Medications, particularly cytotoxic drugs, can also result in increases of urinary solutes. For example, chemotherapeutic agents destroy cells and cause an increase in nucleic acid breakdown. As a result, the uric acid concentration in the blood and urine is increased. Because uric acid is seven times less soluble than urate salts, it readily precipitates out of solution if the urine is acidified sufficiently by the distal tubules. Endocrine disorders such as hyperparathyroidism cause reabsorption of calcium from bone and subsequently hypercalcemia and hypercalciuria. Metabolic conditions such as gout (hyperuricemia), inborn errors of metabolism (e.g., cystinuria), or primary oxaluria can also produce urines supersaturated with chemical salts.

Changes in urinary pH play an important role in calculi formation. With the proper pH, even high concentrations of chemicals can remain soluble. Calculi formation is enhanced when a patient loses the normal "acid-alkaline tide" of the body and experiences isohydruria (i.e., a constant and unchanging urinary pH). The inorganic salts—calcium, magnesium, ammonium, phosphate, and oxalate—are less soluble in neutral or alkaline urine. In contrast, organic salts such as uric acid, cystine, and bilirubin are less soluble in acidic urine. Renal tubular acidosis, which is associated with many renal disorders and was discussed earlier in this chapter, is also linked to calculi formation. With RTA, the patient's tubules are unable to acidify the urine (i.e., excrete hydrogen ions), and to compensate, increased amounts of calcium are excreted in the urine. As a result, patients with RTA have an increased chance of forming renal calculi.

Patients with UTIs caused by urea-splitting organisms such as *Proteus, Pseudomonas,* and enterococci produce alkaline urine owing to bacterial conversion of urea to ammonia. As a result, these individuals form magnesium ammonium phosphate stones, also known as *struvite* stones. These stones are usually large, causing bleeding (hematuria), obstruction, and infection without stone passsage.[9] When stones in the renal pelvis become so large that they extend into two or more calyces, they are called *staghorn* stones. This name describes their branching shape, which matches the renal pelvis in which they are formed. Almost without exception, staghorn stones are associated with an upper urinary tract infection.

Urinary stasis (e.g., malformations) enhances renal calculi formation by increasing the chances of supersaturation and precipitation. Nucleation and attachment occur on renal epithelium, other cell surfaces, cellular debris, bacteria, and denatured or aggregated proteins. Once crystal deposition has begun (nucleation), it is only a matter of time until crystal growth results in a clinically symptomatic stone.

The formation of renal stones is most often discovered when the urinary tract becomes obstructed or the stones produce ulceration and bleeding. Small stones can pass from the renal pelvis into the ureters, where they can cause obstruction and produce intense pain, often referred to as *renal colic*. This pain is intense, beginning in the kidney region and radiating forward and downward toward the abdomen, genitalia, or legs. Patients often experience nausea, vomiting, sweating, and a frequent urge to urinate. Large stones unable to pass into the ureter (or urethra) remain in the renal pelvis (or bladder) and are revealed because of the trauma they produce, which usually occurs as hematuria.

Prevention and Treatment. Increasing fluid intake to produce a dilute urine and modifying the diet to eliminate excesses in certain solutes are the two primary approaches to preventing future calculi formation. Oral medications are commonly used to lower urine calcium excretion. Most frequently used are thiazide diuretics, which reduce calcium excretion by increasing calcium reabsorption by proximal tubular cells. Oral phosphate medications as well as citrate therapy may be used to reduce urinary calcium excretion or to bind calcium, respectively. Medications can also be used to convert a solute to a more soluble form. For example, D-penicillamine reduces cystine formation through the competitive production of a soluble salt, whereas allopurinol reduces uric acid formation by altering purine metabolism to form hypoxanthine instead.

Eliminating the causative agent, such as urea-splitting bacteria or an offending drug, may also prevent stone formation. In these cases, administering an appropriate antibiotic long term or discontinuing drug administration (e.g., indinavir, guaifenesin) may be needed.

Once a stone has formed, several techniques are available for its destruction or removal. Extracorporeal shockwave lithotripsy (ESWL)—the use of sound waves to break up the stone in vivo—is often used. If a stone is located in the lower third of a ureter or in the bladder, cystoscopy can be used to remove the stone or to place a stent for drainage. If ESWL is unsuccessful, percutaneous nephrolithotomy (PCNL) is performed. Today, surgical procedures (surgical ureterolithotomy) are rarely necessary or performed.

METABOLIC DISEASES

A routine urinalysis can provide important information regarding metabolic diseases. These diseases vary and may be characterized by increased excretion of a normal urine solute or by the appearance in the urine of a substance that is not normally present. Because some metabolic diseases are linked to lifelong detrimental effects, such as mental retardation or nervous system degeneration, early detection is paramount. Although the urinalysis laboratory may detect or suspect the presence of a particular substance in a patient's urine, more

TABLE 9-10	Qualitative Tests Used to Screen for Metabolic Disorders
Test	**Disorder**
Ferric chloride test	Alkaptonuria (homogentisic acid)
	MSUD
	Melanoma (melanin)
	PKU
Ammoniacal silver nitrite	Alkaptonuria (Homogentisic acid)
Benedict's test	Alkaptonuria (Homogentisic acid)
Nitrosonaphthol test	Tyrosinuria
Hoesch test	Porphyria (porphobilinogen)
Watson-Schwartz test	Porphyria (porphobilinogen)

MSUD, Maple syrup urine disease; *PKU,* phenylketonuria.

accurate quantitative procedures are used to specifically identify them.

Historically, a variety of simple "screening" tests (Table 9-10) were available and were used in clinical laboratories to provide preliminary evidence of metabolic disease. Currently, these "screening" tests are rarely performed because (1) the tests are nonspecific and insensitive, (2) disease prevalence is low with few test requests, and (3) a large amount of time is needed to maintain the reagents and the quality assurance program. Today these disorders are diagnosed using specific, quantitative, and specialized assays often provided by reference laboratories.

Amino Acid Disorders

The liver and the kidneys are actively involved in the metabolism of amino acids. They interconvert amino acids by transamination and degrade them by deamination. The latter results in ammonium ions, which are used to form urea. Urea is subsequently eliminated from the body by the kidneys. Normally, amino acids readily pass the glomerular filtration barrier and are reabsorbed by the proximal tubule. This reabsorption, an active transport mechanism, is threshold limited and is facilitated by membrane-bound carriers.

The three types of **aminoaciduria,** differentiated by their causes, include overflow, no-threshold, and renal aminoacidurias. Overflow aminoaciduria is caused by an increase in the plasma levels of the amino acid(s) such that the renal threshold for amino acid reabsorption is exceeded, and additional amino acids are excreted in the urine. The second type, no-threshold aminoaciduria, also has an overflow mechanism. The difference is that amino acids in this type normally are not reabsorbed by the tubules; any increase in the blood produces an increased quantity in the urine. The third type, renal aminoaciduria, occurs when the plasma levels of amino acids are normal, but because of a tubular defect (congenital or acquired), they are not reabsorbed and appear in the urine in increased amounts.

Aminoacidurias can occur as a primary or a secondary disease. The primary diseases are also known as *inborn errors of metabolism* and result from an inherited defect. Two types of defects are possible: (1) an enzyme may be defective (or deficient) in the specific amino acid metabolic pathway, or (2) tubular reabsorptive dysfunction may occur. Secondary aminoacidurias are induced, most notably by severe liver disease or through generalized renal tubular dysfunction (e.g., Fanconi syndrome).

Cystinosis. Cystinosis is an inherited (autosomal recessive) lysosomal storage disease that results in the intracellular deposition of cystine in the lysosomes of cells throughout the body, particularly the kidneys, eyes, bone marrow, and spleen. The accumulated cystine crystallizes within cells, causing damage and disrupting cellular functions.

Three distinct types of cystinosis are caused by mutations in the same gene but differ in disease severity, age of onset, or clinical presentation.[10] *Nephropathic cystinosis* is the most common and severe form. Accumulated cystine crystallizes within the proximal tubular cells of the nephrons, causing generalized proximal tubular dysfunction and the development of the Fanconi syndrome. Eventually, the distal tubules become involved and patients are unable to concentrate or acidify their urine. The disease is evident during the first year of life with patients also showing growth retardation, rickets, polyuria, polydipsia, dehydration, and acidosis. By 2 years of age, cystine crystals may be present in the cornea of the eye, causing increased light sensitivity. Without treatment—renal dialysis or kidney transplant—patients die by the age of 10 years owing to extensive kidney damage.

A second and rare form known as *intermediate cystinosis* has the same clinical features as nephropathic cystinosis; however the onset of symptoms occurs in adolescence, and the disorder has a slower rate of progression. These individuals develop kidney failure by their late twenties or early thirties. Another rare form is *ocular cystinosis*. Individuals with this form manifest only ocular impairment caused by cystine deposition in the cornea. They do not develop renal or other adverse effects.

Cystinuria. Cystinuria is a disorder characterized by the urinary excretion of large amounts of cystine and the dibasic amino acids—arginine, lysine, and ornithine. It is an inherited autosomal recessive disorder in which the nephrons (i.e., proximal tubular cells) are unable to reabsorb these amino acids. Similarly, these patients have defective intestinal absorption of the same amino acids. Because cystine has a pKa of 8.3, this disorder often becomes evident when cystine crystals appear in urine with a pH ≤8. Note that the dibasic amino acids also present, are soluble regardless of urine pH and remain undetectable in the urine unless amino acid analysis is performed.

Because of its low solubility, in vivo cystine precipitation and renal calculi formation can occur in these patients. Clinical symptoms include hematuria and sudden severe abdominal or low back pain. To prevent cystine stone formation, patients need to alkalinize their urine (diet modification) and stay well hydrated, particularly at night, when the urine becomes the most concentrated and acidic. Treatment to prevent the formation of cystine calculi involves the oral administration of D-penicillamine. This drug diverts cystine metabolism to form penicillamine-cysteine-disulfide, which is highly soluble in urine regardless of pH. However, D-penicillamine is expensive and has several undesirable side effects, including fever, rash, proteinuria, and the possibility of developing the nephrotic syndrome.

Maple Syrup Urine Disease. Maple syrup urine disease (MSUD) is a rare, autosomal recessive inherited disease characterized by the accumulation of branched-chain amino acids—leucine, isoleucine, and valine and their corresponding α-keto acids—in blood, cerebrospinal fluid (CSF), and urine. These acids accumulate because of a deficiency in the enzyme complex (branched-chain α-keto acid dehydrogenase [BCKD]) responsible for their oxidative decarboxylation to acyl coenzyme A derivatives (fatty acids). In the United States, neonatal screening and prenatal screening are routinely performed to detect this inherited disorder.

Leucine, isoleucine, and valine are present in numerous foods. They predominate in protein-rich foods, particularly milk, meat, and eggs, but are also present in lower amounts in flour, cereal, and some fruits and vegetables. Although infants with MSUD appear normal at birth, symptoms begin to appear within the first few weeks of life. Eventually an acute ketoacidosis develops along with vomiting, seizures, and lethargy. If not diagnosed and treated appropriately, brain damage and mental retardation occur; without treatment, death occurs in a few months. The high excretion of keto acids in the urine is responsible for the distinctive maple syrup or caramelized sugar odor associated with this disease. Although assessment of urine odor is not routinely performed with urinalysis, it is customary to notify clinicians of unusual and distinctive findings. Diagnosis of MSUD is made following amino acid analysis of plasma, urine, or CSF using ion exchange chromatography.

Treatment of MSUD consists of dietary restriction of foods that contain branched-chain amino acids, as well as the intake of a special formula that provides the nutrients and protein needed without the offending amino acids. Thiamine supplementation has also shown beneficial effects. To monitor and adjust treatment (i.e., diet and special formula composition), the levels of branched-chain amino acids in the blood are periodically tested. Note that with prompt and lifelong treatment, patients have the potential to lead lives with typical growth and development patterns. Despite treatment, however, some

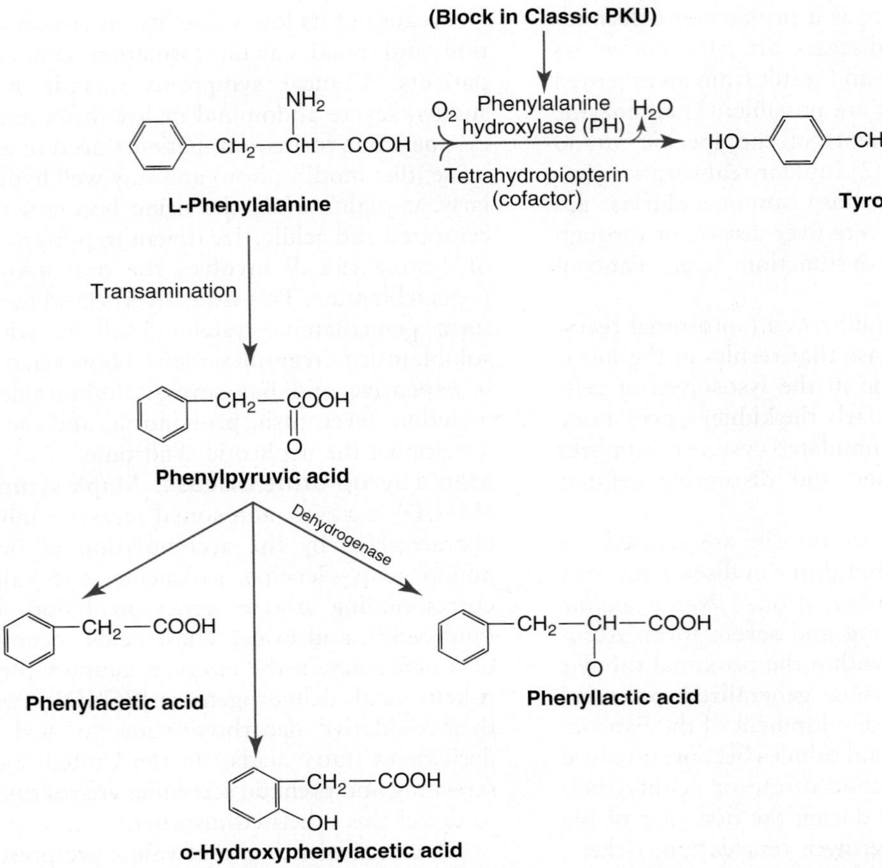

FIGURE 9-2 Major and minor pathways of phenylalanine metabolism.

children have episodes of metabolic crises that can result in mental retardation or spasticity.

Phenylketonuria. Inherited as an autosomal recessive disease, **phenylketonuria** (PKU) is characterized by increased urinary excretion of phenylpyruvic acid (a ketone) and its metabolites. Normally, phenylalanine is converted to tyrosine by the major metabolic pathway depicted in Figure 9-2. However, in classic phenylketonuria, the enzyme phenylalanine hydroxylase is deficient or defective, and the minor metabolic pathway that produces phenylketones is stimulated. Other forms of PKU can result when a defect or decrease occurs in the enzyme cofactor, tetrahydrobiopterin.

Without detection and treatment, PKU results in severe mental retardation. As with other aminoacidurias, affected children appear normal at birth. Nonspecific initial symptoms include delayed development and feeding difficulties such as severe vomiting. Within the infant's first 2 to 3 weeks of life, high plasma levels of phenylalanine cause brain injury, with maximum detrimental effects achieved by 9 months of age.

The urine, sweat, and breath of PKU patients have a characteristic mousy or musty odor, which is caused by the phenylacetic acid in these fluids. Another feature of PKU is decreased skin pigmentation, such that individuals have often noticeably lighter skin, hair, and eyes than

siblings without the disease. This occurs because phenylalanine competitively inhibits the enzyme tyrosinase, which decreases the production of melanin from tyrosine (Figure 9-3).

Screening of all newborns for PKU is mandated in the United States. Blood testing is used because urinary excretion of phenylpyruvic acid does not occur until phenylalanine has accumulated substantially in the plasma, which takes 2 or more weeks. In other words, if urine detection methods were used to screen 2-week-old infants, the detrimental and irreversible effects of PKU would have already taken place.

Treatment for PKU consists of dietary modification to eliminate phenylalanine from the diet. Mental retardation can be avoided completely with early diagnosis and treatment; however, even late detection (e.g., 4 to 6 months old) can often avoid further mental deterioration if adherence to a strict diet is maintained. Attention-deficit hyperactivity disorder (ADHD) is common in patients that do not strictly adhere to a low-phenylalanine diet. Routine testing of patients' plasma is used to monitor compliance with dietary restrictions.

Alkaptonuria. Alkaptonuria is a rare, autosomal recessive disease characterized by the excretion of large amounts of homogentisic acid (HGA), a substance

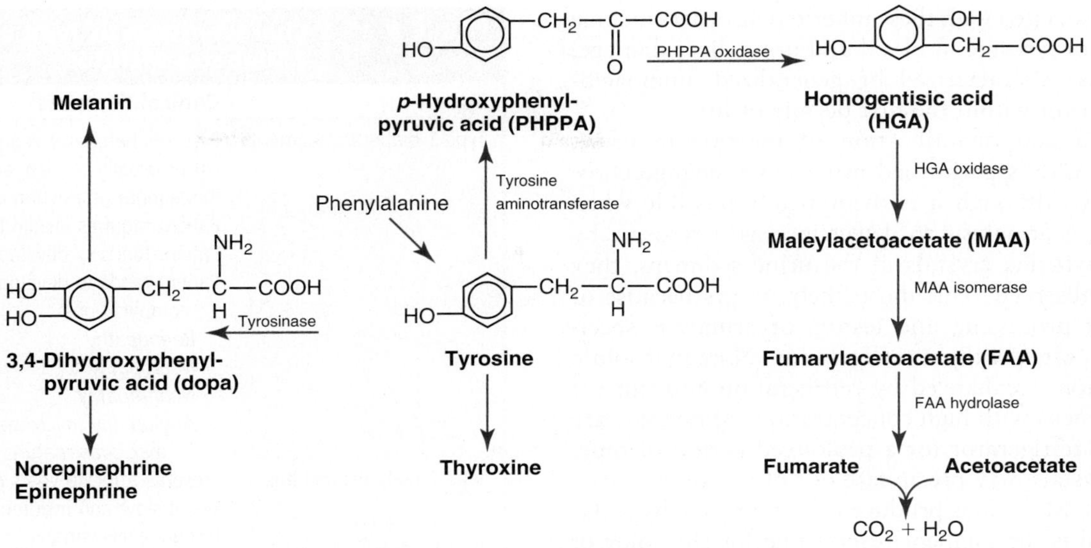

FIGURE 9-3 Pathways of tyrosine metabolism.

not normally present in urine. This disease was called *alkaptonuria* because of the unusual darkening of the urine when alkali is added. In vivo, HGA is normally oxidized to maleylacetoacetic acid by the enzyme homogentisic acid oxidase (see Figure 9-3). When this liver enzyme is deficient or absent, HGA is unable to proceed down the remaining steps of its normal metabolic pathway. As a result, HGA accumulates in the cells and body fluids and is excreted in the urine. HGA polymerizes and binds to collagen in cartilage and other connective tissues to cause an abnormal dark blue or black tissue pigmentation and the development of degenerative arthritis. Alkaptonuria is not usually diagnosed until middle age (30 to 40 years old), when arthritis of the spine and large joints develops and pigmentation in the ears (ochronosis) becomes apparent.

When urine with HGA is exposed to air and sunlight or is alkalinized, it darkens and a fine black precipitate forms. Note that this urine darkening is not unique and requires further investigation and differentiation from other substances that can cause similar changes such as melanin, indican (indoxyl sulfate), and gentisic acid (a salicylate metabolite). Historically, when infants wore cloth diapers that were laundered using strong alkaline soap, the presence of a black pigment on the diaper was suggestive of HGA and provided clinicians with a diagnostic clue. Today with the use of plastic diapers, excretion of HGA usually imparts a pink color to the diaper liner. Consequently, the urinalysis laboratory no longer plays a role in the detection of alkaptonuria unless nonspecific screening tests are available (see Table 9-10). Definitive identification and quantification of homogentisic acid in urine are done using chromatographic methods such as gas chromatography-mass spectrometry (GC-MS) or liquid chromatography-tandem mass spectrometry (LC-MS-MS).

Treatment for alkaptonuria is limited. High doses of vitamin C have been shown to be beneficial and may retard pigment production and the development of arthritis.

Tyrosinuria. Tyrosine is the metabolic precursor of several compounds—melanin, thyroxine, and catecholamines (epinephrine, norepinephrine). Consequently, a defect in one pathway will affect the production of one compound but not another (see Figure 9-3). The predominant tyrosine metabolic pathway leads to the formation of homogentisic acid and the ultimate end-products of carbon dioxide and water.

The presence of an increased amount of tyrosine in the urine, known as **tyrosinuria,** occurs when plasma levels are abnormally high. The high amount of tyrosine readily passes from the bloodstream through the glomeruli and into the renal tubules, where the amount present overwhelms the reabsorptive capacity of the proximal tubular cells. Several causes of tyrosinemia (high plasma tyrosine) are known, but the most frequently encountered is a transient condition in newborns. Other causes include severe liver disease and a rare inherited disorder known as *hereditary tyrosinemia.*

Transient neonatal tyrosinemia is due to the immature liver of infants and inadequate liver enzymes to metabolize tyrosine. As the liver matures, normal enzyme levels are established and the tyrosinemia resolves within 4 to 8 weeks. A similar mechanism is responsible for the tyrosinemia associated with *severe liver disease,* namely, insufficient enzyme synthesis due to diseased and nonfunctioning hepatocytes.

Two rare inherited tyrosinemias called type I and type II, have been identified. Type I, also known as *tyrosinosis,* is caused by a defect in the enzyme fumaryl acetoacetate hydrolase (FAA). Type II tyrosinemia is caused by a defect in the enzyme tyrosine aminotransferase.

Findings associated with these inherited disorders include high levels of tyrosine in blood and urine, liver damage, renal disease characterized by generalized aminoaciduria, and death within the first decade of life.

Detection and quantification of tyrosine in urine, plasma, or CSF is performed using ion exchange chromatography. Although it is theoretically possible when performing a urinalysis to detect increased tyrosine by observing tyrosine crystals in the urine sediment, they are rarely observed. This most likely occurs because of the prompt processing and testing of urinalysis specimens today, often without refrigeration. Note that solute crystallization is enhanced by refrigeration and time; if urine specimens with high concentrations of tyrosine are stored in a refrigerator for a prolonged period of time, tyrosine crystals may precipitate out of solution.

Melanuria. Melanin is produced from tyrosine by melanocytes and is the pigment responsible for the color of hair, skin, and eyes. When inherited defects result in defective melanin production, hypomelanosis or albinism results. Increased production of melanin and its colorless precursors (e.g., 5,6-dihydroxyindole) will cause an increase in the urinary excretion of melanin, or **melanuria.** This occurs with malignant neoplasms of melanocytes (i.e., melanoma) in the skin, mucous membranes, or retina. When melanin and its precursors are present in urine, the urine color darkens with exposure to air or sunlight. The degree of darkening varies with melanin concentration and exposure time; in extreme cases, urine can turn black. Note that other substances can cause a similar color change (e.g., homogentisic acid), and further investigation is required to specifically identify the substance involved.

Carbohydrate Disorders

Glucose and Diabetes Mellitus. Diabetes mellitus is not a single disorder but a group of disorders that affect the metabolism of carbohydrate, fat, and protein. It is characterized by chronic hyperglycemia and glucosuria, both of which provide evidence of the impaired ability to utilize glucose. Diabetes mellitus develops when defects in (1) insulin production, (2) insulin action, or (3) both are present.

Diabetes mellitus is classified as type 1 or type 2 (Table 9-11). Type 1 diabetes was previously called insulin-dependent diabetes mellitus or juvenile-onset diabetes and accounts for 5% to 10% of all diagnosed cases. Type 1 diabetes mellitus can occur at any age; however, most individuals have symptoms before 40 years of age. Type 1 diabetes mellitus develops when the immune system destroys the pancreatic β-cells responsible for the production of insulin and often presents suddenly as an acute illness with ketoacidosis. Other classic symptoms include polyuria, polydipsia, ketonuria, and rapid weight loss. These individuals require insulin by injection or an insulin pump to maintain

TABLE 9-11	Characteristics of Type 1 and Type 2 Diabetes Mellitus	
Type	**Clinical Features**

Type 1 diabetes mellitus	Presents before 40 years of age
	Onset usually sudden, acute
	Inadequate production of insulin
	Patient requires insulin injections
	Patient tends to develop ketoacidosis
	Patient tends to develop complications:
	  Retinopathy
	  Neuropathy
	  Nephropathy
	  Angiopathy (microvasculature and macrovasculature)

Type 2 diabetes mellitus	Presents after 40 years of age Onset slow and insidious Insulin levels variable Dietary regimens, exercise, and oral medications aid in control of hyperglycemia Obesity common Angiopathy of macrovasculature common

normal blood glucose levels. Known risk factors for the development of type 1 diabetes mellitus include autoimmune disorders, genetic inheritance, and environmental factors.

Type 2 diabetes mellitus was previously called *non–insulin-dependent diabetes mellitus* or *adult-onset diabetes.* It usually presents after 40 years of age and accounts for 90% to 95% of all diagnosed cases. Although obesity is common and is often associated with type 2 diabetes mellitus, it is not found in all type 2 patients. Type 2 diabetes mellitus progresses slowly and is often initially detected during a routine wellness screening, or during testing for other clinical concerns. In the early stages, the peripheral tissues are "insulin resistant"—unable to use insulin properly. With time, the pancreas gradually loses its ability to produce sufficient insulin to overcome the insulin resistance, and hyperglycemia develops. Many individuals with type 2 diabetes do not require exogenous insulin and are able to control their blood glucose by following a careful diet, increasing their physical activity (e.g., walking 2.5 hours per week), and taking oral medications.

Diabetic individuals can develop numerous complications involving the eyes (retinopathy), nerves (neuropathy), blood vessels (angiopathy), and kidneys (nephropathy). Two studies have provided landmark results regarding the treatment of diabetes and the development of complications: they are the Diabetes Control and Complications Trial for type 1 diabetic people and the United Kingdom Prospective Diabetes Study for those with type 2 diabetes.[2,3] These research studies found that improved blood glucose control benefits all diabetic individuals and reduces the risk for developing microvascular complications (eye, kidney, or nerve disease). In other studies involving diabetic complications, close control of blood pressure reduced the development of cardiovascular disease (heart disease and stroke) and microvascular disease.

Currently, diabetes is the leading cause of blindness among working-age persons, of end-stage renal disease, and of nontraumatic limb amputations.[11] Diabetes increases the risks for cardiac, cerebral, and peripheral vascular disease. Table 9-11 summarizes clinical features associated with type 1 and type 2 diabetes mellitus.

Polydipsia and polyuria are two classic symptoms associated with inadequately controlled diabetes mellitus. When this occurs, the urine appears dilute (pale yellow or colorless), but it has a high specific gravity because of the large amount of glucose present. Glucosuria indicates that the reabsorptive capacity of the tubules for glucose has been exceeded. At the same time, the body turns to fat metabolism for its energy needs, which results in the formation of ketones that will also be excreted and detected in the urine.

Galactosemia. Normally, the monosaccharide galactose is rapidly metabolized to glucose, and minimal amounts are present in the blood or urine. Lactose, a disaccharide composed of glucose and galactose, is the principal dietary source. Galactosemia with **galactosuria** is associated most often with three rare inherited autosomal recessive disorders that cause an enzyme in the galactose metabolic pathway to be defective or deficient. Because of the enzyme defect, galactose and galactose 1-phosphate accumulate in the blood and are metabolized by alternate pathways to galactitol or galactonate. Galactose 1-phosphate, galactitol, and galactonate are the compounds responsible for the clinical manifestations of these diseases.

The three enzymes responsible for galactosemia are galactose 1-phosphate uridylyltransferase (GALT), galactokinase (GALK), and uridine diphosphate galactose-4-epimerase (GALE). Type I galactosemia (or GALT deficiency or defect) is the classic and most common form of galactosemia. In this disorder, galactonate is the primary end-product of the abnormal metabolism, although galactitol is also abnormally increased. Soon after lactose ingestion, infants with GALT deficiency present with failure to thrive (delayed growth and development), vomiting, jaundice (liver involvement), and diarrhea. Hepatomegaly is a common finding, and the liver damage can progress to cirrhosis. Other complications can include sepsis and shock. Cataracts (due to galactitol) may be present, although this finding is most often associated with type II galactosemia.

The predominant clinical feature of type II galactosemia due to GALK deficiency is cataracts. They are present shortly after birth and result from the persistent high level of galactitol in the bloodstream. Type III

galactosemia due to GALE deficiency is extremely rare and is most common in the Japanese population. Clinical symptoms of type III vary from mild to severe depending on the degree of GALE deficiency and include cataracts, failure to thrive, and liver and kidney disease.

With GALT deficiency, if milk feedings are continued, edema, ascites, splenomegaly, and bleeding can lead rapidly to death. With GALK and GALE deficiencies, the patient can be asymptomatic. In untreated galactosemia patients, long-term consequences include severe mental retardation, delayed language development, and ovarian failure in females. Even with early intervention and dietary restrictions, developmental delay (reduced IQ) remains a consequence of galactosemia.

Prenatal detection of galactosemia can be done using cultured amniotic cells or chorionic villus samples, or by quantification of galactitol in amniotic fluid. Many states (and countries) mandate blood screening of infants for type I galactosemia or GALT deficiency. Note that false-positive and false-negative results are possible. Infants or children with cataracts should also be tested. Urine testing is a rapid and economical means of screening for abnormally increased amounts of galactose. It is a standard laboratory practice used to routinely screen for reducing substances in urine specimens from children younger than 2 years old. If a reducing substance is present while glucose and ascorbic acid are not, then additional testing is needed to identify the reducing substance present. Disease is confirmed using enzymatic assays, chromatography, and molecular methods on blood or cultured fibroblasts.

Diabetes Insipidus

Diabetes insipidus (DI) derives its name *diabetes* from the copious amounts of urine (polyuria) that this disorder produces. The term *insipidus* refers to the bland taste of the urine produced. In contrast, the term *mellitus* means sweet and is used to describe the disorder characterized by polyuria with glucose in the urine (i.e., diabetes mellitus).

Diabetes insipidus can be separated into two types based on the defect responsible: neurogenic and nephrogenic. In health, antidiuretic hormone (ADH), also known as *vasopressin,* is synthesized in the hypothalamus but stored and released from the posterior pituitary. Neurogenic DI occurs when synthesis and release of ADH are reduced. In contrast, nephrogenic DI presents with normal synthesis and release of ADH but with defective renal tubular response to ADH. With both types of DI, water is not reabsorbed by the renal tubules (regardless of bodily needs), causing polyuria and polydipsia. DI can be induced by compulsive water drinking or by the use of certain drugs (e.g., lithium, demeclocycline).

The copious amount of urine produced by DI patients appears dilute and has a low specific gravity, unlike that

Glycine + Succinyl-CoA

↓ ALA synthase
(rate limiting step)

δ-Aminolevulinic acid (ALA)

↓ ALA dehydratase

Porphobilinogen (PBG)

Porphyrin precursors

↓ PBG deaminase

Uroporphyrinogen (UPG)

↓

Coproporphyrinogen (CPG) → Oxidation → Porphyrins

↓

Protoporphyrinogen

← Fe²⁺

↓ Ferrochelatase

Heme

FIGURE 9-4 Schematic diagram of heme synthesis.

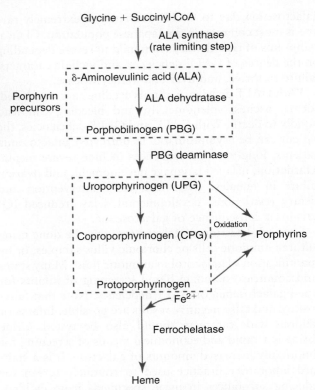

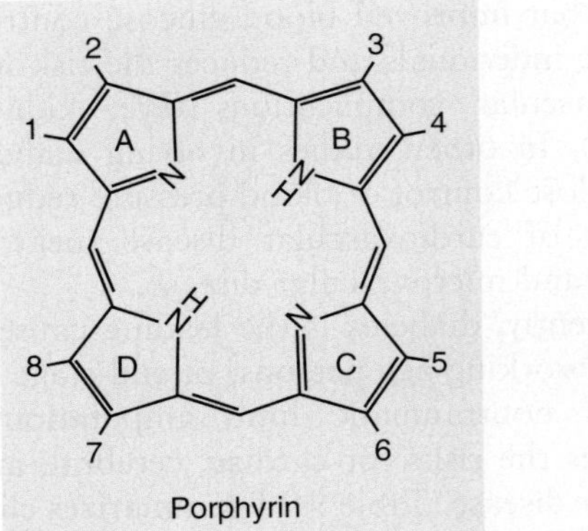

FIGURE 9-5 The basic structure of porphyrins.

of diabetes mellitus patients. DI patients are unable to produce a concentrated urine even when fluids are restricted. Note that dehydration can be life threatening because the plasma can rapidly become hypertonic and patients can go into shock. As long as DI patients are able to replace the large amount of water being excreted, they remain healthy with a normal plasma osmolality (tonicity).

Porphyrias

Porphyrin precursors (porphobilinogen, δ-aminolevulinic acid) and porphyrins (uroporphyrin, coproporphyrin, protoporphyrin) are intermediate compounds that form during the production of heme (Figure 9-4). Disorders associated with the accumulation of one or more of these compounds are collectively termed **porphyrias**. The different porphyrins are derived by the addition of organic groups in the eight peripheral positions on its four pyrrole rings (Figure 9-5). Normally, heme synthesis is so closely regulated that only trace amounts of porphyrins form. They are spontaneous and irreversible oxidation products of the respective porphyrinogens. Once porphyrins form, they cannot reenter the heme synthetic pathway; they have no biological function and are excreted.

The porphyrin precursors and porphyrins differ with respect to their polarity and therefore their solubility in body fluids. Porphobilinogen and δ-aminolevulinic acid—porphyrin precursors—appear principally in urine

because they are rapidly removed from the blood by the kidneys (i.e., low renal threshold). Similarly, uroporphyrin is excreted almost exclusively in the urine; coproporphyrin, being of intermediate solubility, is excreted in both urine and feces; and protoporphyrin, the least water soluble, is excreted only in feces.

The porphyrin precursors (porphobilinogen and δ-aminolevulinic acid) and the porphyrinogens (uroporphyrinogen, coproporphyrinogen, protoporphyrinogen) are colorless, nonfluorescent compounds. In contrast, their oxidative forms (uroporphyrin, coproporphyrin, protoporphyrin) are dark red or purple and intensely fluorescent. Porphobilin, the oxidative form of porphobilinogen, is red. As a result, a urine specimen that contains porphobilinogen can take on a reddish appearance over time because of the photo-oxidation of porphobilinogen to porphobilin. This process takes significant time, and with the rapid handling and processing of urine specimens in laboratories, this subtle color change is rarely observed. In addition, numerous substances can cause a urine to appear reddish. However, when a red-tinged urine tests negative for the presence of blood, and when diet (e.g., beets) and medications have been ruled out, porphyria should be considered.

The porphyrins and heme are produced by all mammalian cells; however, the major sites of synthesis are the bone marrow and the liver. As discussed in Chapter 7 with porphobilinogen, porphyria is inherited or can be an acquired disorder, that is characterized by an increased urinary excretion of porphyrin precursors or porphyrins (Table 9-12). These disorders reflect a deficiency or inhibition of an enzyme required in heme biosynthesis. As intermediate compounds accumulate behind the pathway defect, their concentrations increase in blood, feces, or urine. Porphyrias can be classified as hepatic or erythropoietic based on the site of the metabolic abnormality; however, classification based on clinical presentation is often more practical and useful (Table 9-13).

All porphyrias are rare, with porphyria cutanea tarda (PCT) being the most common type found in North America. All show autosomal dominant inheritance with the exception of congenital erythropoietic porphyria

TABLE 9-12	Classification of Porphyrias	
Disorder	**Enzyme Deficient**	**Inheritance**
Inherited		
ALAD-Deficiency Porphyria (ADP)	δ-aminolevulinic dehydratase (ALAD)	Autosomal recessive
Acute intermittent porphyria (AIP)	Porphobilinogen deaminase (PBGD), formerly called *uroporphyrinogen I synthase*	Autosomal dominant
Congenital erythropoietic porphyria (CEP)	Uroporphyrinogen III cosynthase	Autosomal recessive
Erythropoietic protoporphyria (EPP)	Ferrochelatase	Autosomal dominant
Hereditary coproporphyria (HCP)	Coproporphyrinogen oxidase	Autosomal dominant
Hepatoerythropoietic porphyria (HEP)	Uroporphyrinogen decarboxylase (UROD)	Autosomal recessive
Variegate porphyria (VP)	Protoporphyrinogen oxidase	Autosomal dominant
Acquired		
Porphyria cutanea tarda (PCT)	Uroporphyrinogen decarboxylase (UROD)	Most often an acquired disorder; "familial PCT" autosomal dominant
Coproporphyrinuria	Caused by lead poisoning, tyrosinemia, alcoholism, drugs (e.g., sedatives, hypnotics)	None
Protoporphyrinemia	Caused by lead poisoning, iron deficiency anemias	None

TABLE 9-13	Summary of Porphyria Characteristics					
			Porphyrins Increased			
Clinical Presentation	**Disorder**	**Onset**	**Urine**	**Blood**	**Fecal**	
Neurologic symptoms	ALAD-deficiency porphyria (ADP)	Acute	ALA	ZPP		
	Acute intermittent porphyria (AIP)	Acute	ALA, PBG, UP			
Neurologic and cutaneous symptoms*	Hereditary coproporphyria (HCP)	Acute	ALA, PBG, CP		CP	
	Variegate porphyria (VP)	Acute	ALA, PBG, CP		CP, PP	
Cutaneous symptoms (photosensitivity)	Congenital erythropoietic porphyria (CEP)	Chronic	UP, CP	EP, ZPP	P	
	Hepatoerythropoietic porphyria (HEP)	Chronic	UP, CP	EP, ZPP	P	
	Erythropoietic protoporphyria (EPP)	Chronic		EP	PP	
	Porphyria cutanea tarda (PCT)	Chronic	UP, 7C-P			

*Note that only some patients develop cutaneous symptoms.
ALA, δ-Aminolevulinic acid; *CP*, coproporphyrin; *EP*, erythrocyte porphyrin; *P*, porphyrins; *PBG*, porphobilinogen; *PP*, protoporphyrin; *UP*, uroporphyrin; *ZPP*, zinc protoporphyrin; *7C-P*, 7-carboxyl porphyrin.

(CEP) and δ-aminolevulinic acid dehydratase (ALAD)-deficiency porphyria, two of the rarest forms of porphyria. Acquired or induced disorders are generally classified into one of two types: those that result in the accumulation and excretion of coproporphyrin in the urine, and those that result in the accumulation of protoporphyrin in the blood and its excretion in feces. Chronic lead poisoning can cause the development of both features, whereas other disorders, such as iron deficiency anemia or tyrosinemia, are associated with only one of these features. Induced porphyria-like disorders also produce excesses of other porphyrins or porphyrin precursors to varying degrees.

Clinically, the porphyrias manifest themselves differently. Disorders that result in accumulation of the precursors (porphobilinogen and D-aminolevulinic acid) present with primarily neurologic symptoms, because these substances are neurotoxins. In contrast, when porphyrins are the major accumulation products,

photosensitivity is the distinguishing clinical feature. When porphyrins absorb light, they cause toxic free radicals to form; this causes cutaneous lesions (e.g., extensive blistering or bullous lesions) or a burning sensation with an inflammatory skin reaction.

Diagnosis of porphyria is based on the quantity and type of porphyrin precursors or porphyrins in the blood, urine, and feces. Chapter 7 discusses briefly tests used historically in the urinalysis laboratory to detect increased excretion of porphobilinogen. Measurement of specific enzyme activities may be required or re-testing during an acute attack may be necessary because the levels of porphyrin precursors and porphyrins can return to normal.

Clinically, porphyrias that present primarily with neurologic symptoms can be difficult to diagnose unless a family history provides a clue. For example, the symptoms associated with acute intermittent porphyria (AIP) are similar to those with gastrointestinal or mental health problems. In an acute presentation, patients with AIP often have abdominal pain, nausea, constipation, depression, muscle weakness, hypertension, and tachycardia, as well as a variety of neuropsychiatric problems such as hysteria, psychosis, or seizures.

Acute porphyria episodes can be initiated by the ingestion of drugs, particularly barbiturates and oral contraceptives. Other precipitating agents include ingestion of alcohol, stress, hormonal changes, starvation, and infection. Some of these same factors, most notably a history of excessive alcohol ingestion, can also induce chronic porphyrias.

In all cases of porphyria, treatment consists of identifying and removing any precipitating factors. In acute porphyrias, supportive measures include maintaining fluid and electrolyte balance and using analgesics to relieve pain. Patients with AIP benefit from intravenous infusion of hematin, which inhibits the activity of δ-aminolevulinic acid synthetase: the rate-limiting step in heme synthesis. (See Porphobilinogen in Chapter 7 for more discussion of the heme biosynthetic pathway.) Patients with a porphyria characterized by photosensitivity must avoid direct sunlight and use barrier skin lotions that provide protection from the ultraviolet rays of the sun.

STUDY QUESTIONS

1. Which of the following statements about renal diseases is true?
   A. Glomerular renal diseases are usually immune mediated.
   B. Vascular disorders induce renal disease by increasing renal perfusion.
   C. All structural components of the kidney are equally susceptible to disease.
   D. Tubulointerstitial renal diseases usually result from antibody-antigen and complement interactions.

2. In glomerular diseases, morphologic changes in the glomeruli include all of the following except
   A. cellular proliferation.
   B. erythrocyte congestion.
   C. leukocyte infiltration.
   D. glomerular basement membrane thickening.

3. When all renal glomeruli are affected by a morphologic change, this change is described as
   A. diffuse.
   B. focal.
   C. differentiated.
   D. segmental.

4. In glomerular renal disease, glomerular damage results from
   A. deposition of infectious agents.
   B. a decrease in glomerular perfusion.
   C. changes in glomerular hemodynamics.
   D. toxic substances induced by immune complex formation.

5. Clinical features that are characteristic of glomerular damage include all of the following except
   A. edema.
   B. hematuria.
   C. proteinuria.
   D. polyuria.

6. Which of the following disorders frequently occurs following a bacterial infection of the skin or throat?
   A. Acute glomerulonephritis
   B. Chronic glomerulonephritis
   C. Membranous glomerulonephritis
   D. Rapidly progressive glomerulonephritis

7. Which of the following disorders is characterized by cellular proliferation into Bowman's space to form cellular "crescents"?
   A. Chronic glomerulonephritis
   B. Membranous glomerulonephritis
   C. Minimal change disease
   D. Rapidly progressive glomerulonephritis

8. Which of the following disorders is the major cause of the nephrotic syndrome in adults?
   A. IgA nephropathy
   B. Membranoproliferative glomerulonephritis
   C. Membranous glomerulonephritis
   D. Rapidly progressive glomerulonephritis

9. Which of the following glomerular diseases is the major cause of the nephrotic syndrome in children?
   A. IgA nephropathy
   B. Minimal change disease
   C. Membranous glomerulonephritis
   D. Rapidly progressive glomerulonephritis

10. Which of the following statements regarding IgA nephropathy is true?
   A. It often follows a mucosal infection.
   B. It is associated with the nephrotic syndrome.
   C. It is characterized by leukocyte infiltration of the glomeruli.
   D. It often occurs secondary to systemic lupus erythematosus.

11. Eighty percent of patients who develop chronic glomerulonephritis previously had some type of glomerular disease. Which of the following disorders is implicated most frequently in the development of chronic glomerulonephritis?
   A. IgA nephropathy
   B. Membranous glomerulonephritis
   C. Poststreptococcal glomerulonephritis
   D. Rapidly progressive glomerulonephritis

12. Chronic renal failure often develops in each of the following diseases except
   A. amyloidosis.
   B. diabetes mellitus.
   C. diabetes insipidus.
   D. systemic lupus erythematosus.

13. Which of the following features characterize the nephrotic syndrome?
    1. Proteinuria
    2. Edema
    3. Hypoalbuminemia
    4. Hyperlipidemia
    A. 1, 2, and 3 are correct.
    B. 1 and 3 are correct.
    C. 4 is correct.
    D. All are correct.

14. When a patient has the nephrotic syndrome, microscopic examination of their urine sediment often reveals
    A. granular casts.
    B. leukocyte casts.
    C. red blood cell casts.
    D. waxy casts.

15. Which of the following has not been associated with acute tubular necrosis?
    A. Antibiotics
    B. Galactosuria
    C. Hemoglobinuria
    D. Surgical procedures

16. Which formed element in urine sediment is characteristic of toxic acute tubular necrosis and aids in its differentiation from ischemic acute tubular necrosis?
    A. Collecting tubular cells
    B. Granular casts
    C. Proximal tubular cells
    D. Waxy casts

17. Which of the following disorders is characterized by the urinary excretion of large amounts of arginine, cystine, lysine, and ornithine?
    A. Cystinosis
    B. Cystinuria
    C. Lysinuria
    D. Tyrosinuria

18. Generalized loss of proximal tubular function is a characteristic of
    A. Fanconi's syndrome.
    B. nephrotic syndrome.
    C. renal glucosuria.
    D. renal tubular acidosis.

19. Which of the following changes is not associated with renal tubular acidosis?
    A. Decreased glomerular filtration rate
    B. Decreased renal tubular secretion of hydrogen ions
    C. Decreased proximal tubular reabsorption of bicarbonate
    D. Increased back-diffusion of hydrogen ions in the distal tubules

20. Which of the following disorders is considered a lower urinary tract infection?
    A. Cystitis
    B. Glomerulonephritis
    C. Pyelitis
    D. Pyelonephritis

21. Most urinary tract infections are caused by
    A. yeast, such as *Candida* spp.
    B. gram-negative rods.
    C. gram-positive rods.
    D. gram-positive cocci.

22. Which of the following formed elements when present in urine sediment is most indicative of an upper urinary tract infection?
    A. Bacteria
    B. Casts
    C. Erythrocytes
    D. Leukocytes

23. The most common cause of chronic pyelonephritis is
    A. cystitis.
    B. bacterial sepsis.
    C. drug-induced nephropathies.
    D. reflux nephropathies.

24. Eosinophiluria, fever, and skin rash are characteristic clinical features of
    A. acute pyelonephritis.
    B. acute interstitial nephritis.
    C. acute glomerulonephritis.
    D. chronic glomerulonephritis.

25. Cessation of the administration of a drug is the fastest and most effective treatment for
    A. acute pyelonephritis.
    B. acute interstitial nephritis.
    C. acute glomerulonephritis.
    D. chronic glomerulonephritis.

26. Yeast is considered part of the normal flora in each of the following locations except in the
    A. gastrointestinal tract.
    B. oral cavity.
    C. urinary tract.
    D. vagina.

27. Acute renal failure can be caused by all of the following except
    A. hemorrhage.
    B. acute tubular necrosis.
    C. acute pyelonephritis.
    D. urinary tract obstruction.

28. Which of the following statements about chronic renal failure is true?
    A. It can be reversed by appropriate treatment regimens.
    B. It eventually progresses to end-stage renal disease.
    C. It is monitored by periodic determinations of renal blood flow.
    D. Its onset involves a sudden decrease in the glomerular filtration rate.

29. Isosthenuria, significant proteinuria, and numerous casts of all types describes the urinalysis findings from a patient with
    A. acute renal failure.
    B. acute tubular necrosis.
    C. chronic renal failure.
    D. renal tubular acidosis.
30. Approximately 75% of the renal calculi that form in patients contain
    A. calcium.
    B. cystine.
    C. oxalate.
    D. uric acid.
31. The formation of renal calculi is *enhanced* by
    A. an increase in urine flow.
    B. the natural "acid-alkaline tide" of the body.
    C. increases in protein in the urine ultrafiltrate.
    D. increases in chemical salts in the urine ultrafiltrate.
32. An overflow mechanism is responsible for the aminoaciduria present in
    A. cystinosis.
    B. cystinuria.
    C. tyrosinuria.
    D. phenylketonuria.
33. Which of the following hereditary diseases results in the accumulation and excretion of large amounts of homogentisic acid?
    A. Alkaptonuria
    B. Melanuria
    C. Phenylketonuria
    D. Tyrosinuria
34. Which of the following substances oxidizes with exposure to air, causing the urine to turn brown or black?
    A. Melanin
    B. Porphyrin
    C. Tyrosine
    D. Urobilinogen
35. Which of the following diseases is related to tyrosine production or metabolism?
    1. Tyrosinuria
    2. Melanuria
    3. Phenylketonuria
    4. Alkaptonuria
    A. 1, 2, and 3 are correct.
    B. 1 and 3 are correct.
    C. 4 is correct.
    D. All are correct.

36. Which of the following diseases can result in severe mental retardation if not detected and treated in the infant?
    1. Phenylketonuria
    2. Maple syrup urine disease
    3. Galactosuria
    4. Alkaptonuria
    A. 1, 2, and 3 are correct.
    B. 1 and 3 are correct.
    C. 4 is correct.
    D. All are correct.
37. Which of the following is a characteristic feature of type 2 diabetes mellitus?
    A. Daily insulin injections are necessary.
    B. Onset of the disease is usually sudden.
    C. Strong tendency to develop ketoacidosis.
    D. The disease usually presents after 40 years of age.
38. Which of the following abnormalities is not a clinical feature of an infant with galactosuria?
    A. Cataract formation
    B. Liver dysfunction
    C. Mental retardation
    D. Polyuria
39. Galactose is produced in the normal metabolism of
    A. fructose.
    B. glucose.
    C. lactose.
    D. sucrose.
40. Which of the following features is not a characteristic of diabetes insipidus?
    A. Polyuria
    B. Polydipsia
    C. Increased production of antidiuretic hormone
    D. Urine with a low specific gravity
41. Porphyria is characterized by
    A. increased heme degradation.
    B. increased heme formation.
    C. decreased globin synthesis.
    D. decreased iron catabolism.
42. Which of the following statements regarding porphyrin and porphyrin precursors is true?
    1. Porphyria can be inherited or induced.
    2. Porphyrin precursors are neurotoxins.
    3. Porphyrins can be dark red or purple.
    4. Porphyrin precursor accumulation causes skin photosensitivity.
    A. 1, 2, and 3 are correct.
    B. 1 and 3 are correct.
    C. 4 is correct.
    D. All are correct.

CASE 9-1

A 30-year-old woman is seen by her physician. She has a temperature of 101° F and reports nausea and headache, with flank (below ribs and above ileac crest) tenderness and pain. When asked, she states that urination is sometimes painful, that she must urinate much more frequently than usual, and that she has a sensation of urgency. A random, midstream clean catch urine specimen is collected for a routine urinalysis and culture.

Results

Physical Examination	Chemical Examination	Microscopic Examination
Color: yellow	SG: 1.010	RBC/hpf: 0-2
Clarity: cloudy	pH: 6.5	WBC/hpf: 25-50
Odor: —	Blood: trace	Casts/lpf: 0-2 granular;
	Protein: 30 mg/dL	2-5 WBC
	SSA: 1+	Epithelials: few SE cells/hpf
	LE: positive	Crystals/hpf: few CaOx
	Nitrite: positive	Bacteria/hpf: moderate
	Glucose: negative	
	Ketones: negative	
	Bilirubin: negative	
	Urobilinogen: normal	
	Ascorbic acid: negative	

1. List any abnormal or discrepant urinalysis findings.
2. Select the most probable diagnosis.
   A. Normal urinalysis
   B. Yeast infection
   C. Upper urinary tract infection (upper UTI)
   D. Lower urinary tract infection (lower UTI)
3. Which single microscopic finding is most helpful in differentiating an upper UTI from a lower UTI?
   A. Red blood cells
   B. White blood cells
   C. Casts
   D. Bacteria
   E. Epithelial cells
4. Another name for this condition is
   A. urethritis.
   B. acute cystitis.
   C. acute pyelonephritis.
   D. acute interstitial nephritis.
5. State two physiologic mechanisms that can lead to the development of this condition.
6. Suggest a reason for the trace blood result yet a normal number of red blood cells (0 to 2 per hpf) observed microscopically.
7. At this patient's level of hematuria, is the blood that is present most likely contributing to the reagent strip protein result of 30 mg/dL? Explain briefly.

CaOx, Calcium oxalate; *hpf,* high-power field; *LE,* leukocyte esterase; *lpf,* low-power field; *RBC,* red blood cell; *SSA,* sulfosalicylic acid precipitation test; *SE,* squamous epithelial; *WBC,* white blood cell.

CASE 9-2

A 58-year-old male is seen in the emergency department and reports intermittent severe pain that radiates from his right side to his abdomen and groin area (renal colic). He has a frequent need to urinate with little or no urine output. Other complaints include a cold that he has been self-treating with over-the-counter medications and vitamin supplements for longer than a week.

Results

Physical Examination	Chemical Examination	Microscopic Examination
Color: pink	SG: >1.030	RBC/hpf: 10-25
Clarity: slightly	Refractometry: 1.035	WBC/hpf: 5-10
cloudy	pH: 5.5	Casts/lpf: 0-2 hyaline
Odor: —	Blood: negative	Epithelials: few TE
	Protein: trace	cells/hpf
	SSA: trace	Crystals/hpf: many CaOx
	LE: negative	Bacteria/hpf: few
	Nitrite: positive	
	Glucose: negative	
	Ketones: negative	
	Bilirubin: negative	
	Urobilinogen: normal	

1. List any abnormal or discrepant urinalysis findings.
2. For each discrepancy, list a test that could be performed to confirm or deny the cause for the discrepancy.
3. Based on the information provided, which of the following is the most probable cause of this patient's condition?
   A. Renal calculi
   B. Urinary tract infection
   C. Acute glomerulonephritis
   D. Drug-induced acute interstitial nephritis
4. State at least three factors that could influence the development of this patient's condition.

CaOx, Calcium oxalate; *hpf,* high-power field; *LE,* leukocyte esterase; *lpf,* low-power field; *RBC,* red blood cell; *SSA,* sulfosalicylic acid precipitation test; *SE,* squamous epithelial; *WBC,* white blood cell.

CASE 9-3

A 14-day-old baby girl is admitted to the hospital with lethargy, diarrhea, vomiting, and difficulty in feeding. Physical examination reveals jaundice, an enlarged liver, and neurologic abnormalities (e.g., increased muscular tonus). No blood group incompatibility is found. She has lost 1.8 lb since birth. The infant is fitted with a collection bag to obtain a urine specimen. The collection takes place over several hours, and the baby's urine is sent to the laboratory for routine urinalysis.

Results

Physical Examination	Chemical Examination	Microscopic Examination
Color: amber	SG: 1.025	RBC/hpf: 0-2
Clarity: cloudy	pH: 8.0	WBC/hpf: 0-2
Odor: —	Blood: negative	Casts/lpf: 0-2 hyaline;
Yellow foam	Protein: trace	0-2 granular
noted.	SSA: 1+	Epithelials: few SE cells/lpf
	LE: negative	Crystals/hpf: moderate
	Nitrite: negative	triple
	Glucose: negative	phosphate
	Clinitest: 1000 mg/dL	Bacteria/hpf: few
	Ketones: negative	
	Bilirubin: positive	
	Ictotest: positive	
	Urobilinogen: normal	

1. List any abnormal or discrepant urinalysis findings.
2. Which results may have been modified by the specimen collection conditions?
3. What substance is most likely causing the yellow coloration of the foam?
4. What is the most likely explanation for the discrepancy in the glucose screening results?
5. What is a possible diagnosis for this patient? How could this diagnosis be confirmed?
6. Does this patient have a urinary tract infection? Why or why not?

hpf, High-power field; *LE,* leukocyte esterase; *lpf,* low-power field; *RBC,* red blood cell; *SSA,* sulfosalicylic acid precipitation test; *SE,* squamous epithelial; *WBC,* white blood cell.

CASE 9-4

A 6-year-old boy is brought to the hospital emergency department by his mother. This morning after his bath, she noticed that his scrotum appeared swollen. In addition, for the past several days her son has been has been tired—that is, definitely not his active self—and has been complaining of a headache. Physical examination is unremarkable except for mild peripheral edema of the eyelids, scrotum, and lower limbs. No skin rash or fever is present. During the examination, the boy reveals that he "doesn't need to go potty much anymore." The previous week, the boy had a routine wellness physical and received a booster of the diphtheria-pertussis-tetanus vaccine. The following blood tests and routine urinalysis were obtained:

Urinalysis Results

Physical Examination	Chemical Examination	Microscopic Examination
Color: dark yellow	SG: 1.030	RBC/hpf: 0-2
Clarity: clear	pH: 6.0	WBC/hpf: 0-2
Odor: —	Blood: negative	Casts/lpf: 0-2 hyaline
White foam that	Protein: 500 mg/dL	Epithelials: none seen
does not dissipate	SSA: 3+	Crystals/hpf: few
was noted.	LE: negative	amorphous
	Nitrite: negative	urates
	Glucose: negative	Bacteria: none seen
	Ketones: negative	
	Bilirubin: negative	
	Urobilinogen: normal	

Blood Results	Reference Range
Sodium: 136 mmol/L	136-145 mmol/L
Potassium: 4.2 mmol/L	3.5-5.0 mmol/L
Glucose: 92 mg/dL	70-105 mg/dL
Urea nitrogen: 25 mg/dL	11-23 mg/dL
Creatinine: 0.8 mg/dL	0.6-1.2 mg/dL

Blood Results	Reference Range
Total protein: 4.8 g/dL	6.0-8.0 g/dL
Albumin: 1.3 g/dL	3.5-5.5 g/dL
Cholesterol: 282 mg/dL	<200 mg/dL
Triglyceride: 255 mg/dL	<150 mg/dL

1. List any abnormal or discrepant urinalysis findings.
2. What urinary substance is responsible for the white foam noted during the urinalysis?
3. If the glomerular filtration barrier loses its "shield of negativity," which plasma protein is usually lost first? Explain your selection.
4. Explain the physiologic processes responsible for the edema exhibited in this patient.
5. The proteinuria in this patient should be classified as
   A. glomerular proteinuria.
   B. tubular proteinuria.
   C. overflow proteinuria.
   D. postrenal proteinuria.
6. Based on the patient's symptoms (edema) and laboratory results (proteinuria, hypoalbuminemia, hyperlipidemia), select the most probable disorder.
   A. acute glomerulonephritis.
   B. acute pyelonephritis.
   C. acute renal failure.
   D. nephrotic syndrome.

   By exclusion, it was determined this patient had minimal change disease that presented as (see answer to question 6), and he was treated promptly with corticosteroids (i.e., oral prednisone). In 8 days, his urine output increased significantly, and his urine protein result decreased to 30 mg/dL. A routine urinalysis another 24 hours later was negative for urine protein.

hpf, High-power field; *LE,* leukocyte esterase; *lpf,* low-power field; *RBC,* red blood cell; *SSA,* sulfosalicylic acid precipitation test; *WBC,* white blood cell.

CASE 9-5

Two days previous, a 26-year-old woman saw her primary care physician, and it was determined that she had a urinary tract infection. A conventional 10-day regimen of ampicillin was prescribed. Today, she returns to the clinic with a fever and urticarial rash on her chest, back, face, and hands. The following routine urinalysis is obtained:

Urinalysis Results

Physical Examination	Chemical Examination	Microscopic Examination
Color: dark yellow	SG: 1.015	RBC/hpf: 5-10
Clarity: cloudy	pH: 6.5	WBC/hpf: 10-25
Odor: —	Blood: small	Casts/lpf: 0-2 WBC; 0-2 RTE; 2-5 granular
	Protein: 100 mg/dL	
	LE: positive (1+)	Epithelials: moderate RTE cells/hpf; few TE cells/hpf; few SE cells/lpf
	Nitrite: negative	
	Glucose: negative	
	Ketones: negative	
	Bilirubin: negative	Crystals/hpf: few urates
	Urobilinogen: normal	Bacteria/hpf: few

1. List any abnormal or discrepant urinalysis findings.
2. A cytospin preparation of the urine sediment is performed and stained using Hansel stain. A differential white cell count of the sediment reveals 12% eosinophils. Based on this finding and the urinalysis results, the most likely diagnosis is
   A. acute glomerulonephritis.
   B. acute interstitial nephritis.
   C. acute pyelonephritis.
   D. nephrotic syndrome.
3. The proteinuria in this patient should be classified as
   A. glomerular proteinuria.
   B. tubular proteinuria.
   C. overflow proteinuria.
   D. postrenal proteinuria.
4. Which microscopic findings indicate that the inflammatory process is in the kidneys?
5. State three reasons why the nitrite test is negative despite the presence of bacteria in the urine sediment.

hpf, High-power field; *LE*, leukocyte esterase; *lpf*, low-power field; *RBC*, red blood cell; *RTE*, renal tubular epithelial; *SE*, squamous epithelial; *TE*, transitional epithelial; *WBC*, white blood cell.

CASE 9-6

A 43-year-old woman with a 15-year history of systemic lupus erythematosus is transferred to a university hospital because of significant deterioration of renal function. The following routine urinalysis is obtained on admission:

Urinalysis Results

Physical Examination	Chemical Examination	Microscopic Examination
Color: brown	SG: 1.010	RBC/hpf: 25-50; dysmorphic forms present
Clarity: cloudy	pH: 7.0	
Odor: —	Blood: large	WBC/hpf: 5-10
	Protein: 100 mg/dL	Casts/lpf: 0-2 RBC; 5-10 granular; 0-2 hyaline
	LE: negative	
	Nitrite: negative	
	Glucose: negative	
	Ketones: negative	Epithelials: few TE cells/hpf
	Bilirubin: negative	Crystals/hpf: few CaOx
	Urobilinogen: normal	Bacteria: none seen

1. List any abnormal or discrepant urinalysis findings.
2. What substance most likely accounts for the brown color of this urine?
3. State two reasons to explain why the leukocyte esterase test is negative despite increased numbers of white blood cells in the urine sediment.
4. At this patient's level of hematuria, is the blood that is present contributing to the reagent strip protein result? Explain briefly.
5. List the microscopic finding(s) that indicate whether hematuria/hemorrhage is occurring in the nephrons?
6. The proteinuria in this patient should be classified as
   A. glomerular proteinuria.
   B. tubular proteinuria.
   C. overflow proteinuria.
   D. postrenal proteinuria.
7. Based on the information provided and the results obtained, the most likely diagnosis is
   A. acute glomerulonephritis.
   B. acute interstitial nephritis.
   C. acute pyelonephritis.
   D. nephrotic syndrome.
8. Briefly describe a physiologic mechanism to account for the development of this patient's condition (as cited in question 7).

CaOx, Calcium oxalate; *hpf*, high-power field; *LE*, leukocyte esterase; *lpf*, low-power field; *RBC*, red blood cell; *TE*, transitional epithelial; *WBC*, white blood cell.

REFERENCES

1. de Wardener HE: The kidney, ed 5, New York, 1985, Churchill Livingstone.
2. Diabetes Control and Complications Trial Research Group: The effect of intensive treatment of diabetes on the development and progression of long-term complications of insulin-dependent diabetes mellitus. N Engl J Med 329:927, 1993.
3. Turner RC, Holman RR, Cull CA, et al: Intensive blood-glucose control with sulphonylureas or insulin compared with conventional treatment and risk of complications in patients with type 2 diabetes (UKPDS 33). Lancet 352:837, 1998.
4. Anderson RJ, Schrier RW: Acute tubular necrosis. In Diseases of the kidney, ed 5, Boston, 1993, Little, Brown & Company.
5. Cotran RS, Leaf A: Renal pathophysiology, ed 3, New York, 1985, Oxford University Press.
6. Sharfuddin AA, Molitoris BA: Pathophysiology of acute kidney injury. In Alpern RJ, Hebert SC, editors: The kidney, ed 4, Amsterdam, 2008, Elsevier Inc.
7. Khan SR, Glenton PA, Backov R, Talham DR: Presence of lipids in urine, crystals and stones: implications for the formation of kidney stones. Kidney Int 62:2062, 2002.
8. Coe FL, Parks JH, Evan A, Worcester E: Pathogenesis and treatment of nephrolithiasis. In Alpern RJ, Hebert SC, editors: The kidney, ed 4, Amsterdam, 2008, Elsevier Inc.
9. Hruska K: Renal calculi (nephrolithiasis). In Goldman L, Bennett JC, editors: Cecil textbook of medicine, ed 21, Philadelphia, 2000, WB Saunders.
10. Gahl WA, Thoene JG, Schneider JA. Cystinosis. N Engl J Med 347:111, 2002.
11. Sherwin RS: Diabetes mellitus. In Goldman L, Bennett JC, editors: Cecil textbook of medicine, ed 21, Philadelphia, 2000, WB Saunders.

Fecal Analysis

LEARNING OBJECTIVES

After studying this chapter, the student should be able to:

1. Describe the composition and formation of normal feces.
2. Describe the effect of abnormal intestinal water reabsorption on the consistency of feces.
3. Classify the condition of diarrhea according to the physiologic mechanisms involved.
4. Differentiate between secretory and osmotic diarrhea using the fecal osmolality.
5. Identify at least three causes of secretory and osmotic diarrhea.
6. Compare and contrast the mechanisms of maldigestion and malabsorption and the relationship of each to diarrhea.
7. Differentiate steatorrhea from diarrhea and discuss the physiologic conditions that result in steatorrhea.
8. Describe the following types of fecal collections and give an example of a test requiring each type:
   - A random stool collection, with and without dietary restrictions
   - A 3-day fecal collection, with and without dietary restrictions
9. Describe the macroscopic characteristics of normal feces.
10. List the major causes of abnormal fecal color, consistency, and odor.
11. State the primary purpose of the microscopic examination for fecal leukocytes.
12. Discuss the qualitative assessment of fecal fat using a microscopic examination and the clinical utility of quantitative fecal fat tests.
13. List at least five causes of blood in feces and state the importance of fecal occult blood detection.
14. Discuss the advantages and disadvantages of the different indicators used on commercial slide tests for fecal occult blood.
15. Compare and contrast the following methods for the detection of fecal blood:
    - Slide tests
    - Quantitative chemical tests
    - Immunologic assays
    - Radiometric assays
16. Describe the chemical principle used for screening feces or vomitus for fetal hemoglobin.
17. Discuss the effect that disaccharidase deficiency has on fecal characteristics and formation.
18. State two methods for the qualitative detection of abnormal quantities of fecal carbohydrates.
19. State the purpose and describe the principle of the xylose absorption test.

CHAPTER OUTLINE

Fecal Formation
Diarrhea
Steatorrhea
Specimen Collection
   Patient Education
   Specimen Containers
   Type and Amount Collected
   Contaminants to Avoid
   Gas Formation

Macroscopic Examination
   Color
   Consistency and Form
   Mucus
   Odor
Microscopic Examination
   Fecal Leukocytes
   Fecal Fat, Qualitative
   Meat Fibers

Chemical Examination
   Fecal Blood
   Fetal Hemoglobin in Feces (Apt Test)
   Quantitative Fecal Fat
   Fecal Carbohydrates

KEY TERMS

acholic stools Pale, gray, or clay-colored stools. They occur when production of normal fecal pigments—stercobilin, mesobilin, and

urobilin—is partially or completely inhibited.
constipation Infrequent and difficult bowel movements, compared with an individual's

normal bowel movement pattern. The fecal material produced consists of hard, small, often spherical masses.

diarrhea An increase in the volume, liquidity, and frequency of bowel movements compared with the normal bowel movement pattern of an individual.

disaccharidase deficiency A lack of sufficient enzymes (disaccharidases) to metabolize disaccharides in the small intestine. These deficiencies can be hereditary or acquired (e.g., resulting from diseases, drug therapy).

malabsorption Inadequate intestinal absorption of processed foodstuffs despite normal digestive ability.

maldigestion An inability to convert foodstuffs in the gastrointestinal tract into readily absorbable substances.

melena Excretion of dark or black stools caused by the presence of large amounts (50 to 100 mL/day) of blood in the feces. The coloration is due to hemoglobin oxidation by intestinal and bacterial enzymes in the gastrointestinal tract.

occult blood Small amounts of blood, not visually apparent, in the feces.

steatorrhea The excretion of greater than 6 g/day of fat in the feces.

urobilins Orange-brown pigments responsible for the characteristic color of feces. Specifically, stercobilin, mesobilin, and urobilin, which result from spontaneous intestinal oxidation of the colorless tetrapyrroles: stercobilinogen, mesobilinogen, and urobilinogen.

Examination of feces provides important information that aids in the differential diagnosis of various gastrointestinal tract disorders, which range from maldigestion and malabsorption to bleeding or infestation by bacteria, viruses, or parasites. Hepatic and biliary conditions that result in decreased bile secretion, as well as pancreatic diseases that cause insufficient digestive enzymes, also are identifiable by fecal analysis. By far the test that currently is most commonly performed on feces is the chemical test for occult, or hidden, blood. Occult blood is recognized as the earliest and most frequent initial symptom of colorectal cancer. Fecal blood testing is recommended to be performed routinely on all individuals 50 years of age and older. Bleeding anywhere in the gastrointestinal tract, from the mouth to the anus, can result in a positive fecal blood test; additional follow-up testing is required, however, to identify the specific cause of the bleeding. Fecal analysis is also valuable for determining the presence of increased fecal lipids (steatorrhea) and in the differential diagnosis of diarrhea. This chapter discusses the macroscopic, microscopic, and chemical examinations of feces often performed in the laboratory. For fecal reference intervals, see Appendix B.

FECAL FORMATION

Normally, about 100 to 200 g of fecal material is passed each day. The feces consist of undigested foodstuffs (e.g., cellulose), sloughed intestinal epithelium, intestinal bacteria, gastrointestinal secretions (e.g., digestive enzymes), bile pigments, electrolytes, and water. Because of the slow movement of fecal material in the large intestine, it normally takes 18 to 24 hours for the contents presented to it by the small intestine to be excreted as feces.

The function of the small intestine includes the digestion and absorption of foodstuffs, whereas the principal function of the large intestine is the absorption of water, sodium, and chloride. Approximately 9000 mL of fluid enters the gastrointestinal tract from food, water, saliva, gastric secretions, bile, pancreatic secretions, and small intestinal secretions. Only 500 to 1500 mL actually enters the large intestine each day, however, with a final excretion of only about 150 mL of fluid in normal feces. Because the large intestine has a limited ability to absorb liquid (up to about 2700 mL), a volume of fluid presented to it that exceeds this capacity causes watery stools (diarrhea). Similarly, if water absorption is inhibited, or if inadequate time is allowed for the absorption process, diarrhea results. In contrast, stationary bowel contents (or decreased intestinal motility) permit increased water absorption, resulting in **constipation.** Fecal specimens from constipated individuals are typically small, hard, often spherical masses (scybala) that are often difficult and painful to pass.

Fermentation by intestinal bacteria in the large intestine results in the production of intestinal gas or flatus and is normally produced at a rate of about 400 to 700 mL/day. Some carbohydrates are not digested completely by intestinal enzymes (e.g., brown beans) and are readily metabolized by intestinal bacteria to produce large amounts of gas. Increased gas production and its incorporation into the feces can result in foamy and floating stools. Although these stools can be normal, they are often produced by patients with lactose intolerance and steatorrhea.

DIARRHEA

Diarrhea is defined as an increase in the volume, liquidity, and frequency of bowel movements compared with an individual's normal bowel movement pattern. Diarrhea can be classified into three types: secretory diarrhea, osmotic diarrhea, and diarrhea caused by intestinal hypermotility (Table 10-1). With secretory and osmotic diarrhea, the presence of an unabsorbed solute draws and retains water in the intestinal lumen. The origin of this osmotically active solute differs. Secretory diarrhea results from increased intestinal secretion of a solute; osmotic diarrhea results from ingestion of an osmotically active solute (e.g., lactose).

TABLE 10-1	Classification of Diarrhea	
Type	**Mechanism**	**Common Causes**
Secretory diarrhea	Increased solute secretions by the intestine cause increased fluid volume sent to the large intestine; the resultant fluid volume exceeds the absorptive capacity of the large intestine.	Enterotoxin-producing organisms (e.g., *Vibrio cholerae, Salmonella, Shigella, Escherichia coli, Clostridium, Staphylococcus,* protozoa) Mucosal involvement (e.g., viral gastroenteritis, ulcerative colitis, drugs) Neoplasms Drugs or hormones (e.g., caffeine, prostaglandin, vasoactive intestinal peptide)
Osmotic diarrhea	Increased quantities of osmotically active solutes remain in the intestinal lumen, causing additional secretions of water and electrolytes into the lumen; the resultant fluid volume exceeds the absorptive capacity of the large intestine.	Maldigestion (e.g., lactase deficiency, lipase deficiency) Malabsorption of nonelectrolytes (e.g., mucosal disease) Laxative action of some drugs (e.g., antacids, sorbitol, tetracycline, lincomycin) Parasitic infestations (e.g., giardiasis, strongyloidiasis) Surgical procedures (e.g., small bowel resection)
Intestinal hypermotility	An increase in intestinal motility decreases the time allowed for the intestinal absorptive processes.	Secretory and osmotic diarrhea Parasympathetic nerve activity Laxatives (e.g., castor oil) Emotions (e.g., stress) Cardiovascular drugs (e.g., digitalis, quinidine)

Differentiating these two conditions requires determination of the fecal osmolality, fecal sodium, and fecal potassium levels. Using the fecal sodium and potassium results, a "calculated" fecal osmolality is determined using Equation 10-1.

Equation 10-1

$$\text{Calculated fecal osmolality} = 2 \times (Na^+_{fecal} + K^+_{fecal})$$

If the difference (i.e., osmotic gap) between measured and calculated fecal osmolality exceeds 20 mOsm/kg, the patient is experiencing osmotic diarrhea. If measured and calculated fecal osmolalities agree within 10 to 20 mOsm/kg, the patient is experiencing secretory diarrhea.

Secretory diarrhea is characteristic of infestation with various enterotoxin-producing organisms. These microbes release substances that stimulate electrolyte-rich intestinal secretions. Similarly, damage to intestinal mucosal due to drugs or disease can also cause secretory diarrhea.

Osmotic diarrhea accompanies conditions characterized by maldigestion or malabsorption. **Maldigestion,** the inability to convert foodstuffs into readily absorbable substances, most often results from various pancreatic and hepatic diseases. With these disorders, the pancreatic digestive enzymes or bile salts needed for fat emulsification and lipase activation are deficient or lacking. The absence of other digestive enzymes, such as disaccharidases (e.g., lactase) in the small intestine, can also result in maldigestion. In contrast, intestinal **malabsorption** is characterized by normal digestive ability but inadequate intestinal absorption of the already processed foodstuffs. Some parasitic infestations, mucosal diseases (e.g., celiac sprue, tropical sprue, ulcerative colitis), hereditary diseases (e.g., disaccharidase deficiencies),

surgical procedures, and drugs can cause malabsorption and osmotic diarrhea. In summary, maldigestion and malabsorption present an abnormally increased quantity of foodstuffs to the large intestine. These osmotically active substances (i.e., the foodstuffs) cause the retention of large quantities of water and electrolytes in the intestinal lumen and the excretion of a watery stool or diarrhea.

Intestinal hypermotility results in diarrhea when the transit time for intestinal contents is too short to allow normal intestinal absorption to occur. Normally, intestinal motility is stimulated by intestinal distention. Foodstuffs that are bulky, such as dietary fiber, produce a natural laxative effect because of the intestinal distention they cause. Intestinal motility can also be altered by chemicals, nerves, hormones, and emotions. Laxatives (e.g., castor oil) and parasympathetic nerve activity increase intestinal motility, whereas sympathetic nerve activity decreases intestinal motility. During secretory and osmotic diarrhea, the increased lumen fluid causes intestinal distention, thereby increasing intestinal motility and compounding the diarrheal condition.

When severe, diarrhea decreases the blood volume (hypovolemia) and disrupts the acid-base balance of the body. The large fluid loss and accompanying electrolyte depletion (particularly sodium, bicarbonate, and potassium) can result in metabolic acidosis.

STEATORRHEA

Normally, fecal excretion of fat consists of less than 7 g per day. This fat originates from several sources: the diet, gastrointestinal secretions, bacterial by-products of metabolism, and sloughed intestinal epithelium. Note

TABLE 10-2	Comparison of Diarrhea and Steatorrhea				
Condition	Fecal Characteristics	Fecal Volume	Fecal Frequency	Cause	Clinical Features
Diarrhea	Watery; odor normal or unremarkable	Increased	Increased	Disruption in water and electrolyte absorption	Water and electrolyte imbalance; acidosis; hypovolemia
Steatorrhea	Greasy; foul odor; spongy consistency	Increased	Normal or increased	Maldigestion or malabsorption of dietary fat	Malnutrition; weight loss

that the amount of dietary fat ingested has a minor effect on the total quantity of fecal lipids excreted; in addition, the types of lipid (fatty acid salts, neutral fat) excreted can vary significantly from the dietary fat ingested.[1]

Fecal fat excretion that exceeds 7 g per day is called **steatorrhea** and is a common feature of patients with malabsorption syndromes. Steatorrheal fecal specimens are characteristically pale, greasy, bulky, spongy, or pasty and are extremely foul smelling. They vary in fluidity and may float or be foamy because of the presence of large amounts of gas within them. This latter feature is not particularly significant because normal stools may also contain gas.

Differentiation of steatorrhea from diarrhea is clinically important (Table 10-2). Although macroscopic examination of the feces can be highly suggestive of steatorrhea, some diarrheal conditions can make differentiation difficult. Therefore to diagnose steatorrhea, a fecal fat determination is performed (see "Chemical Examination"). Any condition that alters fat digestion or fat absorption will present with steatorrhea (Table 10-3).

Conditions producing steatorrhea can occur simultaneously with diarrhea. For appropriate patient management to begin, the cause of the diarrhea, steatorrhea, or both must be identified. Usually, this is achieved by following an algorithm similar to that in Figure 10-1. Because a definitive diagnosis may not be readily apparent, a good patient history is invaluable. The patient history can provide information that directly relates to the cause of the patient's condition (e.g., diet, environment, recent exposure or contacts). For example, following the algorithm in Figure 10-1 to a negative stool culture rules out specific bacteria but does not exclude parasites, viruses, or other inflammatory conditions. A good patient history can reveal significant information such as a visit to a foreign country, exposure to a contaminated water source, ingestion of herbs that can be cathartic, or recent intake of fresh oysters.

SPECIMEN COLLECTION

Patient Education

Unlike urination, individuals have limited control in the timing of their fecal excretion. In addition, collecting fecal specimens is highly undesirable by most individuals,

TABLE 10-3	Causes of Steatorrhea
Type	Cause
Maldigestion	*Decreased pancreatic enzymes*
	Pancreatitis
	Cystic fibrosis
	Pancreatic cancer
	Zollinger-Ellison syndrome
	Ileal resection
	Decreased bile acid micelle formation
	Hepatocellular disease (severe)
	Bile duct obstruction; biliary cirrhosis
	Bile acid deconjugation caused by stasis (e.g., strictures, blind loop syndrome, diabetic visceral neuropathy)
Malabsorption	*Damaged intestinal mucosa*
	Celiac disease
	Tropical sprue
	Biochemical defect: abetalipoproteinemia
	Lymphatic obstruction
	Lymphoma
	Whipple's disease

and it is postulated to be at least partially responsible for the high noncompliance rate (50% to 90%) in collecting fecal specimens for occult blood testing observed in studies of colorectal cancer.[2] In light of these facts, patient education regarding the importance of testing and proper collection of fecal specimens is of utmost importance. Verbal and written instructions should be provided to patients along with an appropriate specimen container.

Specimen Containers

Fecal specimen containers vary depending on the amount of specimen to be collected. Essentially any clean, non-breakable container that is sealable and leakproof is acceptable. For specimen collections over multiple days, large containers such as paint cans frequently are used. Single, random collections can be placed in routine urine collection cups or other suitable containers. For some tests, the entire stool is not required for analysis, and the patient must be instructed regarding the portion of the stool to sample or transport to the laboratory. Some commercial fecal collection kits are available for

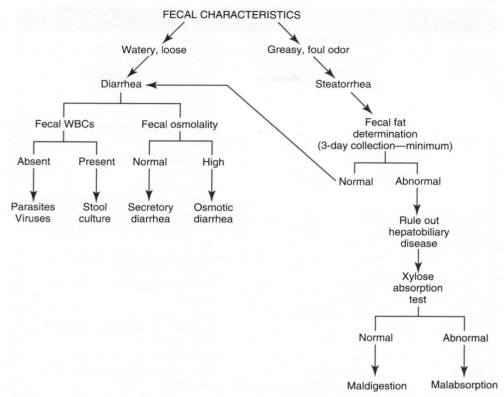

FECAL CHARACTERISTICS

FIGURE 10-1 An algorithm to aid in the evaluation of diarrhea and steatorrhea. *WBC,* White blood cell.

the recovery of feces after they are passed into the toilet onto a sheet of floating tissue paper. These kits have greatly facilitated fecal collection by patients. After sampling a portion of the feces, the patient can flush the remainder.

Type and Amount Collected

The type and amount of specimen collected vary with the test to be performed. Fecal analysis for occult blood, white blood cells, or qualitative fecal fat requires only a small amount of a randomly collected specimen. In contrast, quantitative tests for the daily fecal excretion of any substance usually require a 2- or 3-day fecal collection. Multiple day collections are necessary because the daily excretion of feces does not correlate well with the amount of food ingested by the patient in the same 24-hour period. In addition, to ensure an optimum fecal specimen, dietary restrictions may be necessary before the collection (e.g., tests for occult blood and quantitative fecal fat).

Contaminants to Avoid

Contamination of the fecal specimen with urine, toilet tissue, or toilet water must be avoided. The detection of protozoa can be adversely affected by contaminating urine, and the strong cleaning or deodorizing agents used in toilets can interfere with chemical testing. Patients

must also be instructed to avoid (1) contaminating the exterior of collection containers, and (2) applying too much sample to a collection device or slide.

Gas Formation

Fecal specimens produce gas because of bacterial fermentation in vivo and in vitro. Therefore closed containers of fecal specimens should be covered with a disposable tissue or toweling and slowly opened. This covering retards spattering of fecal matter should gas buildup cause the sudden release of fecal contents when the container is opened.

MACROSCOPIC EXAMINATION

Color

The macroscopic examination of feces involves visual assessment of color, consistency, and form. Other notable substances within the feces include mucus and undigested matter. The normal brown color of feces results from bile pigments. When conjugated bilirubin is secreted as bile into the small intestine, it is hydrolyzed back to its unconjugated form. Intestinal anaerobic bacteria subsequently reduce it to the three colorless tetrapyrroles collectively called the *urobilinogens:* stercobilinogen, mesobilinogen, and urobilinogen. These urobilinogens spontaneously oxidize in the intestine to

TABLE 10-4	Fecal Macroscopic Characteristics	
	Characteristic	**Cause**
Color	Clay-colored or gray, pale yellow, or white	Posthepatic obstruction
		Barium (ingestion or enema)
	Red	Blood (from lower GI tract)
		Beets
		Food dyes
		Drugs (e.g., BSP dye, rifampin)
	Brown	Normal
	Black	Blood (from upper GI tract)
		Iron therapy
		Charcoal ingestion
		Bismuth (e.g., medications, suppositories)
	Green	Green vegetables (e.g., spinach)
		Biliverdin (during antibiotic therapy)
Consistency	Formed	Normal
	Hard	Constipation (i.e., scybalum)
	Soft	Increased fecal water
	Watery	Diarrhea, steatorrhea
Form	Cylindrical	Normal
	Narrow, ribbon-like	Bowel obstruction
		Intestinal narrowing (e.g., strictures)
	Small, round	Constipation
	Bulky	Steatorrhea
Other	Foamy, floating	Increased gas incorporated into feces
	Greasy, spongy	Steatorrhea
	Mucus	Constipation, straining
		Disease (e.g., colitis, villous adenoma)

BSP, Bromsulphalein; *GI*, gastrointestinal.

produce the **urobilins**—stercobilin, mesobilin, and urobilin—which are orange-brown and impart color to the feces. With conditions in which bile secretion into the small intestine is inhibited partially or completely, the color of the feces changes. Pale or clay-colored stools, also termed **acholic stools,** are characteristic of these posthepatic obstructions. Be aware that similarly colored fecal specimens resulting from barium sulfate contamination can be obtained following a diagnostic procedure to evaluate gastrointestinal function (e.g., barium enema). Unusual fecal colors can also be encountered following the ingestion of certain foodstuffs or medications, or as a result of the presence of blood. Table 10-4 summarizes macroscopic characteristics of feces and Table 10-5 provides reference intervals for various tests performed.

Consistency and Form

The consistency of feces ranges from loose and watery stools (diarrhea) to small, hard masses (constipation). Normal feces are usually formed masses; soft stools indicate an increase in fecal water content. The latter can be normal, can be related to laxatives, or can accompany gastrointestinal disorders. A patient history helps the health care provider determine whether the patient has noticed a change in the consistency of his stools. Feces

TABLE 10-5	Fecal Reference Intervals
Physical Examination	
Color	Brown
Consistency	Firm, formed
Form	Tubular, cylindrical
Chemical Examination	
Total fat, quantitative (72-hour specimen)	<6 g/day and <20% of stool
Osmolality	285 to 430 mOsm/kg H_2O
Potassium	30 to 140 mEq/L
Sodium	40 to 110 mEq/L
Microscopic Examination	
Fat, Qualitative Assessment	
Neutral fat	Few globules present per high-power field
Total fat	<100 fat globules (diameter ≤4 microns) per high-power field
Leukocytes (qualitative)	None present
Meat and vegetable fibers (qualitative)	Few

may be bulky because of undigested foodstuffs or increased gas in the stool. Undigested substances such as seed casings, vegetable skins, or proglottids from intestinal parasites may also be apparent. Normal stools are formed, cylindrical masses; in contrast, the excretion of long, ribbon-like stools may indicate intestinal obstruction or lumen narrowing as a result of strictures.

Mucus

Mucus, a translucent gelatinous substance, is not present in normal feces. When present, mucus can vary dramatically from a small amount to the massive quantities associated with a villous adenoma (a tumor of the colon). Mucus has been associated with benign conditions, such as straining during bowel movements or constipation, and with gastrointestinal diseases such as colitis, intestinal tuberculosis, ulcerative diverticulitis, bacillary dysentery, neoplasms, and rectal inflammation.

Odor

The normal odor of feces results from the metabolic by-products of the intestinal bacterial flora. If the normal flora is disrupted or the foodstuffs presented to the flora change dramatically, a change in fecal odor may be noticed. For example, steatorrhea results in distinctively foul-smelling feces because of the bacterial breakdown of undigested lipids.

MICROSCOPIC EXAMINATION

Microscopic examination of the feces is performed on a portion of a stool suspension and can aid in differentiating the cause of diarrhea or in screening for steatorrhea. Microscopically, white blood cells and undigested foodstuffs such as fats, meat fibers, and vegetable fibers can be identified. Although this examination is only qualitative, it is easy to perform and can provide diagnostically useful information.

Fecal Leukocytes

The presence of fecal leukocytes (white blood cells) or pus (an exudate containing white blood cells) aids in the differential diagnosis of diarrhea. Generally, when the intestinal wall is infected or inflamed, fecal leukocytes are present in an inflammatory exudate. In contrast, if the mucosal wall is not compromised, fecal leukocytes are usually not present. Table 10-6 lists disorders in which a microscopic examination for fecal leukocytes aids in the differential diagnosis of diarrhea. Normally, leukocytes are not present in feces; hence the presence of even a small number (one to three per high-power field) indicates an invasive and inflammatory condition. To enhance the identification of leukocytes in feces, wet preparations can be stained using Wright's or methylene blue stain.

Fecal Fat, Qualitative

The presence of an increased amount of fat in feces can be indicated macroscopically and confirmed microscopically and chemically. Steatorrhea (fecal fat excretion that exceeds 7 g/day) is a common feature of maldigestion or malabsorption. Although a qualitative assessment for fecal fat can be performed microscopically, quantitative determinations of fecal fat are used to definitively diagnose steatorrhea.

A simple two-slide qualitative procedure can be used to detect increased fat in feces. This assessment relies on the characteristic orange to red coloration of neutral fat (triglycerides) when a fecal suspension is stained with Sudan III, Sudan IV, or Oil Red O stain. In this procedure, neutral fats are detected when several drops of ethanol (95%) are added to a suspension of feces on a microscope slide. Next, stain is added, a coverslip is applied, and the wet preparation is observed microscopically for the presence of characteristically staining fat globules (Figure 10-2). In health, feces contain less than 60 globules of neutral fat per high-power field.

On a second slide, another aliquot of the fecal suspension is acidified with acetic acid and heated. This slide provides an estimation of the total fecal fat content: neutral fats plus fatty acids and fatty acid salts (soaps). Acidification hydrolyzes soaps to their respective fatty

TABLE 10-6	Disease Differentiation Based on the Presence of Fecal Leukocytes (WBCs)
WBCs Present	**WBCs Absent**
Ulcerative colitis	Amebic colitis
Bacillary dysentery	Viral gastroenteritis
Ulcerative diverticulitis	
Intestinal tuberculosis	
Abscesses or fistulas	

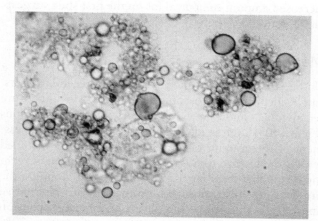

FIGURE 10-2 Numerous globules of neutral fat stained with Sudan III. The orange-red coloration is characteristic. Fat present in fecal suspension during qualitative fecal fat microscopic examination. Brightfield microscopy, 200×.

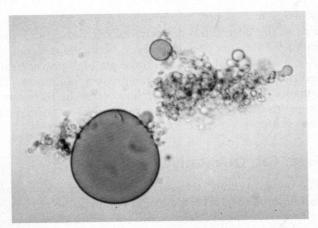

FIGURE 10-3 Large globule of neutral fat stained with Sudan III. The orange-red coloration is characteristic. Brightfield microscopy, 200×.

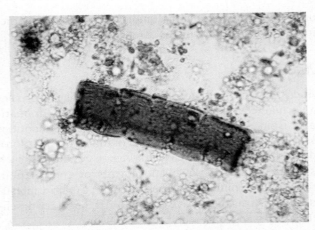

FIGURE 10-4 Meat fiber (note striations on fiber) present in fecal suspension during qualitative fecal fat microscopic examination. Brightfield microscopy, 400×.

acids, and heating causes the fatty acids to absorb the stain. Because fatty acids and their salts (soaps) are present in normal feces, an increased number of orange-red–staining fat globules is observed on the second slide compared with the first. The number of fat globules present and their size (diameter) are important. Normally, fewer than 100 globules per high-power field are observed, and they should not exceed 4 mm in diameter (about half the size of a red blood cell).[3] Increased numbers of globules, as well as extremely large globules (i.e., 40 to 80 mm), are common with steatorrhea (Figure 10-3). Maldigestion can often be differentiated from malabsorption by evaluating the results obtained from the two slides. A normal amount of fecal neutral fat (on the first slide) compared with an increased amount of total fat (on the second slide) indicates intestinal malabsorption. In other words, the increased fat present consists of primarily fatty acids and soaps that were not absorbed by the small intestine. In contrast, an increased amount of neutral fat on the first slide suggests maldigestion.

Meat Fibers

Undigested foodstuffs, such as meat and vegetable fibers, can be identified microscopically in feces. Meat fibers are rectangular and have characteristic cross-striations (Figure 10-4). Often identification and qualitative assessment of the amount of meat fibers present are included with a qualitative fecal fat examination. During screening of the first fecal fat slide for neutral fat globules, the presence of meat fibers is estimated. An alternative approach is to apply a few drops of a fecal suspension to a slide and stain it with a solution of eosin in 10% alcohol. Increased numbers of fecal meat fibers (creatorrhea) correlate with impaired digestion and the rapid transit of intestinal contents.

CHEMICAL EXAMINATION

Fecal Blood

Bleeding anywhere in the gastrointestinal (GI) tract from the mouth (bleeding gums) to the anus (hemorrhoids) can result in detectable blood in the feces. Because fecal blood is a common and early symptom of colorectal cancer, annual screening is recommended by the American Cancer Society on all individuals older than 50 years of age. Of all GI tract cancers, more than 50% are colorectal, and early detection with treatment is directly related to a good prognosis.[4] In addition to cancer, bleeding gums, esophageal varices, ulcers, hemorrhoids, inflammatory conditions, and various drugs that irritate the intestinal mucosa (e.g., aspirin, iron supplements) can cause blood in the feces. When present in large amounts, fecal blood can be macroscopically apparent. With bleeding in the lower GI tract, bright red blood can coat the surface of the stools; in contrast, bleeding in the upper GI tract often causes the stool to appear darker or mahogany-colored. The excretion of dark or black stools resulting from the presence of large amounts of fecal blood (50 to 100 mL/day) is called **melena**. The dark fecal coloration is caused by the degradation of hemoglobin (heme oxidation) by intestinal and bacterial enzymes.

In health, less than 2.5 mL of blood is lost each day in the feces (or approximately 2 mg of hemoglobin per gram of stool). Any increase in fecal blood is significant and requires further investigation to discover its source. A small amount of blood in feces is often not visually apparent and is referred to as **occult blood.**

Other complicating factors to the detection of fecal occult blood are that (1) bleeding in the GI tract is usually intermittent and (2) patients are resistant when it comes to collecting a fecal sample. Note that if bleeding is not occurring at the time of sample collection, the

TABLE 10-7   Fecal Occult Blood Tests

Test	Principle	Advantages	Disadvantages
Guaiac-based	Based on the pseudoperoxidase activity of heme to oxidize colorless guaiac in the presence of hydrogen peroxide to form a blue color	1. Inexpensive 2. Test fast and easy to perform 3. Extensively studied	1. Dietary restrictions required 2. Medication restrictions required 3. False-negative owing to vitamin C intake or hemoglobin degradation 4. Manual method only
Immunochemical-based	Antibody/antigen: Labeled antihuman antibodies to the globin portion of *undegraded* human hemoglobin bind; hemoglobin-antibody complexes are detected visually (manual) or photometrically (automated)	1. No dietary or medication restrictions 2. High specificity; detects *only* undegraded human hemoglobin 3. Test fast and easy to perform 4. Some iFOBTs are automated	1. False-negative owing to hemoglobin degradation 2. Higher cost compared to gFOBT
Porphyrin-based	Fluorescence quantitation of heme-derived porphyrins	1. No dietary restrictions from fruits or vegetables 2. Quantitative assessment of fecal blood; not affected by hemoglobin degradation	1. Test is labor-intensive and time-consuming. 2. False-positive owing to ingestion of red meat (nonhuman heme)

gFOBT, Guaiac-based fecal occult blood tests.

test may be negative regardless of which test is used. To maximize the detection of fecal blood and the correct identification of individuals that need follow-up testing (e.g., colonoscopy), sample collection must be easy to enhance patient compliance, and the occult blood test used must be sensitive and specific.

The two methods that predominate to detect fecal occult blood are guaiac-based tests and immunochemical tests. These tests are primarily used to screen for colorectal cancers that cause bleeding in the lower GI tract (i.e., colon). A third test based on fluorescence is less common and is primarily used to detect an upper GI bleed. Table 10-7 provides a summary of fecal occult blood tests.

Guaiac-Based Fecal Occult Blood Tests. Guaiac-based fecal occult blood tests (gFOBTs) are based on the pseudoperoxidase activity of the heme moiety of hemoglobin. In the presence of an indicator and hydrogen peroxide, the heme moiety catalyzes oxidation of the indicator, which results in a color change (Equation 10-2).

Equation 10-2

$$H_2O_2 + \underset{\text{(colorless)}}{\text{Guaiac}} \xrightarrow[\text{or peroxidase}]{\text{Pseudoperoxidase*}} \underset{\text{(colored)}}{\text{Oxidized}} \text{Indicator} + H_2O$$

*Possible pseudoperoxidases and peroxidases: hemoglobin, myoglobin, bacterial peroxidases, and fruit and vegetable peroxidases.

Because any substance with peroxidase or pseudoperoxidase activity can catalyze the reaction to produce positive results, the less sensitive indicator guaiac is specifically used for fecal testing. Dietary restrictions are necessary to avoid (1) the pseudoperoxidase activity of myoglobin and hemoglobin in meats and fish, and (2) the natural peroxidases from ingested fruits and

TABLE 10-8   Ingested Substances Associated With Erroneous Guaiac-Based Fecal Occult Blood Tests

False-Positive Results	False-Negative Results
Red or rare cooked meats and fish	Ascorbic acid
Vegetables,* such as turnips, broccoli, cauliflower, horseradish	
Fruits,* such as cantaloupe, bananas, pears, plums	
Drugs, such as aspirin and other gastrointestinal irritants	

*Adequate cooking can destroy the peroxidase activity of vegetables and fruits.

vegetables (Table 10-8). Although the sensitivity of these tests has been adjusted to account for the normal amount of fecal blood and for peroxidases from intestinal bacteria, false-positives can still occur.

A typical gFOBT consists of guaiac-impregnated paper that is enclosed in a rigid cardboard holder or slide. When using these slide-based tests, the collection of 3 fecal samples is the standard of practice to maximize test sensitivity. Patients are instructed to sample several portions of a single stool specimen or, ideally, to collect fecal material from stool samples on 3 different days. The patient opens the "front" of the slide, applies fecal material to the exposed paper using an applicator stick, closes the slide, and returns (or mails) the slide to the laboratory for testing. In the laboratory, the "back" of the slide is opened to reveal the guaiac-impregnated paper *behind* the fecal specimen, and developer (hydrogen peroxide) is applied. If hemoglobin or any other pseudoperoxidase

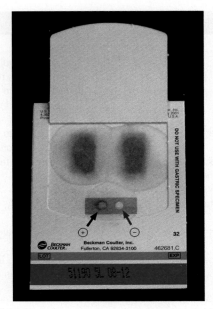

FIGURE 10-5 Positive guaiac-based fecal occult blood test.

or peroxidase is present in adequate amounts, the indicator is oxidized, causing the development of a blue color on the paper (Figure 10-5). The intensity of the color is proportional to the amount of enzymatic activity present. An internal positive and negative control area ensures that the test performed properly.

Numerous factors can interfere with a gFOBT. Improper specimen collection includes the application of too much or not enough fecal material or the use of feces that has been contaminated with toilet water. Specimen contamination with menstrual blood or hemorrhoidal blood is another source of interference. Medications can also interfere. Drugs such as salicylates (aspirin), nonsteroidal anti-inflammatory drugs (NSAIDs), iron supplements, warfarin, and antiplatelet agents can cause upper GI tract bleeding, which can result in a positive test. In contrast, antacids and ascorbic acid (vitamin C) can interfere with the chemical reaction on the test slide and have the potential to cause false-negative results. False-negative results can also be produced when (1) the peroxide developer is expired, (2) slides are defective (e.g., expired), or (3) the fecal specimen or prepared slide is stored for an extended period before testing (e.g., >6 days).

When hemoglobin is degraded, it loses its pseudoperoxidase activity and is no longer detectable by a gFOBT. Note that heme degradation can occur (1) within the intestinal tract, (2) during storage of the fecal specimen, or (3) after it has been applied to the gFOBT slide. Studies have also shown that false-positive results are obtained if fecal specimens on the slides are hydrated with water before testing.[5] Therefore, the American Cancer Society recommends that slides be tested within 6 days of collection and *not* be rehydrated before testing. Lastly, some studies have revealed poor patient compliance with the dietary restrictions and collection of multiple fecal samples.

Immunochemical Fecal Occult Blood Tests. Immunochemical tests for fecal occult blood use polyclonal antihuman antibodies directed against the globin portion of undegraded human hemoglobin. These methods are highly specific and do not have interference from dietary foodstuffs or medications that adversely affect a gFOBT. Because digestive and bacterial enzymes degrade hemoglobin as it passes through the GI tract, blood from an upper GI bleed (esophageal, gastric) is not usually detected by immunochemical fecal occult blood tests (iFOBTs). Hence, these tests are more specific for bleeding in the lower GI tract (i.e., cecum, colon, and rectum).

Numerous iFOBT tests are available world-wide and the collection devices for iFOBTs vary with the manufacturer. For example, a collection card similar to that of a gFOBT is used by the Hemoccult ICT test (Beckman Coulter Inc., Fullerton, CA). Whereas, a small collection bottle with an enclosed sample probe is used by the OC FIT-Chek test (occult fecal immunochemical test; Polymedco, Inc., Cortlandt Manor, NY). Patients apply fecal material to the collection devices—to the sample area of the card (Hemoccult ICT) or by scraping the surface of the stool until feces covers the grooved portion of the sample probe (OC FIT). The collection devices are closed and returned to the laboratory for testing.

In the laboratory, testing is performed either manually or using a fully automated system. In iFOBTs, antihuman hemoglobin antibodies bind to undegraded hemoglobin in the sample and the means for detecting the presence of hemoglobin-antibody complexes vary. Detection may be automated and photometric (OC FIT) or may be manual and visual—observing the presence of the test and control "lines" (Hemoccult ICT).[6]

A distinct advantage of iFOBTs is that no diet or medication restrictions are needed. Therefore, patients can immediately begin the specimen collection phase instead of waiting days until they change their diet or medication routine. It is believed that being able to immediately collect the fecal sample after seeing their physician enhances patient compliance. A disadvantage of the iFOBT is its increased cost compared with the gFOBT. Hence despite the greater specificity (fewer false-positive tests) of iFOBT tests for GI bleeding, gFOBT currently predominates in colorectal cancer screening protocols.

Porphyrin-Based Fecal Occult Blood Test. The detection as well as quantitation of fecal blood can be done using the HemoQuant test (SmithKline Diagnostics, Sunnyvale, CA). This test is based on the chemical conversion of heme to intensely fluorescent porphyrins. The test enables detection and quantitation of the total amount of hemoglobin in feces—the portion that exists as intact hemoglobin, as well as the portion that has been converted to porphyrins in the intestine. Note that with upper GI bleeds or when specimen storage is prolonged, the major fraction of fecal hemoglobin in a specimen can be in the form of heme-derived porphyrins. Because HemoQuant measures only heme and heme-derived porphyrins, it is not affected by many of the factors that interfere with other FOBTs. However, hemoglobin from nonhuman sources such as red meats can cause a false-positive result. The HemoQuant test is more expensive, time-consuming, and labor-intensive compared with other FOBTs. Currently, it is primarily performed by reference laboratories and has specialized and limited clinical utility.

Fetal Hemoglobin in Feces (Apt Test)

The presence of blood in the stool, emesis, or gastric aspirate from a newborn infant requires investigation. This blood may have come from the GI tract of the neonate or could be maternal blood that was ingested during delivery. Differentiation between these two sources is crucial. A qualitative assessment of the blood source can be done and is based on the alkaline resistance of fetal hemoglobin. This test is also known as the *Apt test* after its developer, L. Apt.[7]

The specimen must contain fresh "red" blood, such as a fresh, bloody stool specimen or a soiled, bloody diaper. Black, tarry stools are not acceptable because they indicate that hemoglobin degradation to hematin has occurred. With the Apt test, a suspension of the specimen (e.g., feces, emesis, gastric aspirate) is made using water and is centrifuged to clear the pink supernatant of particulate matter. Five-milliliter aliquots of the resultant pink supernatant are transferred into two tubes. One tube is used as a "reference" to evaluate color changes in the second or "alkaline" tube. To the "alkaline" tube, 1 mL of sodium hydroxide (0.25 mol/L) is added, the tube is mixed, and the color of the liquid is observed for at least 2 minutes. If the original pink color changes to yellow or brown within 2 minutes, the hemoglobin present in the specimen is maternal hemoglobin (Hb A). If the pink color remains, the hemoglobin present is fetal hemoglobin (Hb F). Note that control specimens should be analyzed each time a specimen is tested. Positive controls can be made using infant peripheral or cord blood, and negative controls can be prepared using an adult blood sample.

Quantitative Fecal Fat

A quantitative determination of fecal fat is the definitive test for steatorrhea. Although this chemical test confirms that abnormal quantities of dietary lipids are being eliminated, it does not identify the cause of the increased excretion. For 3 days before specimen collection, as well as during the collection period, patients must limit their fat intake to 100 to 150 grams of fat per day. In addition, they must not use laxatives, synthetic fat substitutes (e.g., Olestra), or fat-blocking nutritional supplements. It is important that during collection, patients do not contaminate the specimen with mineral oils, lubricants, or creams, which can cause false-positive results.

During specimen collection, the patient collects all feces excreted for 2 to 3 days in large, preweighed collection containers (e.g., paint cans). In the laboratory, the entire fecal collection is weighed and homogenized (e.g., using a mechanical shaker). A portion of the homogenized fecal specimen is removed for chemical analysis of the lipid content by gravimetry, titrimetry, or nuclear magnetic resonance spectroscopy. Gravimetric and titrimetric methods use a solvent extraction to remove the lipids from the fecal sample. In the titrimetric method, neutral fats and soaps are converted to fatty acids before extraction.[8] The resultant solution of fatty acids is extracted and titrated with sodium hydroxide. Because the titrimetric method is unable to recover medium-chain fatty acids completely, it measures approximately 80% of the total fecal lipid content. In contrast, the gravimetric method extracts and quantifies all fecal lipids present. In the nuclear magnetic resonance method, the fecal sample is first microwave-dried and then is analyzed by hydrogen nuclear magnetic resonance spectroscopy (^{1}H NMR). This method is fast and accurate and produces results comparable with those attained by the gravimetric reference method.[9]

Fecal fat content is reported as grams of fat excreted per day, with a normal adult excreting 2 to 7 g/day. If the fecal fat excretion is borderline, or if a standard fat diet (100 to 150 g/d) is not used (e.g., with small children), determining the coefficient or percentage of fat retention is helpful. To determine this parameter, careful recording of dietary intake is required, and Equation 10-3 is used.

Equation 10-3

$$\text{Percent fat retention} = \frac{\text{Dietary fat} - \text{Fecal fat}}{\text{Dietary fat}} \times 100$$

Normally, children (3 years old and older) and adults absorb at least 95% of the dietary fat ingested. Values less than 95% indicate steatorrhea in these individuals.

Fecal Carbohydrates

When the enzymes (disaccharidases) necessary for conversion of disaccharides into monosaccharides in the small intestine are insufficient or lacking, the disaccharides are not absorbed and pass into the large intestine. Because these unhydrolyzed disaccharides are osmotically active, they cause large amounts of water to be retained in the intestinal lumen, resulting in an osmotic diarrhea.

Hereditary **disaccharidase deficiency** is uncommon but should be considered and ruled out in infants who have diarrhea and fail to gain weight. Secondary disaccharidase deficiency caused by disease (e.g., celiac disease, tropical sprue) or drug effects (e.g., oral neomycin, kanamycin) is an acquired condition, usually affects more than one disaccharide, and is only temporary. Lactose intolerance in adults is common, particularly in African and Asian populations. These individuals were able to digest lactose adequately as children but progressively developed an inability to do so as adults. Consequently, for these individuals, the ingestion of lactose results in bloating, flatulence, and explosive diarrhea. These clinical manifestations of disaccharidase deficiency result from intestinal bacteria actively fermenting lactose in the intestinal lumen. This fermentation results in the production of large amounts of intestinal gas and diarrheal stools with a characteristically decreased pH (of approximately 5.0 to 6.0). Normally, feces are alkaline (pH greater than 7.0) because of pancreatic and other intestinal secretions. A rapid qualitative fecal pH can be obtained by testing the supernatant of a diarrheal stool using pH paper. Diarrheal stools can also be screened for the presence of carbohydrates (or reducing sugars) using the Clinitest tablet test (Siemens Healthcare Diagnostics Inc., Deerfield, IL), as discussed in Chapter 7. Although the Clinitest is not advocated for use on fecal specimens by the manufacturer (i.e., U.S. Food and Drug Administration approval has not been requested), its use in detecting fecal reducing substances is wide and is documented in the literature.[10] To perform the Clinitest on feces, a 1:3 dilution of the supernatant from a diarrheal stool is used. Fecal excretion of reducing substances greater than 250 mg/dL is considered to be abnormal. A positive Clinitest indicates the presence of a reducing substance but does not identify the substance being excreted. Note that this method does not detect sucrose because it is not a reducing sugar. To quantitate or specifically identify the sugar(s) present in fecal material, chromatographic or specific chemical methods must be used.

The most diagnostic test for determining an intestinal enzyme deficiency (e.g., lactase deficiency) involves specific histochemical examination of the intestinal epithelium. A more convenient approach is to perform an oral tolerance test using specific sugars (e.g., lactose, sucrose). An oral tolerance test involves the ingestion of a measured dose of a specific disaccharide (e.g., lactose, sucrose) by the patient. If the patient has adequate amounts of the appropriate intestinal disaccharidase (e.g., lactase), the disaccharide (e.g., lactose) is hydrolyzed to its corresponding monosaccharides (e.g., glucose and galactose), which are absorbed into the patient's bloodstream. An increase in blood glucose greater than 30 mg/dL above the patient's fasting glucose level indicates adequate enzyme activity (e.g., lactase); an increase less than 20 mg/dL above the patient's fasting glucose level indicates deficiency of the enzyme.

The presence of carbohydrates in feces can also occur as the result of inadequate intestinal absorption.

To differentiate carbohydrate malabsorption from carbohydrate maldigestion, a xylose absorption test is performed. Xylose is a pentose that does not depend on liver or pancreatic function for digestion and is readily absorbed in the small intestine. Normally, xylose is not present at significant levels in the blood, and the body does not metabolize it. In addition, xylose readily passes through the glomerular filtration barrier and is excreted in the urine. The xylose absorption test involves the patient's ingestion of a dose of xylose, followed by the collection of a 2-hour blood sample and a 5-hour urine specimen. The concentration of xylose is measured in the blood and urine. Depending on the size of the initial oral dose, at least 16% to 24% of the ingested dose of xylose is normally excreted by adults.

STUDY QUESTIONS

1. Which of the following substances is not a component of normal feces?
   A. Bacteria
   B. Blood
   C. Electrolytes
   D. Water
2. All of the following actions can result in watery or diarrheal stools except
   A. decreased intestinal motility.
   B. inhibition of water reabsorption.
   C. inadequate time allowed for water reabsorption.
   D. an excessive volume of fluid presented for reabsorption.
3. Lactose intolerance caused by the lack of sufficient lactase primarily presents with
   A. steatorrhea.
   B. osmotic diarrhea.
   C. secretory diarrhea.
   D. intestinal hypermotility.
4. Which of the following tests assists most in the differentiation of secretory and osmotic diarrhea?
   A. Fecal fat
   B. Fecal carbohydrates
   C. Fecal occult blood
   D. Fecal osmolality
5. The inability to convert dietary foodstuffs into readily absorbable substances is called intestinal
   A. inadequacy.
   B. hypermotility.
   C. malabsorption
   D. maldigestion.
6. Intestinal motility is stimulated by each of the following except
   A. castor oil.
   B. dietary fiber.
   C. intestinal distention.
   D. sympathetic nerve activity.

7. Which of the following conditions is characterized by the excretion of greasy, pale, foul-smelling feces?
   A. Steatorrhea
   B. Osmotic diarrhea
   C. Secretory diarrhea
   D. Intestinal hypermotility

8. The daily amount of fat excreted in the feces is normally less than
   A. 0.7 g.
   B. 7.0 g.
   C. 70 g.
   D. 700 g.

9. Which of the following tests is used to diagnose steatorrhea?
   A. Fecal fat
   B. Fecal carbohydrates
   C. Fecal occult blood
   D. Fecal osmolality

10. Which of the following statements about feces is TRUE?
    A. The normal color of feces is primarily due to urobilinogens.
    B. The amount of feces produced in 24 hours correlates poorly with food intake.
    C. The normal odor of feces is usually due to metabolic by-products of intestinal protozoa.
    D. The consistency of feces is primarily determined by the amount of fluid intake.

11. Fecal specimens may be tested for each of the following *except*
    A. fat.
    B. blood.
    C. bilirubin.
    D. carbohydrates.

12. Which of the following substances is responsible for the characteristic color of normal feces?
    A. Bilirubin
    B. Hemoglobin
    C. Urobilins
    D. Urobilinogens

13. Which of the following statements about fecal tests is true?
    A. A fecal fat determination identifies the cause of steatorrhea.
    B. A fecal leukocyte determination aids in differentiating the cause of diarrhea.
    C. A fecal Clinitest identifies the enzyme deficiency that prevents sugar digestion.
    D. A fecal blood screen aids in differentiating bacterial from parasitic infestations.

14. Which of the following types of fat readily stain with Sudan III or Oil Red O stain?
    1. Fatty acids
    2. Cholesterol
    3. Soaps (fatty acid salts)
    4. Neutral fats (triglycerides)
    A. 1, 2, and 3 are correct.
    B. 1 and 3 are correct.
    C. 4 is correct.
    D. All are correct.

15. Which of the following types of fat require acidification and heat before they stain with Sudan III or Oil Red O stain?
    1. Fatty acids
    2. Cholesterol
    3. Soaps (fatty acid salts)
    4. Neutral fats (triglycerides)
    A. 1, 2, and 3 are correct.
    B. 1 and 3 are correct.
    C. 4 is correct.
    D. All are correct.

16. With the two-slide qualitative fecal fat determination, the first slide produces a normal amount of staining fat present, whereas the second slide, following acid addition and heat, produces an abnormally increased amount of fat. These results indicate
    A. malabsorption.
    B. maldigestion.
    C. parasitic infestation.
    D. disaccharidase deficiency.

17. Mass screening in adults for fecal occult blood is performed primarily to detect
    A. ulcers.
    B. hemorrhoids.
    C. colorectal cancer.
    D. esophageal varices.

18. Which of the following dietary substances can cause a false-negative guaiac-based fecal occult blood slide test?
    A. Fish
    B. Red meat
    C. Ascorbic acid
    D. Fruits and vegetables

19. Which of the following actions can cause a false-positive guaiac-based fecal occult blood slide test?
    A. Rehydration of the specimen on the slide before testing
    B. Degradation of hemoglobin to porphyrin
    C. Storage of fecal specimens before testing
    D. Storage of slides with the specimen already applied

20. Select the true statement about fecal occult blood tests (FOBTs)?
    A. Guaiac-based FOBTs are more specific than immunochemical-based FOBTs.
    B. Guaiac-based FOBTs are more expensive than immunochemical-based FOBTs.
    C. Dietary restrictions are not required when immunochemical-based FOBTs are used.
    D. Hemoglobin from nonhuman sources (e.g., red meat) can cause false-positive results when immunochemical-based FOBTs are used.

21. Which of the following conditions can result in the excretion of small amounts of occult blood in the feces?
    1. Hemorrhoids
    2. Bleeding gums
    3. Peptic ulcers
    4. Intake of iron supplements
    A. 1, 2, and 3 are correct.
    B. 1 and 3 are correct.
    C. 4 is correct.
    D. All are correct.

22. Which of the following statements regarding the test for fetal hemoglobin in feces (the Apt test) is TRUE?
    A. Any adult hemoglobin present should resist alkali treatment.
    B. The Apt test is used to differentiate various hemoglobinopathies in the newborn.
    C. Hemoglobin degraded to hematin usually produces a positive test result.
    D. A pink color following alkali treatment indicates the presence of fetal hemoglobin.

23. Which of the following are clinical manifestations of a disaccharidase deficiency?
    1. A positive fecal Clinitest
    2. Constipation and gas
    3. A fecal pH of 5.0
    4. A positive fecal occult blood test
    A. 1, 2, and 3 are correct.
    B. 1 and 3 are correct.
    C. 4 is correct.
    D. All are correct.

24. Which of the following tests can differentiate inadequate carbohydrate metabolism from inadequate carbohydrate absorption?
    A. Fecal Clinitest
    B. Xylose absorption test
    C. Oral carbohydrate tolerance tests
    D. Carbohydrate thin-layer chromatography

CASE 10-1

A 45-year-old traveling salesman sees his physician and reports diarrhea, weight loss, and back pain for the past month. Physical examination reveals yellowing of the sclera of the eyes (jaundice) but no hepatomegaly or splenomegaly. Further tests support a diagnosis of pancreatic cancer. The results of a routine urinalysis, 72-hour stool collection for fecal fat, stool for *Salmonella/Shigella* culture and ova and parasites, and xylose absorption follow.

Urinalysis Results

Physical Examination	Chemical Examination	Microscopic Examination
Color: amber	SG: 1.015	RBC/hpf: 0-2 cells
Clarity: slightly cloudy	pH: 5.5	WBC/hpf: 0-2 cells
	Blood: negative	Casts/lpf: 0-2 hyaline;
Odor: —	Protein: negative	2-5 granular
Yellow foam noted.	LE: negative	Epithelials: few TE/hpf
	Nitrite: negative	
	Glucose: negative	
	Ketones: negative	
	Bilirubin: large	
	Ictotest: positive	
	Urobilinogen: normal	

Fecal Macroscopic Examination	Fecal Microscopic Examination	Fecal Chemical Examination
Color: pale, clay-colored (acholic)	Leukocytes: absent	Fat: 10 g/day
Consistency: watery, greasy		
Form: bulky		

Microbiological Examination

Stool cultures: negative for *Salmonella, Shigella, Campylobacter,* enteropathogenic *Escherichia coli,* and *Yersinia.*
Ova and parasites: negative for ova, cysts, and parasites.

Blood Chemistry Results

Xylose absorption test: normal

1. List any abnormal results.
2. This patient's condition should be classified as
    A. oncotic diuresis.
    B. osmotic diarrhea.
    C. secretory diarrhea.
    D. intestinal hypermotility.
3. What is the term used for an increased amount of fat in the feces?
4. The most likely mechanism responsible for this patient's diarrhea is
    A. malabsorption.
    B. maldigestion.
    C. malexcretion.
    D. malsecretion.
5. Explain the physiologic mechanisms responsible for the increased fat and acholic stools excreted by this patient.
6. Why is this patient's urine urobilinogen result normal and not decreased?

---

hpf, High-power field; *LE,* leukocyte esterase; *lpf,* low-power field; *RBC,* red blood cell; *TE,* transitional epithelial; *WBC,* white blood cell.

CASE 10-2

A 23-year-old woman sees her physician and reports headache, nausea, fever, and diarrhea for the past week. She first experienced the diarrhea shortly after a summer picnic. She currently has five to six bowel movements each day. The stool does not appear bloody. A stool specimen is collected and the following test results obtained:

Fecal Macroscopic Examination	Fecal Microscopic Examination	Fecal Chemical Examination
Color: brown	Leukocytes: present	Sodium: 65 mmol/L
Consistency: watery		Potassium: 98 mmol/L
		Osmolality: 340 mOsm/kg

Microbiological Examination of Stool
    Culture: *Salmonella* sp. present.
Ova and parasites: negative for ova, cysts, and parasites.

1. List any abnormal results.
2. Determine the "calculated" fecal osmolality using the formula:
   Osmolality $= 2 \times (Na^+_{fecal} + K^+_{fecal})$.
3. Based on the difference between observed and calculated osmolality, this patient's condition would be classified as
   A. oncotic diuresis.
   B. osmotic diarrhea.
   C. secretory diarrhea.
   D. intestinal hypermotility.

CASE 10-3

A 60-year-old woman is seen by her physician for a routine annual examination. Her only complaints are a lack of stamina and that she tires easily. Routine urinalysis and hematology tests are performed. She is sent home with instructions and supplies to collect three different fecal specimens for the detection of occult blood.

Urinalysis: normal

Hematologic Test Results	Reference Range	Fecal Occult Blood Test
Hemoglobin: 9.8 g/dL	Female: 12-16.0 g/dL	Specimen #1: positive
Hematocrit: 36%	Female: 38%-47%	Specimen #2: positive
		Specimen #3: positive

1. List any abnormal results.
2. Ingestion of which of the following substances can cause a false-positive guaiac-based fecal occult blood test?
   1. Fish
   2. Bananas
   3. Cauliflower
   4. Vitamin C
   A. 1, 2, and 3 are correct.
   B. 1 and 3 are correct.
   C. 4 is correct.
   D. All are correct.

3. List at least two compounds other than hemoglobin that contain the heme moiety.
4. Which of the following conditions could account for the occult blood results obtained?
   1. Ulcers
   2. Bleeding gums
   3. Hemorrhoids
   4. Colorectal cancer
   A. 1, 2, and 3 are correct.
   B. 1 and 3 are correct.
   C. 4 is correct.
   D. All are correct.
5. Which of the following tests could assist in differentiating an upper GI bleed from a lower GI bleed?
   A. Apt test
   B. Guaiac-based fecal occult blood test
   C. Immunochemical-based fecal occult blood test
   D. Porphyrin-based fecal occult blood test
6. In this case, the limited information and data suggest
   A. melena.
   B. creatorrhea.
   C. gastrointestinal bleeding.
   D. pancreatic cancer.

REFERENCES

1. Kao YS, Liu FJ: Laboratory diagnosis of gastrointestinal tract and exocrine pancreatic disorders. In Henry JB, editor: Clinical diagnosis and management by laboratory methods, ed 18, Philadelphia, 1991, WB Saunders.
2. Vernon SW: Participation in colorectal cancer screening: a review. J Natl Cancer Inst 89:1406, 1997.
3. Drummey GD, Benson JA, Jones GM: Microscopical examination of the stool for steatorrhea. N Engl J Med 264:85, 1961.
4. Mandel JS, Church TR, Bond JH, et al: The effect of fecal occult-blood screening on the incidence of colorectal cancer. N Engl J Med 343:1603, 2000.
5. Ahlquist DA, McGill DB, Schwartz S, et al: HemoQuant: a new quantitative assay for fecal hemoglobin. Ann Intern Med 101:297, 1984.
6. Hemoccult ICT immunochemical fecal occult blood test: Product instructions, Fullerton, CA, May 2008, Beckman Coulter Inc.
7. Apt L, Downey WS: Melena neonatorium: swallowed blood syndrome—a simple test for the differentiation of adult and fetal hemoglobin in bloody stools. J Pediatr 47:5, 1955.
8. Van de Kamer JH, Ten Bokel Huinink H, Weyers HW: Rapid method for the determination of fat in feces. J Biol Chem 177:347, 1949.
9. Korpi-Steiner N, Ward JN, Kumar V, McConnell JP: Comparative analysis of fecal fat quantitation via nuclear magnetic resonance spectroscopy (^{1}H NMR) and gravimetry. Clin Chim Acta 400:33, 2009.
10. Heisig DG, Threatte GA, Henry JB: Laboratory diagnosis of gastrointestinal tract and pancreatic disorders. In Henry JB, editor: Clinical diagnosis and management by laboratory methods, ed 20, Philadelphia, 2001, WB Saunders.

Seminal Fluid Analysis

LEARNING OBJECTIVES

After studying this chapter, the student should be able to:

1. Discuss the composition of seminal fluid and briefly describe the function of each of the following structures in seminal fluid formation:
   - Epididymis
   - Interstitial cells of Leydig
   - Prostate gland
   - Seminal vesicles
   - Seminiferous tubules
2. Outline the maturation of sperm (spermatozoa) and identify the morphologic structures in which each maturation phase occurs.
3. Summarize the collection of seminal fluid for analysis, including the importance of timing and recovery of the complete specimen.
4. Describe the performance of the physical examination (appearance, volume, and viscosity) of seminal fluid and the results expected from a normal specimen.
5. Describe the procedures used to evaluate the following characteristics of sperm in seminal fluid, state the

normal range for each parameter, and relate each function to male fertility:
   - Agglutination
   - Concentration
   - Morphology
   - Motility
   - Viability
6. Identify and describe the morphologic appearance of normal and abnormal forms of spermatozoa.
7. Discuss the origin and clinical significance of cells other than sperm in the seminal fluid.
8. Discuss briefly the role of quantifying the following biochemical substances in seminal fluid and identify the structure evaluated by each substance:
   - Acid phosphatase
   - Citric acid
   - Fructose
   - pH
   - Zinc

CHAPTER OUTLINE

Physiology
Specimen Collection
Physical Examination
   Appearance
   Volume
   Viscosity

Microscopic Examination
   Motility
   Concentration and Sperm Count
   Postvasectomy Sperm Counts
   Morphology
   Vitality

Cells Other Than Spermatozoa
   Agglutination
Chemical Examination
   pH
   Fructose
   Other Biochemical Markers

KEY TERMS

epididymis A long, coiled, tubular structure attached to the upper surface of each testis that is continuous with the vas deferens. The epididymis is the site of final sperm maturation and the development of motility. Sperm are concentrated and stored here until ejaculation.

interstitial cells of Leydig Cells located in the interstitial space between the seminiferous tubules of the testes. These cells produce

and secrete the hormone testosterone.

liquefaction The physical conversion of seminal fluid from a coagulum to a liquid following ejaculation.

prostate gland A lobular gland surrounding the male urethra immediately after it exits the bladder. The prostate is an accessory gland of the male reproductive system and is testosterone dependent. It

produces a mildly acidic secretion rich in citric acid, enzymes, proteins, and zinc that is added to ejaculates.

seminal fluid (also called *semen*) A complex body fluid that transports sperm. Seminal fluid is composed of secretions from the testes, epididymis, seminal vesicles, and prostate gland.

seminal vesicles Paired glands that secrete a slightly alkaline fluid, rich in fructose, into the ejaculatory duct. Most of the fluid in the ejaculate originates in the seminal vesicles.

seminiferous tubules Numerous coiled tubules located in the testes. The seminiferous tubules are collectively the site of spermatogenesis. Immature and immotile sperm are released into the seminiferous tubular lumen and are carried by its

secretions to the epididymis for maturation.

sperm (also called *spermatozoa*) Male reproductive cells.

vasectomy A procedure in which both vas deferens are surgically severed and at least one end of each is sealed. It is a male sterilization procedure because it prevents sperm from becoming part of the ejaculate.

viscosity A measure of fluid flow or its resistance to flow. Low-viscosity fluids (e.g., water) flow freely and form discrete droplets when expelled drop by drop from a pipette. In contrast, high-viscosity fluids (e.g., corn syrup) flow less freely and do not form discrete droplets; rather they momentarily form threads or strings when expelled from a pipette.

Seminal fluid or semen is a complex body fluid used to transport **sperm** or spermatozoa. It is analyzed routinely to evaluate infertility and to follow up after a vasectomy to ensure its effectiveness. Other reasons for analysis include the evaluation of semen quality for donation purposes and forensic applications (e.g., DNA analysis, detection of semen). Familiarity with the male reproductive tract and its various functions facilitates understanding of the physical, microscopic, and biochemical abnormalities that can occur in semen.

PHYSIOLOGY

Semen is composed primarily of secretions from the testes, epididymis, seminal vesicles, and prostate gland, with a small amount derived from the bulbourethral glands. The biochemical composition of semen is complex. Although the specific functions of some components (e.g., fructose) are known, the functions of others (e.g., prostaglandins) remain uncertain. The testes are paired glands suspended in the scrotum and located outside the body (Figure 11-1). Their external location

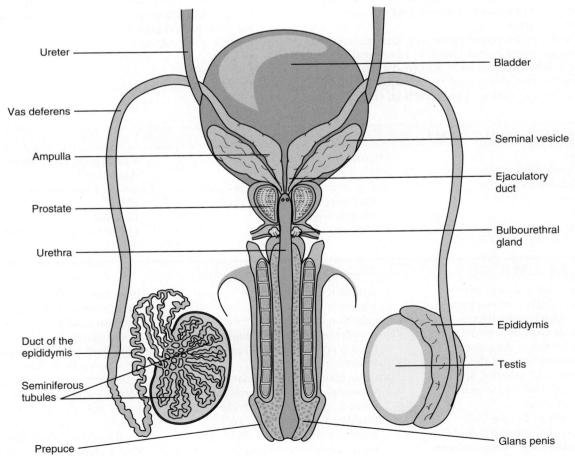

FIGURE 11-1 A schematic diagram of the male reproductive tract.

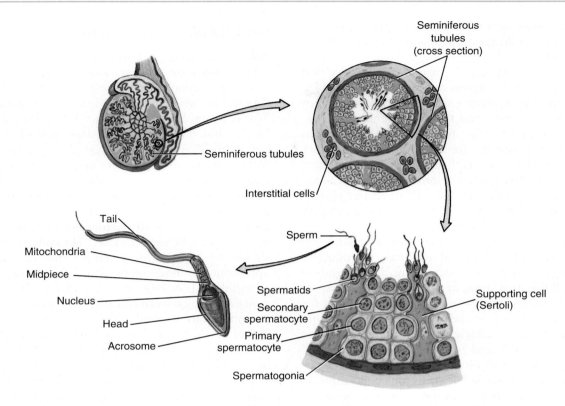

FIGURE 11-2 A schematic diagram of spermatogenesis from germ cells in the seminiferous tubules. *(From Applegate E: The anatomy and physiology learning system, ed 4, Philadelphia, 2011, Saunders.)*

allows for the lower organ temperature necessary for sperm formation.

The testes perform both an exocrine function by the secretion of sperm and an endocrine function by the secretion of testosterone. These two functions are interdependent and are regulated by two pituitary hormones: follicle-stimulating hormone and luteinizing hormone. The cells responsible for these two functions are distinctly different. Sperm production is regulated by Sertoli cells in the **seminiferous tubules,** whereas production and secretion of the male sex hormone, testosterone, is the responsibility of the **interstitial cells of Leydig,** which are located in the *interstitium* of the testes, between the seminiferous tubules.

Sertoli cells of the seminiferous tubular epithelium have several functions. Because of their tight interconnections, they essentially form a barrier that separates the epithelium into two distinct compartments: the basal compartment (i.e., germ cell layer) and the adluminal compartment (i.e., epithelium nearest the tubular lumen). As this barrier or gatekeeper, they limit the movement of chemical substances from the blood into the tubular lumen—playing a role in supplying nutrients, hormones, and other substances necessary for normal spermatogenesis. They also control the movement of spermatocytes from the germ cell layer into the adluminal compartment, and last, they continuously produce a fluid that

carries the newly produced immotile sperm into the lumen of the seminiferous tubules and on to the epididymis.

The *epithelium* of the numerous coiled seminiferous tubules consists of Sertoli and germ cells. The undifferentiated germ cells (spermatogonia) continuously undergo mitotic division to produce more germ cells. At the same time, some of them move slowly toward the tubular lumen, changing in size and undergoing meiotic (reduction) division until they form spermatids. Figure 11-2 depicts spermatogenesis in the seminiferous tubular epithelium with all stages of spermatogenesis depicted. Spermatogonia (germ cells) evolve into spermatocytes, then spermatids. With nuclear modification and cellular restructuring, spermatids ultimately differentiate into immotile sperm.

When Sertoli cells release sperm into the lumen of the seminiferous tubules, they are nonmotile and still immature. Luminal fluid from Sertoli cells carries the sperm into the tubular network of the **epididymis,** where they undergo final maturation and become motile. The epididymis also adds carnitine and acetylcarnitine to the lumen fluid. Although the exact function of these chemicals remains to be elucidated, abnormal levels of them have been associated with infertility. Other functions of the epididymis include the concentration of sperm by the absorption of lumen fluid and their storage until ejaculation. Following a **vasectomy,** the epididymis is the site of leukocyte infiltration and phagocytization of accumulated sperm.

The epididymis ultimately forms a single duct that joins the vas deferens. The vas deferens is a thick-walled muscular tube that transports sperm from the epididymis to the ejaculatory duct, and the dilated end of the vas deferens is located inferior to the bladder. Secretions from the seminal vesicles are added at the ejaculatory duct. Both ejaculatory ducts then pass through the prostate gland and empty into the prostatic urethra along with secretions from the prostate. All structures preceding the prostate gland are paired (e.g., two ejaculatory ducts, two seminal vesicles, two testes).

The **seminal vesicles** and the **prostate gland** are considered accessory glands of the male reproductive system and are testosterone dependent. They produce and store fluids that provide the principal transport medium for sperm. Seminal vesicle fluid accounts for approximately 70% of the ejaculate and is high in flavin. Flavin imparts the characteristic gray or opalescent appearance to semen and is responsible for its green-white fluorescence under ultraviolet light.[1] Another characteristic of seminal vesicle fluid is its high concentration of fructose, believed to serve as a nutrient for spermatozoa. The various proteins secreted by the seminal vesicles play a role in coagulation of the ejaculate, whereas the function of prostaglandins remains under investigation. (Prostaglandins were originally thought to be a prostatic gland secretion, hence their misnaming.)

Prostatic fluid secretions account for approximately 25% of the ejaculate volume. The principal components of this milky, slightly acidic fluid are citric acid; enzymes, particularly acid phosphatase and proteolytic enzymes; proteins; and zinc. Semen is unique in its high concentration of the enzyme acid phosphatase. Hence acid phosphatase activity can be used to positively identify the presence of this body fluid. Proteins and some enzymes in prostatic secretions play a role in coagulation of the ejaculate, whereas the proteolytic enzymes are responsible for its liquefaction. Zinc is primarily added to semen by the prostate gland; however, the testes and sperm also contribute zinc. Semen zinc levels can be used to evaluate prostate function; a decreased level is associated with prostate gland disorders.

In summary, semen is a highly complex transport medium for sperm. The paired seminal vesicles and the single prostate gland are the major fluid contributors to semen. Sperm produced by the testes are matured and concentrated in the epididymis, and make up only a small percentage of an ejaculate. Dilution of sperm by the relatively large volume of seminal fluid at ejaculation enhances sperm motility. Without adequate dilution, sperm motility is significantly reduced. The entire process of spermatogenesis and maturation (i.e., from primary spermatocyte to mature motile spermatozoon) takes approximately 90 days.

SPECIMEN COLLECTION

Because sperm concentration in normal seminal fluid can vary significantly, two or more samples should be analyzed to evaluate male fertility. Specimen collections should take place within a 3-month period and at least 7 days apart. Sexual abstinence for at least 2 days (48 hours), but not exceeding 7 days, should precede the collection. The patient collects the specimen through masturbation, and the entire ejaculate is collected in a clean, wide-mouth sterile plastic or glass container. Although some plastic containers are toxic to spermatozoa, others are not. Sterile urine specimen or similar containers are often satisfactory but the laboratory must evaluate them before their use.[2] The collection container should be kept at room temperature or warmed (to approximately body temperature) before the collection to avoid the possibility of cold shock to the sperm. The container can be warmed easily by holding it next to the patient's body or under the arm for several minutes before the collection. This technique can also be used to control the temperature of specimens being transported in cold climates. Specimen containers and request forms must be labeled with the patient's name, the period of sexual abstinence, and the date and time of specimen collection. The time of actual specimen collection is crucial in evaluating liquefaction and sperm motility.

During specimen collection, lubricants and ordinary condoms should not be used because they have spermicidal properties. For patients unable to collect a specimen through masturbation, special nonspermicidal (e.g., Silastic) condoms can be provided for specimen collection.

The collection of seminal fluid requires sensitivity and professionalism. Written and verbal instructions should be provided to the patient, as well as a comfortable and private room near the laboratory. If the specimen is to be collected elsewhere and delivered to the laboratory, clearly written instructions regarding specimen transport conditions must be provided. Specimens must be received in the laboratory within 1 hour following the collection, and they must be protected from extreme temperatures, that is, maintained between 20° C and 40° C.[3] If these criteria are not met, the specimen will not be satisfactory for sperm function tests and an abnormally low sperm motility can result. Because the ejaculate differs in its composition, only complete collections are acceptable for analysis. Patient instructions must state this clearly, and patients should be asked whether any portion of the specimen was not collected. When a portion of the initial ejaculate is not collected, the sperm concentration will be falsely decreased, and owing to a reduction in prostate secretions, the pH is falsely increased and the coagulum will fail to liquefy. Conversely, when the last portion of an ejaculate is missing (primarily seminal vesicle fluid), the semen volume will be decreased, the sperm concentration falsely increased, and the pH falsely decreased, and a coagulum will not form.

TABLE 11-1	Semen Characteristics Associated With Fertility	
Parameter	Reference Interval*	Lower Reference Limit[†]
Physical Examination		
Appearance	Gray-white, opalescent, opaque	
Volume	2-5 mL	1.5 mL (1.4-1.7)
Viscosity/liquefaction	Discrete droplets (watery) within 60 minutes	
Microscopic Examination		
Motility	50% or more with moderate to rapid linear (forward) progression	40% (38-42)
Concentration	20 to 250 $\times$ 10^6 sperm per mL	15 $\times$ 10^6 sperm per mL
Morphology	14% or more have normal morphology	4% normal forms
Vitality	75% or more are alive	58% (55-63)
Leukocytes	Less than 1 $\times$ 10^6 per mL	
Chemical Examination		
pH	7.2-7.8	$\geq$7.2
Acid phosphatase (total)	$\geq$200 U per ejaculate at 37° C (p-nitrophenylphosphate)	
Citric acid (total)	$\geq$52 μmol per ejaculate	
Fructose (total)	$\geq$13 μmol per ejaculate	$\geq$13 μmol per ejaculate
Zinc (total)	$\geq$2.4 μmol per ejaculate	$\geq$2.4 μmol per ejaculate

*Based on the strict criteria evaluation recommended by the World Health Organization (1999) for assessing sperm morphology for fertility purposes.
[†]The one-sided 5th centile lower reference limit recommended by the WHO (2010) for assessing semen characteristics.

As with all body fluids, seminal fluid represents a potential biohazard and must be handled accordingly. Because seminal fluid can contain infectious agents such as hepatitis virus, human immunodeficiency virus, herpes virus, and others, all personnel must adhere to Standard Precautions (see Chapter 2) when handling these specimens.

PHYSICAL EXAMINATION

Appearance

Normal semen is gray-white and opalescent in appearance. A brown or red hue may indicate the presence of blood, whereas yellow coloration has been associated with certain drugs. If large numbers of leukocytes are present, the semen appears more turbid with less translucence. When the specimen appears almost clear, the sperm concentration is usually low. Mucus clumps or strands can be present. Semen has a distinctive odor that is sometimes described as musty. Although infections in the male reproductive tract can modify this odor, a change is rarely noted or reported. Table 11-1 (and Appendix B) summarizes the semen characteristics (physical, microscopic, and chemical parameters) associated with fertility.

Semen is a homogeneous viscous fluid that immediately coagulates after ejaculation to form a coagulum. Within 30 minutes, the coagulum liquefies (becomes watery). The actual time of specimen collection must be known to evaluate *liquefaction*. Although liquefaction can take longer, any delay beyond 60 minutes is considered abnormal and must be noted. Because complete liquefaction is necessary to perform analysis, semen specimens that do not liquefy completely can be chemically treated (see Appendix C, Semen Pretreatment Solution). Following normal liquefaction, undissolved gel–like granules or particles can be present in the specimen, with a small amount considered normal.

Volume

The physical and microscopic analyses of seminal fluid should take place immediately following liquefaction or within 1 hour after collection (for specimens collected away from the laboratory). Specimen volume is measured to one decimal place (0.1 mL) using a *sterile* serologic pipette (5.0 mL or 10.0 mL). If a semen culture for bacteria is requested, the volume measurement should be performed first using sterile technique. Normally, a complete ejaculate collection recovers 2 to 5 mL of seminal fluid. Volumes less than and greater than this range are considered abnormal and have been associated with infertility.

Viscosity

After complete liquefaction, the **viscosity** of the semen is evaluated using a Pasteur pipette and observing the droplets that form when the fluid is allowed to fall by gravity. A normal specimen is watery and forms into discrete droplets. Abnormal viscosity or fluid thickness is indicated by the formation of a string or thread greater than 2 cm in length.[3] A high mucus content can increase the viscosity. Other conditions associated with increased viscosity include the production of antisperm antibodies and oligoasthenospermia (i.e., decreased concentration and motility of sperm).[4-7]

Grading viscosity varies among laboratories. Numeric terms can be used, with 0 indicating a normal, watery (i.e., forms discrete drops) specimen, and 4 indicating a specimen with gel-like consistency.[8] An alternate reporting format uses descriptive terms, such as normal, slightly viscous (thick), moderately viscous, and extremely viscous (unable to be aspirated into the pipette).

TABLE 11-2	Sperm Motility Grading Criteria
0	Immotile
1	Motile, without forward progression
2	Motile, with slow nonlinear or meandering progression
3	Motile, with moderate linear (forward) progression
4	Motile, with strong linear (forward) progression

MICROSCOPIC EXAMINATION

As in other laboratory areas, the standardization of procedures and techniques is necessary to enhance the precision and reproducibility of semen analysis. Once achieved, this standardization enables intralaboratory and interlaboratory comparisons of data. Appropriate quality control measures must also be in place whenever applicable. The World Health Organization publication *WHO Laboratory Manual for the Examination and Processing of Human Semen* is an excellent reference for any laboratory performing semen analysis.[3] Microscopic examination includes the determination of sperm motility, concentration, morphology, and viability; the concentration of other cells present; and the presence of sperm agglutination. Some laboratories use a single stain for the evaluation of several parameters, such as eosin-nigrosin stain for sperm vitality, morphology, and the identification of other cells, whereas others use different stains that specifically enhance each parameter to aid in the identification and evaluation of sperm and other cells.

Motility

Motility is one of the most important characteristics of sperm because immotile sperm, even in high concentrations, are unable to reach and fertilize an ovum. Traditionally, the evaluation of sperm motility has been assessed subjectively by experienced technologists. Today, computerized systems that use electro-optical techniques or videography have been developed for semen evaluation. This advanced technology enables objective evaluation of sperm motility and morphology; however, the cost of the equipment precludes many laboratories from acquiring it.

Without an automated system, sperm motility is evaluated subjectively and semiquantitatively using phase-contrast microscopy (brightfield microscopy can also be used with appropriate condenser adjustments). After complete liquefaction, the semen sample is mixed well to ensure homogeneity. A consistent volume of each specimen is evaluated by pipetting a fixed volume (e.g., 10 or 20 µL) of semen onto a microscope slide using a calibrated positive-displacement pipette. The sample is covered with a coverslip of predetermined size (e.g., 18 × 18 mm), and the slide is allowed it to settle for about 1 minute before evaluation. To enhance the accuracy and precision of results, wet mounts of each sample should be prepared and evaluated in duplicate.

Because sperm motility is affected adversely by temperature, some laboratories control the temperature of the microscope slide at 37° C using an air curtain incubator.[8] Others perform the analysis at room temperature (i.e., 22 ± 2° C).

Initially, each wet mount is screened to ensure uniformity in sperm movement throughout the preparation. Next, sperm motility is graded subjectively from 0 to 4 under 200× (or 400×) magnification. Table 11-2 shows typical grading criteria used to evaluate sperm motility. Some laboratories use a manual cell counter and evaluate the motility characteristics in 100 sperm, whereas others grade the sperm encountered in 6 to 10 high-power fields (400×).

The speed and forward progression of each sperm are evaluated. In normal semen evaluated within 60 minutes of collection, 50% or more of the sperm will show moderate to strong linear or forward progression. The practice in some laboratories of reassessing sperm motility at additional time intervals serves no purpose and has no clinical significance. Physiologically or in vivo, sperm leave the seminal fluid within minutes following ejaculation and enter the cervical mucus. Therefore, motility on a microscope slide at later time intervals is irrelevant.

Concentration and Sperm Count

For fertility purposes, the actual number of sperm is not as important as other characteristics. This fact is supported by studies of fertile men despite low sperm counts (fewer than 1 million per milliliter).[9] The concentration of sperm in an ejaculate is considered normal when 20 to 250 million per milliliter of sperm are present; values less than or greater than this range are considered abnormal and are associated with infertility. The variation in the sperm concentration within a single individual can be significant and depends partially on the period of sexual abstinence but can also be affected by viral infection and stress. For these reasons, multiple semen specimens should be evaluated to reliably assess the quantity and quality of an individual's sperm.

Manually, the concentration of sperm is determined by using a hemacytometer after preparing an appropriate dilution of the semen. Frequently, a 1:20 dilution is prepared. If during initial microscopic examination, the sperm concentration is noted to be exceptionally high or low, a new dilution can be prepared and mounted. All dilutions should be made using a calibrated positive-displacement pipette to deliver the semen quantitatively to a premeasured amount of diluent (see Appendix C for diluents). Note that a hematology white blood cell

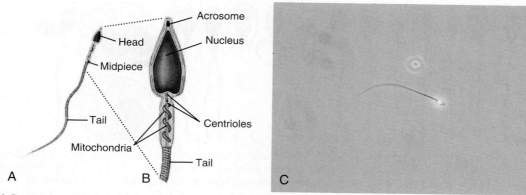

FIGURE 11-3 Spermatozoon or sperm. **A,** A schematic of a mature sperm. **B,** An enlarged view of head and midpiece. **C,** A photomicrograph of a single sperm using phase-contrast microscopy, 400×. (**A** and **B** from Thibodeau GA, Patton KT: Anatomy and physiology, ed 5, St Louis, 2003, Mosby.)

pipette is not accurate for use with seminal fluid because of its viscosity and should not be used.[3] After the hemacytometer is filled with the well-mixed dilution of semen, it is placed in a humidifying chamber and allowed to settle for 3 to 5 minutes before counting. The type of hemacytometer, the specimen dilution used, and the areas counted determine the conversion factor necessary to obtain the concentration of sperm in millions per milliliter (see Chapter 18 for procedural details).

Several alternative manual counting methods have been developed, such as the Makler chamber (Mid-Atlantic Diagnostics, Mt Laurel, NJ), Horwell, Cell VU chambers (Millennium Sciences, NY), Microcell slides (Conception Technologies, San Diego, CA), and Leja slides (Leja, The Netherlands). Studies vary in their outcomes—some supporting the manual hemacytometer method as the method of choice for sperm counting, other studies found better accuracy and precision using an alternative counting chamber.[4,5,10] Regardless of the method used, the dilution of the semen is always a potential source for error and requires the utmost attention to ensure accurate and reproducible technique. The counting of motile sperm and high sperm concentrations have also been identified as two sources of error. Therefore the World Health Organization (WHO) states that the "validity of these alternative counting chambers must be established by checking chamber dimensions, comparing results with the improved Neubauer haemocytometer method, and obtaining satisfactory performance as shown by an external quality control program.[3] In contrast to sperm concentration (sperm per milliliter), the sperm count is the total number of sperm present in the entire ejaculate. This value, often requested by clinicians, is calculated by multiplying the sperm concentration (sperm/mL) by the total volume of the ejaculate.

Equation 11-1

$$\text{Sperm count} = \text{Sperm concentration (sperm/mL)} \times \text{Volume of ejaculate (mL)}$$

Postvasectomy Sperm Counts

Following a vasectomy, the sperm count in semen ideally should be zero—no sperm present (azoospermia)—within 12 weeks after the procedure. However, studies have shown that *nonmotile* sperm can be present for as long as 21 months post vasectomy regardless of the number of ejaculations. It is postulated that the persistence or reappearance of *nonmotile* sperm in semen collections results from the release of *nonviable* residual sperm in the seminal vesicles and the abdominal portion of the vas deferens. Studies have further demonstrated that despite the presence of low numbers ($<1 \times 10^6$) of *nonmotile* sperm post vasectomy, these individuals have a very low risk of causing pregnancy (i.e., comparable with azoospermic men).[11]

In clinical practice, most men ($\approx 66\%$) demonstrate azoospermia within 12 weeks, regardless of the number of ejaculations. Note that the most important feature is not the number of sperm present post vasectomy but the status of their motility. The presence of even a single "motile" spermatozoon is evidence of an unsuccessful vasectomy (i.e., recanalization of the vas deferens has occurred), whereas low numbers of "immotile" sperm can persist for months in some men ($\approx 33\%$).[11]

Morphology

Sperm morphology, like motility, is routinely assessed subjectively. Hence this qualitative determination is subject to intralaboratory and interlaboratory variations. To minimize these variations, standardized procedures and grading criteria must be established by each laboratory and adhered to by all laboratorians. Because the technical ability to identify and classify various morphologic forms requires experience, new staff members must be trained appropriately and their initial work reviewed to ensure accuracy and consistency in reporting. Sperm morphology is complicated by the wide

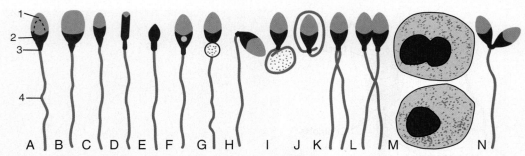

FIGURE 11-4 Sperm morphology. **A,** Normal spermatozoon: *1,* acrosome; *2,* postacrosomal cap; *3,* midpiece; *4,* tail. **B,** Large head. **C,** Tapered head. **D,** Tapered head with acrosome deficiency. **E,** Acrosomal deficiency. **F,** Head vacuole. **G,** Midpiece defect—cytoplasmic extrusion mass. **H,** Bent tail. **I** and **J,** Coiled tails. **K,** Double tail. **L,** Pairing phenomenon. **M,** Sperm precursors (spermatids). **N,** Double-headed (bicephalic) sperm.

variation in abnormal forms that can be encountered, and an inexperienced observer can easily miss subtle abnormalities in sperm. The computerized systems used to assess sperm motility can also evaluate sperm morphology.

Sperm morphometry—measurement of the sperm head length, width, circumference, and area—enables the generation of objective data. To be considered normal, sperm must meet strict criteria regarding their size and shape, which can be determined by computerized systems or manually using a microscope with a calibrated ocular micrometer.

Human sperm have three distinct areas: head, midpiece, and tail. When viewed from the side, sperm appear to be arrowhead shaped (Figure 11-3). When viewed from the top, normal human sperm have oval heads that are 2.5 to 3.5 μm in width and 4.0 to 5.0 μm in length. Only sperm lying flat should be evaluated and their head length-to-width ratio should be 1.50 to 1.75. Spermatozoa with values outside these ranges are considered abnormal, and studies have shown statistically significant differences in the head length-to-width ratios of sperm from ejaculates of fertile and infertile men.[6]

The midpiece, located immediately behind the head, is 6 to 7.5 μm long and is thicker than the tail, but not greater than 1 μm in width. The tail should be slender, uncoiled, and at least 45 μm long. When a "basic" morphology evaluation is performed, each spermatozoon (single sperm cell) is identified simply as normal or abnormal with the percent of normal forms reported. If a "complete" morphology evaluation is performed, then each spermatozoon is classified using five categories: normal, head defects, midpiece defects, tail defects, and cytoplasmic droplet present. Cytoplasmic droplets are usually located in the midpiece region and are considered abnormal if this region is greater than one-third the area of a normal sperm head. The head can contain vacuoles, but they are not considered abnormal unless they occupy more than 20% of the head. Note that a single spermatozoon can have multiple defects, and each defect is

documented. Figure 11-4 depicts a normal spermatozoon and a variety of abnormal forms.

To manually evaluate sperm morphology, smears of fresh semen are made, air dried, and stained. The smears can be made similar to those for traditional blood smears by placing a drop (10 to 15 μL) of semen near one end of a clean microscope slide. Using the edge of another slide, the drop is allowed to spread along the edge of the second slide, and then the edge of the second slide is moved forward, dragging the semen sample across the surface of the first slide and producing a smear. An alternate technique involves placing the second slide over the first and allowing the semen to spread between them. Once spreading is complete, the slides are pulled apart and allowed to air dry. Staining enhances the visualization of sperm morphology and enables the identification and differentiation of white blood cells, epithelial cells of the urethra, and immature spermatogenic cells (i.e., spermatids, spermatocytes, and spermatogonia). Giemsa, Wright's, and Papanicolaou stains are frequently used. These stains differ with respect to complexity and turnaround time, hence laboratories select the stain that best suits their needs and resources.

Using oil immersion (1000×) and an area of the slide where sperm are evenly distributed, 200 sperm are classified. Note that morphologically abnormal sperm are found in all semen specimens. Abnormalities may involve all or only one region of the spermatozoon and can affect its size, shape, or both. In addition, numerous sperm variations are found within a single ejaculate. Although some morphologic abnormalities have been associated with particular disorders (e.g., tapered heads with varicocele), most abnormalities are nonspecific.

The reference range associated with normalcy varies with the criteria and the rigor used to evaluate sperm morphology. In some laboratories, a normal sperm morphology of 50% or greater is considered "normal." However, when strict evaluation criteria are used for fertility purposes as in studies of fertile and subfertile individuals, the number of sperm with normal

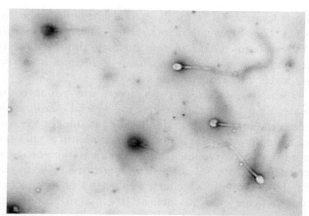

FIGURE 11-5 Sperm vitality using eosin-nigrosin (Blom's) stain. White sperm were alive; pink-stained sperm were dead. Brightfield microscopy, 400×.

morphology is significantly lower. In these studies, normal sperm morphology of less than 5% is a strong predictor of infertility, whereas fertility is associated with normal sperm morphology values of 12% to 15% or greater.[12] Between fertile and subfertile individuals, wide overlap exists in the percentage of sperm with normal morphology. Other variables, particularly sperm concentration and progressive motility, combined with sperm morphology provide the greatest predictive value in assessing male fertility.

Vitality

Vital staining of a fresh semen smear enables rapid differentiation of live and dead sperm. Because dead sperm have damaged plasma membranes, these cells take up stain; living sperm do not (Figure 11-5). When a large percentage of immotile sperm are observed, this evaluation determines whether the sperm are immotile because they are dead or because of a structural abnormality (e.g., defective flagellum).

Eosin alone or an eosin-nigrosin (a modification of Blom's technique) combination is frequently used to determine sperm vitality. Using brightfield or phase-contrast microscopy and 1000× (or 400×), 100 sperm on a stained smear are evaluated. The percentage of dead sperm cells should not exceed the percentage of immotile sperm. In other words, if 65% of the sperm in a semen specimen are dead, the motility cannot exceed 35%. Hence the vitality evaluation provides a convenient quality or cross-check of the motility evaluation. In fresh normal semen, 50% or more of the sperm are alive.

Cells Other Than Spermatozoa

An ejaculate is a complex mixture biochemically and cellularly. Ejaculates normally contain cells other than sperm, such as urethral epithelial cells, white blood cells (WBCs), and immature spermatogenic cells (i.e., spermatids, spermatocytes, and spermatogonia), as well as particulate matter and cellular debris. The spermatogenic cells can be difficult to differentiate from WBCs because of size and nuclear pattern similarities. A peroxidase stain can aid in this evaluation because neutrophils are peroxidase-positive cells, whereas lymphocytes and spermatogenic cells are peroxidase-negative cells. However, owing to the carcinogenicity of the chemicals used in many peroxidase stains and the special handling required, Wright's stain may be preferred.

The presence of greater than 1 million WBCs per milliliter of ejaculate indicates an inflammatory process, most often involving the male accessory glands (e.g., seminal vesicle, prostate). However, a normal WBC count does not rule out infection. Note that the concentrations of WBC and spermatogenic cells can be determined after the sperm count using the same hemacytometer preparation (see Chapter 18). When the concentrations of these cells exceed 1 million per milliliter, a stained smear (e.g., Wright's stain, peroxidase stain) of the fresh ejaculate is evaluated. Using this smear, the numbers of WBCs and immature spermatogenic cells are counted in the same fields used to count 100 mature sperm. With the sperm count (S) and by using the following equation, the concentration (C) of these cell types (N) is determined (Equation 11-2)[3]:

Equation 11-2

$$C = \frac{N \times S}{100}$$

Immature spermatogenic cells are present in the semen when they are exfoliated prematurely from the germinal epithelium of the seminiferous tubules. Distinguishing between an increase in WBCs and an increase in immature spermatogenic cells is necessary to evaluate infection and infertility.

Red blood cells normally are not present in seminal fluid. If their presence is apparent during various aspects of the microscopic evaluation, it should be reported. Similarly, the finding of bacteria in semen should be reported. Bacteria do not normally reside in the male reproductive tract. However, collection of semen by masturbation makes bacterial contamination difficult to avoid.

Agglutination

Agglutination, the sticking together of *motile* sperm, is evident by microscopic examination of a wet preparation. Although some clumping of immotile sperm may occur in normal semen specimens, the observation of distinct head-to-head, head-to-tail, or tail-to-tail orientation of sperm is associated with the presence of sperm-agglutinating antibodies. Clumping of sperm with other entities, such as mucus and other cell types, is not identified as agglutination. The extent of true agglutination is often graded as "few," "moderate," or "many." Even a small amount of true agglutination is significant and indicates the need for further evaluation.

Immunoglobulin G and immunoglobulin A antibodies bound to sperm have been identified and correlated with reduced fertility. This is known as immunologic infertility; the man or the woman can produce antisperm antibodies, and the source can be identified. When the man is producing them, the antibodies are present on the surface of the sperm before intercourse; when the woman is producing them, the sperm are coated with antibodies after they enter the cervical mucus.

Macroscopic and microscopic tests are available to detect and determine the immunoglobulin class of sperm antibodies ([Ig]G, IgA).[3] Both tests produce comparable results, but the mixed agglutination reaction (MAR) test is rapid (≈3 minutes) and easy to perform, whereas the immunobead test is time-consuming (≈45 minutes), technically more complicated, and more expensive. The cutoff values for these tests vary between laboratories. The WHO defines agglutination as clinically significant (abnormal) when antisperm antibodies coat 50% or more of the spermatozoa, whereas other institutions use lower cutoffs (e.g., 20%, 10%).[13]

CHEMICAL EXAMINATION

pH

The pH of fresh normal semen is alkaline and ranges from 7.2 to 7.8. Fresh specimens with a pH less than 7.2 can be obtained from individuals with abnormalities of the epididymis, the vas deferens, or the seminal vesicles. In contrast, fresh specimens exceeding pH 7.8 suggest an infection in the male reproductive tract. Specimens not tested within 1 hour of collection can show changes in the pH for several reasons. An increase in pH can occur because of loss of carbon dioxide; conversely, a decrease in pH can occur because of the accumulation of lactic acid, particularly in specimens with a high sperm count.[2]

Despite the limited usefulness of a seminal fluid pH, the measurement is easy to determine and is usually included in a seminal fluid analysis. Commercial pH paper strips with a range from 4.0 to 10.0 should be used and results recorded to the nearest 0.1 pH unit. Appropriate quality control solutions should be used to ensure the accuracy of the pH strips.

Fructose

The determination of fructose in semen is a commonly performed chemical test. Because fructose is produced and secreted by the seminal vesicles, its presence in semen reflects the secretory function of this gland and the functional integrity of the ejaculatory ducts and vas deferens.

The fructose level is most often determined when the sperm count reveals azoospermia (i.e., no sperm). Obstruction of the ejaculatory ducts or abnormalities of the seminal vesicles or vas deferens can cause low fructose levels and azoospermia.

Normally, semen fructose levels are equal to or greater than 13 μmol per ejaculate. Several quantitative, spectrophotometric procedures are available for fructose determinations. A rapid and easy *qualitative* tube test based on the development of an orange-red color in the presence of fructose can also be performed.[2] With this test, failure of the specimen to develop an orange-red color indicates the absence of fructose. Although this technique is qualitative, relies on the visual assessment of color, and lacks sensitivity to decreased fructose levels, its ease of performance and rapid turnaround time make it a useful tool.

Other Biochemical Markers

Quantitative determinations of zinc and citric acid levels in semen can be used to evaluate the secretory function of the prostate gland. The usefulness of zinc and citric acid measurements as markers of biochemical function is ongoing; clinicians are attempting to establish correlations with disease processes (e.g., low zinc levels with prostatitis). Quantitation of zinc can be performed by spectrophotometric or atomic absorption spectroscopy techniques. In normal semen, the total zinc concentration is equal to or greater than 2.4 mmol per ejaculate.

Citric acid, the major anion in semen, can be quantitated using spectrophotometric methods.[1] Decreased levels indicate dysfunction of the prostate gland. The total citric acid concentration in normal semen is equal to or greater than 52 mmol per ejaculate.

Acid phosphatase activity is a useful marker to assess the secretory function of the prostate gland. Normally, seminal fluid contains 200 units of enzyme activity or more per ejaculate, whereas other body fluids contain insignificant amounts. Because of this uniquely high concentration, prostatic acid phosphatase measurements are often used to determine whether semen is present in vaginal fluid specimens obtained from women following an alleged rape or sexual assault. Even washings of the skin or stained clothing can reveal significant levels of prostatic acid phosphatase, which positively identifies the presence of semen.

Other biochemical substances are being investigated in an attempt to identify and establish specific markers for male reproductive tract abnormalities. For example, L-carnitine and α-glucosidase are being evaluated as indicators of epididymal function, whereas specific lactate dehydrogenase isoenzymes of sperm are being examined for their clinical use in the evaluation of male fertility.

STUDY QUESTIONS

1. Seminal fluid analysis is routinely performed to evaluate which of the following?
   A. Prostate cancer
   B. Postvasectomy status
   C. Penile implant status
   D. Premature ejaculation

2. Which of the following structures contribute(s) secretions to semen?
   1. Epididymis
   2. Prostate gland
   3. Seminal vesicles
   4. Seminiferous tubules
   A. 1, 2, and 3 are correct.
   B. 1 and 3 are correct.
   C. 4 is correct.
   D. All are correct.

3. Which of the following structures performs an endocrine and an exocrine function?
   A. Testes
   B. Epididymis
   C. Prostate gland
   D. Seminal vesicles

4. The primary function of semen is to
   A. nourish the spermatozoa.
   B. coagulate the ejaculate.
   C. transport the spermatozoa.
   D. stimulate sperm maturation.

5. Match the number of the structure to the feature that best describes it. Only one structure is correct for each feature.

Descriptive Feature	Structure
___ A. Produces and secretes testosterone	1. Bulbourethral gland
___ B. Site of spermatogenesis	2. Ejaculatory duct
___ C. Concentrates and stores sperm	3. Epididymis
___ D. Secretes fluid rich in zinc	4. Interstitial cells of Leydig
___ E. Secretes fluid high in fructose	5. Prostate gland
___ F. Transports sperm to the ejaculatory duct	6. Seminal vesicles
	7. Seminiferous tubules
	8. Vas deferens

6. Which of the following is a requirement when collecting semen specimens?
   A. The patient should abstain from sexual intercourse for at least 2 days following the collection.
   B. Only complete collections of the entire ejaculate are acceptable for analysis.
   C. A single semen specimen is sufficient for the evaluation of male fertility.
   D. Semen specimens must be evaluated within 3 hours following collection.

7. Which of the following conditions adversely affects the quality of a semen specimen?
   A. The use of Silastic condoms
   B. The time of day the collection is obtained
   C. The collection of the specimen in a glass container
   D. The storage of the specimen at refrigerator temperatures

8. Which of the following statements regarding semen is true?
   A. Semen usually coagulates within 30 minutes after ejaculation.
   B. For semen to liquefy before 60 minutes is abnormal.
   C. Following liquefaction, the viscosity of normal semen is similar to that of water.
   D. Following liquefaction, the presence of particulate matter is highly indicative of a bacterial infection.

9. Which of the following statements regarding the manual evaluation of sperm motility is *not* true?
   A. Sperm motility most often is graded subjectively.
   B. Sperm motility is affected adversely by temperature.
   C. Sperm motility assesses speed and forward progression.
   D. Sperm motility should be evaluated initially and at 2 hours after collection.

10. Which of the following statements regarding sperm concentration is true?
    A. Sperm concentration within a single individual is usually constant.
    B. Sperm concentration depends solely on the period of abstinence.
    C. In a normal ejaculate, sperm concentration ranges from 20 to 250 million per milliliter.
    D. For fertility purposes, sperm concentration is more important than sperm motility.

11. Which of the following statements regarding sperm morphology is true?
    A. Sperm morphology is usually evaluated using a peroxidase stain.
    B. Stained smears of fresh semen can be used to evaluate sperm morphology.
    C. Sperm morphology is evaluated using 400× (high-power) magnification.
    D. Normal semen contains at least 80% sperm with normal morphology.

12. Which of the following parameters directly relates to and provides a check of the sperm motility evaluation?
    A. Agglutination evaluation
    B. Concentration determination
    C. Morphology assessment
    D. Vitality assessment

13. Microscopically, immature spermatogenic cells are often difficult to distinguish from
   A. bacteria.
   B. erythrocytes.
   C. leukocytes.
   D. epithelial cells.

14. A semen pH greater than 7.8 is associated with
   A. premature ejaculation.
   B. obstruction of the vas deferens.
   C. abnormal seminal vesicle function.
   D. infection of the male reproductive tract.

15. Fructose in semen assists in the evaluation of which of the following?
   1. The secretory function of the seminal vesicles
   2. The functional integrity of the epididymis
   3. The functional integrity of the vas deferens
   4. The secretory function of the prostate gland
   A. 1, 2, and 3 are correct.
   B. 1 and 3 are correct.
   C. 4 is correct.
   D. All are correct.

16. Which of the following substances can be used to evaluate the secretory function of the prostate gland?
   A. Carnitine
   B. Fructose
   C. pH
   D. Zinc

17. The concentration of which of the following substances can be used to positively identify a fluid as seminal fluid?
   A. Acid phosphatase
   B. Citric acid
   C. Fructose
   D. Zinc

CASE 11-2

A semen specimen is collected by a 45-year-old man for evaluation of a vasectomy performed 12 weeks earlier.

Semen Analysis

Physical Examination
   Color: white
   Volume: 3 mL
   Liquefaction: 40 minutes
   Viscosity: 0 (watery)

Microscopic Examination
   Motility: 50%
   Concentration: 1×10^6 sperm/mL
   Morphology: 80% normal
   Vitality: 60%
   Leukocytes: 2×10^6 cells/mL
   Other: moderate bacteria

1. List any abnormal or discrepant results.
2. Do any of the results obtained suggest improper specimen collection or laboratory error?
3. After an appropriate time interval, how many sperm should be present in seminal fluid following a successful vasectomy?

REFERENCES

1. Kjeldsberg CR, Knight JA: Body fluids, ed 2, Chicago, 1986, American Society of Clinical Pathologists Press.
2. Amelar RD, Dubin L: Semen analysis. In Amelar RD, Dubin L, Walsh PC, editors: Male infertility, Philadelphia, 1977, WB Saunders.
3. World Health Organization: WHO laboratory manual for the examination and processing of human semen, ed 5, Geneva, Switzerland, 2010, World Health Organization.
4. Tomlinson M, Turner J, Powell G, et al: One step disposable chambers for sperm concentration and motility assessments: how do they compare with the World Health Organization's recommended methods? Hum Reprod 16:121, 2001.
5. Keel BA, Quinn P, Schmidt CF, et al: Results of the American Association of Bioanalysts national proficiency testing programme in andrology. Hum Reprod 15:680, 2000.
6. Katz DF, Overstreet JW, Samuels SJ, et al: Morphometric analysis of spermatozoa in the assessment of human male fertility. J Androl 7:203, 1986.
7. Mendeluk FL, Flecha G, Castello PR, Bregni C: Factors involved in the biochemical etiology of human seminal plasma hyperviscosity. Journal of Andrology, 21:262, 2000.
8. Overstreet JW, Katz DF, Hanson FW, Fonseca JR: A simple inexpensive method for the objective assessment of human sperm movement characteristics. Fertil Steril 31:162, 1979.
9. Barfield A, Melo J, Coutinho E, et al: Pregnancies associated with sperm concentrations below 10 million/mL in clinical studies of a potential male contraceptive method, monthly depot medroxyprogesterone acetate and testosterone esters. Contraception 20:121, 1979.
10. Lu J, Chen F, Xu H, Huang Y, Lu N: Comparison of three sperm-counting methods for the determination of sperm concentration in human semen and sperm suspensions. Lab Medicine 38(4):232, 2007.
11. De Knijff DW, Vrijhof HJ, Arends J, Janknegt RA: Persistence or reappearance of nonmotile sperm after vasectomy: does it have clinical consequences? Fertil Steril 67:332, 1997.
12. Ombelet W, Bosmans E, Janssen M, et al: Semen parameters in a fertile versus subfertile population: a need for change in the interpretation of semen testing. Hum Reprod 12:987, 1997.
13. Marconi M, Nowotny A, Pantke P, et al: Antisperm antibodies detected by mixed agglutination reaction and immunobead test are not associated with chronic inflammation and infection of the seminal tract. Andrologia 40:227, 2008.

CASE 11-1

A 36-year-old man and his 32-year-old wife are undergoing an evaluation for infertility. A semen specimen is collected at home and is brought to the laboratory for routine testing.

Semen Analysis

Physical Examination
   Color: gray
   Volume: 4.5 mL
   Liquefaction: 50 minutes
   Viscosity: 0 (watery)

Microscopic Examination
   Motility: 70%
   Concentration: 15×10^6 sperm/mL
   Morphology: 70% normal
   Vitality: 60%
   Leukocytes: 0.8×10^6 cells/mL

1. List any abnormal or discrepant results.
2. Do any of the results obtained suggest improper specimen collection or laboratory error?
3. Are any of the results obtained associated with male infertility?
4. Based on these results, what chemical test should be performed to evaluate the functional integrity of the seminal vesicles and ejaculatory ducts?

BIBLIOGRAPHY

Amelar RD: The semen analysis. In Infertility in men: diagnosis and treatment, Philadelphia, 1966, FA Davis.

Barrosos G, Mercan R, Oxgur K, et al: Intra- and inter-laboratory variability in the assessment of sperm morphology by strict criteria: impact of semen preparation, staining techniques and manual versus computerized analysis. Hum Reprod 14:2036, 1999.

Freund M: Standards for the rating of human sperm morphology. Int J Fertil 11:97, 1966.

Jeyendran RS: Sperm collection and processing: a practical guide, New York, 2003, Cambridge University Press.

Keel BA, Quinn P, Schmidt CF, et al: Results of the American Association of Bioanalysts national proficiency testing programme in andrology. Hum Reprod 15:680, 2000.

Makler A: The improved ten-micrometer chamber for rapid sperm count and motility evaluation. Fertil Steril 33:337, 1980.

Overstreet JW, Katz DF: Semen analysis. Urol Clin North Am 14:441, 1987.

Tomlinson MJ, Kessopoulou E, Barratt CL: The diagnostic and prognostic value of traditional semen parameters. J Androl 20:588, 1999.

World Health Organization (WHO) laboratory manual for the examination of human semen and sperm-cervical mucus interaction, ed 4, New York, 1999, Cambridge University Press.

Amniotic Fluid Analysis

KEY TERMS

erythroblastosis fetalis A hemolytic disease of the newborn that results from a blood group incompatibility between mother and infant.

fluorescence polarization An analytical technique based on the change in polarization observed in fluorescent light emitted compared with the incident polarized fluorescent light. Observed changes in light polarization result from the molecular size of the fluorophore-tagged complex. Large molecules cannot randomly orient as rapidly as small molecules. Hence fluorophores tagged to large molecular complexes emit more

fluorescence in the same polarized plane as the initial incident light than fluorophores tagged to small molecular complexes.

lamellar bodies Cytoplasmic storage granules that contain pulmonary surfactant and are secreted into the alveolar lumen by fetal type II pneumocytes that line the lungs. When electron microscopy is used, these granules have a characteristic layered or onion-like appearance, hence the name "lamellar" bodies. They begin to appear in amniotic fluid at 20 to 24 weeks' gestation.

meconium A dark green gelatinous or mucus-like material representing swallowed amniotic

fluid and intestinal secretions excreted by the near-term or full-term infant. The infant normally passes meconium as the first bowel movement shortly after birth.

oligohydramnios A decreased amount (<800 mL) of amniotic fluid in the amniotic sac.

polyhydramnios (also called *hydramnios*) An abnormally increased amount (>1200 mL) of amniotic fluid in the amniotic sac. Polyhydramnios is often associated with malformations of the fetal central nervous system (i.e., neural tube defects) or gastrointestinal tract.

With the use of ultrasound, amniocentesis is now a common and safe obstetric procedure. Advancements in technology have provided new technical methods and clinical applications for amniotic fluid analysis. The study of amniotic fluid is performed primarily for three reasons: (1) to enable antenatal diagnosis of genetic and congenital disorders early in fetal gestation (15 to 18 weeks), (2) to assess fetal pulmonary maturity later in the pregnancy (32 to 42 weeks), and (3) to estimate and monitor the degree of fetal distress caused by isoimmunization or infection.

By far the most frequently performed tests on amniotic fluid in the clinical laboratory are used to assess fetal pulmonary maturity and fetal distress, which are discussed in this chapter. The specialized laboratory techniques required to detect numerous and varied genetic and metabolic disorders using amniotic fluid are beyond the scope and intent of this text and therefore are not discussed.

PHYSIOLOGY AND COMPOSITION

Function

Amniotic fluid is the liquid medium that bathes a fetus throughout its gestation (Figure 12-1). The amnion, a membrane composed of a single layer of cuboidal epithelial cells, surrounds the fetus and is filled with this fluid. Amniotic fluid protects the fetus while enabling fetal movement and plays an important role in numerous biochemical processes. Fetal cells and many biochemical compounds, such as electrolytes, nitrogenous compounds, proteins, enzymes, lipids, and hormones, are present in the amniotic fluid. Although studies have investigated many substances as potential biochemical markers of disease, few substances (e.g., phospholipids) have demonstrated reliable clinical utility and value.

Formation

The dynamics of amniotic fluid formation and its composition change throughout fetal gestation. Initially, amniotic fluid is produced by the amnion and the placenta, and its composition is similar to that of a dialysate of plasma. However, as gestation progresses, the fetus plays more of an active role in the composition of the fluid. Water and solutes exchange between the fetus and its surrounding medium through several mechanisms: (1) intestinal absorption following fetal swallowing of amniotic fluid; (2) capillary exchange in the pulmonary system, as the alveoli of the fetal lungs are bathed with amniotic fluid; and (3) fetal urination. Early in gestation (before keratinization of the skin), a transudate passes through the skin of the fetus and makes a small contribution to the amniotic fluid volume. Because of fetal respiration in utero, the fetal pulmonary surfactants produced by alveolar cells of the fetal lungs mix with and can be evaluated using amniotic fluid.

In the later stages of pregnancy, fetal swallowing and urination play a major role in the volume and composition of the amniotic fluid. The fetus swallows amniotic fluid, removing water and electrolytes, and replaces them through urination with metabolic by-products such as urea, creatinine, and uric acid. At the same time, a similar exchange occurs between the amniotic fluid and the maternal plasma. The maternal plasma removes metabolic waste products and replenishes them with water, nutrients, and electrolytes. This ongoing, dynamic

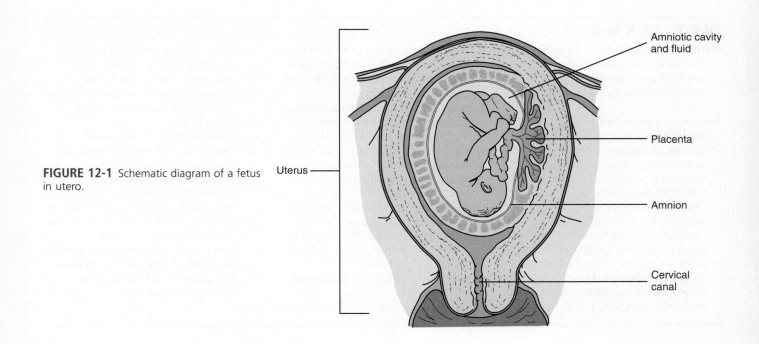

FIGURE 12-1 Schematic diagram of a fetus in utero.

Uterus

Amniotic cavity and fluid

Placenta

Amnion

Cervical canal

equilibrium results in complete exchange of the amniotic fluid volume every 2 to 3 hours.[1] The presence of a neural tube defect causes fetal cerebrospinal fluid to also contribute substances to the amniotic fluid. In such cases, alpha-fetoprotein and acetylcholinesterase are two biochemical markers used to identify these defects.

Volume

The volume of amniotic fluid increases steadily throughout pregnancy, from approximately 25 to 50 mL at 12 weeks' gestation to a volume of 800 to 1200 mL at 37 weeks' gestation.[2] Abnormally increased amounts of amniotic fluid (>1200 mL), termed **polyhydramnios,** are associated with decreased fetal swallowing and often indicate congenital fetal malformations. Abnormally decreased amounts of amniotic fluid (<800 mL), termed **oligohydramnios,** occur with congenital malformations and other conditions, such as premature rupture of the amniotic membranes.

SPECIMEN COLLECTION

Timing of and Indications for Amniocentesis

Amniotic fluid is collected transabdominally or vaginally with simultaneous ultrasonic examination. Use of real-time ultrasonography allows the clinician to identify a maternal tapping site that will yield amniotic fluid and at the same time avoid injury to the fetus or the placenta. Transabdominal amniocentesis is preferred because vaginal amniocentesis is associated with an increased risk of infection, can result in contamination of the fluid with vaginal cells and bacteria, and can adversely affect results obtained using fetal lung maturity tests.

Typically, amniocentesis is performed after 14 weeks' gestation; however, the purpose of performing the procedure dictates when it is done (Table 12-1). For example,

TABLE 12-1	Indications for Amniocentesis
When to Perform Amniocentesis	**Indications**
14-18 weeks	Mother ≥35 years Parent has known chromosomal abnormality Previous child with chromosomal abnormality Previous child with neural tube defect Parent is carrier of a metabolic disorder Elevated maternal alpha-fetoprotein (suspect neural tube defect)
20-42 weeks	Assessment of fetal distress due to: • Blood group incompatibility (e.g., Rh) • Infection Assessment of fetal lung maturity

an amniocentesis to detect neural tube defects or genetic abnormalities is usually performed at 15 to 18 weeks' gestation. This allows sufficient time for the performance of chromosomal and biochemical studies, which may include culturing of fetal cells, as well as time for consideration of pregnancy termination if the fetus is determined to be abnormal.

Amniocentesis later in pregnancy is primarily used to assess the pulmonary and overall health status of the fetus. Tests can determine the maturity of the fetal pulmonary system by analyzing surfactants in the amniotic fluid. If results indicate an immature fetal pulmonary system, elective delivery can be postponed and corticosteroids (betamethasone) that promote lung development can be given, or attempts made to suppress premature labor. In late pregnancy, amniocentesis may be performed to assess fetal status owing to toxemia, diabetes mellitus, or isoimmunization by Rhesus (Rh) factor. At times, these conditions necessitate early termination of a pregnancy and the delivery of a premature infant.

Collection and Specimen Containers

Using aseptic technique, a physician pierces the abdominal and uterine walls with a long, sterile needle and aspirates approximately 10 to 20 mL of amniotic fluid into several sterile syringes. A series of numbered syringes (usually two or three) are used to prevent contamination of the entire collection with blood that can be encountered initially. The blood can result from piercing a blood vessel in the abdominal wall, uterus, placenta, umbilical cord, or fetus. Ideally, the amniotic fluid shows no evidence of blood.

Immediately following its collection, the amniotic fluid should be carefully transferred into sterile plastic containers for transport to the laboratory. Glass containers should be avoided because cells will adhere to glass. Amber-colored containers or aluminum foil should be used to protect the fluid from light; this prevents photo-oxidation of bilirubin, if present. When cytogenetic or microbial studies are to be performed, amniotic fluid must be processed aseptically.

Specimen Transport, Storage, and Handling

Transportation of amniotic fluid specimens to the laboratory should occur as soon as possible to ensure the preservation of cellular and biochemical constituents. Note that storage temperature and handling (e.g., centrifugation) will vary with the tests requested and the protocols used by the laboratory performing the test.

Specimens for cell culture and chromosomal studies must be maintained at body or room temperature. Similarly, those for fetal lung maturity (FLM) testing are usually stable for 16 to 24 hours at room temperature.

Some laboratories may prefer that amniotic fluid samples be refrigerated. When bilirubin analysis is requested, the specimen must be protected from light at the bedside by wrapping the collection tube in foil or using an amber-colored container.

Depending on the FLM tests performed, amniotic fluid may (L/S ratio) or may not (e.g., fluorescence polarization) be centrifuged. Note that the speed and duration of centrifugation can alter the composition of the amniotic fluid supernatant and pellet significantly. Low centrifuge speeds are used to recover fetal cells from amniotic fluid for cell culture. For spectrophotometric assays (e.g., ΔA_{450}), a high speed is used to maximally clear the supernatant of turbidity. Another approach used to remove residual turbidity is to filter the amniotic fluid; however, this can significantly reduce the amount of sample available for testing.

Differentiation From Urine

At times it may be necessary to determine whether the fluid collected is amniotic fluid or whether it is urine aspirated from the bladder. Physical examination alone cannot distinguish between these fluids because they can have the same appearance. However, their chemical compositions are distinctly different for several analytes. Amniotic fluid contains glucose and a significant amount of protein (approximately 2 to 8 g/L), and, until late pregnancy, the creatinine concentration is similar to that of normal plasma. In contrast, urine has essentially no protein or glucose and contains characteristically high concentrations of urea and creatinine (50 to 100× those of plasma). Therefore, these chemical constituents can be used to positively determine the identity of the fluid collected. For example, if a reagent strip test were used, positive results for glucose and protein would identify the fluid as amniotic fluid. However, because diabetes and renal disease can cause protein and glucose to be present in urine, the creatinine or urea concentration of the fluids should also be determined.

It should be noted that in late pregnancy (≥37 weeks' gestation), the use of creatinine levels to distinguish between urine and amniotic fluid is more challenging. Fetal renal function has begun and contributes creatinine to the amniotic fluid. At this stage, the creatinine concentration in amniotic fluid can be two to three times that of normal plasma or up to 3.9 mg/dL (345 μmol/L). If a creatinine value greater than 4 mg/dL (354 μmol/L) is obtained, this indicates that the fluid is either urine or amniotic fluid contaminated with urine.

PHYSICAL EXAMINATION

Color

The physical examination of amniotic fluid should take place immediately after its receipt in the laboratory. This examination consists of a visual assessment of the color and turbidity of the fluid. Normally, amniotic fluid is colorless or pale yellow. Distinctive yellow or amber coloration is associated with the presence of bilirubin; a green color indicates the presence of meconium. **Meconium** is a gelatinous or mucus-like material that forms in the fetal intestine as the result of swallowed amniotic fluid and fetal intestinal secretions. Biliverdin is responsible for its dark green color. Normally, full-term infants do not have a bowel movement in utero but excrete meconium as their first bowel movement after birth. However, fetal distress can cause premature release of meconium into the amniotic fluid.

Blood contamination causes amniotic fluid to appear anywhere from pale pink to red. If blood is present in an amniotic fluid sample, the specimen should be centrifuged immediately to remove any intact red blood cells before hemolysis occurs. Hemolysis causes the formation of oxyhemoglobin, which can interfere with several biochemical tests.

Turbidity

All amniotic fluid is turbid to some degree depending on the stage of pregnancy. Early in pregnancy, little particulate matter is present and the fluid is not very turbid. As pregnancy progresses, increased amounts of fetal cells, hair, and vernix are sloughed and remain suspended in the amniotic fluid. Two techniques that can be used to remove the particulate matter causing the turbidity are centrifugation and filtration.

CHEMICAL EXAMINATION

Fetal Lung Maturity Tests

When premature delivery is anticipated or desired because of fetal distress or other complications, ensuring that the fetus will be viable outside of the mother's uterus is important. To assess fetal maturity and potential viability, tests that evaluate the functional status of the fetal lungs predominate because the pulmonary system is one of the last organ systems to mature. Note that fetal lung maturity (FLM) testing on amniotic fluid when gestation is less than 32 weeks is not performed because all FLM test results will indicate immaturity.[3]

Respiratory distress syndrome (RDS) is the most common cause of death in the newborn and is a primary concern when a preterm delivery is imminent. RDS results from insufficient production of surfactant at the alveolar surfaces in the newborn's lungs. Normally, alveolar epithelial cells of the lungs (type II pneumocytes) produce and secrete phospholipids (90%) and proteins (10%) in the form of **lamellar bodies**.[4] These lamellar bodies release their "surface active" compounds, also known as *surfactants,* into the alveolar air space. Surfactants act in two ways: They alter the surface tension of the alveoli, preventing their collapse during expiration, and they reduce the amount of pressure needed to reopen them during inspiration. Gluck and associates discovered the correlation between fetal lung maturity and the concentrations of specific phospholipids in amniotic fluid.[5] More recently, it has been recognized that the probability of developing RDS is best determined using two factors: the results of FLM tests and the gestational age of the fetus at the time of testing.[3] From several studies, a table has been developed to guide clinicians in making individualized risk-benefit decisions for preterm delivery using gestational age and the fetal lung maturity value.[6]

The American College of Obstetrics and Gynecology (ACOG) recommends a sequential or "cascade" approach to FLM testing. With this approach, a "mature" result using any of the common FLM tests is strongly predictive for the absence of RSD.[7] In other words, a series of FLM tests can be performed until a mature result is obtained or all testing options have been used (Table 12-2). A rapid test, such as the fluorescence polarization method or a lamellar body count, should be performed first. In late pregnancy (>35 weeks' gestation), the rapid immunochemical test used to detect phosphatidylglycerol (PG) can be used. Additional testing is required when initial test results (1) are indeterminate, (2) are at the cutoff value, or (3) indicate immaturity. The availability of FLM tests and the cascade protocol used vary among laboratories. The cutoff values for FLM tests have been selected to reduce the risk of delivering infants with immature lungs. However, a "mature" result from an FLM test does not completely eliminate the possibility of RDS. In other words, the predictive value of a negative test (i.e., a mature result) is high (95% to 100%) for all available FLM tests; however, the predictive value of a positive test (i.e., an immature result and the presence of RDS) is low (23% to 61%) and varies with the FLM test used.[3]

Lecithin/Sphingomyelin Ratio. In fetal lungs, phospholipids are required to decrease the surface tension within the alveoli and in doing so, prevent alveolar collapse and enable gas exchange. Lecithin is the major pulmonary surfactant that performs this function. Sphingomyelin, a phospholipid found in numerous cell membranes, is also present, but its functional role has yet to be established. Studies of phospholipid concentrations in amniotic fluid have revealed that until approximately 33 weeks' gestation, the fetal pulmonary system produces lecithin and sphingomyelin in relatively equal concentrations. However at 34 to 36 weeks' gestation, the concentration of lecithin significantly increases, whereas that of

TABLE 12-2	Fetal Lung Maturity Tests				
Test	**Principle**	**Effects of Blood and Meconium**	**Advantages**	**Disadvantages**
Fluorescence polarization	Competitive binding of fluorescent probe to albumin and surfactant; polarization of probe	• Blood and meconium cause *erroneous* results	Simple, rapid, reliable	Requires specialized instrument Historic; no longer available
Lamellar body counts	Automated cell counter (hematology analyzers) enumerates lamellar bodies in amniotic fluid using the platelet channel	• Blood *falsely decreases* count • Meconium causes minimal *increase in* counts[3,4]	• Simple, rapid, reliable • Inexpensive—uses available instrumentation	No consensus on clearly established cutoff value that predicts RDS[3]
Foam stability index (FSI)	Amniotic fluid shaken vigorously with varying concentrations of ethanol; index is the highest concentration with a stable layer of bubbles at meniscus	• Blood and meconium cause *falsely increased* results	Simple, rapid	• Reproducibility is technically challenging • Requires clean glassware and absolute ethanol
Phosphatidylglycerol (PG)	Agglutination test: agglutination of PG using polyclonal anti-PG antibodies; qualitative results	None	• Simple, rapid, reliable • Can use vaginal pool collections	• Applicable only at ≥35 weeks' gestation • High "false" immaturity rate
	Thin-layer chromatography	None	Reference method	• Technically difficult and labor-intensive • Time-consuming • Expensive
Lecithin/sphingomyelin ratio	Thin-layer chromatography	• Blood *falsely lowers* ratio • Meconium *falsely increases* ratio	Reference method	• Technically difficult, labor-intensive • Time-consuming • Expensive

RDS, Respiratory distress syndrome.

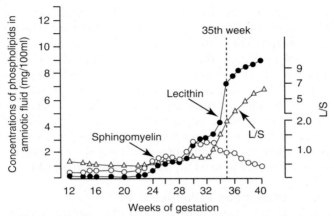

FIGURE 12-2 Changes in the concentrations of lecithin and sphingomyelin and changes in the lecithin/sphingomyelin ratio during normal pregnancy. *(Adapted from Gluck L, Kulovich MV: Lecithin/sphingomyelin ratios in amniotic fluid in normal and abnormal pregnancies. Am J Obstet Gynecol 115:539, 1973.)*

sphingomyelin remains relatively constant or decreases (Figure 12-2). These observations led to the calculation of the lecithin/sphingomyelin (L/S) ratio, which has become clinically valuable in evaluating fetal lung maturity or fetal pulmonary status.

An L/S ratio less than 2.0 is associated with immaturity of the fetal pulmonary system, whereas one equal to or greater than 2.0 indicates maturity. These values are determined using thin-layer chromatography (TLC) to quantify the relative concentrations of each phospholipid. Numerous variations of the original TLC procedure exist. Therefore, assessment of fetal lung maturity requires a comparison of the L/S ratio obtained to the reference criteria established by the laboratory performing the test.

The presence of blood in amniotic fluid can decrease a mature result, whereas it can increase an immature result.[3] Consequently, an L/S ratio that indicates maturity despite using a bloody amniotic fluid specimen has clinical value. However, the reverse (i.e., an immature result on a bloody specimen) does not have value. Meconium-contaminated amniotic fluid should not be used. Although lecithin and sphingomyelin are not present in meconium, the L/S ratio obtained when meconium-contaminated specimens are used is unreliable and must be interpreted with caution, if performed.

The L/S ratio is a better predictor of the maturity of fetal lungs than of immaturity. In other words, some infants (2% to 5%) with an L/S ratio greater than 2.0 still develop RDS, despite having a "mature" L/S ratio. In contrast, 30% to 40% of infants with an L/S ratio between 1.5 and 2.0 do not develop RDS and are falsely identified by the L/S ratio as having an "immature" pulmonary system.

Phosphatidylglycerol. Phosphatidylglycerol (PG), a phospholipid that enhances the spread of surfactants across the alveolar surface, normally is not detectable in amniotic fluid until 35 weeks' gestation. PG can be measured using similar TLC procedures as for L/S ratios or by an agglutination slide test—Amniostat-FLM test (Irvine Scientific, Santa Ana, CA). This immunochemical test uses polyclonal anti-PG antibodies to agglutinate the microscopic PG-containing lamellar bodies in amniotic fluid into macroscopically visible agglutinates or clusters. Results are reported as negative (immature), or as low positive (mature) or high positive (mature), based on the size of agglutinates and the degree of background clearance. The agglutination test is simple to perform and takes a minimal amount of time (<30 minutes) compared with the more labor-intensive TLC procedure.

Even though PG detection tests are specific for PG, they produce a high number of false-negative results (i.e., identifying fluids as immature when in fact there is maturity). Therefore, a positive PG slide test is clinically valuable, indicating pulmonary maturity, whereas a negative test provides no useful information. PG detection tests are reliable and have a distinct advantage in that results are not affected by the presence of blood or meconium. In addition, test results obtained using vaginal pool collections of amniotic fluid are valid.[3] One disadvantage of PG tests is that they cannot be used until late pregnancy (>35 weeks' gestation).

Foam Stability Index. The foam stability index (FSI) or "shake test" is based on the physical or functional characteristics that surfactants impart to amniotic fluid. In other words, if adequate surfactants are present in the amniotic fluid, a foam can be produced by shaking the fluid vigorously with ethanol, and the bubbles remain stable at the air-liquid interface in the tube. Because this indirect assessment of surfactant concentration is rapid and easy to perform, it is used when other methods are not available.

Determining the FSI involves mixing equal volumes of amniotic fluid with differing volumes of ethanol, followed by vigorous shaking. The concentration of ethanol in each tube represents the possible index values, ranging from 0.43 to 0.55. The highest concentration of ethanol with a stable foam present is the FSI for that specimen. A stable foam is one in which the bubbles remain around the entire meniscus of the tube 15 minutes after shaking. An FSI of 0.48 or greater correlates with fetal lung maturity.

A significant disadvantage of the FSI is the inaccurate results obtained when blood or meconium contaminates the amniotic fluid. These substances cause a falsely high or "mature" index value, when in fact the amount of functional pulmonary surfactant present is inadequate. Therefore a "mature" FSI (i.e., 0.48 or greater) obtained on a contaminated specimen is of no clinical value; in contrast, an "immature" index on a contaminated specimen is clinically useful, indicating inadequate pulmonary surfactant.

Fluorescence Polarization Assay. The fluorescence polarization assay used to assess fetal lung maturity is no longer manufactured. TDx-FLM II (Abbott Laboratories, Abbott Park, IL), assay was based on the microviscosity of amniotic fluid, which is related directly to the quantity of pulmonary surfactants present. The TDx-FLM II test used **fluorescence polarization** to evaluate the amount of pulmonary surfactant relative to albumin. In the assay, a fluorophore (i.e., fluorescent dye) was mixed with the amniotic fluid and associated with both albumin and the surfactant liposomes (i.e., aggregated of phospholipids) present. Fluorophores associated with albumin are not able to rotate as freely as fluorophores associated with the surfactant liposomes. Consequently, the measured fluorescence polarization was high when amniotic fluid contained low levels of surfactants.

The surfactant/albumin ratio was determined by comparing the fluorescence polarization value obtained for the sample to a standard curve derived using calibrators of known surfactant/albumin content. Surfactant/albumin ratios less than 40 mg/g indicated immature lungs, and values greater than 55 mg/g indicated mature lungs. Values between 40 mg/g and 55 mg/g were considered indeterminate and indicated the need for additional FLM testing.[3,8,9]

Specimens contaminated with blood or meconium could not be analyzed using this method because results were adversely affected (see Table 12-2).

Lamellar Body Counts. The pulmonary surfactants are stored in **lamellar bodies.** Under electron microscopy, they have a characteristic layered or onion-like appearance, hence their name. The secretion of lamellar bodies into the alveolar lumen begins at 20 to 24 weeks' gestation. By the third trimester, they are present in the amniotic fluid at concentrations ranging from 50,000 to 200,000 per microliter.

Lamellar body counts (LBCs) can be rapidly and reliably obtained using the platelet channel of an automated hematology cell counter. Amniotic fluid contaminated with blood should not be used. Depending on the amount of blood present, it can cause an increased LBC resulting from the presence of blood platelets, or a decreased LBC from trapping of lamellar bodies in the clot matrix.[3] The presence of meconium can cause an increase in the LBC, but this is considered minimal.[10] Several advantages of LBC include (1) the small sample volume needed (≈0.5 mL), (2) the short turnaround time, and (3) the low cost. Studies comparing LBC with the L/S ratio and the PG test have shown LBC to be a reliable screening test to assess fetal lung maturity.[11,12]

The LBC will vary with the laboratory's instrumentation and protocol for specimen preparation. Amniotic fluid specimens should be mixed gently (2 minutes on tube rocker) but not centrifuged.[3] Note that FLM studies using LBC vary regarding the use of centrifugation; therefore laboratories must establish and validate their own cutoffs for maturity. When uncentrifuged samples are used, LBCs greater than 50,000/µL are considered

mature, and those less than 15,000/µL are considered immature.[13] When the LBC value is below the fetal lung maturity cutoff for the laboratory, additional FLM testing using alternate methods is necessary.[14]

Amniotic Fluid Bilirubin (or ΔA450 Determination)

Normally throughout fetal gestation, the bilirubin concentration in amniotic fluid is low and essentially undetectable (≈10 to 30 mg/dL). During normal red blood cell (RBC) destruction in the fetus, unconjugated bilirubin is produced and is removed rapidly by the placenta into the maternal circulation. Because the fetus has an immature liver, when a hemolytic disease process causes increased and persistent hemolysis of fetal erythrocytes, the production of unconjugated bilirubin increases significantly. As a result, an increased amount of unconjugated bilirubin enters the amniotic fluid through a mechanism that remains unclear, and its presence is detectable spectrophotometrically.

Hemolytic disease of the newborn, or **erythroblastosis fetalis,** occurs when maternal antibodies cross the placenta into the fetal circulation and destroy large numbers of fetal RBCs. Isoimmune diseases can involve any blood group antigen. They indicate that, at some point during the current pregnancy or a previous one, the maternal circulation was exposed to fetal blood cells and developed an antibody against them. The most commonly encountered fetal hemolytic disease results from sensitization of an Rh-negative mother to the $Rh_0(D)$ antigen. It can be prevented by the administration of $Rh_0(D)$ immune globulin (RhoGAM) to Rh-negative mothers, typically at 28 weeks' gestation and within 72 hours after childbirth. The immune globulin prevents the mother's immune system from becoming sensitized to fetal Rh antigen.

The amount of bilirubin in amniotic fluid is directly related to the severity of hemolysis, and serial bilirubin measurements are used to monitor these conditions. When normal amniotic fluid is scanned spectrophotometrically from 350 to 580 nm, the spectral curve obtained is essentially a straight line that gradually decreases in absorbance between 365 and 550 nm (Figure 12-3, A). Bilirubin has maximum absorbance at 450 nm. Therefore as the concentration of bilirubin in amniotic fluid increases, the absorbance of the spectral curve at 450 nm also increases proportionately (Figure 12-3, B). The ΔA_{450}, or the change in absorbance at 450 nm, is obtained by drawing a straight baseline for the spectral curve between 365 and 550 nm and calculating the difference in absorbance at 450 nm (Figure 12-3, C).

From numerous studies performed in the 1950s and 1960s, a relationship between the ΔA_{450} of amniotic fluid and the severity of hemolytic disease was established.[15] By using a semilogarithmic plot of ΔA_{450} values versus

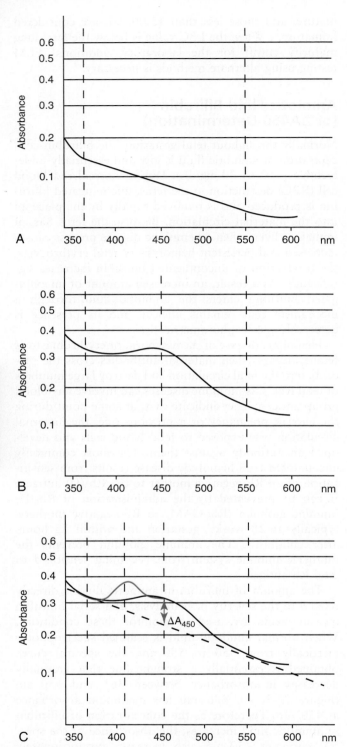

FIGURE 12-3 The determination of A_{450} in amniotic fluid. **A,** Normal amniotic fluid. **B,** Amniotic fluid with a bilirubin peak at 450 nm. **C,** Amniotic fluid with a bilirubin peak at 450 nm and contaminated with oxyhemoglobin, which peaks at 412 nm. The dashed line indicates the baseline drawn between the linear portions of the curve (i.e., between 365 and 550 nm). The red line indicates oxyhemoglobin absorbance.

the fetal gestational age, three zones were determined to represent the severity of hemolytic disease that the fetus is experiencing in utero (Figure 12-4). Note that the ΔA_{450} values indicated by each zone decrease with increasing fetal gestational age. Therefore the gestational age must be known before the ΔA_{450} can be evaluated. See typical reference intervals provided in Table 12-3 and Appendix B.

The ΔA_{450} values that fall into zone I are considered normal, representing a minimally affected fetus. Zone II, the middle zone, indicates moderate hemolysis. However, if serial determinations indicate that values are in zone II and are increasing, then marked hemolysis is taking place. Values in the uppermost region, zone III, indicate that the fetus is experiencing severe hemolysis and will die without intervention.

When an immunologic incompatibility between the fetus and the mother is suspected, amniocentesis is initially performed at 22 weeks' gestation and is repeated at periodic intervals thereafter. A decreasing ΔA_{450} in subsequent determinations is a good prognostic sign, whereas equivalent or increasing values indicate worsening of fetal health status.

Amniotic fluid specimens contaminated with blood generally are not acceptable because of interference caused by oxyhemoglobin absorbance peaks at 412 and 540 nm (see Figure 12-3, C). However, if bloody specimens are processed immediately and the blood is removed before significant hemolysis has taken place, the spectral curve obtained may not be significantly affected. The magnitude of oxyhemoglobin contamination can be determined by calculating the differences in absorbance at 412 nm. If significant overlap of the oxyhemoglobin and bilirubin absorbance curves is evident, the ΔA_{450} results are not valid. Similarly, meconium-contaminated amniotic fluid specimens are not acceptable for ΔA_{450} measurements because meconium absorbs maximally between 350 and 400 nm. Falsely low ΔA_{450} results are obtained using specimens contaminated with blood and meconium because these substances interfere when drawing the spectral baseline. Another source of error in bilirubin detection is not protecting the specimen from light immediately after collection and throughout transport and processing. Loss of bilirubin due to light exposure also causes falsely low ΔA_{450} values.

STUDY QUESTIONS

1. Which of the following is *not* a function of the amniotic fluid surrounding a developing fetus?
   A. Amniotic fluid provides protection of the fetus.
   B. Amniotic fluid enables fetal movement.
   C. Amniotic fluid is a medium for oxygen exchange.
   D. Amniotic fluid is a source of water and solute exchange.

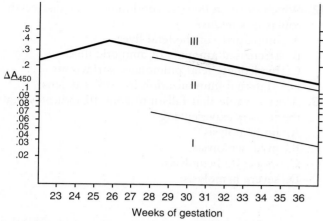

FIGURE 12-4 Liley's three-zone chart (with modification) for the interpretation of amniotic fluid A_{450} values. The dark line extending from 22 to 38 weeks' gestation represents the upward revision of the "danger line" by Irving Umansky. *(Redrawn from Reid DE, Ryan KJ, Benirschke K: Principles and management of human reproduction, Philadelphia, 1972, WB Saunders.)*

TABLE 12-3	Amniotic Fluid Reference Intervals
Physical Examination	
Color	Colorless to pale yellow
Clarity	Clear to slightly turbid*
Chemical Examination	
ΔA_{450} determination	
27 weeks' gestation	<0.065
30 weeks' gestation	<0.052
35 weeks' gestation	<0.035
40 weeks' gestation	<0.022
Lecithin/sphingomyelin ratio (mature)	>2.0

*Turbidity increases with gestational age.

2. Amniocentesis is usually performed at 15 to 18 weeks' gestation to determine which of the following conditions?
   A. Fetal distress
   B. Fetal maturity
   C. Genetic disorders
   D. Infections in the amniotic fluid

3. Through which of the following mechanism(s) does solute and water exchange occur between the fetus and the amniotic fluid?
   1. Fetal swallowing of the amniotic fluid
   2. Transudation across the fetal skin
   3. Fetal urination into the amniotic fluid
   4. Respiration of amniotic fluid into the fetal pulmonary system
   A. 1, 2, and 3 are correct.
   B. 1 and 3 are correct.
   C. 4 is correct.
   D. All are correct.

4. Select the term used to describe a decreased volume of amniotic fluid present in the amniotic sac.
   A. Anhydramnios
   B. Hydramnios
   C. Oligohydramnios
   D. Polyhydramnios

5. Amniotic fluid specimens are immediately protected from light to preserve which of the following substances?
   A. Bilirubin
   B. Fetal cells
   C. Meconium
   D. Phospholipids

6. Which of the following substances, when present in amniotic fluid, is affected adversely by refrigeration?
   A. Bilirubin
   B. Fetal cells
   C. Protein
   D. Phospholipids

7. When processing amniotic fluid, high centrifugation speeds are used to clear the fluid of turbidity for
   A. bilirubin analysis.
   B. culturing of fetal cells.
   C. meconium detection.
   D. phospholipid analysis.

8. Analysis for which of the following substances can aid in the differentiation of amniotic fluid from urine?
   1. Urea
   2. Glucose
   3. Creatinine
   4. Protein
   A. 1, 2, and 3 are correct.
   B. 1 and 3 are correct.
   C. 4 is correct.
   D. All are correct.

9. Which of the following statements about amniotic fluid is true?
   A. Amniotic fluid is normally clear and colorless.
   B. Normally amniotic fluid contains fetal hair, cells, and vernix.
   C. Amniotic fluid and urine can be differentiated by a physical examination of the fluid.
   D. When contaminated with meconium, amniotic fluid takes on a yellow or amber coloration.

10. Which of the following is *not* a test to evaluate the surfactants present in the fetal pulmonary system?
    A. ΔA_{450}
    B. Lecithin/sphingomyelin ratio
    C. Phosphatidylglycerol detection
    D. Foam stability index

11. Which of the following test results would indicate fetal lung immaturity?
    1. A lecithin/sphingomyelin ratio of less than 2.0
    2. A lecithin/sphingomyelin ratio of more than 2.0
    3. A lecithin/sphingomyelin ratio of more than 2.0, with phosphatidylglycerol absent
    4. A lecithin/sphingomyelin ratio of less than 2.0, with phosphatidylglycerol present
    A. 1, 2, and 3 are correct.
    B. 1 and 3 are correct.
    C. 4 is correct.
    D. All are correct.

12. Which of the following conditions can cause erythroblastosis fetalis?
    A. Immaturity of the fetal liver
    B. Decreased amounts of amniotic fluid
    C. Inadequate fetal pulmonary surfactants
    D. Maternal immunization by fetal antigens

13. A ΔA_{450} value that falls into zone III indicates that the fetus is experiencing
    A. no hemolysis.
    B. mild hemolysis.
    C. moderate hemolysis.
    D. severe hemolysis.

CASE 12-1

A 32-year-old pregnant woman is seen by an obstetrician for the first time during her third pregnancy. She thinks she is around 33 weeks' gestation. She is from a Third World country and 3 months ago relocated to the United States with her husband and family. A patient history reveals that she has two children—a boy 7 years old and a girl 5 years old. Both births were normal and uncomplicated; however, she states that her daughter had become yellow shortly after birth and that she was given a blood transfusion.

Routine prenatal blood work is performed. The mother is determined to be type O Rh-negative and an antibody screen reveals the presence of an anti-$Rh_0(D)$. Her antibody titer is positive to a 1:32 dilution. Her husband is determined to be type A Rh-positive. To assess and monitor the severity of the suspected hemolytic process taking place, weekly amnioceneses are scheduled.

Amniotic Fluid Results

33 Weeks' Gestation	34 Weeks' Gestation	35 Weeks' Gestation
ΔA_{450}: 0.200	ΔA_{450}: 0.245	Lecithin: 4.7 mg/dL
L/S ratio: 1.1	L/S ratio: 1.5	Sphingomyelin: 2.3 mg/dL
PG: absent	PG: absent	PG: present

Spectrophotometer scan for ΔA_{450} determination at 35 weeks' gestation

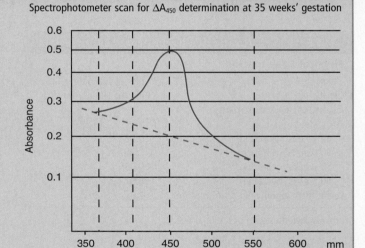

1. Calculate the ΔA_{450} for the amniotic fluid specimen obtained at 35 weeks' gestation using the spectrophotometer scan provided.
2. Using the chart in Figure 12-4, determine the zone in which the ΔA_{450} value falls at 35 weeks.
3. Describe the clinical implications that accompany a result in this zone.
4. Using the values for lecithin and sphingomyelin provided at 35 weeks, calculate the lecithin/sphingomyelin ratio.
5. Based on the fetal lung maturity tests performed each week, state whether the fetal lungs are mature or immature.

L/S ratio, Lecithin/sphingomyelin ratio; *PG,* phosphatidylglycerol.

REFERENCES

1. Greene MF, Fencl MdeM, Tulchinsky D: Biochemical aspects of pregnancy. In Tietz NW, editor: Fundamentals of clinical chemistry, ed 3, Philadelphia, 1987, WB Saunders.
2. Clinical and Laboratory Standards Institute (CLSI): Analysis of Body Fluids in Clinical Chemistry: approved guideline, CLSI Document C49-A, Wayne, PA, 2007, CLSI.
3. American College of Obstetricians and Gynecologists: Practice Bulletin No. 97: Fetal lung maturity. Obstet Gynecol 112:717, 2008.
4. Grenache DG, Gronowski AM: Fetal lung maturity. Clin Biochem 39:1, 2006.
5. Gluck L, Kulovich MV, Borer RC, et al: Diagnosis of the respiratory distress syndrome by amniocentesis. Am J Obstet Gynecol 109:440, 1971.
6. Pinette MG, Blackstone J, Wax JR, et al: Fetal lung maturity indices: a plea for gestational age-specific interpretation—a case study and discussion. Am J Obstet Gynecol 187:1721, 2002.
7. American College of Obstetricians and Gynecologists: Educational Bulletin No. 230: Assessment of fetal lung maturity. Int J Gynecol Obstet 56:191, 1996.
8. Kesselman EJ, Figuera R, Garry D, Maulik D: The usefulness of the TDx/TDxFLx fetal lung maturity II assay in the initial evaluation of fetal lung maturity. Am J Obstet Gynecol 188:1220, 2003.
9. Fantz CR, Powell C, Karon B, et al: Assessment of the diagnostic accuracy of the TDx-FLM II to predict fetal lung maturity. Clin Chem 48:761, 2002.
10. Dubin SB: Characterization of amniotic fluid lamellar bodies by resistive-pulse counting: relationship to measures of fetal lung maturity. Clin Chem 35:612, 1989.
11. Greenspoon JS, Rosen DJD, Roll K, et al: Evaluation of lamellar body number density as the initial assessment in a fetal lung maturity test cascade. J Reprod Med 40:260, 1995.
12. Dilena BA, Ku F, Doyle I, et al: Six alternative methods to the lecithin/sphingomyelin ratio in amniotic fluid for assessing fetal lung maturity. Ann Clin Biochem 34:106, 1997.
13. Neerhof MG, Dohnal JC, Ashwood ER, et al: Lamellar body counts: a consensus on protocol. Obstet Gynecol 97:318, 2001.
14. DeRoche ME, Ingardia CJ, Guerette PJ, et al: The use of lamellar body counts to predict fetal lung maturity in pregnancies complicated by diabetes mellitus. Am J Obstet Gynecol 187:908, 2002.
15. Liley AW: Liquor amnii analysis in the management of pregnancy complicated by rhesus sensitization. Am J Obstet Gynecol 82:1359, 1961.

Cerebrospinal Fluid Analysis

LEARNING OBJECTIVES

After studying this chapter, the student should be able to:

1. Describe the formation of cerebrospinal fluid (CSF) and state at least three functions that the CSF performs.
2. Describe the procedure for lumbar puncture and the proper collection technique for CSF.
3. Discuss the importance of timely processing and testing of CSF and state at least three adverse effects of time delay on CSF specimens.
4. State the physical characteristics of normal CSF and discuss how each characteristic can be modified in disease states.
5. Discuss the clinical importance of the microscopic examination of CSF.
6. Compare and contrast the concentrations of the following constituents of CSF in health and in disease states:

- Albumin
- Glucose
- Immunoglobulin G
- Lactate
- Total protein

7. Describe briefly protein electrophoretic patterns of CSF and the abnormal presence of oligoclonal banding.
8. Calculate the CSF/serum albumin index and the CSF/immunoglobulin G index and state the clinical importance of each index.
9. Discuss the proper microbiological examination of CSF and its importance in the diagnosis of infectious diseases of the central nervous system.
10. Explain briefly the role of CSF immunologic tests in the diagnosis of meningitis.

CHAPTER OUTLINE

Physiology and Composition
Specimen Collection
Physical Examination
Microscopic Examination
   Total Cell Count
   Red Blood Cell (Erythrocyte)
      Count

White Blood Cell (Leukocyte)
   Count
   Differential Cell Count
Chemical Examination
   Protein
   Glucose
   Lactate

Microbiological Examination
   Microscopic Examination of CSF
      Smears
   Culture
Immunologic Methods

KEY TERMS

blood-brain barrier The physiologic interface between the vascular system and cerebrospinal fluid. Changes in the blood-brain barrier can result in changes in the normal chemical and cellular composition of the cerebrospinal fluid.

cerebrospinal fluid The normally clear, colorless fluid present between the arachnoid (or arachnoidea) and the pia mater in the brain and spinal cord. This fluid is formed primarily by selective secretions of plasma by the choroid plexus into the ventricles and to a lesser extent from intrathecal synthesis by ependymal cells.

choroid plexus The highly vascular folds of capillaries, nerves, and ependymal cells in the pia mater. Located in the four ventricles of the brain, the choroid plexus actively synthesizes cerebrospinal fluid.

intrathecal Within the spinal cord or subarachnoid space.

meninges The three membranes that surround the brain and spinal cord. The innermost membrane is the pia mater, the outermost membrane is the dura mater, and the centrally located membrane is the arachnoid (or arachnoidea).

meningitis Inflammation of the meninges.

oligoclonal bands Multiple discrete bands in the γ region noted during electrophoresis of plasma or other body fluids (e.g., cerebrospinal fluid).

pleocytosis The presence of a greater than normal number of cells in cerebrospinal fluid.

stat An abbreviation for the Latin word *statim*, which means "immediately."

subarachnoid space The space between the arachnoid (or arachnoidea) and the pia mater.

ventricles The four fluid-filled cavities in the brain lined with ependymal cells. The choroid plexus is located in the ventricles.

xanthochromia The pink, orange, or yellowish discoloration of supernatant cerebrospinal fluid following centrifugation.

PHYSIOLOGY AND COMPOSITION

Cerebrospinal fluid (CSF) bathes the brain and spinal cord. CSF is produced primarily (70%) from secretions into the four **ventricles** of the brain by the highly vascular **choroid plexus** (vascular fringe–like folds in the pia mater). The ependymal cells that line the brain and spinal cord also play a minor role in the production of CSF. The formation of CSF can be described as a selective secretion from plasma, not as an ultrafiltrate. This is evidenced by higher CSF concentrations of some solutes (e.g., sodium, chloride, magnesium) and lower CSF concentrations of other solutes (e.g., potassium, total calcium) compared with plasma. If simple ultrafiltration were responsible for CSF production, these solute concentration differences would not exist.

The brain and spinal cord are surrounded by three membranes, collectively termed the **meninges.** The tough outermost membrane, the dura mater, is next to the bone. The arachnoid (also called *arachnoidea*), or middle layer, derives its name from its visual resemblance to a spider web. The innermost membrane, the pia mater, adheres to the surface of the neural tissues (Figure 13-1). Cerebrospinal fluid flows in the space between the arachnoidea mater and the pia mater, called the **subarachnoid space,** where it bathes and protects the delicate tissues of the central nervous system. From its initial formation in the ventricles, the CSF circulates to the brainstem and spinal cord, principally through pressure changes caused by postural, respiratory, and circulatory pressures (Figure 13-2). The CSF eventually flows in the subarachnoid

space to the top outer surface of the brain, where projections of the arachnoid membrane called *arachnoid granulations* are present. These projections have small one-way valvelike structures that allow the CSF to enter the bloodstream of the large veins of the head. Cerebrospinal fluid formation, circulation, and reabsorption into the blood make up a dynamic process that constantly turns over about 20 mL each hour.[1] If the flow path between production and reabsorption of CSF into the blood is obstructed for any reason, CSF accumulates, producing hydrocephalus; intracranial pressure can increase, causing brain damage, mental retardation, or death if left untreated. Normally, the total volume of CSF in an adult ranges from 85 to 150 mL. The volume in neonates is significantly smaller, ranging from 10 to 60 mL.

The CSF protects and supports the brain and spinal cord and provides a medium for the transport and exchange of nutrients and metabolic wastes. The capillary endothelium in contact with CSF enables the transfer of substances from the blood into the CSF and vice versa. This capillary endothelium differs from the endothelium in other tissues by the presence of tight junctions between adjacent endothelial cells. These tight junctions significantly reduce the extracellular passage of substances from the blood plasma into the CSF. In other words, all substances that enter or leave the CSF must pass through the membranes and cytoplasm of the capillary endothelial cells. This modulating interface between the blood and the CSF is called the **blood-brain barrier** and accounts for the observed concentration differences of electrolytes, proteins, and other solutes. An example of the selectivity and effectiveness of this blood-brain barrier is the failure of some antibiotics (e.g., penicillins), given intravenously, to enter the CSF, although these antibiotics freely penetrate all other tissues of the body.

In healthy individuals, the chemical composition of CSF is regulated closely and includes low-molecular-weight proteins. Changes in the chemical composition or in the cellular components can aid in the diagnosis of disease. Protein, glucose, and lactate are routinely measured in CSF. Although numerous other parameters (e.g., sodium, potassium, chloride, magnesium, pH, P_{CO_2}, enzymes) have been evaluated for clinical use, they have yet to prove their diagnostic value. In addition to chemical analysis, CSF is routinely cultured for microbial organisms, examined microscopically to evaluate the cellular components, and tested for the presence of specific

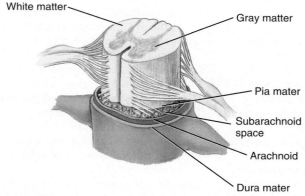

FIGURE 13-1 A schematic representation of the spinal cord and the meninges that surround it. *(From Applegate E: The anatomy and physiology learning system, ed 4, Philadelphia, 2011, Saunders.)*

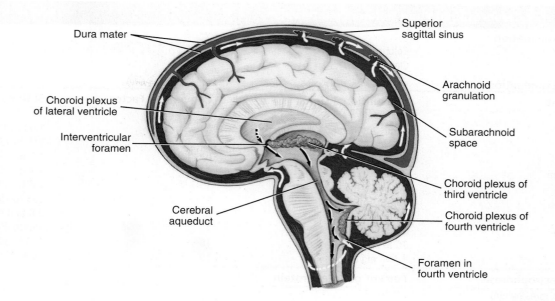

FIGURE 13-2 A schematic representation of the brain and spinal cord, including the circulation of the cerebrospinal fluid. *(From Applegate E: The anatomy and physiology learning system, ed 4, Philadelphia, 2011, Saunders.)*

antigens. These cytologic, microbiological, and immunologic studies can provide valuable diagnostic information. For CSF reference intervals, see Table 13-1 or Appendix B.

SPECIMEN COLLECTION

Cerebrospinal fluid specimens are collected specifically for the diagnosis or treatment of disease (Box 13-1). Although the lumbar puncture principally used to obtain CSF specimens is fairly routine, it involves significant patient discomfort and can cause complications. Therefore once a CSF specimen has been collected, it is imperative that it is properly labeled and handled at the bedside and in the laboratory.

Usually a physician performs a lumbar puncture in the third or fourth lumbar interspace (or lower) in adults or the fourth or fifth interspace in children (Figure 13-3). The puncture site selection can vary if an infection is present at the preferred site. A locally infected site must be avoided to prevent introduction of the infection into the central nervous system. The lumbar puncture procedure is performed aseptically after thorough cleansing of the patient's skin and the application of a local anesthetic. The spinal needle is advanced into the lumbar interspace, and often a pop is heard on penetration of the dura mater. Immediately after the dura mater has been entered and before any CSF has been removed, the physician takes the initial or "opening" pressure of the CSF using a manometer that attaches to the spinal needle. Normal CSF pressures for an adult in a lateral recumbent position range from 50 to 180 mm Hg, with slightly

| BOX 13-1 | Indications and Contraindications for Lumbar Puncture and Cerebrospinal Fluid Examination |

Indications
- *Infections*
  - Meningitis
  - Encephalitis
  - Brain abscess
- *Hemorrhage*
  - Subarachnoid
  - Intracerebral
- *Neurologic Disease*
  - Multiple sclerosis
  - Guillain-Barré syndrome
- *Malignancy*
  - Leukemia
  - Lymphoma
  - Metastatic carcinoma
- *Tumor*
  - Brain
  - Spinal cord
- *Treatments*
  - Chemotherapy
  - Anesthetics
  - Radiographic contrast media
  - Antibiotic therapy

Contraindications
- Infections
- Septicemia
- Systemic infection
- Localized lumbar infection

higher pressures obtained from individuals in a sitting position. If the pressure is in the normal range, up to 20 mL of CSF (approximately 15% of the estimated total CSF volume) can be removed safely. If the CSF pressure is less than or greater than normal, only 1 to 2 mL should be removed. Because the total volume of CSF is significantly smaller in infants and children, proportionately smaller volumes are collected from them. After the CSF has been removed and before the spinal needle has been withdrawn, the physician takes the "closing" CSF pressure, which should be 10 to 30 mm

TABLE 13-1	Cerebrospinal Fluid Reference Intervals*			
Physical Examination				
Color	Colorless			
Clarity	Clear			
Chemical Examination				
Component	**Conventional Units**	**Conversion Factor**		**SI Units**
Electrolytes				
Calcium	2.0 to 2.8 mEq/L	0.5		1.00 to 1.40 mmol/L
Chloride	115 to 130 mEq/L	1		115 to 130 mmol/L
Lactate	10 to 22 mg/dL	0.111		1.1 to 2.4 mmol/L
Magnesium	2.4 to 3.0 mEq/L	0.5		1.2 to 1.5 mmol/L
Potassium	2.6 to 3.0 mEq/L	1		2.6 to 3.0 mmol/L
Sodium	135 to 150 mEq/L	1		135 to 150 mmol/L
Glucose	50 to 80 mg/dL	0.5551		2.8 to 4.4 mmol/L
Total protein	15 to 45 mg/dL	10		150 to 450 mg/L
Albumin	10 to 30 mg/dL	10		100 to 300 mg/L
IgG	1 to 4 mg/dL	10		10 to 40 mg/L
Protein Electrophoresis	**Percent of Total Protein**			
Transthyretin (prealbumin)	2% to 7%			
Albumin	56% to 76%			
α_1-Globulin	2% to 7%			
α_2-Globulin	4% to 12%			
β-Globulin	8% to 18%			
γ-Globulin	3% to 12%			
Microscopic Examination				
Component	**Conventional Units**	**Conversion Factor**		**SI Units**
Neonates (<1 year old)	0 to 30 cells/µL	10^6		0 to 30 $\times$ 10^6 cells/L
1 to 4 years old	0 to 20 cells/µL	10^6		0 to 20 $\times$ 10^6 cells/L
5 to 18 years old	0 to 10 cells/µL	10^6		0 to 10 $\times$ 10^6 cells/L
Adults (>18 years old)	0 to 5 cells/µL	10^6		0 to 5 $\times$ 10^6 cells/L
Differential Cell Count	**Percent of Total Count**			
Neonates				
Lymphocytes	5% to 35%			
Monocytes	50% to 90%			
Neutrophils	0% to 8%			
Adults				
Lymphocytes	40% to 80%			
Monocytes	15% to 45%			
Neutrophils	0% to 6%			

*For cerebrospinal fluid specimens obtained by lumbar puncture.

Hg less than the opening pressure. Both CSF pressure values and the amount of CSF removed are recorded in the patient's chart.

As CSF is collected, it is dispensed into three (or more) sequentially labeled sterile collection tubes. The first tube is used for chemical and immunologic testing, because any minimal blood contamination resulting from vessel injury during the initial tap normally does not affect these results. The second tube is used for microbial testing, and the third tube is reserved for the microscopic examination of cellular components (i.e., red and white blood cell counts and cytologic studies). If only a small amount of CSF is obtained and a single collection tube must be used, the ordering physician prioritizes the tests desired. With these low-volume specimens, the microbiology laboratory receives the specimen first, to ensure culturing of a sterile specimen. Cell counts, followed by chemical and immunologic testing, should immediately follow the microbiological examination.

The examination and testing of CSF should take place as soon as possible after collection. Therefore in most institutions, tests ordered on CSF specimens are considered **stat**. Delay in testing can cause inaccurate results, such as falsely low cell counts caused by the lysis of white blood cells or falsely high lactate levels caused by glycolysis. In addition, the recovery of viable microbial organisms is jeopardized. When delay is unavoidable, each CSF collection tube must be stored at the temperature that best ensures recovery of the constituents of interest (Table 13-2). Any CSF remaining after the initial tests have been performed can be frozen and saved for possible future chemical or immunologic studies.

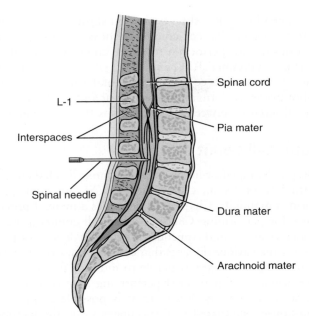

FIGURE 13-3 A schematic representation of a lumbar puncture procedure.

TABLE 13-2	Cerebrospinal Fluid Specimen Handling and Storage Temperature	
Tube #1	Chemical, immunology, serology	Frozen (−15° C to −30° C)
Tube #2	Microbiological studies	Room temperature (19° C to 26° C)
Tube #3	Cell counts and cytology studies	Refrigerated (2° C to 8° C)

PHYSICAL EXAMINATION

Normal CSF is clear and colorless, with a viscosity similar to that of water. Increased viscosity, although rare, can occur as a result of metastatic, mucin-secreting adenocarcinomas. Abnormally increased amounts of fibrinogen in CSF caused by a compromised blood-brain barrier can result in clot formation. Fine, delicate clots can form a thin film or pellicle on the surface of CSF after it has been stored at refrigerator temperatures for 12 or more hours. Most often, clot formation is associated with a traumatic puncture procedure, in which blood and plasma proteins contaminated the CSF. Rarely, no blood is present in the CSF, and clots form as a result of elevated CSF protein levels with conditions such as Froin's syndrome or suppurative or tuberculous meningitis, or as a result of subarachnoid obstruction. Despite the various possibilities for clot formation, clots rarely are encountered even in patients with pathologic conditions. If present, however, clot formation must be noted and reported.

The clarity or turbidity of CSF depends on its cellularity. **Pleocytosis,** an increase in the number of cells in CSF, causes the CSF to appear cloudy to varying degrees. A

BOX 13-2	Causes of Xanthochromia in Cerebrospinal Fluid

Hemorrhage, subarachnoid or intracerebral
Hyperbilirubinemia
Hypercarotenemia
Meningeal melanoma
Normal neonate*
Protein concentration exceeding 150 mg/dL
Previous traumatic tap

*Xanthochromia in neonates results from a combination of increased bilirubin and increased protein due to immaturity in the blood-brain barrier.

cloudy CSF specimen is associated with a white blood cell count greater than 200 cells/mL or a red blood cell count exceeding 400 cells/mL. Similarly, microorganisms or an increased protein content can produce cloudy CSF specimens. Cerebrospinal fluid clarity can be graded semiquantitatively from 0 (clear) to 4+ (newsprint cannot be read through the fluid) using standardized criteria to ensure consistency in reporting. Occasionally, the CSF may appear oily because of the presence of radiographic contrast media.

Although normal CSF is colorless, in disease states it often appears xanthochromic. Although **xanthochromia** literally means a yellow discoloration, this term is applied to a spectrum of CSF discolorations, including pink, orange, and yellow. A pink supernatant after centrifugation results from oxyhemoglobin, a yellow supernatant results from bilirubin, an orange supernatant results from a combination of these, and a brownish supernatant results from methemoglobin formation. High concentrations of other substances, such as carotene, and protein in concentrations greater than 150 mg/dL can cause xanthochromic CSF specimens, as can conditions such as meningeal melanoma or collection of the CSF 2 to 5 days after a traumatic tap (Box 13-2).

Gross blood in CSF is visually apparent, and determining its source requires differentiation between a traumatic puncture procedure and a subarachnoid or intracerebral hemorrhage. Several observations can aid in making this differentiation (Table 13-3). A traumatic tap results in the greatest amount of blood collected in the first specimen tube. Hence a visual assessment or a comparison of the red blood cell (RBC) count between tube 1 and tube 3 (or 4) will show a significant difference (decrease). In contrast, a hemorrhage results in a homogeneous distribution of red blood cells throughout all collection tubes. Second, following centrifugation of the CSF, a colorless supernatant indicates a traumatic tap, whereas a xanthochromic supernatant reveals a hemorrhage because about 1 to 2 hours are needed for red blood cells to lyse in CSF.[2] The lysis of red blood cells observed in CSF is not osmotically induced because plasma and CSF are osmotically equivalent, rather it is speculated that the lack of sufficient CSF proteins and lipids needed to stabilize red blood cell membranes

TABLE 13-3	Features That Aid in Differentiating Hemorrhage From Traumatic Tap	
Traumatic Tap	**Hemorrhage**	
Amount of blood decreases or clears progressively from first to last collection tube	Amount of blood the same in all collection tubes	
Streaking of blood in CSF during collection	Blood evenly dispersed during collection	
CSF may clot	CSF does not clot owing to defibrination in vivo	
Usually no xanthochromia	Xanthochromia present	
No hemosiderin present	Presence of hemosiderin-laden macrophages (siderophage)	

CSF, Cerebrospinal fluid.

causes the lysis. Because lysis can occur in vivo or in vitro, timely processing and testing of CSF specimens are necessary. Once red blood cell lysis has occurred in CSF, xanthochromia, initially resulting from oxyhemoglobin and later from bilirubin, will be evident for as long as 4 weeks. Last, when the microscopic examination of CSF reveals macrophages with phagocytosed red blood cells, a hemorrhage has taken place. These erythrophagocytic cells can persist for 4 to 8 weeks following a hemorrhage; they stain positive for hemosiderin and may include hematoidin crystals.

Because a CSF specimen is collected into three or more specimen tubes and all tubes may not be sent to the same laboratory, the testing laboratory personnel must examine and individually assess each tube for color, clarity, and volume.

MICROSCOPIC EXAMINATION

The CSF of adults normally contains a small number of white blood cells (WBCs), specifically, lymphocytes and monocytes at 0 to 5 cells/μL. Similarly low numbers of WBCs (0 to 10 cells/μL) are expected in children, whereas healthy neonates can have up to 30 WBCs/μL, with monocytes predominating.

In contrast, RBCs are not normally present in CSF. When present, RBCs most often represent CSF contamination with peripheral blood during the lumbar puncture procedure. Rarely, RBCs are present because of a recent (within 1 or 2 hours) subarachnoid or cerebral hemorrhage.

Cell counts on CSF must be performed as soon as possible to ensure valid results. At room temperature, 40% of the WBCs in CSF will lyse in 2 hours.[3] If the specimen is refrigerated, WBC lysis can be reduced significantly to approximately 15%, but not completely prevented. Similarly, RBCs do not demonstrate significant lysis at 4° C; therefore the CSF collection tube for cell counts should be refrigerated if the count must be delayed for any reason.

Depending on the testing institution, different approaches to CSF cell counts are possible. Some laboratories do not perform a total cell count; instead, they perform individual RBC and WBC counts. The sum of these two counts is equivalent to a total cell count. Other laboratories perform a total cell count and a WBC count; the difference between these counts is the RBC count.

Total Cell Count

Despite being labor-intensive and technically challenging with low precision, cell counts on CSF are often performed manually. Chapter 18 describes a manual procedure for performing CSF and other cell counts using a hemacytometer and Appendix C provides details for preparing the various diluents that can be used. Commercial control materials are available to monitor the technical performance of personnel performing manual hemacytometer cell counts. However, it is possible to prepare "in-house" simulated CSF specimens using the method developed by Lofsness and Jensen.[4] These simulated specimens can be used (1) as quality control samples, (2) as samples for training, or (3) for competency assessment of laboratory personnel.

Total cell counts on CSF are usually made using well-mixed, undiluted CSF. Because of the low viscosity and protein content of CSF, cells settle within 1 minute after filling the hemacytometer chambers. When counting clear CSF, Kjeldsberg recommends counting all nine large squares on both sides of the hemacytometer.[5] When the number of cells in the nine squares exceeds 200 or is crowded or overlapping, the CSF should be diluted with saline. Dilutions vary according to the concentrations of cells present. Sometimes an initial dilution may be selected based on the visual appearance of the fluid, ranging from a 1:10 dilution for a slightly cloudy specimen to a 1:10,000 dilution for bloody specimens.

Automation of CSF cell counts significantly increases analytical precision and reduces turnaround time. However, because the number of cells in CSF is normally low (<5 cells/μL in adults or <30 cells/μL in children), many electronic impedance-based cell counters cannot be used because the instrument's background count produces values higher than these "normal" cell counts. This is an issue especially when most of the CSF samples actually tested in the laboratory have low cell counts in the normal range.

Some automated systems currently available for CSF cell counting are the ADVIA 120 and ADVIA 2120 hematology analyzers (Siemens Healthcare Diagnostics, Deerfield, IL), Sysmex XE-5000 hematology analyzers (Sysmex Corporation, Mundelein, IL), and the Iris iQ200 with Body Fluids Module (Iris Diagnostics, Chatsworth, CA). Studies using these analyzers indicate agreement with the manual hemacytometer method, and the best correlations are obtained at high cell counts.[6-8] The ADVIA and Sysmex analyzers enumerate and differentiate cells using flow cytometry, whereas the iQ200 enumerates and differentiates RBCs and nucleated cells using flow cell digital imaging. Note that neither automated system can identify pathologic cell types such as neoplastic cells, siderophages, and lipophages. (See Chapter 17 for additional discussion of automated body fluid analysis.)

Red Blood Cell (Erythrocyte) Count

RBC counts provide little diagnostically useful information. They may be performed to aid in the differentiation of a recent hemorrhage from a traumatic puncture procedure, as previously discussed. Another application of the RBC count is to correct the WBC count and total protein determinations obtained from a CSF specimen known to be contaminated with peripheral blood. These calculated "corrections" have limited accuracy, usually overcorrect the counts, assume that all of the RBCs present result from contamination, and have little clinical use. Therefore this chapter does not describe these corrections in detail; readers are referred to the bibliography for additional information.

As with the total cell count, well-mixed, undiluted CSF is used for the RBC count unless the number of cells present requires dilution because of overlapping and crowding of cells. Because the differentiation between small lymphocytes and crenated erythrocytes can be difficult in unstained wet preparations, some laboratories eliminate this count, replacing it with the difference obtained between the total cell count and the WBC count.

White Blood Cell (Leukocyte) Count

Increased WBC counts in CSF are associated with diseases of the central nervous system and with a variety of other conditions (Table 13-4). The WBC count can vary significantly depending on the causative agent. Often the highest WBC counts (greater than 50,000 cells/mL) in CSF occur with bacterial meningitis. However, the same condition may show no pleocytosis in some patients.[9]

To enhance the visualization of white blood cell nuclei and to eliminate any RBCs present, the CSF is treated with glacial acetic acid before the hemacytometer chambers are filled, and 3 to 5 minutes is allowed for RBC lysis. With the WBC nuclei more readily apparent, the WBCs are counted and may be classified as mononuclear or polymorphonuclear cells. Note that classification of WBCs during this count, known as a "chamber differential," has poor precision and is unsatisfactory for reporting; however, it provides a preliminary indication of the cell types present. When WBC numbers are such that a dilution is required for accurate counting, an acetic acid and stain (e.g., crystal violet) mixture can be used as the diluent; this enhances visualization and facilitates classification of the WBCs.

Differential Cell Count

Techniques. The differential cell count provides useful diagnostic information. Normally, lymphocytes and monocytes predominate in the CSF, with the percentages of each differing for adults and neonates (Table 13-5). A normal range for children 2 months old to 18 years old has yet to be established because of limited data. Before cytocentrifuge techniques were used, any neutrophils present were considered abnormal. Currently, with the increased cell recovery obtained using cytospin preparations, neutrophil counts of less than 10% are considered normal.[10]

Performing a differential count of the cells present in CSF requires the laboratorian to (1) concentrate the cells, (2) prepare a smear of the concentrate on a microscope slide, and (3) stain the slide preparation with Wright's stain. Several techniques are available, but the preferred and most widely used method is cytocentrifugation. This technique is rapid and technically simple to perform and produces "cytospin" slides that show good cellular recovery. (See Chapter 18, "Body Fluid Analysis: Manual Hemacytometer Counts and Differential Slide Preparation," for additional discussion.)

When a differential cell count is performed using a cytospin slide or concentrated smear, the entire slide should be scanned first using a low-power objective (10×). This scan will provide an overview of the cellularity of the specimen and will aid in detecting abnormalities such as plasma cells, macrophages, hemosiderin-laden macrophages, malignant cells, or cell clumps that can be few in number (Figure 13-4). Next, the differential cell count is performed using a 50× or a 100× oil objective.

Pleocytosis

Neutrophils. With bacterial **meningitis**, as many as 90% of the WBCs present in the CSF can be neutrophils (Figure 13-5, *B*). Neutrophilic pleocytosis also occurs in early viral, fungal (Figure 13-5, *A*), tubercular, and parasitic infections, as well as with noninfectious conditions (see Table 13-4). Although pronounced neutrophilic pleocytosis frequently occurs in bacterial meningitis, only a small percentage of neutrophils (≈10%) may be present with other infectious agents. Noninfectious conditions associated with an increased number of neutrophils in the CSF include subarachnoid or intracerebral hemorrhage, repeated lumbar punctures, and intrathecal administration of drugs or radiographic contrast media.

Lymphocytes. An increased number of lymphocytes in the CSF is associated with viral, tuberculous, fungal, and syphilitic meningitis. Although initially these conditions may show a mixture of cells (i.e., neutrophils, lymphocytes, monocytes, and plasma cells), in later stages of the disease, lymphocytes predominate (Figures 13-6 and 13-7). Lymphocytes in CSF can become activated in the same way as those in peripheral blood. As a result, a variety of lymphoid cells can be present in the CSF. They can range in size from small, typical cells to

TABLE 13-4	Cell Types and Causes of Cerebrospinal Fluid Pleocytosis	
Predominant Cell Type	**Infectious Causes**	**Noninfectious Causes**
Neutrophils	Meningitis • Bacterial • *Early* viral, tuberculous, fungal • Amebic encephalomyelitis Cerebral abscess	Hemorrhage • Subarachnoid • Intracerebral Central nervous system infarct Tumor Repeated lumbar puncture Intrathecal treatment (e.g., drugs, myelography)
Lymphocytes	Meningitis • Viral • Tuberculous • Fungal • Syphilitic HIV infection and AIDS Partially treated bacterial meningitis Parasitic infestations	Multiple sclerosis Guillain-Barré syndrome Lymphoma Drug abuse
Monocytes	Meningitis • Tuberculous • Fungal	Tumors
Plasma cells	Same disorders associated with increased lymphocytes, particularly tuberculous and syphilitic meningitis	Multiple sclerosis Guillain-Barré syndrome
Eosinophils	Parasitic infestations *Coccidioides immitis* Fungal infections Idiopathic eosinophilic meningitis	Allergic reaction to: • Intracranial shunts • Radiographic contrast media • Intrathecal medications Lymphoma, leukemia Contamination with blood
Macrophages	Tuberculous meningitis Fungal meningitis	Response to RBCs and lipid in CSF resulting from: • Hemorrhage • Brain abscess, contusion, infarction • Blood contamination following lumbar puncture Treatments: • Intrathecal medications • Radiographic contrast media • Brain irradiation
Malignant cells • Blasts		Leukemia Lymphoma
• Tumor cells		Central nervous system tumors (medulloblastoma) Metastatic tumors (e.g., lung, breast, gastrointestinal tract, melanoma)

AIDS, Acquired immunodeficiency syndrome; *CSF*, cerebrospinal fluid; *HIV*, human immunodeficiency virus; *RBC*, red blood cell.

TABLE 13-5	Normal Cerebrospinal Fluid Differential Count*		
Age	**Lymphocytes**	**Monocytes**	**Neutrophils**
Neonates (0 to 2 mo)	5% to 35%	50% to 90%	0% to 8%
Children (2 mo to 18 yr)	Not yet established	Not yet established	Not yet established
Adults (>18 yr)	40% to 80%	15% to 45%	0% to 6%

*Data apply to cerebrospinal fluid differential counts using a cytospin preparation technique.

large cells with basophilic cytoplasm (a transformed lymphocyte or immunoblast). Along with reactive and plasmacytoid lymphocytes, lymphocytes are often found in patients with viral meningitis. Reactive lymphs can be quantitated or simply stated as present. Table 13-4 lists other conditions demonstrating CSF-lymphocytic pleocytosis.

Plasma Cells. Plasma cells normally are not present in CSF; therefore their presence should always be noted. They may be seen in acute viral and chronic inflammatory conditions—many of the same conditions that result in lymphocytic pleocytosis. In some cases of multiple sclerosis, the presence of plasma cells may be the only CSF abnormality.

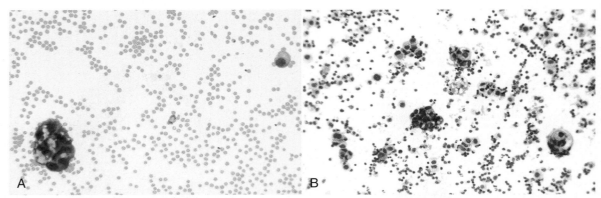

FIGURE 13-4 Low-power fields of view of cerebrospinal fluid (CSF) with tumor cell clumps. **A,** Rare tumor clump with numerous red blood cells (RBCs). **B,** Numerous cells with rare tumor clump. *(Courtesy Charlotte Janita.)*

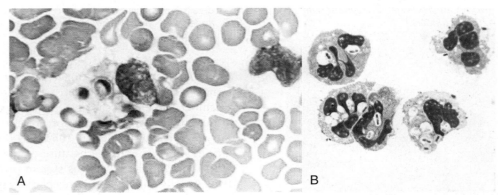

FIGURE 13-5 A, Macrophage with intracellular yeast (cerebrospinal fluid [CSF], ×1000). **B,** Bacteria engulfed by neutrophils (CSF, ×1000). *(**A,** Courtesy Charlotte Janita. **B,** From Carr JH, Rodak BF: Clinical hematology atlas, ed 3, St Louis, 2008, Saunders.)*

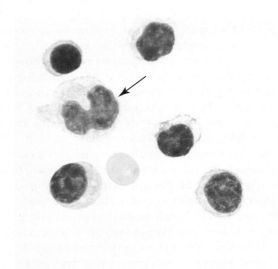

FIGURE 13-6 Normal lymphocytes with monocyte *(arrow)* and red blood cell (RBC) (cerebrospinal fluid [CSF], ×1000). *(From Carr JH, Rodak BF: Clinical hematology atlas, ed 3, St Louis, 2008, Saunders.)*

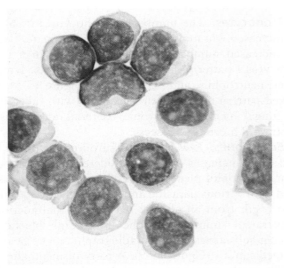

FIGURE 13-7 Reactive lymphocytes (cerebrospinal fluid [CSF], ×1000). *(From Carr JH, Rodak BF: Clinical hematology atlas, ed 3, St Louis, 2008, Saunders.)*

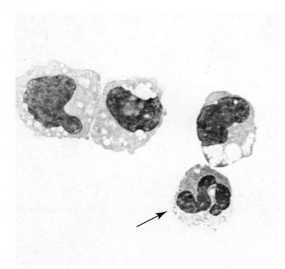

FIGURE 13-8 Monocytes and a single neutrophil (cerebrospinal fluid [CSF], ×1000). *(From Carr JH, Rodak BF: Clinical hematology atlas, ed 3, St Louis, 2008, Saunders.)*

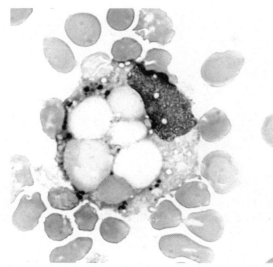

FIGURE 13-10 Macrophage with engulfed (intracellular) red blood cells (RBCs); can also be called an *erythrophage. (From Carr JH, Rodak BF: Clinical hematology atlas, ed 3, St Louis, 2008, Saunders.)*

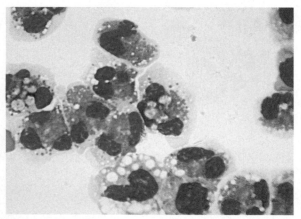

FIGURE 13-9 Eosinophilia in cerebrospinal fluid (CSF). *(Courtesy Charlotte Janita.)*

Monocytes. The number of monocytes in CSF can be increased, but monocytes rarely predominate. Usually an increased number of monocytes occur in a mixed pleocytosis pattern with other cell types (i.e., lymphocytes, neutrophils, and plasma cells) (Figure 13-8). This mixed pattern may be seen in patients with tuberculous or fungal meningitis, chronic bacterial meningitis, or rupture of a cerebral abscess.

Eosinophils. Few eosinophils are seen in normal CSF, and small increases are not considered clinically significant. Eosinophil pleocytosis (10% or greater) is associated with various parasitic and fungal infections and can also result from an allergic reaction to malfunctioning intracranial shunts or to the intrathecal injection of foreign substances such as radiographic contrast media or medications (Figure 13-9). A form of meningitis that results in eosinophil pleocytosis has also been described; when a causative agent or pathogen is not identified, the term used is *idiopathic eosinophilic meningitis.*[11]

Macrophages. Macrophages in CSF originate from monocytes and possibly from stem cells located in the reticuloendothelial tissue of the arachnoid and pia mater. Although macrophages are not present in normal CSF, they frequently are found following hemorrhage and various other conditions because of their active phagocytic ability. Central nervous system procedures such as myelography and pneumoencephalography can stimulate an increase in monocytes and macrophages in the CSF that can persist for 2 to 3 weeks following the procedure. Macrophages are capable of phagocytosing other cells, such as RBCs and WBCs, and other substances such as lipids, pigments, and microorganisms. Following a subarachnoid or cerebral hemorrhage, recently phagocytosed RBCs are readily apparent in macrophages. The engulfed RBCs rapidly lose their pigmentation, forming vacuoles in the cytoplasm of these large cells (Figure 13-10). The presence of hemosiderin (i.e., brown- or black-pigmented granules from RBC hemoglobin) is observed best with iron staining of a cytospin preparation (Figure 13-11). In addition to hemosiderin formation, which takes 2 to 4 days, hematoidin crystals can eventually develop. These yellow or red, often parallelogram-shaped, crystals are similar in chemical composition to bilirubin and do not contain iron. Hematoidin crystals can be present extracellularly or in the cytoplasm of macrophages (intracellular) (Figure 13-12).

The presence of a small number of erythrophagocytic macrophages does not always indicate a hemorrhage. If a second lumbar puncture is performed within 8 to 12 hours of a previous puncture, peripheral blood that entered the CSF during the initial procedure can be responsible for stimulating the observed activity. However, if hematoidin crystals are present or iron staining reveals hemosiderin-laden macrophages (siderophages),

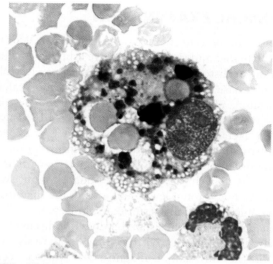

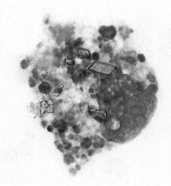

FIGURE 13-12 Siderophage with intracellular hematoidin crystal (cerebrospinal fluid [CSF], ×1000). *(From Rodak BF, Fristma GA, Doig K: Hematology: clinical principles and applications, ed 3, St Louis, 2007, Saunders.)*

FIGURE 13-11 Hemosiderin-laden macrophage; also called a *siderophage. (From Carr JH, Rodak BF: Clinical hematology atlas, ed 3, St Louis, 2008, Saunders.)*

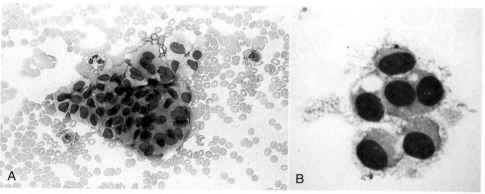

FIGURE 13-13 Clumps of ependymal or choroid plexus cells. **A,** Cerebrospinal fluid (CSF), ×200. **B,** CSF, ×500. **(A,** *From Rodak BF, Fristma GA, Doig K: Hematology: clinical principles and applications, ed 3, St Louis, 2007, Saunders.* **B,** *Courtesy Charlotte Janita.)*

a hemorrhage in the central nervous system most likely occurred. Note that these siderophages can persist for 2 to 8 weeks. Macrophages also actively phagocytose lipids that may be present in the CSF as a result of injury, abscess, or infarction in the central nervous system. These lipid-laden macrophages are often termed *lipophages* and display a foamy cytoplasm with the nucleus often pushed to one side.

Other Cells. Ependymal or choroid plexus cells occasionally can be seen singularly or in clumps (Figure 13-13). These cells are similar in size to a small lymphocyte and have round to oval nuclei. Their cytoplasm is moderate to abundant and light gray when stained using Wright's stain. Microscopically, it is impossible to differentiate ependymal cells from choroid plexus cells. These cells may also be called *ventricular lining cells* or *ependymal-choroid cells.* They are frequently seen in patients with ventricular or cisternal taps or shunts. In these cases, their presence is not clinically significant, but

it is important to be familiar with their cytologic characteristics so they can be differentiated from malignant cells.

Other cells such as squamous epithelial cells, chondrocytes (cartilage cells), cells originating from bone marrow contamination, spindle-shaped cells, neurons, and astrocytes can also be observed in CSF.

Malignant Cells. Malignant cells can be present in the CSF as a result of a primary central nervous system tumor (e.g., medulloblastoma) or of metastasis. Most commonly seen are metastatic tumor cells from melanoma, and lung, breast, or gastrointestinal tract cancers. Leukemia, particularly acute lymphoblastic leukemia and acute myeloblastic leukemia, as well as lymphoma, can also result in the presence of malignant cells in the CSF. In patients with lymphoma and acute lymphoblastic leukemia with meningeal infiltration, increased numbers of lymphoblasts are present in the CSF (Figure 13-14); in patients with acute myeloblastic leukemia, readily

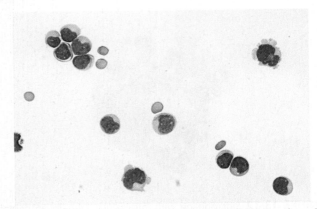

FIGURE 13-14 Lymphoblasts in cerebrospinal fluid (lymphoma).

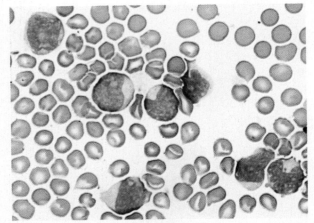

FIGURE 13-15 Myeloblasts in cerebrospinal fluid (acute myelogenous leukemia).

identifiable and uniform myeloblasts are seen (Figure 13-15). The leukemic and lymphoma lymphoblasts are characteristically uniform in size, shape, and appearance, in contrast to transformed reactive lymphocytes in lymphoid-stimulating conditions that show a significant variation in the types of cells present. The actual number of lymphoblasts present is not of diagnostic importance; even small numbers are clinically significant. Because drugs used in chemotherapy do not pass the blood-brain barrier, malignant cells that enter the central nervous system can proliferate unchecked in the CSF. As a result, most patients with acute lymphoblastic leukemia (≈80%) and acute myeloblastic leukemia (approximately 60%) develop central nervous system involvement at some stage during the disease.[5]

Malignant tumor cells can appear singly or as cell clumps in CSF. When clumps of cells are present, it is important to positively identify and differentiate malignant cells from clumps of normal choroid plexus cells and from ependymal cells that line the ventricles. These normal cells of the central nervous system closely resemble malignant cells in size, shape, and appearance, but they have no clinical significance. In contrast, malignant cells are always of diagnostic importance.

CHEMICAL EXAMINATION

Although numerous chemical constituents of CSF have been evaluated and studied, few have established clinical usefulness. Historically, although numerous electrolytes and acid-base indicators—such as chloride, calcium, magnesium, pH, and Pco_2—were analyzed, these analytes now have little clinical value. Instead, assays of glucose, lactate, and various proteins in CSF predominate, providing substantive diagnostic information. This chapter does not discuss those chemical tests with limited clinical use, such as glutamine quantitation, which reflects CSF ammonia levels and aids in the diagnosis of hepatic encephalopathy resulting from Reye's syndrome, viral hepatitis, or cirrhosis, and it does not discuss lactate dehydrogenase activity with isoenzyme analysis, which aids in the differential diagnosis of various central nervous system disorders.

Protein

The bulk of CSF protein (more than 80%) is derived from the transport of plasma proteins (via pinocytosis) through the capillary endothelium in the choroid plexus and meninges; the rest of the protein results from intrathecal synthesis.[12] Because of this transport process of proteins, normally only low-molecular-weight proteins are present in the CSF. Electrophoresis, after concentrating CSF (80 to 100 times), normally reveals only the presence of transthyretin (previously called *prealbumin*), albumin, and transferrin. Trace amounts of immunoglobulin G (IgG), a high-molecular-weight protein (molecular weight 160,000), can also be demonstrated electrophoretically in some normal CSF specimens.

Total Protein. The total amount of protein in the CSF varies with the age of the individual and the site from which the CSF is obtained. The protein content of CSF obtained from the lumbar region is greater than that obtained from the cisterna or ventricles. In general, CSF total protein concentrations ranging from 15 to 45 mg/dL (150 to 450 mg/L) are considered normal, although infants and adults older than 40 years often have higher protein concentrations.

The CSF total protein is most commonly determined to assess the integrity of the blood-brain barrier and to indicate pathologic conditions of the central nervous system. Increased CSF total protein can result from one of four different mechanisms: (1) CSF contamination with peripheral blood during the puncture procedure; (2) altered capillary endothelial exchange (change in the blood-brain barrier); (3) decreased reabsorption into the venous blood; or (4) increased synthesis in the central nervous system. Because of the high concentration of proteins in the blood plasma compared with CSF (≈1000:1), a traumatic tap can result in significant false elevation of the CSF total protein. Formulas to correct for the contribution of plasma protein to CSF after a traumatic tap use the RBC count obtained from the same collection tube. As mentioned earlier, however, these RBC-based formulas overestimate the correction, are rough estimates at best, and are not clinically useful.

Changes in the permeability of the blood-brain barrier and decreased reabsorption at the arachnoid villi occur with numerous disorders, such as bacterial, viral, and other forms of meningitis; cerebral infarction; hemorrhage; endocrine disorders; and trauma. Obstruction to the flow of CSF caused by tumors, disk herniation, or abscess prevents the normal circulation of fluid, which enhances water reabsorption in the spinal cord and results in increased CSF protein. Last, the infiltration of the central nervous system with immunocompetent cells that synthesize immunoglobulins can also result in an increased total protein determination (e.g., in multiple sclerosis, neurosyphilis).

Decreased CSF total protein can result from (1) increased reabsorption through the arachnoid villi because of increased intracranial pressure, or (2) loss of fluid because of trauma (e.g., a dural tear) or invasive procedures (e.g., pneumoencephalography).

Several methods are available to determine CSF total protein. Test selection is dictated by the limited sample volume and the need for sensitivity because CSF protein concentrations are normally low (15 to 45 mg/dL). Turbidimetric procedures based on the precipitation of protein are often used. For a comprehensive discussion of the methods available, including the advantages and disadvantages of each, the reader should consult a textbook in clinical chemistry.

Albumin and Immunoglobulin G. Because albumin is not synthesized in the central nervous system, all albumin present in CSF results from passage across the blood-brain barrier, assuming no contamination occurs during the puncture procedure. Therefore albumin can be used as a reference protein to monitor the permeability of the blood-brain barrier. Permeability is evaluated by determining the CSF/serum albumin index, which is the ratio of the CSF albumin concentration to the serum albumin concentration (Equation 13-1). Note that the concentration units differ: Albumin in CSF is reported in milligrams per deciliter, whereas serum albumin is reported in grams per deciliter. A CSF/serum albumin index less than 9 is considered normal. Index values between 9.0 and 14.0 represent minimal impairment of the blood-brain barrier, index values between 15 and 100 represent moderate to severe impairment of the barrier, and index values that exceed 100 indicate a complete breakdown of the barrier.[12]

Equation 13-1

$$\text{CSF/serum albumin index} = \frac{\text{Albumin}_{CSF} \text{ (mg/dL)}}{\text{Albumin}_{Serum} \text{ (g/dL)}}$$

In contrast to albumin, IgG is a large-molecular-weight protein that is normally present in minute amounts (approximately 1 mg/dL) in the CSF. In some pathologic conditions, increased CSF IgG can result from increased production within the central nervous system or from increased transport from the blood plasma. To specifically identify those conditions characterized by increased intrathecal synthesis, albumin is used as a reference protein, and the following formula is used to determine the CSF IgG index:

Equation 13-2

$$\text{CSF IgG index} = \frac{\text{IgG}_{CSF} \text{ (mg/dL)}}{\text{IgG}_{Serum} \text{ (g/dL)}} \times \frac{\text{Albumin}_{Serum} \text{ (g/dL)}}{\text{Albumin}_{CSF} \text{ (mg/dL)}}$$

As with albumin, the concentration units of IgG differ with specimen type. Because this calculation depends on determinations of the albumin and IgG concentrations, any analytical error is magnified. Therefore it is imperative to use accurate and precise quantitative immunochemical methods (e.g., nephelometry) to determine the albumin and IgG concentrations. A typical reference interval for the IgG index is 0.30 to 0.70 (this range varies with the technical methods used and the patient population). Values greater than this range are associated with increased intrathecal production of IgG, whereas values less than this range indicate a compromised blood-brain barrier. Because about 90% of patients with multiple sclerosis have an IgG index greater than 0.70, this index is diagnostically sensitive for this disease. However, other inflammatory disorders of the central nervous system can cause increased IgG synthesis, which limits the specificity of the index for multiple sclerosis. Regardless, the CSF IgG index is a diagnostically useful tool and is frequently used.

Protein Electrophoresis. Protein electrophoresis reveals the composition and distribution of proteins in CSF. An abnormal distribution of proteins can be present in CSF (see Table 13-1) despite a normal total protein content. Because of its low protein content, CSF must be concentrated 80- to 100-fold before electrophoresis. This is most often done using commercial concentrating devices.

Four protein bands predominate in a normal CSF pattern: transthyretin (TTR), albumin, and two distinct transferrin bands (Figure 13-16, *A*). In addition, faint bands of α_1-antitrypsin and IgG may be present. The second transferrin band, also known as τ (tau) transferrin, migrates in the β_2 region and is a sialic acid–deficient form of transferrin synthesized almost exclusively in the central nervous system (CNS). Because it is a protein unique to CSF, when a CSF electrophoretic pattern is compared with a serum electrophoretic pattern from the same individual, τ transferrin will not be present in the serum pattern. Normally, serum, nasal fluid, middle ear fluid, saliva, and sputum do not contain τ transferrin. Therefore, the presence of τ transferrin in a fluid or discharge positively identifies it as CSF, which assists in the diagnosis of CSF rhinorrhea or otorrhea (i.e., the discharge of CSF through the nose or ears, respectively).[13]

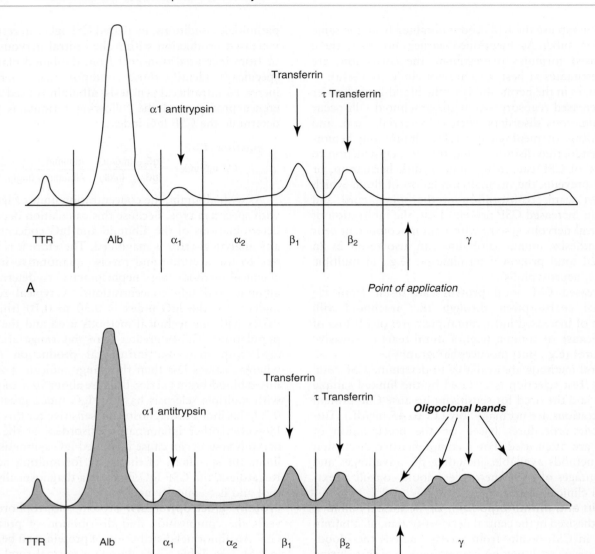

FIGURE 13-16 Cerebrospinal fluid protein patterns using high-resolution electrophoresis. **A,** A "normal" cerebrospinal fluid protein pattern. The presence in the β_2-region of τ transferrin, a protein unique to cerebrospinal fluid, is noteworthy. **B,** An "abnormal" cerebrospinal fluid protein pattern demonstrating the presence of oligoclonal bands in the γ region. These bands will not be present on electrophoresis of the patient's serum. *TTR,* Transthyretin (previously called *prealbumin*).

Electrophoresis of CSF is performed primarily to detect **oligoclonal bands** in the γ-region (Figure 13-16, *B*). Oligoclonal banding can vary significantly from a few faint discrete bands to many intense bands. Their presence in CSF and concomitant absence in serum is highly indicative of multiple sclerosis. Because IgG can pass the blood-brain barrier, simultaneous electrophoretic analysis of serum and CSF is necessary. Some lymphoproliferative disorders also produce oligoclonal banding, but the bands are present in both serum and CSF. In these cases, if only CSF is analyzed, an inaccurate diagnosis could be made. Among patients with multiple sclerosis, 90% demonstrate CSF oligoclonal bands at some time in the course of their disease. Although these bands aid in the diagnosis of multiple sclerosis, their presence or intensity does not correlate with a particular stage of disease, nor can they be used to predict disease progression. In addition, other central nervous system disorders, such as subacute sclerosing panencephalitis, neurosyphilis, bacterial and viral meningitis, and acute necrotizing encephalitis, can also demonstrate CSF oligoclonal banding. As a result, CSF oligoclonal banding alone cannot be considered pathognomonic for multiple sclerosis. Instead, a protocol consisting of laboratory tests and a clinical assessment of neurologic dysfunction is used to diagnose multiple sclerosis.

Myelin Basic Protein. Myelin, a primarily lipid substance (70%), surrounds the axons of nerves and is necessary for proper nerve conduction. The remaining 30% of myelin is made up of proteins, one of which is myelin basic protein. With multiple sclerosis and other demyelinating diseases, the myelin sheaths undergo degradation and release myelin basic protein into the CSF, where it can be detected using sensitive immunoassays. Detection of myelin basic protein is not specific for multiple sclerosis, and the protein is present only during acute exacerbation of the disease. Myelin basic protein determinations, therefore, are used primarily to follow the course of disease or to identify those individuals with multiple sclerosis who do not show oligoclonal banding (≈10%).

Glucose

The CSF glucose concentration is in a dynamic equilibrium with glucose in the blood plasma. Two mechanisms account for glucose in the CSF: (1) active transport by endothelial cells, and (2) simple diffusion along a concentration gradient that exists between the blood plasma and the CSF. Because of the time involved for these processes to occur, a CSF glucose value reflects the plasma glucose concentration 30 to 90 minutes preceding collection of the fluid. Accurately interpreting CSF glucose values requires a plasma glucose drawn 0 to 60 minutes preceding the lumbar puncture, preferably a fasting level. Normally, CSF glucose ranges from 50 to 80 mg/dL (2.75 to 4.40 mmol/L), which is approximately 60% to 70% of the plasma concentration. If a CSF/plasma glucose ratio is calculated, normal values average 0.6.

Increased CSF glucose levels are found following hyperglycemia and traumatic puncture procedures (because of peripheral blood contamination) but have no diagnostic significance. In contrast, low CSF glucose values (less than 40 mg/dL) are associated with numerous conditions such as hypoglycemic states, meningitis, and infiltration of the meninges with metastatic or primary tumor. More than 50% of meningitis cases have a low CSF glucose level. The mechanism for the low CSF glucose level observed is twofold: decreased or defective transport across the blood-brain barrier, and increased glycolysis within the central nervous system.

Lactate

Lactate is normally present in CSF at concentrations ranging from 10 to 22 mg/dL (1.1 to 2.4 mmol/L), and its CSF concentration is essentially unrelated to that of blood plasma. Increased CSF lactate levels result from anaerobic metabolism within the central nervous system because of tissue hypoxia or decreased oxygenation of the brain. Any condition that impairs the blood supply or the transport of oxygen to the central nervous system results in increased CSF lactate levels. Numerous conditions that produce high CSF lactate levels include low arterial Po_2, cerebral infarction, cerebral arteriosclerosis, intracranial hemorrhage, hydrocephalus, traumatic brain injury, cerebral edema, and meningitis.

Determination of CSF lactate can assist in differentiating meningitis caused by bacterial, fungal, or tuberculous agents from viral meningitis. In viral meningitis, the lactate level rarely exceeds 25 to 30 mg/dL; in contrast, other forms of meningitis usually produce CSF lactate levels greater than 35 mg/dL. It is interesting to note that increased CSF lactate levels are closely associated with low CSF glucose levels, and that together these parameters may be a better diagnostic indicator of bacterial meningitis than either parameter alone.

MICROBIOLOGICAL EXAMINATION

The microbiology laboratory plays a key role in the diagnosis and selection of treatment for meningitis. If a limited volume of CSF is obtained, most often microbiological studies take precedence over all other studies. With identification of the causative agent responsible for meningitis, appropriate antibiotic therapy can begin. Gram staining and other microscopic techniques may reveal the causative agent; a CSF culture can assist in diagnosis but more often confirms it; detection of microbial antigens in the CSF using immunologic tests greatly aids in the diagnosis of meningitis.

Usually the second CSF collection tube obtained from a puncture procedure is sent to the microbiology laboratory. This tube or any subsequent tube is preferred because it is less likely than the first tube to contain microbial organisms from the puncture site. The CSF for microbial studies must be maintained at room temperature and should be processed immediately to ensure the recovery of viable organisms. Centrifugation of CSF at $1500 \times g$ for 15 minutes produces a sediment from which smears and cultures are prepared.[14]

Microscopic Examination of CSF Smears

Because the microscopic examination of concentrated CSF sediment can provide a rapid presumptive diagnosis of meningitis in 60% to 80% of cases, it is imperative that a skilled microbiologist perform the examination. Routine or cytocentrifuged smears can be prepared, with the latter technique concentrating any organisms present into a well-defined area on the slide, facilitating microscopic examination. Gram-stained smears can be difficult to interpret. False-negatives can occur because of the presence of only a small number of organisms. However, precipitated dye and debris, as well as contaminating organisms from reagents and supplies, can lead to false-positive Gram stain results. Although other stains, such as acridine orange, a fluorescent stain, are being evaluated for their sensitivity, the Gram stain remains the most commonly used stain to identify microorganisms in CSF.

If tuberculous meningitis is suspected, the CSF smear is stained with an acid-fast stain. In suspected cases of fungal meningitis, CSF smears are often evaluated by using Gram stain and by putting together an India ink preparation for *Cryptococcus neoformans*. Because microscopic identification can be insensitive (requires the presence of numerous organisms), immunologic tests are frequently used to assist in the diagnosis of various types of meningitis.

Primary meningoencephalitis due to the amoeba *Naegleria fowleri* is a rare but deadly disease. Diagnosis can be made from the microscopic identification of amoebas in a cytocentrifuged CSF smear stained with Wright's stain. The amoebas are 15 to 20 μm in diameter with a sky blue cytoplasm and a distinct finely granular, violet nucleus. They inhabit warm fresh-water areas and can infect children and young adults who play or relax in these waters.

Culture

The most common causes of meningitis are *Haemophilus influenzae, Neisseria meningitidis,* and *Streptococcus pneumoniae;* however, numerous other bacteria, fungi, parasites, and viruses can be causative agents. Aerobic culturing of CSF enables the isolation of common types of bacteria in 80% to 90% of cases. If antibiotic therapy precedes CSF collection, however, recovery of bacterial isolates from the specimen can be significantly reduced. In suspected cases of tuberculous meningitis, the chance of positive culture increases with repeat CSF cultures. In cases of suspected meningitis, blood cultures should also be performed. These cultures are positive in 40% to 60% of patients with suspected meningitis and often provide the only clue as to the causative agent.[5]

IMMUNOLOGIC METHODS

Several immunologic assays are currently available to detect the presence of microbial antigens in CSF (and in serum). The various techniques used include coagglutination, latex agglutination, immunoassay, and counterimmunoelectrophoresis. In these assays, the reagent containing polyclonal antibodies is combined with CSF; if the microbial antigen is present, a positive test result is obtained. As monoclonal antibodies are developed, the sensitivity and specificity of these assays will improve.

Currently, immunologic tests can be used to detect several bacterial and fungal organisms that cause meningitis. The latex slide agglutination test for *Cryptococcus* antigen is widely used because of its high sensitivity (60% to 99%) and specificity (80% to 99%). In addition, this test serves as a good prognostic indicator, with increasing titers suggesting spread of the disease and decreasing titers associated with response to treatment. Similarly, immunologic assays for *Coccidioides immitis, Mycobacterium tuberculosis, Haemophilus influenzae, Neisseria meningitidis, Streptococcus pneumoniae,* and group B streptococci are available. Although these assays generally are rapid and easy to perform, they do not have equivalent diagnostic value. Sensitivity and specificity

vary with each assay, and false-positive nonspecific reactions and false-negative reactions can occur. Consequently, CSF Gram stain and culture remain the standard for the diagnosis of bacterial and fungal meningitis.

At times to assist in the diagnosis of neurosyphilis, a request for a venereal disease research laboratory (VDRL) test on CSF may be received. Although the VDRL-CSF test is highly specific for syphilis, it should not be used as a "screening" test because it yields a high percentage of false-negatives (i.e., low sensitivity). In other words, a nonreactive result does not rule out neurosyphilis. Therefore, the VDRL-CSF should be performed only when the patient's serum fluorescent treponemal antibody absorbed test (FTA-ABS) result is reactive (positive).

STUDY QUESTIONS

1. Cerebrospinal fluid (CSF) is produced primarily from
   A. secretions by the choroid plexus.
   B. diffusion from plasma into the central nervous system.
   C. ultrafiltration of plasma in the ventricles of the brain.
   D. excretions from ependymal cells lining the brain and spinal cord.

2. Cerebrospinal fluid is found between the
   A. arachnoid and dura mater.
   B. arachnoid and pia mater.
   C. pia mater and dura mater.
   D. pia mater and choroid plexus.

3. Which of the following statements regarding CSF is true?
   A. Cerebrospinal fluid is constantly produced.
   B. Cerebrospinal fluid is reabsorbed into the blood at the choroid plexus.
   C. Cerebrospinal fluid is essentially composed of diluted plasma.
   D. Cerebrospinal fluid circulates through the brain and spinal cord because of active and passive diffusion processes.

4. Which of the following substances does not normally pass through the blood-brain barrier?
   A. Po_2
   B. Albumin
   C. Glucose
   D. Fibrinogen

5. During a lumbar puncture procedure, the first collection tube of CSF removed should be used for
   A. chemistry tests.
   B. cytologic studies.
   C. hematologic tests.
   D. microbiological studies.

6. Which of the following is not an analytical concern when the processing and testing of CSF are delayed?
   A. The viability of microorganisms
   B. The lability of the immunoglobulins
   C. The lysis of leukocytes and erythrocytes
   D. Alterations in the chemical composition
7. Pleocytosis is a term used to describe
   A. an increased number of cells in the CSF.
   B. a pink, orange, or yellow CSF specimen.
   C. an increased protein content in the CSF caused by cellular lysis.
   D. inflammation and sloughing of cells from the choroid plexus.
8. All of the following can cause xanthochromia in CSF except
   A. high concentrations of protein.
   B. high concentrations of bilirubin.
   C. increased numbers of leukocytes.
   D. erythrocytes from a traumatic tap.
9. In CSF, which of the following findings indicates a traumatic puncture?
   A. The presence of erythrophagocytic cells in the CSF
   B. Hemosiderin granules within macrophages in the CSF sediment
   C. An uneven distribution of blood in the CSF collection tubes
   D. A xanthochromic supernatant following CSF centrifugation
10. How many leukocytes are normally present in the CSF obtained from an adult?
    A. 0 to 5 cells/mL
    B. 0 to 10 cells/mL
    C. 0 to 20 cells/mL
    D. 0 to 30 cells/mL
11. Which of the following cells can be present in small numbers in normal CSF?
    A. Erythrocytes
    B. Lymphocytes
    C. Macrophages
    D. Plasma cells
12. Which of the following cell types predominate in CSF during a classic case of bacterial meningitis?
    A. Lymphocytes
    B. Macrophages
    C. Monocytes
    D. Neutrophils
13. Which of the following cell types predominate in CSF during a classic case of viral meningitis?
    A. Lymphocytes
    B. Macrophages
    C. Monocytes
    D. Neutrophils

14. When choroid plexus cells and ependymal cells are present in CSF, they
    A. are often clinically significant.
    B. represent the demyelination of nerve tissue.
    C. can closely resemble clusters of malignant cells.
    D. indicate breakdown of the blood-brain barrier.
15. All of the following proteins are normally present in the CSF except
    A. albumin.
    B. fibrinogen.
    C. transthyretin.
    D. transferrin.
16. Which of the following events does not result in an increased CSF total protein?
    A. A traumatic puncture procedure
    B. Alterations in the blood-brain barrier
    C. Trauma to the central nervous system, resulting in fluid loss
    D. Decreased reabsorption of CSF into the peripheral blood
17. Which of the following proteins in the CSF is used to monitor the integrity of the blood-brain barrier?
    A. Albumin
    B. Transthyretin
    C. Transferrin
    D. Immunoglobulin G
18. An immunoglobulin G index greater than 0.70 indicates
    A. intrathecal synthesis of immunoglobulin G.
    B. a compromised blood-brain barrier.
    C. active demyelination of neural proteins.
    D. increased transport of immunoglobulin G from plasma into the CSF.
19. An unknown fluid can be positively identified as CSF by determining the
    A. lactate concentration.
    B. albumin concentration.
    C. presence of oligoclonal banding on electrophoresis.
    D. presence of carbohydrate-deficient transferrin on electrophoresis.
20. Which of the following statements about oligoclonal bands is false?
    A. In the CSF, these bands indicate increased intrathecal concentrations of immunoglobulin G.
    B. The bands usually correlate with the stage of disease and can be used to predict disease progression.
    C. The bands are often present in the CSF and serum of individuals with a lymphoproliferative disease.
    D. The bands are often present in the CSF but not in the serum of individuals with multiple sclerosis.

21. Which of the following statements about CSF glucose is false?
    A. Increased CSF glucose values are diagnostically significant.
    B. Glucose enters the CSF by active transport and simple diffusion.
    C. Decreased CSF glucose values reflect a defective blood-brain barrier and increased glycolysis.
    D. CSF glucose values reflect the plasma glucose concentration 30 to 90 minutes preceding collection.

22. Normal CSF lactate levels (less than 25 mg/dL) are commonly found in patients with
    A. bacterial meningitis.
    B. fungal meningitis.
    C. tuberculous meningitis.
    D. viral meningitis.

23. Which of the following procedures frequently provides a rapid presumptive diagnosis of bacterial meningitis?
    A. A blood culture
    B. A CSF culture
    C. A CSF Gram stain
    D. Immunologic tests on CSF for microbial antigens

24. India ink preparations and microbial antigen tests on CSF can aid in the diagnosis of
    A. bacterial meningitis.
    B. fungal meningitis.
    C. tuberculous meningitis.
    D. viral meningitis.

CASE 13-1

A 4-year-old girl is brought to the emergency room by her parents. She is lethargic, reports that her head hurts, and shows signs of stiffness in her neck. Her mother states that she has had "a temperature" for the past 2 days; her current temperature is determined to be 104° C. She is admitted to the hospital, where blood is drawn and a lumbar puncture performed. Cerebrospinal fluid and pertinent blood chemistry results follow.

1. List any abnormal results.
2. Calculate the CSF/plasma glucose ratio.
3. These results are most consistent with a preliminary diagnosis of
   A. viral meningitis.
   B. bacterial meningitis.
   C. Guillain-Barré syndrome.
   D. acute lymphocytic leukemia.
4. Does the CSF lactate value assist in determining a diagnosis for this patient?
5. Situation: If Gram stain results are negative (i.e., no organisms seen), would you change the diagnosis selected in #4? Why or why not?
6. Explain briefly the physiologic mechanisms that account for the CSF total protein and glucose values.

Blood Chemistry Results	**Reference Interval**
Glucose, fasting: 90 mg/dL	<110 mg/dL

Cerebrospinal Fluid Results

Physical Examination	Microscopic Examination	Chemical Examination
Color: colorless	Leukocyte count: 7300 cells/μL	Total protein: 130 mg/dL
Clarity: cloudy (3+)	Differential count:	Glucose: 32 mg/dL
Gram stain: results pending	Monocytes: 7%	Lactate: 33 mg/dL
	Lymphocytes: 6%	
	Neutrophils: 87%	

CASE 13-2

A 39-year-old woman noticed numbness in her left leg and difficulty walking approximately 3 months ago. Since that time, the numbness seems to come and go along with episodes of dizziness. More recently, she has experienced numbness on the right side of her face and "blurred" vision in her right eye that comes and goes. She gets tired easily and often feels unsteady while upright and walking. She is admitted to the hospital for tests. Cerebrospinal fluid and pertinent blood chemistry results follow.

Blood Chemistry Results

	Reference Interval
Glucose, fasting: 85 mg/dL	<110 mg/dL
Albumin: 4.6 g/dL	3.5-5.0 g/dL
Immunoglobulin G: 1.4 g/dL	0.65-1.50 g/dL

Cerebrospinal Fluid Results

Physical Examination	Microscopic Examination	Chemical Examination
Color: colorless	Leukocyte count: 3 cells/μL	Total protein: 45 mg/dL
Clarity: clear	Differential count:	Albumin: 28 mg/dL
Gram stain: no organisms seen	Monocytes: 24%	IgG: 12.4 mg/dL
	Lymphocytes: 75%	Glucose: 72 mg/dL
	Neutrophils: 1%	Lactate: 18 mg/dL

1. List any abnormal results.
2. Calculate CSF/serum albumin index as follows:

$$\text{CSF/serum albumin index} = \frac{\text{Albumin}_{CSF}\ (mg/dL)}{\text{Albumin}_{Serum}\ (g/dL)}$$

   (reference interval: < 9.0)

3. Why is the CSF/serum albumin index a good indicator of the integrity of the blood-brain barrier?
4. Calculate the CSF IgG index as follows:

$$\text{CSF IgG index} = \frac{\text{IgG}_{CSF}\ (mg/dL)}{\text{IgG}_{Serum}\ (g/dL)} \times \frac{\text{Albumin}_{Serum}\ (g/dL)}{\text{Albumin}_{CSF}\ (mg/dL)}$$

   (reference interval: 0.30–0.70)

5. Suggest a diagnosis that is consistent with the results obtained and the patient history.
6. Based on the diagnosis chosen, state two additional chemical tests that could be performed to confirm this diagnosis, and indicate the results expected.

REFERENCES

1. McComb JG: Recent research into the nature of cerebrospinal fluid formation and absorption. J Neurosurg 59:369-383, 1983.
2. Marton KI, Gean AD: The spinal tap: a new look at an old test. Ann Intern Med 104:840-848, 1986.
3. Chow G, Schmidley JW: Lysis of erythrocytes and leukocytes in traumatic lumbar punctures. Arch Neurol 41:1084-1085, 1984.
4. Lofsness KG, Jensen TL: The preparation of simulated spinal fluid for teaching purposes. Am J Med Technol 49:493-497, 1983.
5. Aune MW, Becker JL, Brugnara C, et al: Automated flow cytometric analysis of blood cells in cerebrospinal fluid. Am J Clin Pathol 121:690-700, 2004.
6. Strik H, Luthe H, Nagel I, et al: Automated cerebrospinal fluid cytology, limitations and reasonable applications. Analyt Quant Cytol Histol 27:1-7, 2005.
7. Walker TJ, Nelson LD, Dunphy BW, et al: Comparative evaluation of the Iris iQ200 body fluid module with manual hemacytometer count. Am J Clin Pathol 131:333-338, 2009.
8. Fishbein D, Palmer DL, Porter KM: Bacterial meningitis in the absence of pleocytosis. Arch Intern Med 141:1369-1372, 1981.
9. Novak RW: Lack of validity of standard corrections for white cell counts of blood contaminated cerebrospinal fluid in infants. Am J Clin Pathol 82:95-97, 1984.
10. Kuberski T: Eosinophils in the cerebrospinal fluid. Ann Intern Med 91:70-75, 1979.
11. Kjeldsberg CR, Knight JA: Body fluids, ed 3, Chicago, 1993, American Society for Clinical Pathology Press.
12. Grant GH, Silverman LM, Christenson RH: Amino acids and proteins. In Tietz NW, editor: Fundamentals of clinical chemistry, Philadelphia, 1987, WB Saunders.
13. Normasell DE, Stacy EK, Booker CF, et al: Detection of beta-2 transferrin in otorrhea and rhinorrhea in a routine clinical laboratory setting. Clin Diagn Lab Immunol 1:68, 1994.
14. Murray PR, Hampton CM: Recovery of pathogenic bacteria from cerebrospinal fluid. J Clin Microbiol 12:554-557, 1980.

Synovial Fluid Analysis

KEY TERMS

arthritis Inflammation of a joint.
arthrocentesis A percutaneous puncture procedure used to remove synovial fluid from joint cavities.
hyaluronate A high-molecular-weight polymer of repeating disaccharide units secreted by synoviocytes into synovial fluid. Hyaluronate is a salt or ester of hyaluronic acid

that imparts a high viscosity to the fluid and serves as a joint lubricant.
synovial fluid Fluid within joint cavities. Synovial fluid is formed by ultrafiltration of plasma across the synovial membrane and by secretions from synoviocytes.
synoviocytes Cells of the synovial membrane. Two types of

synoviocytes differ on the basis of their physiologic roles. The predominant type is actively phagocytic and synthesizes degradative enzymes; the second type synthesizes and secretes hyaluronate.

PHYSIOLOGY AND COMPOSITION

In areas of the skeleton where friction could develop, such as the joints, bursae, and tendon sheaths, viscous **synovial fluid** is present. Within articulated diarthrodial joints (e.g., the knee), the ends of apposing bones are covered with articular cartilage, the joint space is lined

by a synovial membrane (except in weight-bearing areas), and synovial fluid bathes and lubricates the joint (Figure 14-1). The surface of the synovial membrane surrounding the joint consists of numerous microvilli with a layer, one to three cells deep, of synovial cells called **synovio-cytes** (Figure 14-2). Two types of synoviocytes are present

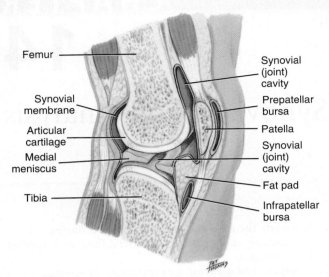

FIGURE 14-1 A schematic representation of the knee: a diarthrodial joint. *(From Applegate E: The anatomy and physiology learning system, ed 4, Philadelphia, 2011, Saunders.)*

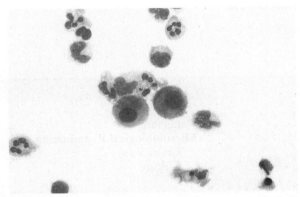

FIGURE 14-2 Synoviocytes in synovial fluid, ×400. Note similarity to mesothelial cells. *(From Rodak BF, Fristma GA, Doig K: Hematology: clinical principles and applications, ed 3, St Louis, 2007, Saunders.)*

TABLE 14-1	Synovial Fluid Reference Intervals*	
Physical Examination		
Total volume	0.1 to 3.5 mL	
Color	Pale yellow	
Clarity	Clear	
Viscosity	High; forms "strings" 4 to 6 cm long	
Spontaneous clot formation	No	
Microscopic Examination		
Erythrocyte count	<2000 cells/mL	
Leukocyte count	<200 cells/mL	
Differential cell count:		
Monocytes and macrophages	≈60%	
Lymphocytes	≈30%	
Neutrophils	≈10%	
Crystals	None present	
Chemical Examination		
Glucose	Equivalent to plasma values[†]	
Glucose: P-SF difference	<10 mg/dL[†]	
Uric acid	Equivalent to plasma values[†]	
Total protein	1 to 3 g/dL	
Lactate	9 to 33 mg/dL[‡]	
Hyaluronate	0.3 to 0.4 g/dL	

*Values for fluid obtained from a knee joint.
[†]Synovial fluid values are equivalent to blood plasma values if obtained from a fasting patient.
[‡]Normal lactate values are assumed to be similar to those in blood and cerebrospinal fluid; actual reference intervals have yet to be established.

in the synovial membrane. The most prevalent type is actively phagocytic and synthesizes degradative enzymes (e.g., collagenases). The second type of synoviocyte synthesizes hyaluronate, a mucopolysaccharide linked with approximately 2% protein. The synoviocytes are loosely organized in the synovial membrane and differ from cells in other lining membranes in that they have no basement membrane, and adjacent synovial cells are not joined with desmosomes. Beneath the synoviocytes is a thin layer of loose connective tissue containing a vast network of blood vessels, lymphatics, and nerves. Variable numbers of mononuclear cells are also found in this connective tissue layer.

Synovial fluid is formed by the ultrafiltration of plasma across the synovial membrane and from secretions by synoviocytes. The resultant viscous fluid serves as a lubricant for the joint and is the sole nutrient source for the metabolically active articular cartilage, which lacks blood vessels, lymphatics, and nerves. The composition of synovial fluid is unique: Its glucose and uric acid concentrations are equivalent to blood plasma levels, whereas its total protein and immunoglobulin concentrations can vary from one-fourth to one-half those of plasma. Table 14-1 (and Appendix B) lists reference values for various characteristics and constituents of normal synovial fluid obtained from a knee joint.

CLASSIFICATION OF JOINT DISORDERS

Arthritis and other joint diseases are common, and laboratory analysis of synovial fluid assists in the diagnosis and classification of these conditions. When synovial fluid is removed from a joint space, laboratory examination enables classification of the disease process into one of four principal categories: noninflammatory, inflammatory, septic, or hemorrhagic. These general classifications aid in differential diagnosis of joint disease and are summarized in Table 14-2. An important note is that (1) these categories partially overlap, (2) several conditions can occur in the joint at the same time, and (3) variations in test results can occur depending on the stage of the disease process. Consequently, these classifications are used only as a guide for the clinician in the evaluation and diagnosis of joint disease. In contrast to the tentative

TABLE 14-2	Classification of Synovial Fluid Based on Laboratory Examination				
Test	Normal	Group I Noninflammatory	Group II Inflammatory	Group III Septic	Group IV Hemorrhagic
Volume, mL	<3.5	>3.5	>3.5	>3.5	>3.5
Color	Pale yellow	Yellow	Yellow-white	Yellow-green	Red-brown
Viscosity	High	High	Low	Low	Decreased
WBC count, cells/μL	<200	<3000	2000 to 100,000[11]	10,000 to >100,000[11]	>5000[11]
Neutrophils	<25%	<25%	>50%	>75%	>25%
Glucose concentration	Approximately equal to plasma level	Approximately equal to plasma level	Less than plasma level	Less than plasma level	Approximately equal to plasma level
Glucose: P–SF* difference	≤10 mg/dL	<20 mg/dL	>20 mg/dL (range, 0 to 80[6])	>40 mg/dL (range, 20 to 100[6])	<20 mg/dL
Culture	Negative	Negative	Negative	Positive	Negative
Associated diseases	—	Osteoarthritis Osteochondritis Osteochondromatosis Traumatic arthritis Neuroarthropathy	Crystal synovitis[†] (gout, pseudogout) Rheumatoid arthritis[‡] Reactive arthritis[§] Systemic lupus erythematosus[¶]	Bacterial infection Fungal infection Mycobacterial infection	Trauma Blood disease (e.g., hemophilia, sickle cell disease) Tumor Joint prosthesis

*The plasma–synovial fluid difference in glucose concentration when specimens are obtained simultaneously.
[†]With chronic or subsiding conditions, crystal synovitis may present as group I.
[‡]Early stages of rheumatoid arthritis may present as group I.
[§]Previously known as Reiter's syndrome.
[¶]Systemic lupus erythematosus may also present as group I.

diagnoses possible on the basis of laboratory findings, a definitive diagnosis is possible when microorganisms are identified (septic arthritis) or crystals are present (crystal synovitis) in the synovial fluid.

SPECIMEN COLLECTION

Synovial fluid is removed by **arthrocentesis,** which is the percutaneous aspiration of fluid from a joint using aseptic technique. Disposable, sterile needles and syringes are used most often to prevent birefringent contaminants associated with the cleaning and resterilization of reusable supplies. If possible, patients should be fasting a minimum of 4 to 6 hours to allow for the equilibration of chemical constituents between plasma and synovial fluid. A blood sample is collected at approximately the same time as the arthrocentesis procedure is performed when determination of the plasma–synovial fluid difference in glucose is requested.

The volume of synovial fluid in a joint varies with the size of the joint cavity and is normally small—about 0.1 to 3.5 mL.[1] Consequently, arthrocentesis of a joint when an effusion (or fluid buildup) is not present can result in a "dry tap"—a small yield of synovial fluid. Sometimes synovial fluid is present only in the aspiration needle; this requires that the contents of the needle be expressed into an appropriate small-volume container or, at times, directly into culture media. Alternatively, the clinician may insert the needle into a sterile cork and transport the entire syringe to the laboratory for processing. However, this practice represents a significant potential biohazard and should be avoided. Note that specimens should not be rejected because of a low volume of fluid. Diagnostic crystals, cell counts with differentials, and microbial growth are possible from a few drops of synovial fluid.

Synovial fluid handling and volume requirements are summarized in Table 14-3. It is recommended by the Clinical Laboratory Standards Institute (CLSI) that the first portion of fluid obtained (tube #1) be placed into a plain red-top tube (no anticoagulant) for chemical and immunologic evaluation. The next portion (tube #2) is collected in an anticoagulant tube for microscopic examinations, and the last portion (tube #3) is placed in a sterile anticoagulant tube for microbiological studies. Because the volume of synovial fluid present can vary significantly, the amount collected and distributed into each collection tube will also vary.

Note that using larger volumes of synovial fluid for cultures can enhance the recovery of microbial organisms; similarly, greater volumes of fluid will increase the numbers of cells recovered for cytologic evaluation. The best anticoagulant for synovial fluid is sodium heparin at approximately 25 units (U) per milliliter of synovial fluid or "liquid" ethylenediaminetetraacetic acid (EDTA). These anticoagulants prevent clotting if fibrinogen is present but do not form crystals. Oxalate and powdered EDTA must be avoided because they can produce crystalline structures that resemble monosodium urate crystals, thereby interfering with microscopic examination for in vivo crystals. For microbial studies, synovial fluid placed in a sterile tube with sodium polyanetholsulfonate

TABLE 14-3	Synovial Fluid Analysis and Specimen Requirements		
Collection Tube Order	**Test**	**Volume**	**Tube Type**
All tubes	**Physical examination**	≈1 mL	
	Color, clarity, viscosity		
#1	**Chemical examination**		
	Lactate, lipids (cholesterol, triglycerides), protein, uric acid	1 to 3 mL	No anticoagulant (red top)
	Glucose	1 to 3 mL	No anticoagulant (red top) or sodium fluoride (gray top)
#2	**Microscopic examination**		
	Total cell count	2 to 5 mL	Sodium heparin* or liquid EDTA
	Differential cell count		
	Crystal identification		
	Cytologic studies (e.g., malignant cells)	5 to 50 mL[†]	Sodium heparin*
#3	**Microbiological studies**		
	Culture	3 to 10 mL[‡]	Sterile tube; no anticoagulant (red top), sodium heparin,* or sodium polyanethole sulfonate (yellow top)

EDTA, Ethylenediaminetetraacetic acid.
*Sodium heparin concentration at 25 U/mL synovial fluid.
[†]No upper limit to the amount of fluid that can be submitted; large volumes of fluid increase the recovery of cellular elements.
[‡]Large fluid volumes may increase the recovery of viable microbial organisms.

(SPS) is also acceptable.[2] Because synovial fluid specimens are often sent to different laboratories for testing, the total volume of fluid removed should be recorded in the patient's chart and on specimen test request forms at the time of fluid collection.

Synovial fluid should be transported and analyzed at room temperature. As with other body fluids, it should be processed and tested as soon as possible after collection. If processing is delayed, several adverse changes can occur: (1) Cells in the synovial fluid can alter the chemical composition, (2) detection of microbial organisms can be jeopardized, and (3) blood cells (white blood cells [WBCs], red blood cells [RBCs]) can lyse. Note that refrigeration adversely affects the viability of microorganisms and could erroneously induce in vitro crystalline precipitation.

Following arthrocentesis, if the health care provider suspects that the fluid obtained is not synovial fluid, a *mucin clot test* or staining using toluidine blue (a metachromatic stain) can be done. The mucin clot test is based on the fact that normal synovial fluid contains no fibrinogen and normally does not clot. By diluting the fluid using dilute acetic acid (2%) in a ratio of one part fluid to four parts acid, hyaluronate will form a clot, which positively identifies the specimen as synovial fluid. The clot that forms typically is graded as good (compact clot, clear solution), fair, or poor (flocculent precipitate, cloudy solution). When toluidine blue is used, a few drops of the suspect fluid are placed onto filter paper followed by 0.2% toluidine blue stain. If synovial fluid is present, the drops of fluid will stain blue.[3] However, a drawback to using toluidine blue stain is that fluids anticoagulated with heparin cannot be evaluated because heparin itself causes strong metachromatic staining and a false-positive result.

PHYSICAL EXAMINATION

Color

The hematology laboratory often performs the physical and microscopic examinations of synovial fluid. The physical examination includes visual assessment for color, clarity, and viscosity. Normally, synovial fluid appears pale yellow or colorless and is clear. Color variations of red and brown are associated with trauma during the arthrocentesis and with disorders that disrupt the synovial membrane, allowing blood to enter the joint cavity, such as joint fracture, tumor, and traumatic arthritis. A traumatic procedure is indicated when the amount of blood in the fluid decreases as collection continues, or when a streak of blood is noticed in the fluid. With some joint disorders, particularly infections, synovial fluid can appear greenish or purulent; with other conditions (e.g., tuberculous arthritis, systemic lupus erythematosus), synovial fluid can appear milky.

Clarity

Numerous substances can modify the clarity of synovial fluid and include WBCs, RBCs, synoviocytes, crystals, fat droplets, fibrin, cellular debris, rice bodies, and ochronotic shards. The specific entity or entities causing the observed turbidity are usually identified by microscopic examination. Some substances are evident upon gross visual examination of synovial fluid. Rice bodies are white, free-floating particles made up of collagen covered by fibrinous tissue.[4] They resemble polished, shiny grains of rice and can vary greatly in size. Although they may be seen in many arthritic conditions, they are observed most commonly with rheumatoid arthritis.

Dark, pepper-like particles called ochronotic shards can be present in synovial fluid from individuals with ochronotic arthropathy, a consequence of alkaptonuria and ochronosis.[5] These pepper-like particles are pieces of pigmented cartilage that has eroded and broken loose into the fluid.

Viscosity

Synovial fluid has high viscosity compared with water because of its high concentration of the mucoprotein **hyaluronate**. This high-molecular-weight polymer of repeating disaccharide units is secreted by synoviocytes and serves as a joint lubricant. During inflammatory conditions, hyaluronate can be depolymerized by the action of the enzyme hyaluronidase, which is present in neutrophils, as well as by some bacteria (e.g., *Staphylococcus aureus*, *Streptococcus pyogenes*, *Clostridium perfringens*). In addition, some disease processes inhibit the production and secretion of hyaluronate by synoviocytes.

Synovial fluid viscosity can be assessed at the bedside by observing the fluid as it is expelled from the collection syringe. A drop of normal synovial fluid forms a string at least 4 cm long before breaking. The viscosity of the fluid is considered abnormally low when the string breaks earlier or forms discrete water-like droplets. Because more accurate viscosity measurements have little diagnostic or clinical value, they are not performed.

The mucin clot test previously described (see "Specimen Collection") is also an indirect measure of viscosity because it indicates the amount of hyaluronate polymerization in the fluid. This test is considered obsolete because similar information can be obtained through more precise procedures.

Clot Formation

Spontaneous clot formation in synovial fluid indicates the abnormal presence of fibrinogen. Because of its high molecular weight (340,000), fibrinogen cannot pass through a normal or healthy synovial membrane. Pathologic processes that damage the synovial membrane or a traumatic atherocentesis with blood contamination can cause fibrinogen to be present in synovial fluid, which will result in clot formation. Therefore, a portion of a synovial fluid collection should always be anticoagulated using sodium heparin or liquid EDTA to prevent potential fibrin clots that interfere with the microscopic examination.

MICROSCOPIC EXAMINATION

With a hemacytometer, a manual microscopic examination is performed using well-mixed, undiluted synovial fluid. See Chapter 18 for procedural details for performing manual cell counts When the fluid is significantly turbid, dilutions must be made using normal saline (0.85%) or another appropriate diluent (see Appendix C). Acetic acid cannot be used because it causes hyaluronate to form a mucin clot and cells to clump; these events interfere with the microscopic examination.

Because synovial fluid has a high viscosity, an extended period of time may be needed for cells to settle in the hemacytometer chamber before counting. To reduce the viscosity and enhance an even distribution of cells in the counting chamber, a hyaluronidase buffer solution (see Appendix C) can be used as the diluent.[6]

Total Cell Count

Normally, the number of RBCs in synovial fluid is fewer than 2000 RBCs/μL. Some RBCs originate from the procedure itself; those resulting from hemorrhagic effusions are usually obvious from their large numbers and the initial red-brown appearance of the fluid. When the number of RBCs present is excessive and they must be eliminated to allow performance of an accurate WBC and differential count, hypotonic saline (0.3%) is used as the diluent because it will selectively lyse the RBCs, while retaining the WBCs.

WBCs are normally present in synovial fluid at cell counts *lower than* 200 WBCs/μL. Although WBC counts greater than 2000 cells/μL are typically associated with bacterial arthritis, leukocytosis can occur with other conditions such as acute gouty arthritis and rheumatoid arthritis. Therefore, a total WBC cell count has limited value in identifying a specific disease process.

Differential Cell Count

Synovial fluid can be concentrated by several techniques; however, cytocentrifugation preserves cellular morphology better than routine centrifugation procedures.[7] Normally, about 60% of synovial fluid WBCs are monocytes or macrophages, approximately 30% are lymphocytes, and approximately 10% are neutrophils.[8] Differential counts have limited clinical value because they can differ not only with the disease process but also with the stage of the disease. A leukocyte differential with more than 80% neutrophils is associated with bacterial arthritis and urate gout, regardless of the total cell count. An increase in the lymphocyte percentage often occurs in the early stages of rheumatoid arthritis, whereas neutrophils predominate in later stages. An increased eosinophil count (greater than 2%) has been associated with a variety of disorders, including rheumatic fever, parasitic infestations, and metastatic carcinoma, and often follows procedures such as arthrography and radiation therapy.

Other cells that can be present in synovial fluid include lupus erythematosus cells; cells with hemosiderin inclusions from a hemorrhagic process; multinucleated cartilaginous cells in patients with osteoarthritis; malignant

TABLE 14-4	Synovial Fluid Crystal Identification, Microscopic Characteristics, and Associated Clinical Conditions	
Crystal	**Microscopic Characteristics***	**Clinical Conditions**
Monosodium urate monohydrate	Fine, needle-like, with pointed ends; strong negative birefringence	Urate arthritis (gouty arthritis)
Calcium pyrophosphate dihydrate	Rodlike or rhombic; weak positive birefringence	Pseudogout (i.e., chondrocalcinosis)
Cholesterol	Flat, platelike, with notched corners; negative birefringence; intensity varies with crystal thickness	Chronic arthritic conditions (e.g., rheumatoid arthritis)
Hydroxyapatite	Requires electron microscopy for visualization; not birefringent	Apatite-associated arthropathies
Corticosteroid	Varies with corticosteroid preparation used	Indicates previous intra-articular injection

*Characteristics of typical crystalline forms; however, other crystalline forms can also be present.

cells in patients with metastatic tumor; and normal synoviocytes from the synovial membrane.

Crystal Identification

One of the most important laboratory tests routinely performed on synovial fluid is microscopic examination for crystals. Identification of some crystals is pathognomonic of a specific joint disease, thereby enabling a rapid definitive diagnosis (Table 14-4). Because temperature and pH changes affect crystal formation and solubility, synovial fluid specimens should be maintained at room temperature and examined as soon as possible after collection. Time delays before microscopic examination can result in a decrease in WBCs (lysis) and in phagocytosis of crystals by WBCs during storage.

Microscope Slide Preparations. Synovial fluid can be viewed microscopically using a cytocentrifuged (or cytospin) slide preparation or a wet preparation. Several advantages are associated with the use of cytospin slides. First, cytocentrifugation concentrates the fluid components in a small area on a slide; this increases the sensitivity of the recovery and the detection of small numbers of crystals. Second, they are permanent slides that can be retained and used for review, training, and competency assessment. Last, cytospin slides can be viewed stained or unstained using polarizing microscopy because the appearance and birefringence of crystals are identical to those observed in wet preparations. The only disadvantage is the initial cost of the cytocentrifuge (see discussion of cytocentrifugation in Chapter 18).

When a "manual" wet preparation is made, a drop of synovial fluid is placed onto an alcohol-cleaned microscope slide, and a coverslip is applied. The specimen should just fill the area beneath the coverslip; too much specimen will cause the coverslip to float. The coverslip edges can be sealed with fingernail polish or melted paraffin to eliminate evaporation, thereby allowing time for an extensive microscopic examination.

Thorough examination of synovial fluid preparations by a skilled microscopist is imperative to ensure visualization and proper identification of synovial fluid crystals. Such examination is necessary because (1) the number of crystals present can vary significantly with disease (i.e., only a few small crystals may be present); (2) the differentiation of crystals is difficult because different types of crystals closely resemble each other; (3) free crystals can become enmeshed in fibrin or debris and can easily be overlooked; and (4) numerous artifacts are birefringent and must be appropriately identified. In addition, synovial fluid findings in infectious arthritis and crystal synovitis can be similar, which makes microscopic examination for crystals an important tool in differentiating these conditions.

Slide preparations are viewed microscopically using direct and compensated polarizing microscopy (see Chapter 1 for discussion of polarizing microscopy). Under polarizing microscopy, birefringent substances appear as bright objects against a black background, and the intensity of their birefringence varies with the substance. For example, monosodium urate and cholesterol crystals are bright and easy to visualize as compared with calcium pyrophosphate dihydrate crystals. Compensated polarizing microscopy (using a red compensator plate) enables the identification and differentiation of positively and negatively birefringent substances based on the different colors produced when the crystals are oriented parallel and perpendicular to the axis of the compensator (Figure 14-3, A).

Monosodium Urate Crystals. Monosodium urate (MSU) crystals in synovial fluid indicate gouty arthritis. Present intracellularly in leukocytes during acute stages of the disease, these needle-like crystals with pointed ends can distend the cytoplasm of WBCs. Free-floating crystals enmeshed in fibrin can also be present. Under polarizing microscopy, monosodium urate crystals are strongly birefringent, appearing bright against a black background. When a red compensator or full-wave plate is used, these negatively birefringent crystals appear yellow when their longitudinal axes are parallel to the axis of the red-compensator plate (Figure 14-3, B) and blue when their longitudinal axes are perpendicular to it (Figure 14-3, C). This characteristic enables the differentiation of MSU crystals from other similarly appearing crystals (e.g., EDTA crystals, betamethasone acetate crystals).

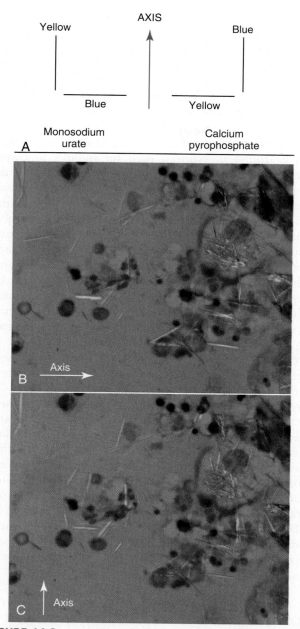

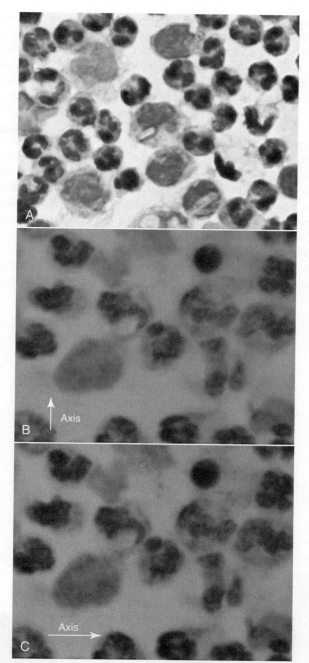

FIGURE 14-3 A, A diagrammatic representation of monosodium urate and calcium pyrophosphate crystals when viewed using polarizing microscopy with a red compensator. The axis indicated is that of the compensator. **B,** Monosodium urate crystals in joint fluid. The crystals with their longitudinal axis parallel to the red compensator plate axis as indicated in the lower left corner are yellow. **C,** With the axis of the red compensator plate perpendicular to the longitudinal axis, the same monosodium urate crystals are blue (polarizing microscopy).

FIGURE 14-4 A, Calcium pyrophosphate dihydrate crystal in joint fluid; brightfield microscopy. **B,** Calcium pyrophosphate dihydrate crystal appears yellow; its axis is perpendicular to the axis of the red compensator plate (polarizing microscopy). **C,** Calcium pyrophosphate dihydrate crystal appears blue; its axis is parallel to that of the red compensator plate (polarizing microscopy).

Calcium Pyrophosphate Dihydrate Crystals. A group of diseases is associated with calcium pyrophosphate dihydrate (CPPD) crystals in synovial fluid. These conditions, often referred to as *pseudogout* or *chondrocalcinosis,* are associated with the calcification of articular cartilages and include degenerative arthritis and arthritides accompanying metabolic diseases (e.g., hypothyroidism, hyperparathyroidism, diabetes mellitus). Several

characteristics enable the differentiation of CPPD crystals from MSU crystals. Calcium pyrophosphate dihydrate crystals are smaller and blunter, rodlike, or rhomboid (Figure 14-4, *A*). With compensated polarizing microscopy, CPPD crystals display weak positive birefringence with their color opposite to that observed for MSU crystals. CPPD crystals are blue when their longitudinal axes are parallel to the red compensator plate and yellow when their longitudinal axes are perpendicular (Figure 14-4, *B* and *C*).

Cholesterol Crystals. Note that cholesterol crystals are best identified using a wet prep or an "unstained" cytospin slide because Wright's staining can cause cholesterol crystals to dissolve. Cholesterol crystals usually appear as flat, rectangular plates with notched corners (Figure 14-5). However, rhomboid or needle-like forms that resemble MSU and CPPD crystals have also been observed in synovial fluid. Under polarizing microscopy, the birefringence of cholesterol crystals varies with the thickness of the crystal. Associated with chronic inflammatory conditions (e.g., rheumatoid arthritis), cholesterol crystals are considered nonspecific and frequently occur in chronic effusions found in other body cavities.

Hydroxyapatite Crystals. Hydroxyapatite crystals are present intracellularly in WBCs and require electron microscopy for visualization. They are tiny, needle-like crystals and are not birefringent. Hydroxyapatite crystals are associated with conditions characterized by calcific deposition and are collectively termed *apatite-associated arthropathies*. Apatite is the principal component of bone and is also present in cartilage. In crystalline form, hydroxyapatite crystals can induce an acute inflammatory reaction similar to that caused by monosodium urate and CPPD crystals.[9]

Corticosteroid Crystals. Because corticosteroid crystals can be found in synovial fluid for months following intra-articular injection, the laboratory must be informed of any injections when requested to do a synovial fluid microscopic examination. Depending on the drug preparation used, corticosteroid crystals can closely resemble monosodium urate or CPPD crystals but yield conflicting results based on their birefringence (Figure 14-6). In fact, laboratories can use betamethasone acetate (Celestone, Soluspan) as a microscopic control material because its crystals closely resemble MSU morphologically and exhibit similar negative birefringence. Corticosteroid crystals have no clinical significance other than indicating previous injection of the drug into the joint.

Artifacts. Numerous artifacts in synovial fluid show birefringence using polarizing microscopy, and differentiating artifacts from crystals is necessary (Figure 14-7). Birefringent artifacts include anticoagulant crystals, starch granules from examination gloves, cartilage and prosthesis fragments, collagen fibers, fibrin, and dust particles. An experienced microscopist is able to differentiate artifacts based on their irregular or indistinct morphologic appearance compared with crystals. Note that anticoagulant-associated crystals (e.g., calcium oxalate, powdered EDTA) can also be phagocytosed by WBCs after collection and storage. Therefore only sodium heparin or liquid EDTA, which do not form crystals, should be used as an anticoagulant for synovial fluid specimens.

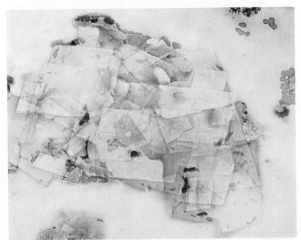

FIGURE 14-5 Cholesterol crystals in joint fluid; brightfield microscopy.

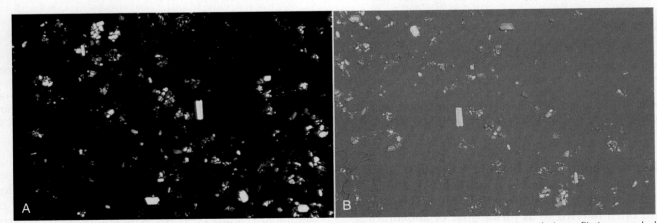

FIGURE 14-6 Synovial fluid with corticosteroid drug (triamcinolone diacetate [Aristocort]) crystals present. Note their conflicting morphology (suggests calcium pyrophosphate dihydrate [CPPD]) and strong negative birefringence (suggests monosodium urate [MSU]). Wet preparation, unstained; polarizing microscopy, 400×. **A,** Many strongly birefringent drug crystals that morphologically resemble CPPD using polarizing microscopy. **B,** Drug crystals with their long axes parallel to that of the red compensator plate are yellow—suggesting MSU crystals. *(From Ringsrud KM, Linne JJ: Urinalysis and body fluids: a color text and atlas, St Louis, 1995, Mosby.)*

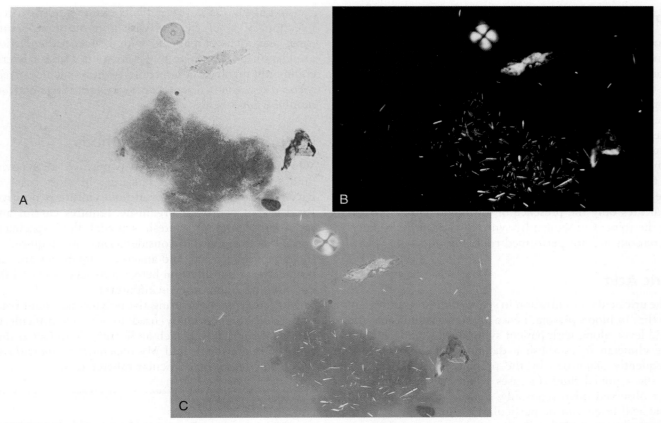

FIGURE 14-7 Synovial fluid with mass of hyaluronate, small monosodium urate (MSU) crystals, starch granule, and fibers. Cytocentrifuged preparation, Wright's stain, 400×. **A,** Brightfield microscopy; starch granule and fiber. Note that no crystals are evident in the pink mass. **B,** Polarizing microscopy; presence of MSU crystals is evident, fibers have strong birefringence, and the starch granule shows a typical Maltese cross-pattern. **C,** Compensated polarizing microscopy; crystals with their long axis perpendicular to the red compensator plate are blue, which indicates that the crystals are MSU. *(From Ringsrud KM, Linne JJ: Urinalysis and body fluids: a color text and atlas, St Louis, 1995, Mosby.)*

CHEMICAL EXAMINATION

Although numerous chemical constituents in synovial fluid can be analyzed, few analytes provide diagnostically useful information. Regardless of joint disease, some analytes such as uric acid maintain the same concentration in synovial fluid as in blood plasma, and they are often monitored using blood plasma measurements. In contrast, joint diseases can cause other analytes (e.g., glucose) to differ in synovial fluid concentration as compared with blood plasma. In these conditions, determination of the plasma–synovial fluid difference can aid in identification and differentiation of the joint disease. Currently, lipid (cholesterol, triglycerides) and enzyme analysis of synovial fluid has limited clinical value in rare cases of joint disorders. Therefore these chemical tests are rarely performed on synovial fluid.

Glucose

To evaluate synovial fluid glucose concentrations, a blood sample must be drawn at the same time that the arthrocentesis is performed. In a normal *fasting* patient, the glucose concentrations in the blood and in synovial fluid are equivalent. In other words, the plasma–synovial fluid glucose difference is less than 10 mg/dL (0.55 mmol/L). Because of the time required in vivo for this dynamic equilibrium to occur, the plasma–synovial fluid glucose difference observed in a *nonfasting* patient can be greater than 10 mg/dL (greater than 0.55 mmol/L).

With various joint diseases, the concentration of glucose in synovial fluid is decreased, which causes an increased plasma–synovial fluid glucose difference. Typically, in noninflammatory and hemorrhagic joint disorders, the plasma–synovial fluid difference is less than 20 mg/dL (less than 1.11 mmol/L). When the difference is greater than 20 mg/dL (greater than 1.11 mmol/L), this is suggestive of septic or inflammatory arthritis. In a nonfasting patient, the synovial fluid glucose is considered significantly low if the glucose concentration of the synovial fluid is less than half that of the plasma glucose value.

Synovial fluid specimens for glucose quantitation should be assayed within 1 hour of collection,[2] or, when quantitation will be delayed, a portion of the specimen should be placed into a sodium fluoride anticoagulant tube (gray top). These precautions will eliminate falsely low glucose values due to the glycolytic activity of WBCs that may be present in the fluid.

Total Protein

Normally, the total protein concentration of synovial fluid is approximately one-third the protein concentration of blood plasma. An increased amount of protein in the synovial fluid results from changes in the permeability of the synovial membrane or from increased synthesis within the joint. A variety of joint diseases (e.g., rheumatoid arthritis, crystal synovitis, septic arthritis) routinely have increased protein levels. However, determination of synovial fluid protein content does not assist in the differential diagnosis of joint disease or in its treatment. Rather, increased total protein in synovial fluid indicates only the presence of an inflammatory process in the joint. Consequently, synovial fluid protein determinations are not performed routinely.

Uric Acid

The uric acid concentration in synovial fluid is equivalent to that in blood plasma, hence an increased plasma uric acid level, along with patient symptoms, usually enables the clinician to establish a diagnosis of gout. Gout is frequently diagnosed by the presence of MSU crystals in the synovial fluid. In cases where MSU crystals are not observed microscopically, plasma or synovial fluid uric acid levels can be particularly valuable. It is worth noting that many individuals with gout may not have an increased plasma uric acid level.

Lactate

Increased synovial fluid lactate concentrations are believed to result from anaerobic glycolysis in the synovium. With severe inflammatory conditions comes an increased demand for energy, and tissue hypoxia can occur. Although the lactate level in synovial fluid can be determined easily, its clinical use remains uncertain. Some conditions of the joint, particularly septic arthritis, have been associated with significantly increased synovial fluid lactate levels. In contrast, gonococcal arthritis presents with normal or low lactate levels. Despite numerous studies, the clinical value of routine lactate quantitation in synovial fluid has yet to be established.

MICROBIOLOGICAL EXAMINATION

Gram Stain

To aid in the differential diagnosis of joint disease, the routine examination of synovial fluid includes a Gram stain and a culture. Gram stains, when positive, provide immediately useful clinical and diagnostic information. Most infectious agents in synovial fluid are bacterial and originate from the blood; other agents in the fluid include fungi, viruses, and mycobacteria. The sensitivity of the Gram stain depends on the organism involved;

approximately 75% of patients with staphylococcal infection, 50% of patients with gram-negative organisms, and 40% of patients with gonococcal infection are identified as positive by Gram stain. Other bacteria commonly involved in infectious arthritis include *Streptococcus pyogenes*, *Streptococcus pneumoniae*, and *Haemophilus influenzae*.

Culture and Molecular Methods

Whether or not the Gram stain is positive, all synovial fluid specimens should be cultured. In most cases of bacterial arthritis, the synovial fluid culture is positive. Recovery of microbial organisms requires careful and rapid processing of a fresh synovial fluid specimen. Special culture media considerations are required if fungal, mycobacterial, and anaerobic organisms are suspected, hence consultation between the clinician and the microbiology laboratory is important.

Molecular methods using the polymerase chain reaction (PCR) are currently used to identify difficult to detect microorganism, such as *Borrelia burgdorferi* that causes Lyme arthritis and *Mycobacterium tuberculosis*, which can cause osteoarticular tuberculosis.

STUDY QUESTIONS

1. Which of the following tasks is a function of synovial fluid?
   1. Providing lubrication for a joint
   2. Assisting in the structural support of a joint
   3. Transporting nutrients to articular cartilage
   4. Synthesizing hyaluronate and degradative enzymes
   A. 1, 2, and 3 are correct.
   B. 1 and 3 are correct.
   C. 4 is correct.
   D. All are correct.

2. Which of the following statements is a characteristic of normal synovial fluid?
   A. Synovial fluid is viscous.
   B. Synovial fluid is slightly turbid.
   C. Synovial fluid is dark yellow.
   D. Synovial fluid forms small clots on standing.

3. Which of the following components is not normally present in synovial fluid?
   A. Fibrinogen
   B. Neutrophils
   C. Protein
   D. Uric acid

4. Which of the following substances will not increase the turbidity of synovial fluid?
   A. Fat
   B. Crystals
   C. Hyaluronate
   D. WBCs

5. Abnormally decreased viscosity in synovial fluid results from
   A. mucin degradation by leukocytic lysosomes.
   B. overproduction of synovial fluid by synoviocytes.
   C. autoimmune response of synoviocytes in joint disease.
   D. depolymerization of hyaluronate by neutrophilic enzymes.

6. A synovial fluid specimen is received in the laboratory 2 hours after collection. Which of the following changes to the fluid will most likely have taken place?
   A. The specimen will have clotted.
   B. The uric acid concentration will have decreased.
   C. Crystals may have precipitated or dissolved.
   D. The lactate concentration will have decreased because of anaerobic glycolysis.

7. Which of the following anticoagulants does not have the potential to precipitate out in crystalline form when used for synovial fluid specimens?
   A. Sodium citrate
   B. Sodium heparin
   C. Lithium heparin
   D. Potassium oxalate

8. A synovial fluid specimen has a high cell count and requires dilution to be counted. Which of the following diluents should be used?
   A. Normal saline
   B. Dilute acetic acid (2%)
   C. Dilute methanol (1%)
   D. Phosphate buffer solution (0.050 mol/L)

9. Which of the following results from synovial fluid analysis indicates a joint disease process?
   A. A few synoviocytes present in the fluid
   B. A WBC count lower than 200 cells/mL
   C. An RBC count lower than 2000 cells/mL
   D. A differential count showing greater than 25% neutrophils

10. Differentiation of synovial fluid crystals, based on their birefringence, is achieved using
    A. transmission electron microscopy.
    B. phase-contrast microscopy.
    C. direct polarizing microscopy.
    D. compensated polarizing microscopy.

11. The microscopic examination of synovial fluid for crystals can be difficult because
    1. numerous artifacts are also birefringent.
    2. few crystals may be present.
    3. free-floating crystals can become enmeshed or hidden in fibrin.
    4. different crystals can closely resemble each other morphologically.
    A. 1, 2, and 3 are correct.
    B. 1 and 3 are correct.
    C. 4 is correct.
    D. All are correct.

12. Which of the following crystals characteristically occurs in patients with gout?
    A. Cholesterol crystals
    B. Hydroxyapatite crystals
    C. Monosodium urate crystals
    D. Calcium pyrophosphate dihydrate crystals

13. In synovial fluid, which of the following crystals is not birefringent?
    A. Cholesterol crystals
    B. Hydroxyapatite crystals
    C. Monosodium urate crystals
    D. Calcium pyrophosphate dihydrate crystals

14. Assuming that a patient is fasting, which of the following analytes is normally present in the synovial fluid in essentially the same concentration as in the blood plasma?
    1. Glucose
    2. Lactate
    3. Uric acid
    4. Protein
    A. 1, 2, and 3 are correct.
    B. 1 and 3 are correct.
    C. 4 is correct.
    D. All are correct.

15. Which of the following findings provides a definitive diagnosis of a specific joint condition?
    A. Staphylococcal bacteria identified by Gram stain
    B. Corticosteroid crystals identified during the microscopic examination
    C. A plasma–synovial fluid glucose difference exceeding 20 mg/dL
    D. Greater than 25 WBCs/µL observed during the microscopic examination

16. Analysis of a synovial fluid specimen reveals the following:
    - Cloudy, yellow-green fluid of low viscosity
    - Total leukocyte count of 98,000 cells/µL
    - Plasma–synovial fluid glucose difference of 47 mg/dL

    Based on the information provided and Table 14-2, this specimen most likely would be classified as
    A. noninflammatory.
    B. inflammatory.
    C. septic.
    D. hemorrhagic.

17. An analysis of a synovial fluid specimen reveals the following:
    - Yellow fluid of high viscosity
    - Total leukocyte count of 300 cells/µL
    - Plasma–synovial fluid glucose difference of 17 mg/dL

    Based on the information provided and Table 14-2, this specimen would most likely be classified as
    A. noninflammatory.
    B. inflammatory.
    C. septic.
    D. hemorrhagic.

CASE 14-1

A 51-year-old man has painful swelling in both knees. He is hospitalized, and an arthrocentesis is scheduled for the following morning. In the morning, a fasting blood sample is drawn for routine chemistry tests. Synovial fluid is aspirated from the right knee and submitted to the laboratory.

Blood Chemistry Results

	Reference Interval
Glucose, fasting: 85 mg/dL	≤110 mg/dL
Uric acid: 12.7 mg/dL	2.6-8.0 mg/dL

Synovial Fluid Results

Physical Examination
- Color: yellow
- Clarity: cloudy
- Viscosity: decreased

Microscopic Examination
- WBC count: 43,000 cells/µL
- Differential count:
  - Monocytes: 24%
  - Lymphocytes: 13%
  - Neutrophils: 63%
  - Crystals: many intracellular needle-shaped crystals; negative birefringence
- Gram stain: no organisms seen; many leukocytes present

Chemical Examination
- Glucose: 55 mg/dL
- Uric acid: 12.4 mg/dL
- Total protein: 4.0 g/dL
- Lactate: 19 mg/dL

1. List any abnormal results.
2. Calculate the plasma–synovial fluid glucose difference.
3. Based on the results obtained, this synovial fluid specimen should be classified as
   A. normal.
   B. noninflammatory (group I).
   C. inflammatory (group II).
   D. septic (group III).
   E. hemorrhagic (group IV).
4. What is the most likely identity of the crystals observed in the synovial fluid?
   A. Cholesterol
   B. Corticosteroid
   C. Hydroxyapatite
   D. Calcium pyrophosphate dihydrate
   E. Monosodium urate
5. These results are most consistent with a diagnosis of
   A. gouty arthritis.
   B. pseudogout.
   C. rheumatoid arthritis.
   D. bacterial infection.
   E. traumatic arthritis, with previous corticosteroid injection.
6. If no crystals were observed in the microscopic examination, would you change the diagnosis? Why or why not?

CASE 14-2

A 37-year-old woman has persistent and painful swelling in her left knee several days following arthroscopic repair of a torn ligament (i.e., medial meniscus). A fasting blood sample is drawn for routine chemistry tests. Arthrocentesis is performed, and the synovial fluid is submitted to the laboratory.

Blood Chemistry Results

	Reference Interval
Glucose, fasting: 79 mg/dL	≤110 mg/dL
Uric acid: 6.2 mg/dL	2.6-8.0 mg/dL

Synovial Fluid Results

Physical Examination
- Color: yellow
- Clarity: cloudy
- Viscosity: decreased

Microscopic Examination
- WBC count: 97,000 cells/µL
- Differential count:
  - Monocytes: 13%
  - Lymphocytes: 5%
  - Neutrophils: 82%
  - Crystals: none present
- Gram stain: gram-positive cocci present; many leukocytes present

Chemical Examination
- Glucose: 35 mg/dL
- Uric acid: 5.9 mg/dL
- Total protein: 5.3 g/dL
- Lactate: 35 mg/dL

1. List any abnormal results.
2. Calculate the plasma–synovial fluid glucose difference.
3. Based on the results obtained, this synovial fluid specimen should be classified as
   A. normal.
   B. noninflammatory (group I).
   C. inflammatory (group II).
   D. septic (group III).
   E. hemorrhagic (group IV).
4. These results are most consistent with a diagnosis of
   A. gouty arthritis.
   B. pseudogout.
   C. rheumatoid arthritis.
   D. bacterial infection.
   E. traumatic arthritis, with previous corticosteroid injection.

CASE 14-3

A 25-year-old professional football player is in an automobile accident. His recovery is complete except for persistent swelling in his left knee. This same knee had been a chronic problem before the accident, and he had received a corticosteroid intra-articular injection 6 months earlier. An arthrocentesis is scheduled, along with the collection of a fasting blood sample for routine chemistry tests. The blood and synovial fluid are submitted to the laboratory.

Blood Chemistry Results

	Reference Interval
Glucose, fasting: 95 mg/dL	≤110 mg/dL
Uric acid: 5.7 mg/dL	2.6-8.0 mg/dL

Synovial Fluid Results

Physical Examination	Microscopic Examination	Chemical Examination
Color: yellow	WBC count: 950 cells/µL	Glucose: 80 mg/dL
Clarity: slightly cloudy	Differential count:	Uric acid: 5.7 mg/dL
Viscosity: normal	Monocytes: 65%	Total protein: 5.5 g/dL
	Lymphocytes: 17%	Lactate: 21 mg/dL
	Neutrophils: 18%	
	Crystals: few needle-shaped crystals; negative birefringence	
	Gram stain: no organisms seen; few leukocytes present	

1. List any abnormal results.
2. Calculate the plasma–synovial fluid glucose difference.
3. Based on the results obtained, this synovial fluid specimen should be classified as
   A. normal.
   B. noninflammatory (group I).
   C. inflammatory (group II).
   D. septic (group III).
   E. hemorrhagic (group IV).
4. Based on the results obtained, what is the most likely identity of the crystals observed in the synovial fluid?
   A. Cholesterol
   B. Corticosteroid
   C. Hydroxyapatite
   D. Calcium pyrophosphate dihydrate
   E. Monosodium urate
5. These results are most consistent with a diagnosis of
   A. gouty arthritis.
   B. pseudogout.
   C. rheumatoid arthritis.
   D. bacterial infection.
   E. traumatic arthritis, with previous corticosteroid injection.

REFERENCES

1. Ropes MW, Rossmeisl EC, Bauer W: The origin and nature of normal human synovial fluid. J Clin Invest 19:795-799, 1940.
2. Clinical and Laboratory Standards Institute (CLSI): Analysis of body fluids in clinical chemistry: approved guideline, CLSI Document C49-A, Wayne, PA, 2007, CLSI.
3. Goldenberg DL, Brandt KD, Cohen AD: Rapid, simple detection of trace amounts of synovial fluid. Arthritis Rheum 16:487-490, 1973.
4. Asik M, Eralp L, Cetik O, Altinel L: Rice bodies of synovial origin in the knee joint. Arthroscopy 17:1-4, 2001.
5. Mannoni A, Selvi E, Lorenzini S, Giorgi M, Airo P, Cammelli D, Andreotti L, Marcolongo R, Porfirio B: Alkaptonuria, ochronosis, and ochronotic arthropathy. Semin Arthritis Rheum 33:239, 2004.
6. Kjeldsberg CR, Knight JA: Synovial fluid. In Body fluids, ed 3, Chicago, 1993, American Society of Clinical Pathologists Press.
7. Villanueva TG, Schumacher HR, Jr: Cytologic examination of synovial fluid. Diagn Cytopathol 3:141-147, 1987.
8. Cohen AS, Goldenberg D: Synovial fluid. In Laboratory diagnostic procedures in the rheumatic diseases, ed 3, New York, 1985, Grune & Stratton.
9. Glasser L: Reading the signs in synovia. Diagn Med 3:35-50, 1980.
10. Carter JD, Hudson AP: Reactive arthritis: clinical aspects and medical management. Rheum Dis Clin N Am 35:21-44, 2009.
11. Clinical and Laboratory Standards Institute (CLSI): Body fluid analysis for cellular composition: approved guideline, CLSI Document H56-A, Wayne, PA, 2006, CLSI.

BIBLIOGRAPHY

Eisenberg JM, Schumacher HR, Davidson PK, Kaufmann L: Usefulness of synovial fluid analysis in the evaluation of joint effusions. Arch Intern Med 144:715-719, 1984.
Gatter RA: A practical handbook of joint fluid analysis, Philadelphia, 1991, Lea & Febiger.
Glasser L: Extravascular biological fluids. In Kaplan LA, Pesce AJ, Kazmierczak SC, editors: Clinical chemistry: theory, analysis, correlation, ed 4, St Louis, 2003, Mosby.
Pal B, Nash J, Oppenheim B, et al: Is routine synovial fluid analysis necessary? Lessons and recommendations from an audit. Rheumatol Int 18:181-182, 1999.
Shmerling RH: Synovial fluid analysis: a critical reappraisal. Rheum Dis Clin North Am 20:503-512, 1994.
Shmerling RH, Delbanco TL, Tosteson ANA, et al: Synovial fluid tests: what should be ordered? JAMA 264:1009-1014, 1990.
Smith GP, Kjeldsberg CR: Cerebrospinal, synovial, and serous body fluids. In Henry JB, editor: Clinical diagnosis and management of laboratory methods, ed 20, Philadelphia, 2001, WB Saunders.

Pleural, Pericardial, and Peritoneal Fluid Analysis

LEARNING OBJECTIVES

After studying this chapter, the student should be able to:

1. Describe the function of serous membranes as it relates to the formation and absorption of serous fluid.
2. Describe four pathologic changes that lead to the formation of an effusion.
3. Discuss appropriate collection requirements for serous fluid specimens.
4. Classify a serous fluid effusion as a transudate or an exudate based on the examination of its physical, microscopic, and chemical characteristics.
5. Compare and contrast chylous and pseudochylous effusions.
6. Correlate the microscopic examination and differential cell count of serous fluid analyses with diseases that affect the serous membranes.
7. Correlate the concentrations of selected chemical constituents of serous fluids with various disease states.
8. Discuss the microbiological examination of serous fluids and its importance in the diagnosis of infectious diseases.

CHAPTER OUTLINE

Physiology and Composition
Specimen Collection
Transudates and Exudates
Physical Examination
Microscopic Examination
   Total Cell Counts
   Differential Cell Count

   Cytologic Examination
Chemical Examination
   Total Protein and Lactate
     Dehydrogenase Ratios
   Glucose
   Amylase

   Lipids (Triglycerides and
     Cholesterol)
   pH
   Carcinoembryonic Antigen
Microbiological Examination
   Staining Techniques
   Culture

KEY TERMS

ascites the excessive accumulation of serous fluid in the peritoneal cavity.

chyle a milky-appearing emulsion of lymph and chylomicrons (triglycerides) that originates from intestinal lymphatic absorption during digestion.

chylous effusion a milky-appearing effusion that persists after centrifugation; its chemical composition includes chylomicrons and an elevated triglyceride level (i.e., greater than 110 mg/dL).

effusion an accumulation of fluid in a body cavity as a result of a pathologic process.

exudate an effusion in a body cavity caused by increased capillary permeability or decreased lymphatic absorption. An exudate is identified by a fluid-to-serum total protein ratio greater than 0.5, a fluid-to-serum lactate dehydrogenase ratio greater than 0.6, or both.

mesothelial cells flat cells that form a single layer of epithelium that covers the surface of serous membranes (i.e., the pleura, pericardium, and peritoneum).

paracentesis a percutaneous puncture procedure used to remove fluid from a body cavity such as from the pleural, pericardial, or peritoneal cavity.

pseudochylous effusion an effusion that appears milky but does not contain chylomicrons and has a low (less than 50 mg/dL) triglyceride content.

serous fluid a fluid that has a composition similar to that of serum.

transudate an effusion in a body cavity caused by increased hydrostatic pressure (i.e., blood pressure) or decreased plasma oncotic pressure. A transudate is identified by a fluid-to-serum total protein ratio of less than 0.5 and a fluid-to-serum lactate dehydrogenase ratio of less than 0.6.

PHYSIOLOGY AND COMPOSITION

The lungs, heart, and abdominal organs are surrounded by a thin, continuous, serous membrane, as well as by the internal surfaces of the body cavity wall. A space or cavity filled with fluid lies between the membrane that covers the organ (visceral membrane) and the membrane that lines the body wall (parietal membrane) (Figure 15-1). Each cavity is separate and is named for the organ or organs it encloses. The lungs are individually surrounded by a pleural cavity, the heart by the pericardial cavity, and the abdominal organs by the peritoneal cavity. The serous membranes that line these cavities consist of a thin layer of connective tissue covered by a single layer of flat **mesothelial cells.** Within the membrane is an intricate network of capillary and lymphatic vessels. Each membrane is attached firmly to the body wall and the organ it surrounds; however, the opposing surfaces of the membrane—despite close contact—are not attached to each other. Instead, the space between the opposing surfaces (i.e., between the visceral and parietal membranes) is filled with a small amount of fluid that serves as a lubricant between the membranes, which permits free movement of the enclosed organ. The cavity fluid is created and is maintained through plasma ultrafiltration in the parietal membrane and absorption by the visceral membrane. The name serous fluid is a general term used to describe fluids that are an ultrafiltrate of plasma with a composition similar to that of serum.

The process of fluid formation and absorption in the pleural, pericardial, and peritoneal cavities is dynamic. Fluid formation is controlled simultaneously by four factors: (1) permeability of the capillaries in the parietal membrane, (2) hydrostatic pressure in these capillaries, (3) oncotic pressure (or colloid osmotic pressure) produced by the presence of plasma proteins within the capillaries, and (4) absorption of fluid by the lymphatic system (Box 15-1). Hydrostatic pressure (i.e., blood pressure) forces a plasma ultrafiltrate to form in the cavity; at the same time, plasma proteins in the capillaries produce a force (oncotic pressure) that opposes this filtration.

The permeability of the capillary endothelium regulates the rate of ultrafiltrate formation and its protein composition. For example, increased permeability of the endothelium will cause increased movement of protein from the blood into the cavity fluid. When this occurs, the now protein-rich fluid in the cavity further enhances the movement of more fluid into the cavity. Such an accumulation of fluid in a body cavity is termed an **effusion** and indicates an abnormal or pathologic process. The lymphatic system, or the fourth component in cavity

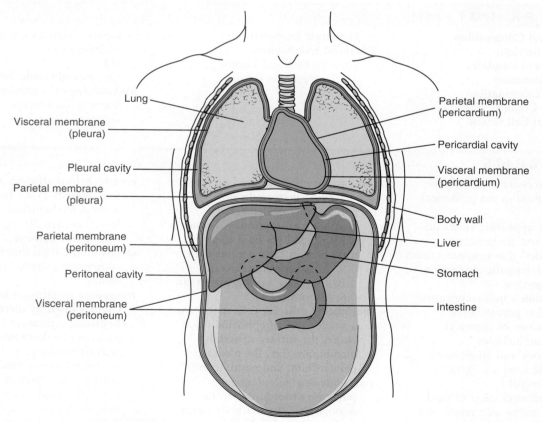

FIGURE 15-1 Parietal and visceral membranes of the pleural, pericardial, and peritoneal cavities. Parietal membranes line the body wall, whereas visceral membranes enclose organs. The two membranes are actually one continuous membrane. The space between opposing surfaces is identified as the body cavity (i.e., pleural cavity, pericardial cavity, peritoneal cavity).

fluid formation, plays a primary role in removing fluid from a cavity by absorption. However, if the lymphatic vessels become obstructed or impaired, they cannot adequately remove the additional fluid, resulting in an effusion. Other mechanisms can cause effusions, and they may occur with a variety of primary and secondary diseases, including conditions that cause a decrease in hydrostatic blood pressure (e.g., congestive heart failure, shock) and those characterized by a decrease in oncotic pressure (i.e., disorders characterized by hypoproteinemia).

A pleural, pericardial, or peritoneal effusion is diagnosed by a physical examination of the patient or on the basis of radiographic, ultrasound, or echocardiographic imaging studies. The collection and clinical testing of pleural, pericardial, and peritoneal fluids play an important role in determining the type of effusion present and in identifying its cause.

SPECIMEN COLLECTION

The term **paracentesis** refers to the percutaneous puncture of a body cavity for the aspiration of fluid. Other anatomically descriptive terms denote fluid collection from specific body cavities. *Thoracentesis*, for example, refers to the surgical puncture of the chest wall into the pleural cavity to collect pleural fluid, *pericardiocentesis* into the pericardial cavity, and *peritoneocentesis* (or abdominal paracentesis) into the peritoneal cavity. The term **ascites** refers to an effusion specifically in the peritoneal cavity, and *ascitic fluid* is simply another name for peritoneal fluid.

Collection of effusions from a body cavity is an invasive surgical procedure performed by a physician using sterile technique. Unlike cerebrospinal fluid and synovial fluid collections, serous fluid collections from effusions in the pleural, pericardial, and peritoneal cavities often yield large volumes of fluid. Consequently, the amount of fluid obtained often exceeds that needed for diagnostic testing. Note that at times, additional or repeat puncture procedures are necessary to remove a recurring effusion from a cavity for therapeutic purposes, such as when the effusion is compressing or inhibiting the movement of vital organs.

Before serous fluid is collected from a body cavity, the laboratory should be consulted to ensure that appropriate collection containers are used and suitable volumes are obtained (Table 15-1). In microbiological studies, the percentage of positive cultures obtained increases when a larger volume of specimen (10 to 20 mL) is used, or when a concentrated sediment from a centrifuged specimen (50 mL or more) is used to inoculate cultures.

Normally, serous fluids do not contain blood or fibrinogen, but a traumatic puncture procedure, a

BOX 15-1	Forces Involved in Normal Pleural Fluid Formation and Absorption
Forces Favoring Fluid Formation	
Hydrostatic pressure (in systemic capillary)	+30 mm Hg
Oncotic pressure (in systemic capillary)	−26 mm Hg
Intrapleural pressure	+5 mm Hg
Net pressure favoring fluid formation in pleural cavity	+9 mm Hg
Forces Favoring Fluid Absorption	
Hydrostatic pressure (in pulmonary capillary)	−11 mm Hg
Oncotic pressure (in pulmonary capillary)	+26 mm Hg
Intrapleural pressure	−5 mm Hg
Net pressure favoring fluid absorption out of pleural cavity	+10 mm Hg

TABLE 15-1	Suggested Serous Fluid Specimen Requirements	
Physical Examination	**Volume**	**Acceptable Containers**
Color and clarity		Recorded at bedside by physician and noted on test request form
Microscopic Examination		
Cell counts, differential	5-8 mL	EDTA
Cytology study (PAP stain, cell block)	50 mL recommended; 15-100 mL*	Plain tube/container, sodium heparin, EDTA
Chemical Examination		
Glucose	3-5 mL	Plain tube, sodium fluoride
Protein, lactate dehydrogenase, amylase, triglyceride, cholesterol, others	5-10 mL	Plain tube, sodium heparin
pH (pleural fluid)	1-3 mL	Heparinized syringe; anaerobically maintained
Microbiological Studies		
Gram stain, bacterial culture	10-20 mL[†]	Sterile container; SPS, none, sodium heparin
Acid-fast stain and culture	15-50 mL[†]	Sterile container; SPS, none, sodium heparin

*No upper limit to the amount of fluid that can be submitted; large volumes of fluid enhance the recovery of cellular elements.
[†]Large fluid volumes may facilitate the recovery of viable microbial organisms.
EDTA, Ethylenediaminetetraacetic acid; *PAP*, Papanicolaou; *SPS*, sodium polyanetholsulfonate.

hemorrhagic effusion, or an active bleed (e.g., from a ruptured blood vessel) can result in serous fluid that appears bloody and clots spontaneously. Therefore to prevent clot formation, which entraps cells and microorganisms, sterile tubes coated with an anticoagulant such as sodium heparin or liquid ethylenediaminetetraacetic acid (EDTA) are used to collect fluid specimens for the microscopic examination and microbiological studies. In contrast, serous fluid for chemical testing is placed into a nonanticoagulant tube (red top), which will allow clot formation when fibrinogen or blood is present. Serous fluids should be maintained at room temperature and transported to the laboratory as soon as possible after collection to eliminate potential chemical changes, cellular degradation, and bacterial proliferation. Note that refrigeration (4° C to 8° C) adversely affects the viability of microorganisms and should not be used for serous fluid specimens. However, serous fluid samples intended for cytology examination are an exception and can be refrigerated at 4° C when storage is necessary.

A blood sample must be collected shortly before or after the paracentesis procedure to enable comparison studies of the chemical composition of the effusion with that of the patient's plasma. These studies enable classification of the effusion (transudate or exudate, chylous or pseudochylous), which assists in diagnosis and treatment. Note that for chemical analysis, the same type of specimen collection tube (nonanticoagulant, sodium heparin) should be used for both the fluid specimen and the blood collection (serum or plasma). In addition, specimen transport and handling conditions should be the same to eliminate result variations due to these potential differences.

TRANSUDATES AND EXUDATES

An effusion, particularly in the pleural or peritoneal cavity, is classified as a **transudate** or an **exudate**. This classification is based on several criteria, including appearance, leukocyte count, and total protein, lactate dehydrogenase, glucose, and bilirubin concentrations; however, because of the overlap between categories, no single parameter differentiates a transudate from an exudate in all patients.[1] Table 15-2 lists parameters and the values associated with transudates and exudates.

Classifying an effusion as a transudate or exudate is important because this information assists the physician in identifying its cause. Transudates primarily result from a systemic disease that causes an increase in hydrostatic pressure or a decrease in plasma oncotic pressure in the parietal membrane capillaries. These changes are noninflammatory and frequently are associated with congestive heart failure, hepatic cirrhosis, and nephrotic syndrome (i.e., hypoproteinemia). Once an effusion has been identified as a transudate, further laboratory testing usually is not necessary.

In contrast, exudates result from inflammatory processes that increase the permeability of the capillary endothelium in the parietal membrane or decrease the absorption of fluid by the lymphatic system. Numerous disease processes such as infections, neoplasms, systemic

TABLE 15-2	Differentiation of Transudates and Exudates	
Parameter	**Transudates**	**Exudates**
Causes	Increased hydrostatic pressure Decreased oncotic pressure	Increased capillary permeability Decreased lymphatic absorption
Physical Examination		
Clarity	Clear	Cloudy
Color	Pale yellow	Variable (yellow, greenish, pink, red)
Clots spontaneously	No	Variable; often yes
Microscopic Examination		
WBC count	<1000 cells/µL (pleural) <300 cells/µL (peritoneal)	Variable, usually >1000 cells/µL (pleural) >500 cells/µL (peritoneal)
Differential count	Mononuclear cells predominate	Early, neutrophils predominate; late, mononuclear cells
Chemical Examination		
Bilirubin ratio (fluid-to-serum)	≤0.6	>0.6
Glucose	Equal to serum level	Less than or equal to serum level
TP concentration	<50% of serum	>50% of serum
TP ratio (fluid-to-serum)	≤0.5	>0.5
LD activity	<60% of serum	>60% of serum
LD ratio (fluid-to-serum)	≤0.6	>0.6
Cholesterol ratio (fluid-to-serum)	≤0.3	>0.3

LD, Lactate dehydrogenase; *TP*, total protein; *WBC*, white blood cell.

disorders, trauma, and inflammatory conditions may cause exudates. Additional laboratory testing is required with exudates, such as microbiological studies to identify pathologic organisms or cytologic studies to evaluate suspected malignant neoplasms.

Table 15-3 summarizes various causes of pleural, pericardial, and peritoneal effusions. Unlike pleural and peritoneal effusions, pericardial effusions usually are not classified as a transudate or an exudate. Most often, pericardial effusions result from pathologic changes of the parietal membrane (e.g., because of infection or damage) that cause an increase in capillary permeability. Hence the majority of pericardial effusions could be considered exudates.

PHYSICAL EXAMINATION

Reference values for the characteristics of normal serous fluid in the pleural, pericardial, and peritoneal cavities are not available because in healthy individuals, the fluid volume in these cavities is small and the fluid is not normally collected. Only effusions are routinely collected and categorized as a transudate or an exudate (see Table 15-2). Transudates are usually clear fluids, pale yellow to yellow, that have a viscosity similar to that of serum. Because transudates do not contain fibrinogen, they do not spontaneously clot. In contrast, exudates are usually cloudy; vary from yellow, green, or pink to red; and may have a shimmer or sheen to them. Because exudates often contain fibrinogen, they can form clots, thus requiring an anticoagulant (e.g., sodium heparin) in the collection tube. The physical appearance of an effusion usually is recorded on the patient's chart by the physician after paracentesis and should be transcribed onto all test request forms. If this information is not provided, the laboratory performing the microscopic examination should document the physical characteristics of the fluid.

A cloudy paracentesis fluid most often indicates the presence of large numbers of leukocytes, other cells, chyle, lipids, or a combination of these substances. In pleural or peritoneal fluid, a characteristic *milky appearance* that persists after centrifugation usually indicates the presence of **chyle** (i.e., an emulsion of lymph and chylomicrons) in the effusion. A **chylous effusion** is caused by obstruction of or damage to the lymphatic system. In the pleural cavity, this can be caused by tumors, often lymphoma, or by damage to the thoracic duct due to trauma or accidental damage during surgery. Chylous effusions in the peritoneal cavity result from obstruction to lymphatic fluid drainage, which can occur with hepatic cirrhosis and portal vein thrombosis. Note that chronic effusions (as seen with rheumatoid arthritis, tuberculosis, and myxedema) can have a similar appearance owing to the breakdown of cellular components, and they have a characteristically high cholesterol content. Consequently because of their visual similarity, chronic effusions often are called **pseudochylous effusions** and are differentiated from true chylous effusions by their lipid composition (i.e., triglycerides, chylomicron content). In a chylous effusion, lipoprotein analysis will show an elevated triglyceride level (i.e., greater than 110 mg/dL) and chylomicrons present, whereas a pseudochylous effusion has a low triglyceride level (less than 50 mg/dL) and no chylomicrons present. Table 15-4 summarizes characteristics features that assist in differentiating chylous and pseudochylous effusions.

Blood can be present in transudates and exudates because of a traumatic paracentesis procedure. As with

TABLE 15-3	Serous Effusions: Types, Mechanism of Formation, and Associated Conditions		
Effusion	**Type**	**Mechanism of Formation**	**Conditions**
Pleural and peritoneal	Transudates	Decreased hydrostatic pressure Decreased oncotic pressure	Congestive heart failure Hepatic cirrhosis Nephrotic syndrome
Pleural and peritoneal	Exudates	Increased capillary permeability	Infection (e.g., bacterial, tuberculous, viral, fungal) Tumors/neoplasms: Pleural: lung and metastatic cancers Peritoneal: hepatic and metastatic cancers Systemic disease (e.g., rheumatoid arthritis, systemic lupus erythematosus) Gastrointestinal disease (e.g., pancreatitis)
		Decreased lymphatic absorption	Tumors/neoplasms (e.g., lymphoma, metastasis) Trauma or surgery
Pericardial	Not categorized as transudate or exudate	Increased capillary permeability due to changes in parietal membrane	Infections (e.g., bacterial, tuberculous, viral, fungal) Cardiovascular disease (e.g., myocardial infarction, aneurysms) Tumors/neoplasms (e.g., metastatic cancers) Hemorrhage Systemic disease (e.g., rheumatoid arthritis, systemic lupus erythematosus)

TABLE 15-4	Differentiation of Chylous and Pseudochylous Effusions	
Parameter	**Chylous Effusion**	**Pseudochylous Effusion**
Physical Examination	Milky	Milky
Chemical Examination Chylomicrons Triglycerides Cholesterol	Present >110 mg/dL (1.2 mmol/L) Usually <200 mg/dL (5.2 mmol/L)	Absent <110 mg/dL (1.2 mmol/L) Usually >200 mg/dL (5.2 mmol/L)
Microscopic Findings	Lymphocytes	Variety of cell types Lipid-laden macrophages Cholesterol crystals*
Conditions	Pleural effusions due to: • Trauma or surgery (caused damage to thoracic duct) • Obstruction of lymphatic system: tumors (lymphomas), fibrosis Peritoneal effusions due to: • Hepatic cirrhosis • Portal vein thrombosis	Chronic diseases such as: • Tuberculosis • Rheumatoid arthritis • Collagen vascular disease

*Presence confirms or establishes fluid as pseudochylous effusion.

other body fluids (e.g., cerebrospinal fluid, synovial fluid), the origin of the blood is determined by the distribution of blood during paracentesis. If the amount of blood decreases during the collection and small clots form, a traumatic tap is suspected. If the blood is homogeneously distributed in the fluid and the fluid does not clot (indicating that the fluid has been defibrinogenated in the body cavity—a process that takes several hours), the patient has a hemorrhagic effusion.

MICROSCOPIC EXAMINATION

The microscopic examination of pleural, pericardial, and peritoneal fluids may include a total cell count of erythrocytes (RBCs) and leukocytes (WBCs), a differential cell count, cytology studies, and, at times, identification of crystals. In the microbiology laboratory, a Gram stain is also performed to aid in the microscopic identification of microbes (see "Microbiological Examination"). As with other body fluids, normal saline must be used as the diluent when cloudy effusions are diluted for cell counting. (See Appendix C for acceptable diluents and their preparation.) Avoid acetic acid diluents because they cause cells to clump, which prevents accurate cell counting. Cell counts can be performed manually using a hemacytometer or an automated analyzer. For details, see Chapter 18, "Body Fluid Analysis: Manual Hemacytometer Counts and Differential Slide Preparation," and Chapter 17, "Automation of Urine and Body Fluid Analysis."

Total Cell Counts

Total RBC and WBC counts have little differential diagnostic value in the analysis of pleural, pericardial, and peritoneal fluids. No single value for a WBC count can be used reliably to differentiate transudates from exudates, hence these counts have limited clinical use. However, WBC counts in transudates are usually less than 1000 cells/μL, whereas those in exudates generally exceed 1000 cells/μL.

With pericardial fluid, a WBC count of greater than 1000 cells/μL is suggestive of pericarditis, whereas an RBC count or hematocrit of the fluid can assist in identifying a hemorrhagic effusion. With pleural fluid, RBC counts can also be used to identify hemorrhagic effusions. However, high RBC counts (greater than 10,000 cells/μL) are frequently associated with neoplasms or trauma of the pleura. With peritoneal fluid, a WBC count exceeding 500 cells/μL with a predominance of neutrophils (greater than 50%) suggests bacterial peritonitis. However, the volume of peritoneal fluid (or ascites) can change significantly because of extracellular fluid shifts, and these fluid shifts can significantly change the cell count obtained. Hence a wide range of WBC counts can be encountered in peritoneal effusions throughout the course of a disease.

Differential Cell Count

Microscope Slide Preparation. A cytocentrifuged-prepared smear of the body fluid is used most often to perform a differential cell count. Cytocentrifugation is easy and fast and enables good cell recovery in a concentrated area of the microscope slide with minimal cell distortion. For additional details, see Chapter 18, "Body Fluid Analysis: Manual Hemacytometer Counts and Differential Slide Preparation."

Cell Differential. The clinical value of a differential leukocyte count varies with the origin of the paracentesis fluid. When the differential is performed, all nucleated cells are counted, including mesothelial cells and malignant cells. Note that before or after the differential examination using high-power oil immersion objectives (50× or 100×), all cytocentrifuged smears should be scanned using a low-power objective (10×) to enhance the detection of abnormalities such as hemosiderin-laden macrophages or malignant cells that can be present singly or in clumps.

In pleural fluid, neutrophils predominate in about 90% of effusions caused by acute inflammation (i.e., exudates). Lymphocytes predominate in 90% of effusions caused by tuberculosis, neoplasms, and systemic diseases. Similarly, in peritoneal fluid, neutrophils predominate (greater than 25%) in most exudates, suggesting bacterial infection. In peritoneal transudates and in exudates caused by decreased lymphatic absorption (e.g., tuberculosis, neoplasms, lymphatic obstruction), lymphocytes predominate. Pericardial fluid differential counts often are not performed because a variety of conditions (e.g., bacterial and viral pericarditis, postmyocardial infarction) can produce the same cell differential, hence a pericardial fluid differential count provides little diagnostic information.

Various cell types are found in pleural, pericardial, and peritoneal fluids and include neutrophils, eosinophils, lymphocytes, monocytes, macrophages, plasma cells, mesothelial cells (the lining cells of the serous membrane), and malignant cells. Most of these cells are easily identifiable in effusions (Figures 15-2 through 15-5). Increased numbers of eosinophils (greater than 10%) have been observed in pleural, pericardial, and peritoneal fluids as a result of a variety of conditions. Although rare, lupus erythematosus (LE) cells (i.e., neutrophils with a phagocytized homogeneous nucleus) may be present in fluids from patients with systemic lupus erythematosus (Figure 15-6).

Mesothelial cells that line the serous membrane are routinely sloughed off and often appear in effusions.

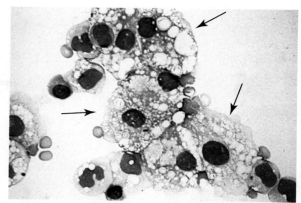

FIGURE 15-3 Macrophages in peritoneal (ascites) fluid. Cytocentrifuged smear, Wright's stain, 500×. *(Courtesy Charlotte Janita.)*

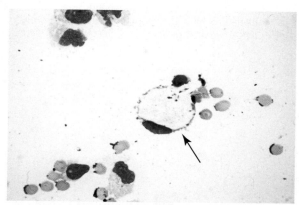

FIGURE 15-4 A signet ring macrophage and some red blood cells (RBCs) in pleural fluid. Cytocentrifuged smear, Wright's stain, 400×. *(Courtesy Charlotte Janita.)*

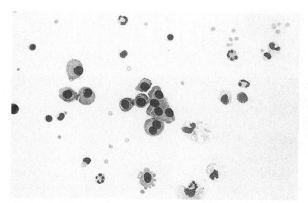

FIGURE 15-2 Mesothelial cells, macrophages, neutrophils, and lymphocytes in peritoneal fluid, Wright's stain, 200×. *(From Rodak BF, Fristma GA, Doig K: Hematology: clinical principles and applications, ed 3, St Louis, 2007, Saunders.)*

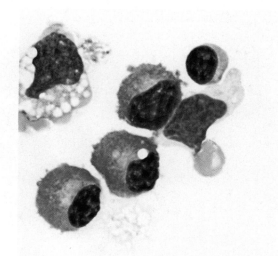

FIGURE 15-5 Plasma cells in pleural fluid (1000×). *(From Carr JH, Rodak BF: Clinical hematology atlas, ed 3, St Louis, 2008, Saunders.)*

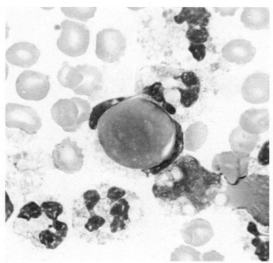

FIGURE 15-6 Lupus erythematosus (LE) cell in pleural fluid, 1000× (Wright's stain). The engulfed homogeneous mass pushes the nucleus of the neutrophil to the periphery of the cell. *(From Carr JH, Rodak BF: Clinical hematology atlas, ed 3, St Louis, 2008, Saunders.)*

They are large cells (12 to 30 μm in diameter) with light gray to deep blue staining cytoplasm (Figure 15-7). Their nuclei are often eccentric with smooth, regular nuclear membranes; the nuclear chromatin pattern is loose and homogeneous; and one to three nucleoli may be present. Often mesothelial cells have abundant cytoplasm, and they sometimes resemble plasma cells. Mesothelial cells can show evidence of phagocytosis—their cytoplasm loses its blue color, and they contain cytoplasmic vacuoles of various sizes. Because they can vary in appearance, such as appearing singly or in clumps, can be multinucleated, and show reactive or degenerative changes, mesothelial cells can be difficult to differentiate from malignant cells and macrophages.

Malignant cells in effusions are common in patients with neoplastic disease, although the number of malignant cells found can vary significantly. These cells can be *monomorphic* (no variation in morphology; all cells look alike) or *pleomorphic* (numerous variations in morphology). Several characteristics aid in identification of

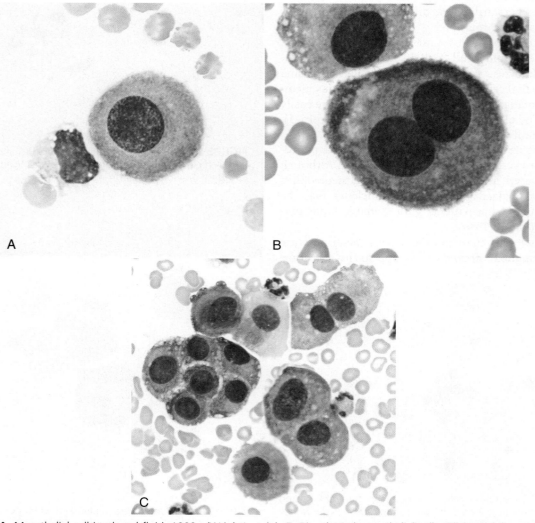

FIGURE 15-7 A, Mesothelial cell in pleural fluid, 1000× (Wright's stain). **B,** Binucleated mesothelial cell with basophilic cytoplasm, pleural fluid, 1000× (Wright's stain). **C,** Clump of mesothelial cells in pleural fluid, 500× (Wright's stain). *(From Carr JH, Rodak BF: Clinical hematology atlas, ed 3, St Louis, 2008, Saunders.)*

malignant cells, in particular, (1) they tend to form cell clumps, (2) their nuclear membrane is irregular or jagged, (3) their nuclear chromatin is distributed unevenly, (4) they contain prominent, frequently multiple nucleoli with irregular membranes, (5) their nuclear-to-cytoplasmic ratio is higher than normal, and (6) their cytoplasm may be basophilic and may contain vacuoles.

Most malignant effusions are caused by metastatic adenocarcinomas (Figure 15-8). Additional characteristics of the malignant cells of adenocarcinomas include the following: (1) They are often present in multiple, round cell aggregates (balls or clumps), (2) they often have large cytoplasmic vacuoles, and (3) large isolated bizarre forms may be present. Note that malignant mesothelioma can be very difficult to differentiate from reactive or malignant mesothelial cells. Therefore proper identification of malignant cells in effusions is crucial and is performed during a cytologic examination by a skilled professional.

Any of the blood cancers, leukemias, or lymphomas can infiltrate body cavities, causing an effusion. In these cases, the use of immunocytochemistry and flow cytometry is valuable in determining an accurate diagnosis.

Cytologic Examination

When malignant disease is suspected, large volumes (10 to 200 mL) of the pleural, pericardial, or peritoneal effusion should be submitted for cytologic examination. The fluid should be concentrated to increase the yield of cells, and a cell block as well as cytocentrifuged smears can be prepared. Cytologic examination is an important, sensitive, and specific procedure in the diagnosis of primary and metastatic neoplasms and is performed by a cytologist or a pathologist.

CHEMICAL EXAMINATION

The chemistry tests selected to evaluate pleural, pericardial, and peritoneal fluids assist the physician in establishing or confirming a diagnosis for the cause of an effusion. Once a diagnosis has been established,

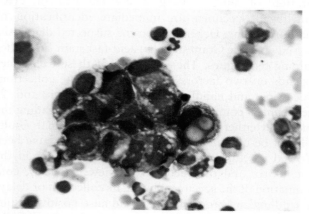

FIGURE 15-8 Adenocarcinoma in peritoneal fluid. Cytocentrifuged smear, Wright's stain, 400×. *(Courtesy Charlotte Janita.)*

appropriate treatment can be initiated, and further testing usually is not required. A specific diagnosis based on laboratory findings from serous fluids is limited to (1) malignancy, when malignant cells are recovered and identified; (2) systemic lupus erythematosus, when characteristic lupus erythematosus cells are found during the microscopic examination; and (3) infectious disease, when microorganisms (e.g., bacteria, fungi) are identified by Gram stain or culture. Several disease processes can occur simultaneously, each contributing to the development of an effusion. Therefore chemistry tests initially classify the effusion as a transudate or an exudate. Transudates usually require no further chemical analysis, whereas exudates are tested further to identify their causative agents or cause. A systematic approach in serous fluid testing greatly facilitates the diagnostic process.

Total Protein and Lactate Dehydrogenase Ratios

No single test can identify specifically the disease process causing effusions in the pleural, pericardial, and peritoneal cavities. Historically, transudates and exudates were classified by the total protein content or specific gravity of the fluid alone. Because of the significant overlap noted when these criteria were used (i.e., exudates with protein content or specific gravity values that were equivalent to those of transudates and vice versa), a better discriminator was needed. Useful tests for classifying a serous fluid as a transudate or an exudate are simultaneous determinations of the serum and serous fluid total protein (TP) concentration and lactate dehydrogenase (LD) activity. From these values, the fluid-to-serum total protein ratio and the fluid-to-serum lactate dehydrogenase ratio can be determined as follows:

Equation 15-1

$$\text{TP ratio} = \frac{TP_{fluid}}{TP_{serum}}$$

Equation 15-2

$$\text{LD ratio} = \frac{LD_{fluid}}{LD_{serum}}$$

These ratios together provide a reliable means to distinguish a transudate from an exudate. If the total protein ratio is less than 0.5 and the lactate dehydrogenase ratio is less than 0.6, the fluid is classified as a transudate. In contrast, exudates are those fluids with a total protein ratio greater than 0.5, a lactate dehydrogenase ratio greater than 0.6, or both.

Glucose

Following appropriate classification, several chemical tests can be used to evaluate exudates further. The tests selected and their usefulness vary with the origin of the fluid. The simultaneous measurement of serum and serous fluid glucose concentrations has limited value. If the serous fluid glucose is less than 60 mg/dL, or if the glucose difference between serum and fluid is greater than 30 mg/dL, an exudative process is identified. Only low fluid glucose levels are clinically significant, and a variety of disease processes are associated with them, particularly rheumatoid arthritis. Other conditions such as bacterial infection, tuberculosis, and malignant neoplasm may also present with decreased fluid glucose levels; however, a normal serous fluid glucose value does not rule out these disorders.

Amylase

The determination of simultaneous serum and fluid amylase levels, particularly in pleural and peritoneal fluids, is clinically useful and has become routine in many laboratories. A serous fluid amylase value that exceeds the established upper limit of normal (for serum specimens) or is 1.5 to 2 times the serum value is considered abnormally increased.[2] These high fluid amylase levels most often occur in effusions caused by pancreatitis, esophageal rupture (salivary amylase), gastroduodenal perforation, and metastatic disease.

Lipids (Triglyceride and Cholesterol)

Because identification of a *chylous effusion* is clinically significant, determining the triglyceride level of a fluid is an important adjunct when evaluating serous fluids. The milky appearance of an effusion does not identify it specifically as a chylous effusion because pseudochylous effusions can have a similar appearance. Therefore, fluid triglyceride levels are used as an additional determining factor. A serous fluid triglyceride value that exceeds 110 mg/dL (1.2 mmol/L) indicates a chylous effusion, whereas a triglyceride value less than 50 mg/dL rules it out. If the triglyceride level is between 50 and 110 mg/dL, lipoprotein electrophoresis can be performed; the presence of chylomicrons identifies a chylous effusion, whereas the absence of chylomicrons indicates a pseudochylous effusion. Chylous effusions are associated with obstruction or damage to the lymphatic system, which can occur with neoplastic disease (e.g., lymphoma), trauma, tuberculosis, and surgical procedures. Pseudochylous effusions are most often encountered with chronic inflammatory conditions (e.g., rheumatoid arthritis). Note that the presence of cholesterol crystals in a serous fluid is diagnostic of a pseudochylous effusion.[3]

The cholesterol level of pleural fluid can be useful for differentiating between a chylous and a pseudochylous effusion. A fluid-to-serum cholesterol ratio of greater than 1.0 indicates a pseudochylous effusion. The cholesterol ratio can also be helpful in identifying a pleural effusion as a transudate or exudate when other chemical results (TP ratio, LD ratio) are equivocal. In these cases,

a fluid-to-serum cholesterol ratio of greater than 0.3 indicates an exudate.[3,4]

pH

With pleural fluid, an abnormally low pH value can help identify patients with parapneumonic effusions (i.e., exudates caused by pneumonia or lung abscess) that require aggressive treatment. Parapneumonic effusions can involve the parietal and visceral membranes, produce pus, and loculate in the pleural cavity. Studies show that if the pleural fluid pH is less than 7.30, despite appropriate antibiotic therapy, the placement of drainage tubes is necessary for resolution of the effusion. In contrast, if the pleural fluid pH exceeds 7.30, the effusion completely resolves following antibiotic treatment alone. An important note is that the collection of pleural fluid specimens for pH measurement requires the same rigorous sampling protocol as the collection of arterial blood gas specimens (i.e., an anaerobic sampling technique using a heparinized syringe, placing the specimen on ice, and immediately transporting it to the laboratory for analysis).

Pericardial and peritoneal fluid pH measurements currently have no clearly established clinical value.

Carcinoembryonic Antigen

The measurement of carcinoembryonic antigen (CEA), a tumor marker, is useful in evaluating pleural and peritoneal effusions from patients who have a previous history or are currently suspected of having a carcinoembryonic antigen–producing tumor. When a CEA measurement is combined with a fluid cytologic examination, the identification of malignant effusions is significantly increased.

MICROBIOLOGICAL EXAMINATION

Staining Techniques

The microbiological examination includes the preparation of smears using a concentrated or cytocentrifuged specimen for immediate identification of microorganisms. Depending on the suspected diagnosis, this may include Gram stain, an acid-fast stain, and other staining techniques. The sensitivity of these techniques depends on two factors: (1) the appropriate collection, processing, and handling of the fluid specimen, and (2) the technical competence of the microscopist reading the smears. If either aspect is substandard, optimal results will not be obtained. In fluid specimens that have been allowed to clot, microorganisms can be caught in the clot matrix and obstructed from view; similarly, contamination of the specimen during its collection or delays in handling and processing can yield false-positive results from in vitro bacterial proliferation. Because of the potential presence of stain precipitates, cellular components, and other debris, smears must be evaluated by appropriately trained and experienced laboratorians. Under the best conditions, a Gram stain is positive in about 30% to 50% of bacterial effusions, whereas acid-fast stains are positive in only 10% to 30% of tuberculous effusions.

Culture

As with smear preparations, the larger the volume of pleural, pericardial, or peritoneal fluid used or the more concentrated the inoculum used, the greater the chances of obtaining a positive culture. Both aerobic and anaerobic cultures should be performed. The sensitivity of a positive culture varies with the origin of the fluid and the organism present. Positive bacterial cultures are obtained in approximately 80% of all bacterial effusions. In contrast, peritoneal tuberculous (or mycobacterial) effusions culture positive in 50% to 70% of cases, pericardial effusions culture positive in about 50% of cases, and pleural tuberculous effusions culture positive in only about 30% of cases.

STUDY QUESTIONS

1. Which of the following statements about serous fluid–filled body cavities is true?
   1. A parietal membrane is attached firmly to the body cavity wall.
   2. Serous fluid acts as a lubricant between opposing membranes.
   3. A serous membrane is composed of a single layer of flat mesothelial cells.
   4. The visceral and parietal membranes of an organ are actually a single continuous membrane.
   A. 1, 2, and 3 are correct.
   B. 1 and 3 are correct.
   C. 4 is correct.
   D. All are correct.

2. Which of the following mechanisms is responsible for the formation of serous fluid in body cavities?
   A. Ultrafiltration of circulating blood plasma
   B. Selective absorption of fluid from the lymphatic system
   C. Diuresis of solutes and water across a concentration gradient
   D. Active secretion by mesothelial cells that line the serous membranes

3. Which of the following conditions enhances the formation of serous fluid in a body cavity?
   A. Increased lymphatic absorption
   B. Increased capillary permeability
   C. Increased plasma oncotic pressure
   D. Decreased capillary hydrostatic pressure

4. The pathologic accumulation of fluid in a body cavity is called
   A. an abscess.
   B. an effusion.
   C. pleocytosis.
   D. paracentesis.

5. Paracentesis and serous fluid testing are performed to
   1. remove serous fluids that may be compressing a vital organ.
   2. determine the pathologic cause of an effusion.
   3. identify an effusion as a transudate or an exudate.
   4. prevent volume depletion caused by the accumulation of fluid in body cavities.
   A. 1, 2, and 3 are correct.
   B. 1 and 3 are correct.
   C. 4 is correct.
   D. All are correct.

6. Thoracentesis refers specifically to the removal of fluid from the
   A. abdominal cavity.
   B. pericardial cavity.
   C. peritoneal cavity.
   D. pleural cavity.

7. Which of the following parameters best identifies a fluid as a transudate or an exudate?
   A. Color and clarity
   B. Leukocyte and differential counts
   C. Total protein and specific gravity measurements
   D. Total protein ratio and lactate dehydrogenase ratio

8. Chylous and pseudochylous effusions are differentiated by their
   A. physical examinations.
   B. cholesterol concentrations.
   C. triglyceride concentrations.
   D. leukocyte and differential counts.

9. Which of the following conditions is most often associated with the formation of a transudate?
   A. Pancreatitis
   B. Surgical procedures
   C. Congestive heart failure
   D. Metastatic neoplasm

10. Match the type of serous effusion most often associated with each pathologic condition.

Pathologic Condition	Type of Serous Effusion
___ A. Neoplasms	1. Exudate
___ B. Hepatic cirrhosis	2. Transudate
___ C. Infection	
___ D. Rheumatoid arthritis	
___ E. Trauma	
___ F. Nephrotic syndrome	

11. Which of the following laboratory findings on an effusion does not indicate a specific diagnosis?
    A. LE cells found during the microscopic examination
    B. A serous fluid glucose concentration less than 60 mg/dL
    C. Microorganisms identified by Gram or acid-fast stain
    D. Malignant cells identified during the microscopic or cytologic examination

12. An abnormally low fluid pH value is useful when evaluating conditions associated with
    A. pleural effusions.
    B. pleural and pericardial effusions.
    C. pericardial and peritoneal effusions.
    D. pleural, pericardial, and peritoneal effusions.

13. A pleural or peritoneal fluid amylase level two times higher than the serum amylase level can be found in effusions resulting from
    A. pancreatitis.
    B. hepatic cirrhosis.
    C. rheumatoid arthritis.
    D. lymphatic obstruction.

14. A glucose concentration difference greater than 30 mg/dL between the serum and an effusion is associated with
    A. pancreatitis.
    B. hepatic cirrhosis.
    C. rheumatoid arthritis.
    D. lymphatic obstruction.

15. Which of the following actions can adversely affect the chances of obtaining a positive stain or culture when performing microbiological studies on infectious serous fluid?
    A. Using a large volume of serous fluid for the inoculum
    B. Storing serous fluid specimens at refrigerator temperatures
    C. Using an anticoagulant in the serous fluid collection container
    D. Concentrating the serous fluid before preparing smears for staining

---

CASE 15-1

A 51-year-old man with a history of tuberculosis is found to have a unilateral pleural effusion. A pleural fluid specimen is obtained by thoracentesis and is sent to the laboratory for evaluation.

Blood Chemistry Results

	Reference Interval
Total protein: 7.0 g/dL	6.0-8.3 mg/dL
Lactate dehydrogenase: 520 U/L	275-645 U/L
Glucose, fasting: 75 mg/dL	≤110 mg/dL

Pleural Fluid Results

Physical Examination	Microscopic Examination	Chemical Examination
Color: yellow	Leukocyte count: 1100 cells/µL	Total protein: 4.2 g/dL
Clarity: cloudy	Differential count:	Lactate dehydrogenase: 345 U/L
Clots present: no	Mononuclear: 93%	Glucose: 55 mg/dL
	Neutrophils: 3%	
	Gram stain: no organisms seen; leukocytes present	

1. Calculate the fluid-to-serum total protein ratio.
2. Calculate the fluid-to-serum lactate dehydrogenase ratio.
3. Classify this pleural fluid specimen as a transudate or an exudate, and state two physiologic mechanisms that can cause this type of effusion.

CASE 15-2

A 48-year-old woman has ascites and pleural effusion. Blood is drawn and a peritoneal fluid specimen is obtained by paracentesis and sent to the laboratory for evaluation.

Blood Chemistry Results

	Reference Interval
Total protein: 6.5 g/dL	6.0-8.3 mg/dL
Lactate dehydrogenase: 300 U/L	275-645 U/L
Glucose, fasting: 82 mg/dL	≤110 mg/dL
Liver function tests*: normal	

Peritoneal Fluid Results

Physical Examination	Microscopic Examination	Chemical Examination
Color: yellow	Leukocyte count: 8 cells/μL	Total protein: 2.9 g/dL
Clarity: clear	Cytologic examination: no malignant cells seen	Lactate dehydrogenase: 125 U/L
Clots present: no	Gram stain: no organisms seen	Glucose: 67 mg/dL

1. Calculate the fluid-to-serum total protein ratio.
2. Calculate the fluid-to-serum lactate dehydrogenase ratio.
3. Classify this peritoneal fluid specimen as a transudate or an exudate, and state two physiologic mechanisms that can cause this type of effusion.

*Alanine aminotransferase, aspartate aminotransferase, γ-glutamyltransferase, alkaline phosphatase, and bilirubin.

REFERENCES

1. Krieg AF, Kjeldsberg CR: Cerebrospinal fluid and other body fluids. In Henry JB, editor: Clinical diagnosis and management of laboratory methods, Philadelphia, 1991, WB Saunders.
2. Kjeldsberg CR, Knight JA: Pleural and pericardial fluids. In Body fluids, ed 2, Chicago, 1986, American Society of Clinical Pathologists Press.
3. Clinical and Laboratory Standards Institute (CLSI): Analysis of body fluids in clinical chemistry: approved guideline, CLSI Document C49-A, Wayne, PA, 2007, CLSI.
4. Valdes L, Suarez APJ, Gonzalez-Juanatey JR, et al: Cholesterol: a useful parameter for distinguishing between pleural exudates and transudates. Chest 99:1097-1102, 1999.

BIBLIOGRAPHY

Glasser L: Extravascular biological fluids. In Kaplan LA, Pesce AJ, Kazmierczak SC, editors: Clinical chemistry: theory, analysis, correlation, ed 4, St Louis, 2003, Mosby.
Heffner JE, Brown LK, Barbieri CA: Diagnostic value of tests that discriminate between exudative and transudative pleural effusions. Chest 111:970-980, 1997.

Kalish RI, Cheskin HS, Blumenfeld TA: Body fluid specimens. In Slockbower JM, Blumenfeld TA, editors: Collection and handling of laboratory specimens, Philadelphia, 1983, JB Lippincott.
Kjeldsberg CR, Knight JA: Peritoneal fluid. In Body fluids, ed 3, Chicago, 1993, American Society for Clinical Pathology Press.
Light RW: Diagnostic principles in pleural disease. Eur Respir J 10:476-481, 1997.
Lossos IS, Breuer R, Intrator O, et al: Differential diagnosis of pleural effusion by lactate dehydrogenase isoenzyme analysis. Chest 111:648-651, 1997.
Meisel S, Shamiss A, Thaler M, et al: Pleural fluid to serum bilirubin concentration ratio for the separation of transudates and exudates. Chest 98:141-144, 1990.
Meyers DG, Meyers RE, Prendergast TW: The usefulness of diagnostic tests on pericardial fluid. Chest 11:1213, 1997.
Smith GP, Kjeldsberg CR: Cerebrospinal, synovial, and serous body fluids. In Henry JB, editor: Clinical diagnosis and management of laboratory methods, Philadelphia, 2001, WB Saunders.

Analysis of Vaginal Secretions

KEY TERMS

bacterial vaginosis noninvasive inflammation of the vagina and upper genital tract most often caused by *Gardnerella vaginalis* in association with anaerobes such as *Mobiluncus* species.

bactericidal capable of killing bacteria.

clue cells squamous epithelial cells with large numbers of bacteria adhering to them. Clue cells appear soft and finely granular with indistinct or "shaggy" cell borders. To be considered a clue cell, bacteria do not need to cover the entire cell, but the bacterial organisms must extend beyond and obscure at least 75% of the cytoplasmic borders of the cell. Clue cells are characteristic of bacterial vaginosis, a synergistic infection involving *Gardnerella vaginalis* and anaerobic bacteria.

dyspareunia pain in the vulva, vagina, or pelvis during or after intercourse. The cause may be disease-related, mechanical, or psychologic.

dysuria pain or difficulty experienced with urination. Dysuria most often is associated with infections of the urinary tract (e.g., urethritis, cystitis). Such "internal" dysuria contrasts with "external" dysuria, which is pain experienced during urination because of the passage of urine over inflamed tissues (e.g., vulva, perineum).

KOH preparation a preparation technique used to enhance the viewing of fungal elements. Secretions obtained using a sterile swab are suspended in saline. A drop of this suspension is placed on a microscope slide, followed

by a drop of 10% KOH. The slide is warmed and is viewed microscopically. KOH destroys most formed elements with the exception of bacteria and fungal elements.

vaginal fornix the arched recesses of the vaginal mucosa that surround the cervix. Of the four recesses, the posterior fornix is deeper than the anterior and lateral (right and left) fornices.

vaginal pool the mucus and cells present in the posterior fornix of the vagina when a female is in a supine position.

vaginitis inflammation of the vagina.

vulvovaginitis inflammation of the vulva and vagina or of the vulvovaginal glands (i.e., Bartholin's glands).

TABLE 16-1	Vaginal Secretion Findings and Associated Conditions				
	Healthy/ Normal*	Candidiasis	Bacterial Vaginosis	Trichomoniasis	Atrophic Vaginitis
Patient complaints	—	Vulvovaginal itching and soreness, discharge, "external" dysuria,[†] dyspareunia	Malodorous discharge	Vulvovaginal soreness, malodorous discharge, "external" dysuria,[†] dyspareunia	Vaginal dryness, dyspareunia
Discharge characteristics	—	White, curdlike	Foul-smelling, thin, gray, homogeneous; adherent to mucosa	Copious, yellow-green, frothy; may be foul-smelling, adherent to mucosa	—
pH	3.8 to 4.5	3.8 to 4.5	>4.5	5.0 to 6.0	5.0 to 7.0
Direct wet mount microscopy findings: *Bacteria*	Large rods[†] predominate	Large rods[†] predominate	Increase in gram-variable coccobacilli; rare to absent large rods[†]	Mixed bacterial flora	Decreased large rods,[†] increase in gram-positive cocci and gram-negative rods
WBCs	Rare to 2+	3+ to 4+	Rare	2+ to 4+	3+ to 4+
Other		Budding yeast, pseudohyphae	Clue cells	Motile trichomonads (60%)	RBCs: 1+ or greater; Parabasal cells present
KOH microscopic examination	Negative	Budding yeast, pseudohyphae	Negative	Negative	Negative
Amine or "whiff" test	Negative	Negative	Positive	Positive, often	Negative
Miscellaneous	—	If microscopy negative, use culture or DNA probe analysis	If results inconclusive, use DNA probe analysis; culture of no value	If microscopy negative, use culture or DNA probe analysis	

KOH, 10% potassium hydroxide; *RBCs*, red blood cells; *WBCs*, white blood cells.
*Values from healthy nonmenstruating women.
[†]External dysuria is pain experienced during urination owing to the passage of urine over inflamed tissue.
[‡]These large (gram-positive) rods are lactobacilli, the predominant microbe in vaginal secretions of healthy individuals.

The most common gynecologic complaints encountered by health care providers are vaginal discharge, vaginal discomfort, and vaginal odor. The three major causes for these symptoms are bacterial vaginosis, candidiasis, and trichomoniasis. Whereas the causative agent for each of these conditions is distinctly different, the clinical presentations can be nonspecific and similar (Table 16-1). Because treatment can differ significantly, determining the causative agent before initiating therapy is important, and in some cases, treating sexual partners is also necessary to avoid reinfection.

These conditions are usually differentiated using a sample of vaginal secretions and a few direct microscopy tests: wet mount examination, amine or "whiff" test, KOH examination, and Gram stain. Despite the fact that these microscopy tests are simple and easy to perform, the accuracy of the results obtained depends directly on the skill and expertise of the microscopist. This fact should not be minimized. If personnel with the necessary technical skills and expertise are not available, testing should be referred to a laboratory with qualified personnel.

The Clinical Laboratory Improvement Act has classified the wet mount examination and the KOH examination of vaginal secretions as provider-performed microscopy tests. The Act also states that when nonlaboratory personnel (i.e., clinical practitioners such as physicians, physician assistants, nurse practitioners, and nurses) perform these tests, the designated laboratory director is responsible for ensuring the accuracy and reliability of the testing performed. Timely and accurate testing of vaginal fluid specimens can identify offending organisms that cause vaginal discharge and discomfort, enabling health care providers to immediately diagnose and treat common causes of vaginitis/vaginosis.

SPECIMEN COLLECTION AND HANDLING

Appropriate collection and handling of vaginal secretion specimens optimizes the recovery and detection of microorganisms and other cellular elements. Based on the presence, absence, or combination of elements observed microscopically, the cause of vaginitis or vulvovaginitis can be determined.

A health care provider collects vaginal secretions during a pelvic examination. A nonlubricated speculum, moistened only with warm water, is used to provide access to the vaginal fornices. Speculum lubricants are avoided because they often contain antimicrobial agents. The specimen collection device is usually a sterile, polyester-tipped (e.g., Dacron) swab on a plastic shaft or, alternatively, a sterile wire loop. Selection of the sampling device is important because cotton has been toxic to *Neisseria gonorrhoeae,* whereas wooden shafts have been toxic to *Chlamydia trachomatis.*[1] The health care provider uses one or more swabs or a collection loop to obtain vaginal secretions from the posterior **vaginal fornix** and the **vaginal pool.**

After collection, the labeled specimen should be transported to the laboratory as soon as possible in a biohazard bag accompanied by a requisition slip. In addition to the standard patient identification information on the request slip, an appropriate medical history should be provided, such as the patient's menstrual status, exposure to sexually transmitted diseases, and use of vaginal lubricants, creams, and douches.

Tests on vaginal secretion specimens should be performed as soon as possible. If a delay in transport or analysis is unavoidable, these specimens should be kept at room temperature. Refrigeration adversely affects the recovery of *N. gonorrhoeae* and the detection of the trophozoite *Trichomonas vaginalis,* whose identification depends on observing its characteristic "flitting" motility. However, for detection of *C. trachomatis* or viruses (e.g., herpes simplex virus), refrigeration is preferred to prevent overgrowth of the normal bacterial flora.

When a health care provider immediately examines the vaginal secretions following collection (i.e., provider-performed microscopy testing), the swab is often placed directly into 0.5 to 1.0 mL of sterile physiologic saline (0.9% NaCl), and the microscopic examinations are performed. An alternate approach is to place a small drop of sterile physiologic saline onto a microscope slide into which the swab of vaginal secretions is directly rolled for microscopic viewing.

pH

The pH of vaginal secretions should be determined using commercial pH paper before the sampling swab is placed into saline. The pH is valuable because it assists in the differential diagnosis of vaginitis (see Table 16-1). A pH greater than 4.5 is associated with bacterial vaginosis, trichomoniasis, and atrophic vaginitis.

Vaginal secretions should have a pH in the range of 3.8 to 4.5. The predominant bacteria in a healthy vagina are lactobacilli, and it is lactic acid, their major metabolic end product, that maintains this normally acidic pH. Studies have demonstrated that some lactobacilli also produce hydrogen peroxide, which further enhances the healthy acidic environment of the vagina. In part, the bactericidal qualities of hydrogen peroxide prevent overgrowth of some indigenous microbes, such as *Gardnerella vaginalis.* In fact, the reduction or absence of hydrogen peroxide–producing lactobacilli is associated with bacterial vaginosis.[2,3]

MICROSCOPIC EXAMINATIONS

Microscopic examinations should be performed as soon as possible on vaginal secretion specimens, particularly for detection of *T. vaginalis,* for which identification depends solely on observing actively motile organisms. The vaginal swab is placed into a tube containing approximately 1.0 mL of sterile physiologic saline (0.9% NaCl) and is agitated or twirled for a few seconds to release the secretions from the swab.

Two microscope slides are typically prepared using the vaginal swab. One slide is used for a direct wet mount examination and the second slide for a 10% KOH preparation and the amine or "whiff" test. Depending on the laboratory protocol, a third slide may also be prepared for Gram stain. Each slide is prepared from the saline suspension made using the vaginal swab. A drop of this suspension is placed onto a clean, labeled microscope slide by using a disposable transfer pipette or, alternatively, by pressing and rolling the moistened swab on the microscope slide to express liquid onto the slide. The wet mount and KOH slides, as well as the slide for Gram stain (if requested), are usually prepared at the same time.

Wet Mount Examination

When preparing the direct wet mount slide, a coverslip is placed on the drop of saline-suspended specimen, taking care not to trap air bubbles. This slide is examined using brightfield or phase-contrast microscopy at low-power (100×) and high-power (400×) magnifications. Low-power magnification is used to assess the overall distribution of the specimen components and to evaluate epithelial cells, such as the number, the type, and whether clumping is present. Subsequently, high-power magnification is used to quantify the elements using criteria similar to those listed in Table 16-2.[4,5] The following elements typically are identified and reported when

TABLE 16-2	Quantification Criteria for Microscopic Examinations	
Results	**Number of Cells/ Organisms**	**Viewing Results Area**
Rare	<10	per slide
Occasional	<1	per 10 hpfs
1+	<1	per hpf
2+	1 to 5	per hpf
3+	6 to 30	per hpf
4+	>30	per hpf

hpf, High-power field.

observed in wet mount preparations of vaginal secretions: red blood cells, white blood cells, predominant bacterial morphotypes, yeast, hyphae/pseudohyphae, trichomonads, clue cells, parabasal cells, basal cells, and squamous epithelial cells.

Blood Cells. In health, white blood cells are present in vaginal secretions and their numbers range from a few observed in an entire preparation to several cells observed in every high-power field of view. This variation is often associated with a woman's menstrual cycle, with increased white blood cells present during ovulation and menses.[6] In contrast, red blood cells usually are not present unless the specimen was collected around or during menstruation. This highlights the need for a current patient history to accompany the results of each vaginal fluid specimen.

Bacterial Flora. The vagina has a complex bacterial flora with the characteristically large rods of lactobacilli accounting for 50% to 90% of the microbes in a healthy vagina.[7] These morphologically distinct, large, nonmotile, gram-positive rods produce lactic acid as their major metabolic waste product, which is principally responsible for the acidic (pH 3.8 to 4.5) environment of a healthy vagina (Figure 16-1). In addition, a subset of these lactobacilli produce hydrogen peroxide, which helps maintain balance in the vaginal flora by preventing the proliferation of other bacteria, in particular, *G. vaginalis* and *Prevotella bivia*. Any decrease in the number of lactobacilli relative to the number of squamous epithelial cells present in the preparation is an indication of an imbalance in the microbial flora. Whereas small numbers of other bacterial morphotypes may be observed in normal vaginal secretions, the presence of increased numbers or a preponderance of them is considered abnormal. These morphotypes include small, nonmotile, gram-variable coccobacilli (e.g., *G. vaginalis*); thin,

curved, gram-variable, motile rods (e.g., *Mobiluncus* spp.); gram-positive cocci (e.g., *Peptostreptococcus* spp., staphylococci, and streptococci); gram-negative cocci (e.g., *Enterococcus* spp.); and gram-negative rods (e.g., *Prevotella* spp., *Porphyromonas* spp., *Bacteroides* spp., coliforms).

Yeast. An occasional yeast or blastoconidium can be present in normal vaginal secretions. Because of the visual similarity of yeast and red blood cells, the KOH preparation, which lyses red blood cells, is useful in distinguishing these two entities. Yeast cells are typically 10 to 12 μm in diameter and are Gram stain positive. Increased numbers (1+ or greater) of yeast or the presence of hyphae or pseudohyphae is considered abnormal and indicates candidiasis (i.e., a fungal or yeast infection) (Figure 16-2).

Epithelial Cells. The vagina is a thick-walled fibromuscular tube lined with stratified squamous epithelium. Therefore when the vaginal mucosa is swabbed during the collection of vaginal secretions, a significant number of squamous epithelial cells are recovered. These cells predominate in wet mounts from a healthy vagina and

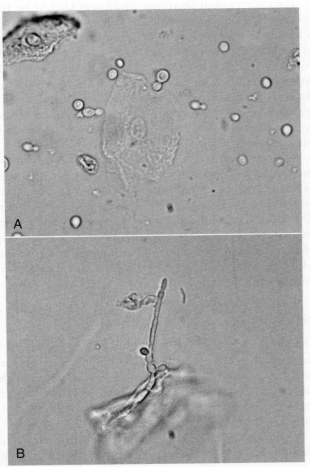

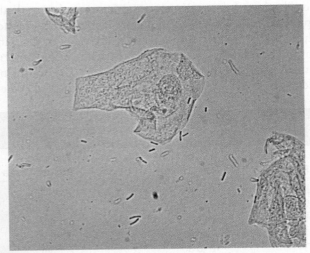

FIGURE 16-1 Large rods characteristic of *Lactobacillus* spp. surrounding a typical squamous epithelial cell from a healthy vagina.

FIGURE 16-2 Yeast and pseudohyphae in the wet mount of a vaginal secretions specimen. **A,** Budding yeast (blastoconidia) and two squamous epithelial cells. **B,** Pseudohyphae.

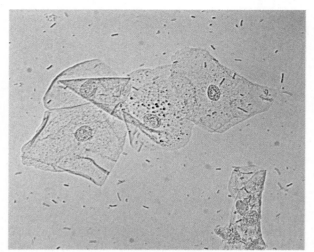

FIGURE 16-3 Several squamous epithelial cells from a healthy vagina. Keratohyalin granulation is most pronounced in the centrally located cell. Numerous large rods characteristic of *Lactobacillus* spp. are also present.

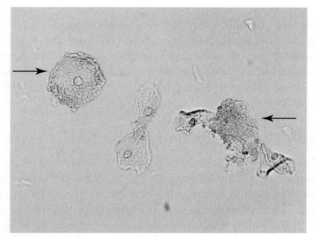

FIGURE 16-4 Two clue cells *(arrows)* and several normal squamous epithelial cells in the wet mount of a vaginal secretions specimen.

are identified easily by their large (30 to 60 mm), thin, flat, flagstone-shaped appearance. They have a small, centrally located nucleus and a large amount of cytoplasm, which becomes finely granulated as the cell ages (Figure 16-3). This intracellular keratohyalin granulation caused by cell degeneration is distinctly different from and must not be confused with the shaggy appearance of **clue cells,** which are formed when numerous bacteria adhere to the membranes of epithelial cells (Figure 16-4; see Figure 8-95). Clue cells, a diagnostic indicator of **bacterial vaginosis,** appear soft and finely stippled with indistinct cellular borders because of the numerous bacteria adhering to them. In these bacteria-laden cells with shaggy-appearing edges, the nuclei may not be visible. To be considered a clue cell, the bacteria do not need to cover the entire cell; however, a significant

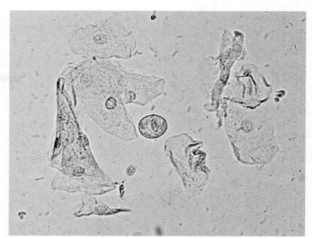

FIGURE 16-5 A single parabasal cell surrounded by numerous squamous epithelial cells.

number of bacterial organisms must extend beyond and obscure visualization of at least 75% of the cytoplasmic borders of the cell. Sometimes these cells are described as "bearded." The skill and expertise of the microscopist prevent the intracellular keratohyalin granulation of normal degenerating squamous cells from being misidentified as adherent bacteria of clue cells. Two microscopic characteristics that facilitate this differentiation is that keratohyalin granules vary in size, and they are usually larger and more refractile than bacteria.

Parabasal cells reside below the surface or luminal squamous epithelium of the vaginal mucosa. Therefore no or at most a few parabasal cells are present in normal vaginal secretions. However, increased numbers may be found during menstruation or in specimens from postmenopausal women. These cells are 15 to 40 μm in diameter and are oval to round with distinct cytoplasmic borders (Figure 16-5). In size and shape, these cells closely resemble transitional epithelial cells of the urinary system; however, their nucleus-to-cytoplasm ratio is smaller, that is, 1:1 to 1:2. Increased numbers of parabasal cells are usually observed in vaginal secretions from women with atrophic vaginitis and desquamative inflammatory vaginitis.

Basal cells, as their name denotes, are derived from the basal layer of the vaginal stratified epithelium (i.e., they rest on the basal lamina). These cells are similar in size to white blood cells, are 10 to 16 μm in diameter, and have a nucleus-to-cytoplasm ratio of 1:2. The presence of basal cells in the wet mount is abnormal. These cells are usually accompanied by numerous white blood cells in vaginal secretion specimens from women with desquamative inflammatory vaginitis.

Trichomonads. Trichomonads are flagellated protozoans that infect and cause inflammation of the vaginal epithelium. They are typically pear or turnip shaped, and their unicellular bodies average 15 mm in length. However, their size can vary from 5 mm to 30 mm in length and their shape from spherical to rectangular or

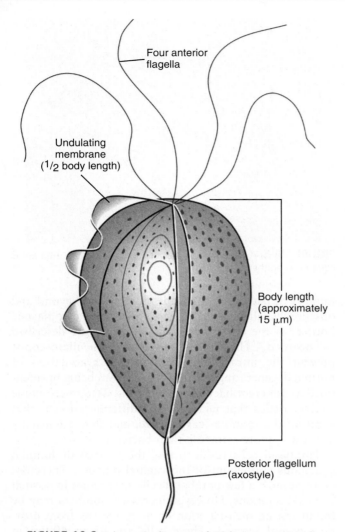

Four anterior
flagella

Undulating
membrane
($^1/_2$ body length)

Body length
(approximately
15 μm)

Posterior flagellum
(axostyle)

FIGURE 16-6 Schematic diagram of *Trichomonas vaginalis*.

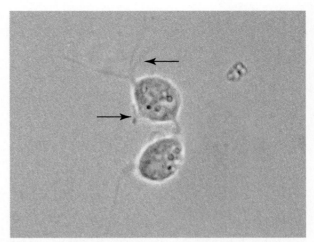

FIGURE 16-7 Two trichomonads. Visible on the upper organism are three of the four anterior flagella *(upper arrow)*, a portion of the undulating membrane *(lower arrow)*, and the posterior axostyle.

sausage-like. *Trichomonas vaginalis* thrive in an oxygen-free (anaerobic) environment and have optimal growth and metabolic function at a pH of 6.0.[8]

Regardless of their size or shape, trichomonads are readily identified by their characteristic flitting or jerky motion. This motion results from four anterior flagella and an undulating membrane that extends halfway down its body. The flagella provide propulsion, while the constant wavelike motion of the undulating membrane imparts a rotary motion to the organism (Figures 16-6 and 16-7). A single posterior axostyle is also present and is believed to play a role in the attachment of the organism to the vaginal mucosa and hence is a potential cause of the tissue damage associated with trichomoniasis. Nonmotile or dead trichomonads are essentially impossible to identify because they closely resemble white blood cells. As trichomonads die, they first lose their motility; later, the undulating membrane ceases. Finally, they "ball up" to look just like white blood cells. Stains are toxic to trichomonads, hence staining wet mounts do

not aid in their identification. Trichomonads are not hardy organisms, and once removed from the vaginal mucosa, they quickly die. Therefore when trichomoniasis is suspected, a wet mount of vaginal secretions should be prepared and examined as soon as possible after collection.

KOH Preparation and Amine Test

The KOH slide is prepared and the amine test is performed by adding 1 drop of 10% KOH directly onto the drop of vaginal secretion suspension on the microscope slide. Immediately, the slide is checked for the release of a "fishy" odor, hence this test is often referred to as the "whiff" test. The distinctive, pungent and foul-smelling odor is *trimethylamine,* a volatilization product of polyamines, which results from the pH change caused by the addition of KOH. During bacterial vaginosis, the microbial flora of the vagina is significantly altered, and the proliferation of microbes that produce polyamines increases. Development of a vaginal discharge (a transudate) and increased exfoliation of epithelial cells are directly related to this increase in polyamine production.[9] Results of the amine or "whiff" test are reported as positive or negative.

Next, a coverslip is placed on the suspension in preparation for the microscopic examination. This slide is typically prepared at the same time as the direct wet mount, but it is set aside to allow the KOH to dissolve epithelial and blood cells in the specimen. If immediate microscopic viewing is necessary, digestion of the cellular elements can be enhanced by gently heating the slide. Digestion of the cellular elements greatly enhances visualization of any fungal elements present. Low-power (100×) magnification is used to screen the preparation, and high-power (400×) magnification is used to identify and enumerate any fungal elements, such as blastoconidia (yeast cells) and pseudohyphae. Although the KOH preparation provides limited information, it remains a valuable aid in detecting and identifying fungal elements and in revealing the presence of increased polyamines by virtue of the amine or "whiff" test.

CLINICAL CORRELATIONS

Bacterial Vaginosis

The most common cause of vaginal infection in women is bacterial vaginosis, which results not from an exogenous pathogen but from an alteration in the normal indigenous bacterial flora of the vagina. Most often in bacterial vaginosis, the lactobacilli present in health are replaced by an overgrowth of *G. vaginalis* and a facultative anaerobe, such as *Mobiluncus* species (e.g., *M. curtisii* or *M. mulieris*). The acidic environment of a healthy vagina, established and maintained by the lactic acid production of lactobacilli, normally limits the proliferation of *G. vaginalis* and other anaerobic bacteria. In addition, some strains of lactobacilli produce hydrogen peroxide, which has bactericidal qualities that prevent the overgrowth of some indigenous microbes.[3] Whereas *G. vaginalis* and *Mobiluncus* species are the most frequently implicated microbes, the overgrowth of other anaerobes has been associated with bacterial vaginosis, including *Prevotella* species, *Peptostreptococcus* species, *Porphyromonas* species, *Propionibacterium* species, *Bacteroides* species, and *Mycoplasma hominis*.[10,11]

Studies of bacterial vaginosis complications have shown increased risk in pregnant women for premature labor and delivery and low-birth-weight infants.[12] In addition, untreated bacterial vaginosis is known to progress to endometritis and pelvic inflammatory disease. Therefore the detection and treatment of bacterial vaginosis are clinically important.

Women with bacterial vaginosis are often asymptomatic, with their only complaint being a malodorous discharge, which is particularly noticeable after intercourse. This unique observation results when the alkaline seminal fluid (pH 7.2 to 7.8) changes the vaginal pH, which leads to volatilization of the polyamines present to *trimethylamine*—the cause of the foul-smelling odor. The vaginal discharge is gray or off-white, thin, and homogeneous. Noticeably absent is vulvovaginal pruritus, soreness, and **dyspareunia,** and the diagnosis of bacterial vaginosis often involves ruling out or eliminating candidiasis or trichomoniasis as the cause.

The single most reliable indicator of bacterial vaginosis is the presence of clue cells in the wet mount examination of vaginal secretions[2] (see Figure 16-4). Typically, the presence of at least one clue cell in each of 10 fields, or identification of one out of five squamous cells as clue cells, is considered "positive" for clue cells. In bacterial vaginosis, the wet mount also reveals that the lactobacilli present in health are rare or absent. Most often they are replaced by the small, gram-variable coccobacilli of *G. vaginalis* and the thin, curved or comma-shaped, gram-variable, motile rods of the anaerobe *Mobiluncus* species. The amine test is characteristically positive, and the KOH preparation examination negative (see Table 16-2). Another notable feature is that white blood cells in the vaginal secretions are rare. This lack of an increase in white blood cells suggests that the microbial organisms involved do not invade the subepithelial tissue. Hence the condition is called *vaginosis* instead of *vaginitis*. The consistency and reliability of these findings have culminated in the classic diagnostic criteria for bacterial vaginosis, which requires the presence of at least three of the following four features: (1) the presence of clue cells, (2) a positive amine test, (3) a vaginal pH greater than 4.5, and (4) a homogeneous vaginal discharge.[13]

If wet mount and amine tests are inconclusive or are not available, DNA probe analysis for *G. vaginalis* can be clinically valuable. Although these tests are comparatively expensive, they are accurate and clinically sensitive and specific for *G. vaginalis*. Culturing vaginal secretions is of no value in establishing a diagnosis of bacterial vaginosis because 50% to 60% of healthy asymptomatic women have a positive culture for *G. vaginalis*. In addition, no threshold has been established to identify clinically significant increases in *G. vaginalis* in vaginal secretions.

The most successful treatment of bacterial vaginosis is orally administered metronidazole. In approximately 30% of cases, bacterial vaginosis recurs most likely because of failure to reestablish the normal microbial balance dominated by lactobacilli in the vagina. One new approach to treatment and recolonization of the vagina is the use of lactobacillus-containing vaginal suppositories. Concurrent treatment of sexual partners is not needed or recommended.

Candidiasis

Vulvovaginal candidiasis is the second most common cause of vaginitis in women. Most adult women have experienced at least one episode of vaginal candidiasis, and many have had several infections. Candidiasis occurs in celibate as well as sexually active women and decreases with age, being less common in postmenopausal women.

Candida albicans is responsible for most (80% to 92%) cases of vulvovaginal candidiasis.[9] However, other *Candida* species, particularly *Candida (Torulopsis) glabrata*, are appearing with increasing frequency, and it is postulated that this is happening because of an increase in self-diagnosis and treatment with over-the-counter antimycotic agents.[14]

Candida albicans and other *Candida* species are part of the normal vaginal flora. Their overproliferation results when a disruption in the vaginal environment (pH) or a change in the bacterial flora occurs. Most episodes of candidiasis occur in women with no known risk or predisposing factors. Two potential initiators of candidiasis are treatment with broad-spectrum antibiotics and oral contraceptive use; however, not all women share this susceptibility. Other clinical conditions that predispose an individual to develop candidiasis include pregnancy, uncontrolled diabetes mellitus, immunosuppression, and human immunodeficiency virus infection. Regardless, candidiasis is a common infection in women and is usually evident by vulvovaginal itching and soreness, external **dysuria,** and a white, curdlike discharge (see Table 16-1).

With candidiasis, the pH of vaginal secretions remains normal (pH 3.8 to 4.5). Typically, a wet mount examination of vaginal secretions reveals an increase in white blood cells and the presence of budding yeast (blastoconidia) and/or pseudohyphae (see Figure 16-2). Depending on the species present, yeast buds can vary in size and shape and in whether pseudohyphae form. The squamous epithelial cells present are often clumped, and lactobacilli are the predominant bacterial morphotype. The amine test is negative, but the KOH preparation examination also reveals budding yeast and/or pseudohyphae. If a wet mount and KOH preparation are not available, or if they produce negative results despite clinical symptoms, a culture or DNA probe analysis for *Candida* species can be performed. Although these two tests are more costly and time consuming, they are reliable and have greater clinical sensitivity and specificity.

Topical antimycotic agents from the family of imidazole derivatives predominate, such as miconazole, clotrimazole, butoconazole, and terconazole. Oral agents appear to be equally effective and include fluconazole, ketoconazole, and itraconazole. Recurrent candidiasis, defined as four or more episodes a year, is a problem for a minority of women and may require long-term (e.g., 6 months) antimycotic suppression therapy. The treatment of sexual partners is not indicated or advised.

Trichomoniasis

Of parasitic gynecologic infections, trichomoniasis caused by *T. vaginalis* is among the most common and affects millions of women worldwide. The disease is sexually transmitted, with human beings as its only known host. In women, trichomonads primarily reside in the vaginal mucosa; in men, they infect the urogenital tract. Infection in women can range from an asymptomatic carrier state to a severe, inflammatory condition. Recurrence is common if a woman's sexual partner is not treated simultaneously because of the fact that approximately 35% of asymptomatic male partners are positive for *T. vaginalis* when tested.[9] Although nonvenereal (nonsexual) transmissions of *T. vaginalis* have occurred, particularly in older women, the mechanism for such infections has not been elucidated clearly.[15,16]

Trichomoniasis in men is usually asymptomatic or presents as urethritis. In the latter cases, usually when tests for *N. gonorrhoeae* and *C. trachomatis* are negative, cultures or DNA probe analysis for *T. vaginalis* is performed, revealing the parasitic infection. Hence untreated male sexual partners can be the source of initial trichomoniasis infection or reinfection if they are not identified and treated with their partners.

In pregnant women, trichomoniasis is a risk factor for preterm rupture of membranes and for premature labor and delivery.[12] Studies have shown that the transmission of human immunodeficiency virus is facilitated in women with trichomoniasis.[17] Hence to reduce these risks in women, the detection and appropriate treatment of trichomoniasis are of paramount importance.

Although approximately 50% of women are asymptomatic, the remaining women complain of a copious, frothy, often malodorous discharge that is yellow to greenish (see Table 16-1). They usually experience soreness of the vulva, external dysuria, and dyspareunia. A pelvic examination often reveals vaginal inflammation, and visually the exocervix is often described as strawberry-like because of numerous punctate hemorrhages.

Of available methods for diagnosing trichomoniasis, the most rapid and economical is a direct wet mount examination of vaginal secretions. However, studies have revealed that motile trichomonads are observed only in 50% to 70% of culture-confirmed cases.[18] An important note is that the skill and expertise of the microscopist directly affect the results of a wet mount microscopic examination. Hence this and other specimen-related factors could be a source of the variation observed in the detection of motile trichomonads.

If a wet mount examination is negative for motile trichomonads yet trichomoniasis is strongly suspected, a culture or DNA probe test should be performed. Both of these tests provide equivalent or greater sensitivity and specificity for the detection of *T. vaginalis* but may be less desirable because of the additional time and cost required.[9,19]

A characteristic and useful feature of *T. vaginalis* infection is an elevation in the pH of the vaginal secretions (i.e., pH 5.0 to 6.0). Wet mount examination also reveals numerous white blood cells, often clumped, and a mixed bacterial flora with lactobacilli usually present but in reduced numbers. In addition, the KOH preparation often produces a positive amine test.

Treatment for *T. vaginalis* infection in women and men consists of metronidazole (or tinidazole). Oral therapy is preferred because it ensures that all potential sites (vagina, urethra, periurethral glands, prostate, and epididymis) that may harbor the organism are treated. Simultaneous treatment of sexual partners is necessary to prevent reinfection. Rarely, treatment failures have been observed because of *T. vaginalis* strains resistant to metronidazole. In such cases, tinidazole or paromomycin has been used successfully.

Atrophic Vaginitis

In perimenopausal and postmenopausal women, the vaginal epithelium changes because of the reduction in estrogen production. These changes include thinning of the vaginal epithelium and decreased glycogen production. As glycogen production in the vagina decreases, so does the presence of lactobacilli and their metabolic by-product lactic acid. These changes can lead to the development of atrophic vaginitis, with mild to moderate conditions being asymptomatic. However on rare occasions, these changes induce significant alterations in the vaginal microflora with overgrowth of nonacidophilic bacteria (e.g., gram-positive cocci, gram-negative rods) and the disappearance of lactobacilli (see Table 16-1).

In the rare severe cases of atrophic vaginitis, women complain of vaginal dryness, vaginal soreness, dyspareunia, and spotting. A pelvic examination reveals a thin, diffusely red vaginal mucosa with little to no vaginal folding.

Vaginal secretions are characteristically alkaline with the pH usually greater than 5.0. A wet mount examination reveals numerous white blood cells and a small number of red blood cells. In addition to the usual squamous epithelial cells, parabasal and to a lesser extent basal cells may be present. The characteristic large rods of lactobacilli are decreased, with numerous cocci (gram-positive) and coliforms (gram-negative rods) predominating. The KOH preparation and amine tests are negative.

Treatment of atrophic vaginitis is easy and involves the replacement of estrogen. Localized replacement using topical vaginal ointments can be used, but recurrence often necessitates the use of a systemic estrogen regimen such as oral or transcutaneous (the patch) replacement.

STUDY QUESTIONS

1. Which of the following devices should be used to collect a sample of vaginal secretions?
   A. Cervical brush on a teflon shaft
   B. Cotton-tipped swab on a wooden shaft
   C. Polyester-tipped swab on a plastic shaft
   D. Wool-tipped swab on a wooden shaft
2. Which of the following organisms is adversely affected if a vaginal secretions specimen is refrigerated?
   A. *Chlamydia trachomatis*
   B. *Candida albicans*
   C. *Gardnerella vaginalis*
   D. *Trichomonas vaginalis*
3. Which range of pH values is associated with secretions from a healthy vagina?
   A. 3.8 to 4.5
   B. 4.5 to 5.8
   C. 5.8 to 6.5
   D. 7.0 to 7.4

4. Which of the following elements is considered abnormal when present in vaginal secretions?
   A. Bacteria
   B. Pseudohyphae
   C. Yeast
   D. White blood cells
5. Which of the following organisms and substances is responsible for the normal pH of the vagina?
   A. *Gardnerella vaginalis* and its metabolic by-product succinic acid
   B. *Lactobacilli* spp. and their metabolic by-product lactic acid
   C. *Mobiluncus* spp. and their metabolic by-product acetic acid
   D. *Prevotella* spp. and their metabolic by-product phenylacetic acid
6. Which of the following statements best describes a clue cell?
   A. Degenerating squamous epithelial cells with distinctive keratohyalin granulation
   B. Budding yeast (e.g., blastoconidia) with small coccobacilli adhering to their surfaces
   C. Squamous epithelial cells with numerous bacteria adhering to their outer cell membranes
   D. White blood cells with numerous bacteria completely covering them such that they appear as floating spherical orbs of bacteria
7. Which of the following vaginal secretion results correlate with health?
   A. pH 3.9; white blood cells, 3+
   B. pH 4.2; white blood cells, 1+
   C. pH 4.8; white blood cells, rare
   D. pH 5.5; white blood cells, 2+
8. Which of the following statements best describes the microbial flora of a healthy vagina?
   A. Large gram-positive rods predominate.
   B. Large gram-positive cocci predominate.
   C. Small gram-negative rods predominate.
   D. Small gram-variable coccobacilli predominate.
9. Which of the following tests is most helpful in differentiating red blood cells from yeast in vaginal secretions?
   A. pH
   B. Amine test
   C. Wet mount examination
   D. KOH preparation and examination
10. Which of the following vaginal secretion findings is most diagnostic for bacterial vaginosis?
    A. pH 5.0
    B. Clue cells
    C. Pseudohyphae
    D. Parabasal cells

11. Which of the following substances is responsible for the foul, fishy odor obtained when the "whiff" test is performed on vaginal secretions?
   A. Lactic acid
   B. Polyamine
   C. Trimethylamine
   D. Hydrogen peroxide

12. Select the condition that correlates best with the following vaginal secretion results:

   pH: 5.9
   Amine test: positive
   KOH examination: negative
   Wet mount examination: bacteria: mixed bacterial flora
   WBC: 4+

   A. Normal, indicating a healthy vagina
   B. Bacterial vaginosis
   C. Candidiasis
   D. Trichomoniasis

13. Select the condition that correlates best with the following vaginal secretion results:

   pH: 4.6
   Amine test: negative
   KOH examination: negative
   Wet mount examination: bacteria: large rods predominate
   WBC: 1+

   A. Normal, indicating a healthy vagina
   B. Bacterial vaginosis
   C. Candidiasis
   D. Trichomoniasis

CASE 16-1

A 49-year-old perimenopausal female is seen by her gynecologist for a routine annual Pap smear. Before the examination, the health care provider asked if she had any concerns, to which the patient stated that she has been noticing a foul vaginal odor, particularly following intercourse with her husband. A sample of her vaginal secretions was collected and the following results obtained.

Vaginal Secretion Results

Wet Mount Examination
   pH: 5.0
Bacteria: rare large rods, few small rods, many coccobacilli
WBCs: rare
Other: clue cells present

KOH Preparation and Examination
   Amine test: positive
   KOH examination: negative

1. Based on the patient information and the vaginal fluid results provided, what is the most likely diagnosis?
2. Discuss the formation of the substance responsible for the foul odor described by this patient.
3. Explain why the foul odor is more noticeable after unprotected intercourse.
4. Briefly describe the development of this disorder in a typical women.
5. When performing vaginal secretion analysis, what is the single most diagnostic finding associated with this condition?
6. Why are so few white blood cells present in this condition?

WBCs, White blood cells.

REFERENCES

1. Woods GL: Specimen collection and handling for diagnosis of infectious diseases. In Henry JB, editor: Clinical diagnosis and management by laboratory methods, ed 20, Philadelphia, 2001, WB Saunders.
2. Eschenbach DA, Davick PR, Williams BL, et al: Prevalence of hydrogen peroxide-producing *Lactobacillus* species in normal women and women with bacterial vaginosis. J Clin Microbiol 27:251-256, 1989.
3. Hillier SL, Krohn MA, Rabe LK, et al: The normal vaginal flora, H_2O_2-producing lactobacilli and bacterial vaginosis in pregnant women. Clin Infect Dis 16(Suppl 4):S273-S281, 1993.
4. Clinical and Laboratory Standards Institute (CLSI): Provider-performed microscopy testing: approved guideline, CLSI Document HS02-A, Wayne, PA, 2003, CLSI.
5. Metzger GD: Laboratory diagnosis of vaginal infections. Clin Lab Sci 11:47-52, 1998.
6. Erlandsen SL, Magney JE: Color atlas of histology, St Louis, 1992, Mosby–Year Book.
7. Redondo-Lopez V, Cook RL, Sobel JD: Emerging role of lactobacilli in the control and maintenance of the bacterial microflora. Rev Infect Dis 12:856-872, 1990.
8. Spence M. Trichomoniasis, Contemp OB/GYN 1992 Nov 132-141.
9. Sobel JD: Vaginitis. N Engl J Med 337:1896-1903, 1997.
10. Koneman EW, Allen SD, Janda WM, et al: Color atlas and textbook of diagnostic microbiology, ed 5, Philadelphia, 1997, Lippincott-Raven.
11. Hill GB: The microbiology of bacterial vaginosis. Am J Obstet Gynecol 169:450-454, 1993.
12. McGregor JA, French JI, Parker R, et al: Prevention of premature birth by screening and treatment for common genital tract infections: results of a prospective controlled evaluation. Am J Obstet Gynecol 173:157-167, 1995.
13. Amsel R, Totten PA, Spiegel CA, et al: Nonspecific vaginitis: diagnostic criteria and microbial and epidemiologic associations. Am J Med 74:14-22, 1983.
14. Fidel PL, Vazquez JA, Sobel JD: *Canidida glabrata*: review of epidemiology, pathogenesis, and clinical disease with comparison to *C. albicans*. Clin Microbiol Rev 12:80-96, 1999.

15. Pearson RD: Other protozoan diseases. In Goldman L, Bennett JC, editors: Cecil textbook of medicine, ed 21, Philadelphia, 2000, WB Saunders.

16. Sparling PF: Introduction to sexually transmitted diseases and common syndromes. In Goldman L, Bennett JC, editors: Cecil textbook of medicine, ed 21, Philadelphia, 2000, WB Saunders.

17. Laga M, Manoka AT, Kivuvu M, et al: Non-ulcerative sexually transmitted diseases as risk factors for HIV-1 transmission in women: result for a cohort study. AIDS 7:95-102, 1993.

18. Krieger JN, Tam MR, Stevens CE, et al: Diagnosis of trichomoniasis: comparison of conventional wet-mount examination with cytologic studies, cultures, and monoclonal antibody staining of direct specimens. JAMA 259:1223-1227, 1988.

19. DeMeo LR, Draper DL, McGregor JA, et al: Evaluation of a deoxyribonucleic acid probe for the detection of *Trichomonas vaginalis* in vaginal secretions. Am J Obstet Gynecol 174:1339-1342, 1996.

BIBLIOGRAPHY

COLA test procedure: direct wet preps, COLA, 9881 Broken Land Parkway, Suite 200, Columbia, MD 21046-1195, Jan 2001, www.cola.org.

COLA test procedure: fern test (amniotic fluid crystallization test), COLA, 9881 Broken Land Parkway, Suite 200, Columbia, MD 21046-1195, Jan 2001, www.cola.org.

COLA test procedure: the potassium hydroxide prep, COLA, 9881 Broken Land Parkway, Suite 200, Columbia, MD 21046-1195, Jan 2001, www.cola.org.

Eschenbach DA, Hillier SL, Critchlow C, et al: Diagnosis and clinical manifestations of bacterial vaginosis. Am J Obstet Gynecol 158:819-828, 1988.

Lossick JC: Epidemiology of urogenital trichomoniasis. In Honigberg BM, editor: *Trichomonads* parasitic in humans, New York, 1990, Springer-Verlag.

Markell EK, Voge M, John DT: Medical parasitology, ed 7, Philadelphia, 1992, WB Saunders.

National Network of STD/HIV Prevention Training Centers: Examination of vaginal wet preps (video): http://depts.washington.edu/nnptc/online_training/wet_preps_video.html. Accessed May 1, 2011.

Automation of Urine and Body Fluid Analysis

LEARNING OBJECTIVES

After studying this chapter, the student should be able to:

1. Describe the principle of reflectance photometry.
2. Discuss and differentiate between semi-automated and fully automated urine chemistry analyzers.
3. State advantages gained by performing automated urine sediment analysis.
4. Compare and contrast the two technologies used to perform fully automated urine microscopy analysis—flow cytometry and flowcell digital imaging.
5. Discuss the advantages and disadvantages of current automated body fluid analyzers.

CHAPTER OUTLINE

Automation of Urinalysis
Urine Chemistry Analyzers
Automated Microscopy Analyzers
Fully Automated Urinalysis Systems

Automation of Body Fluid Analysis
Body Fluid Cell Counts Using Hematology Analyzers
Body Fluid Cell Counts Using iQ200

KEY TERMS

fully automated urinalysis indicates that the entire urinalysis—physical, chemical, and microscopic examinations—is performed by analyzers and results integrated by a computer system to produce a complete urinalysis report. Two analyzers are required, as well as a connectivity system that brings urine samples (in racks) to the sampling position of each analyzer for testing and last to an off-loading area. A urine chemistry analyzer performs the physical and chemical analyses; these are followed by urine particle analysis using a urine microscopy analyzer.

reflectance photometry the detection and quantification of light intensity that scatters from a surface.

semi-automated indicates that some steps are performed manually and others are automated.

semi-automated urinalysis a urinalysis that is partially automated using a reflectance photometry–based analyzer to interpret commercial reagent strip results (i.e., chemical examination). The urine's physical parameters—color and clarity—and the urine microscopic examination results (if performed) are obtained manually.

AUTOMATION OF URINALYSIS

A goal of the urinalysis laboratory is to maximize productivity and testing quality, while keeping costs and turnaround time at a minimum. The first reagent strip tests to determine the chemical composition of urine were developed in the 1950s in an effort to achieve these goals. Since that time, reagent strips have streamlined the chemical examination, significantly reducing the time required and increasing the number of specimens that can be analyzed in a given time period. Efforts next focused on ensuring consistency in reagent strip reading (e.g., color interpretation, timing), reducing the amount of specimen handling, and increasing specimen throughput. These efforts have resulted in the development of instruments that assess reagent strip results and automate evaluation of the physical characteristics of urine. In the early 1980s, automation of the microscopic examination was achieved by the development of a urine microscopy analyzer (i.e., Yellow Iris). Today, automated urine chemistry analyzers and urine microscopy analyzers are available that can be used as standalone instruments or linked together to enable a fully automated urinalysis system.

As with all technology, new analyzers and methods are constantly being developed and modified. The combinations of analyzers or urinalysis workstations available through the collaboration of manufacturers are dynamic and change with time. Note that despite our global economy, instruments that are available in Europe or Asia may not be available in the United States, and vice versa. Although the instruments presented in this chapter are limited to a few of the most commonly encountered in U.S. laboratories at the writing of this chapter, the basic approach to testing and the measurement principles remain applicable.

Urine Chemistry Analyzers

Semi-automation of the chemical examination of urine was developed to standardize the interpretation of reagent strip results. Consistent, unbiased, and accurate color interpretation was the goal when urine chemistry analyzers were developed. All reagent strip reading instruments, regardless of manufacturer, use reflectance photometry to interpret the color formed on each test pad. These **semi-automated** instruments require the user to properly dip the reagent strip and place it onto a platform. After this is done, the instrument automatically performs the remaining steps in the analysis: reading the reaction pads at the appropriate read time and moving the strip to a waste container.

Some manufacturers include a color compensation pad on their reagent strips. The purpose of this pad is to assess urine color and use it when interpreting the colors that develop on each reaction pad. In other words, the instrument modifies test results by essentially subtracting the contribution of urine color from the color change obtained on the test reaction pads. Note that this is possible only when reagent strip results are interpreted using an automated instrument. Consequently, depending on the intended use—manual or automated—reagent strips with or without a color compensation pad are available.

Principle of Reflectance Photometry. Reflectance photometry quantifies the intensity of the colored product produced on the reagent strip reaction pads. When light strikes a matte or unpolished surface (e.g., a reagent strip), some light is absorbed, and the remaining light is scattered or reflected in all directions. The scattered light is known as *diffuse reflectance*. The incident light is usually of one or more wavelengths, whereas only reflected light of a single, specific wavelength is detected. Reflectance photometers are calibrated using reflectance standards such as magnesium carbonate or barium sulfate that "completely" reflect all incident light. Because the potential colors that develop on each reaction pad dictate the wavelengths of light needed for reflectance measurements, each reflectance photometer must have a way of

selecting the appropriate wavelength for each test pad. To obtain the desired wavelength, reflectance photometers use (1) polychromatic light and a series of filters to isolate specific wavelengths, or (2) a series of monochromatic light sources (e.g., light-emitting diodes [LEDs]).

Reflectance measurements are performed at specific wavelengths and are expressed as percent reflectance (% R). The percent reflectance (% R) is the ratio of the test pad reflectance (R_t) compared with the calibration reflectance (R_c), multiplied by the percent reflectivity of the calibration reference, which is usually 100%.

Equation 17-1

$$\% \, R = \frac{R_t}{R_c} \times 100$$

The relationship between concentration and reflectance is not linear. Therefore a microprocessor is needed to apply complex algorithms that convert the relationship to a linear one.

Semi-Automated Chemistry Analyzers. The term **semi-automated urinalysis** indicates that an analyzer is used to interpret the commercial reagent strip results of urine when the chemical examination is performed. The term *semi-automated* indicates that the user performs the remaining steps of the urinalysis—physical examination of color and clarity, as well as the microscopic examination, if performed.

Numerous reagent strip manufacturers are located worldwide, and many market a reflectance photometer for use with their reagent strips. Urine chemistry analyzers commonly used in the United States are listed in Table 17-1. Several semi-automated instruments are shown in Figures 17-1 through 17-3. All instruments are user friendly and include various display and audio prompts to aid in their operation. Most semi-automated systems require the user to (1) press a button to ready the analyzer for analysis, (2) properly dip the reagent strip into a suitable urine sample, (3) blot the strip to remove excess urine, and (4) place the strip onto an intake platform. A microprocessor controls the remaining aspects of testing: It mechanically moves the strip through the instrument; at the appropriate timed interval, reflectance readings are taken; results are adjusted for urine color and are stored by the microprocessor; and last, the strip is moved to a waste container. Patient identifiers, user identification, and the physical parameters of the urine can be manually entered into the analyzer; a barcode reader can be used to identify specimens. Typically, results print out, are stored within the analyzer, or can be transmitted to a laboratory information system (LIS). The quantity of patient and quality control results that can be stored on-board varies with the analyzer. Table 17-2 lists some basic features of semi-automated urine chemistry analyzers. Daily maintenance consists primarily of cleaning the transport platform and areas in contact with the reagent strips and emptying the waste container of used reagent strips.

TABLE 17-1	Selected Urine Chemistry Analyzers	
Manufacturer	**Analyzer**	**Comments**
ARKRAY Inc., Kyoto, Japan	Diascreen 50 AUTION MAX AX-4280, AX-4030	• Semi-automated • Fully automated • Includes color (photometric), clarity (light scatter), specific gravity (refractive index)
Iris Diagnostics, Chatsworth, CA	iChem 100 iChem Velocity	• Semi-automated • Fully automated • Includes color and clarity (transmitted and scattered light), specific gravity (refractive index)
Roche Diagnostics, Indianapolis, IN	URISYS 1800, Criterion II, COBAS u411 URISYS 2400, 1800	• Semi-automated • Fully automated • Includes color (reflectance photometry); SG and clarity by physical determination
Siemens Healthcare Diagnostics Inc., Deerfield, IL	Clinitek 50, 100, 200, 200+, 500, Status, Advantus Clinitek ATLAS	• Semi-automated • Fully automated • Includes color (reflectance photometry), clarity (transmitted and scattered light), specific gravity (refractive index)

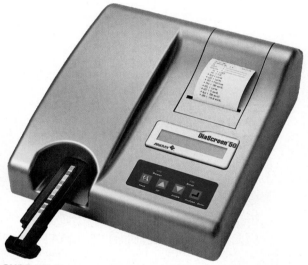

FIGURE 17-1 Diascreen 50 semi-automated urine chemistry analyzer. *(Image courtesy ARKRAY Inc.)*

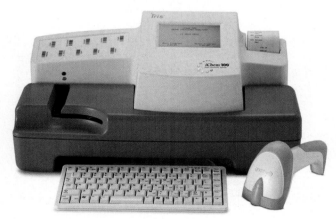

FIGURE 17-2 iChem 100 semi-automated urine chemistry analyzer. *(Image courtesy Iris Diagnostics.)*

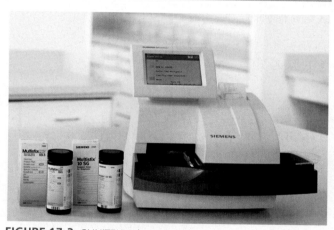

FIGURE 17-3 CLINITEK Advantus semi-automated urine chemistry analyzer. *(Image courtesy Siemens Healthcare Diagnostics Inc.)*

Fully Automated Chemistry Analyzers. When using a *fully automated* urine chemistry analyzer, the user simply places labeled tubes of urine into a sample rack or carousel (Figure 17-4). Testing is initiated by pressing a button on the instrument display or panel. From this point on, the instrument controls movement of the specimen rack, identifies each sample, mixes it, aspirates urine using a sample probe, and dispenses it onto a reagent strip. At the appropriate read time, each reaction is read using the appropriate wavelengths of light for that specific test.

Three fully automated urine chemistry analyzers are shown in Figures 17-5 through 17-7. These instruments also determine the physical characteristics of urine—color, clarity, and specific gravity (SG)—but the methods used to do so vary. To perform urine color assessment, some manufacturers include an additional pad on the reagent strip to determine urine color by reflectance photometry; others use spectrophotometry at multiple wavelengths to assign color. Light transmittance or light

TABLE 17-2	Typical Features of Semi-automated Urine Chemistry Analyzers
Tests performed	Blood, leukocyte esterase, nitrite, protein, glucose, ketone, bilirubin, urobilinogen, pH, specific gravity
Measurement principle	Intensity of color on reagent strip pads measured by reflectance photometry; automatic adjustments made for urine color
Sample handling	User *manually* dips and places strip onto instrument platform.
Sample ID entry	User manually enters, uses a barcode reader, or downloads from LIS.
Results	Printout and on-board data storage; can interface to LIS Color and clarity can be *manually* entered to be included on report and printout.
Daily maintenance	Clean reagent strip platform, empty used reagent strip container

LIS, Laboratory information system.

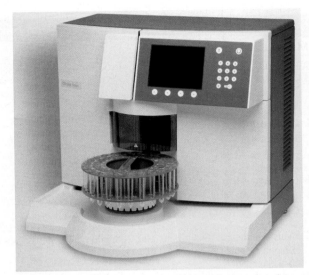

FIGURE 17-5 CLINITEK Atlas, an automated urine chemistry analyzer. *(Image courtesy Siemens Healthcare Diagnostics Inc.)*

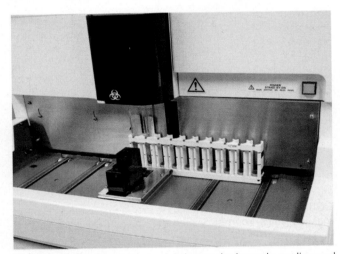

FIGURE 17-4 Rack of specimen tubes at the barcode reading and sampling station on the iChem Velocity.

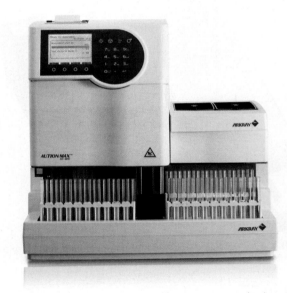

FIGURE 17-6 AUTION Max AX-4030, an automated urine chemistry analyzer. *(Image courtesy ARKRAY Inc.)*

scatter is used to determine urine clarity. Despite the universal availability of an SG reagent strip test, most fully automated chemistry analyzers use refractive index because of its greater accuracy. A microprocessor collates all results—color, clarity, SG, and chemistry tests—which are sent to data storage but are also printed on a report form or are sent to an LIS.

Automated Microscopy Analyzers

Automated urine sediment analyzers assist in decreasing labor costs and increasing productivity in the urinalysis laboratory. Because uncentrifuged urine is used, the time spent in handling and preparing concentrated urine sediment for manual microscopy is eliminated; this also reduces exposure to potential biohazards. Other benefits include increased standardization of the microscopic

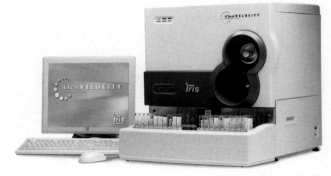

FIGURE 17-7 iChem Velocity fully automated urine chemistry analyzer. *(Image courtesy Iris Diagnostics.)*

examination, which enhances the accuracy and repro-ducibility (precision) of results. Second, because these analyzers are usually interfaced to an LIS, manual data entry is decreased, which reduces the potential for tran-scription errors. Last, significant data storage is available in some instruments such that urinalysis results can be archived and retrieved later for consultations, continuing education, competency assessments, or training purposes (e.g., iQ200 analyzer).

Currently, two automated urine microscopy instru-ments are available and they differ in the technology used to perform the analysis. The Iris iQ200 Microscopy Analyzer is the most recent in a series of automated urine microscopy instruments developed by IRIS Diagnostics Inc. (Chatsworth, CA), the pioneer in urine microscopic instrumentation since the 1980s (Figure 17-8). With the Iris iQ200 analyzer, analysis is based on flowcell digital imaging followed by urine particle recognition using pro-prietary neural network software. The iQ200 uses pat-ented technologies to capture and automatically classify digital images of urine particles.

Urine microscopy analyzers of the second type use flow cytometry to identify and categorize the particles in urine. The UF-1000i analyzer and its predecessor the UF-100 analyzer were developed by Sysmex Corporation (Mundelein, IL) (Figure 17-9). Urine particles are identi-fied and categorized based on forward scatter, fluores-cence, impedance signals (UF-100), and adaptive cluster analysis.[1]

iQ200 Urine Microscopy Analyzer. The iQ200 Micros-copy Analyzer can be purchased as a standalone instru-ment. It is an automated system that performs the microscopic examination of urine, as well as cell counts on body fluids (see "Automation of Body Fluid Analysis").

Before the aspiration of 1 mL of urine, the analyzer mixes the sample. The aspirated urine is immediately sandwiched within a special fluid called *lamina* (iQ Lamina, Iris Diagnostics) that flows through a propri-etary flowcell. The lamina and the flowcell are key to hydrodynamically orienting the particles in the urine. The flow path is at a specific depth of focus that enables precise microscopic viewing. The field of view of the microscope is coupled to a digital video camera, and stroboscopic illumination freezes the particles in motion as they stream past, which ensures blur-free imaging. With each sample, the camera captures 500 frames, digitizes them, and sends them to a computer for pro-cessing (Figure 17-10). Note that the individual parti-cles within each of the 500 frames are isolated as separate images, and the Auto-Particle Recognition (APR; Iris Diagnostics) software classifies each image (Figure 17-11).

The APR software is a highly trained neural network that uses size, shape, contrast, and texture to automati-cally classify each image into one of 12 categories (Table 17-3). Next, the APR software calculates the concentra-tion of each particle present. The results obtained for

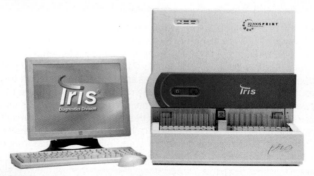

FIGURE 17-8 iQ200 microscopy analyzer. *(Image courtesy Iris Diagnostics.)*

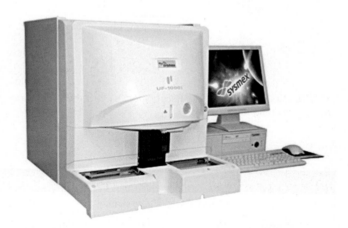

FIGURE 17-9 Sysmex UF1000i analyzer. *(Image courtesy Sysmex Corporation, Mundelein, IL.)*

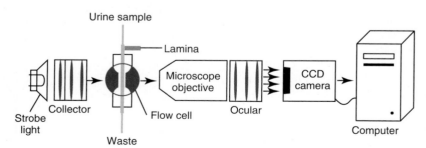

FIGURE 17-10 Diagram of the iQ200 digital flow capture process. *(Image courtesy Iris Diagnostics.)*

each sample are compared with user-defined auto-release criteria, and if the criteria are met, results can be sent to the LIS. If the criteria are not met, or if the option to auto-release reports to the LIS is not used by the laboratory, the results are stored and the user can review them at anytime on the computer monitor.

Using the computer monitor, the user can review results, visually assess the particles present, and subclassify them into the 26 additional categories, as listed in Table 17-3. Subclassification is used to indicate the specific types of crystals, casts, and nonsquamous epithelial cells present, as well as to identify pseudohyphae, trichomonads, or fat (Figure 17-12). Additional free text comments can be added to reports as needed, such as "Ascorbic acid positive" or "Presence of fat confirmed."

The average time required for an experienced user to review urinalysis results from a single urine sample is approximately 30 seconds. However, laboratories can select their own auto-release criteria. When urinalysis results do not exceed these criteria, the results do not require review and are automatically sent to the LIS. Results that exceed user-defined values are available at

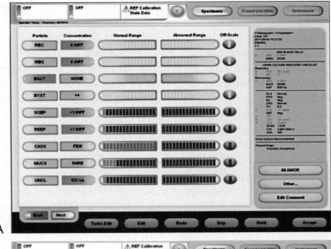

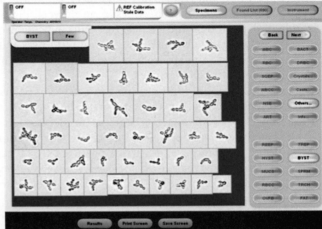

A

B

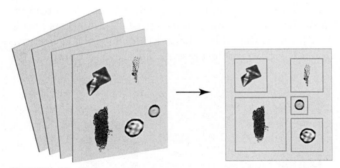

FIGURE 17-11 Auto-Particle Recognition (APR) process. *(Image courtesy Iris Diagnostics.)*

FIGURE 17-12 Displays of iQ200 urinalysis results. **A,** On-screen review of iQ200 results. The results for this sample did not auto-release because the amount of some microscopic elements resided in the "Particle Verification Range" set by the user. These results appear "yellow" and require review as established by this laboratory. Results that appear "green" are in the normal range and those that appear "red" are considered abnormal but do not need verification (as established by the user-defined criteria). When no yellow results are present, results can be automatically released without review or verification. **B,** On-screen display of automatically classified images of budding yeast (BYST). *(Image courtesy Iris Diagnostics.)*

TABLE 17-3	iQ200 Autoclassification and Subclassification Categories for Urine Sediment Particles					
	Blood Cells	**Crystals**	**Casts**	**Epithelial Cells**	**Yeast**	**Others**
Autoclassified *by analyzer*	RBCs WBCs WBC clumps	Unclassified crystals*	Hyaline Unclassified casts*	Squamous Nonsquamous†	Budding yeast	Bacteria Mucus Sperm
Subclassified *by user*	RBC clumps	Amorphous Calcium carbonate Calcium oxalate Calcium phosphate Triple phosphate Uric acid Cystine Tyrosine Leucine Unclassified crystals	Granular Cellular Waxy Broad RBCs WBCs Epithelial cells Fatty Unclassified casts	Transitional Renal	Yeast with pseudohyphae	*Trichomonads* Fat Oval fat bodies

RBCs, Red blood cells; *WBCs,* white blood cells.
*Unclassified crystals and casts can be reported as such, or user can specifically subclassify by type.
†Nonsquamous epithelial cells can be reported as such, or user can specifically subclassify as transitional or renal.

any time for the user to review, subclassify, and forward to the LIS. Therefore the number of reports that actually require user review will vary with the auto-release criteria selected by the laboratory and with its patient population.

Sysmex UF-1000I and UF-100 Flow Cytometers. The UF-1000i analyzer and its predecessor, the UF-100, are instruments that use flow cytometry and impedance to categorize particles in urine on the basis of their size, shape, volume, and staining characteristics. Although the technology in both analyzers is the same, changes have been made in the UF-1000i to enhance the detection of bacteria and improve the classification of white blood cells (WBCs).[1,2] Changes in the UF-1000i analyzer include a separate channel for bacterial analysis and the monitoring of lateral or side scatter, which improves detection of bacteria. In addition, a red semi-conductor laser is used in contrast to the argon laser used in the UF-100 analyzer.

For automated particle analysis, the UF-1000i analyzer requires a 4 mL sample volume; however, if the instrument is used in the manual mode, only 1 mL of urine is required. After aspiration into the analyzer, the urine sample is divided into two channels because the diluent, the staining time, and the staining temperature for sediment analysis differ from those used for bacterial analysis. Urine particles are oriented into a single file by flowcell and laminar flow dynamics. As each channel passes through the flowcell, it is analyzed by a single red semi-conductor laser (λ635 nm), and particles in the urine are categorized on the basis of (1) forward scatter, (2) fluorescence staining characteristics, (3) impedance signals, (4) adaptive cluster analysis, and (5) side scatter, which is specific for detection of bacteria (Figure 17-13).

As with all flow cytometry systems, results are displayed as scattergrams and histograms (Figure 17-14). The UF-1000i is able to report particles as red blood cells (RBCs), WBCs, epithelial cells (squamous), hyaline casts, or bacteria (Table 17-4). Note that the analyzer "flags"

TABLE 17-4	UF-1000i Particle Detection Categories
Particles Enumerated	**Flagged Particles**
RBCs	Nonhyaline (pathologic) casts*
WBCs	Crystals*
Epithelial cells	Small round cells*
Hyaline casts	Yeast
Bacteria	Mucus
	Sperm

RBCs, Red blood cells; *WBCs,* white blood cells.
*Manual microscopic examination by user is required to specifically identify and categorize the type present.

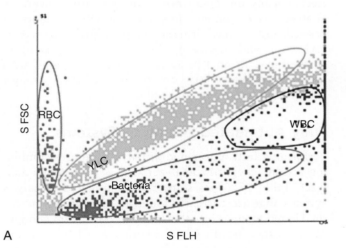

A

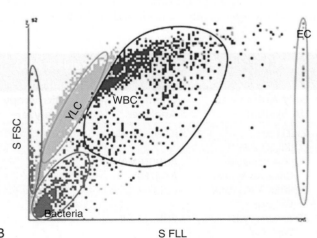

B

FIGURE 17-14 Sysmex UF-1000i urine particle results. **A,** Scattergram of forward scatter (S_FSC) versus fluorescent light intensity-high sensitivity (S_FLH). **B,** Scattergram of forward scatter (S_FSC) versus fluorescent light intensity–low sensitivity (S_FLL). *EC,* Epithelial cells; *RBC,* red blood cells; *WBC,* white blood cells; *YLC,* yeastlike cells. *(Images courtesy Sysmex Corporation, Mundelein, IL.)*

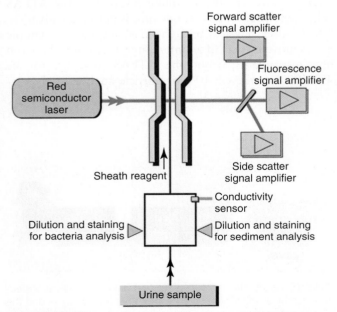

FIGURE 17-13 Diagram of urine particle analysis in the Sysmex UF-1000i. *(Image courtesy Sysmex Corporation, Mundelein, IL.)*

specimens when it detects the presence of the following particles: casts (other than hyaline), crystals, yeast, mucus, small round cells (i.e., transitional or renal cells), or sperm. Determining the specific identity of elements in "flagged" specimens requires a microscopic review of the urine by the user. In other words, to classify nonhyaline casts (granular, cellular, RBC, WBC, crystalline), identify crystals (e.g., calcium oxalate, uric acid, cystine), and categorize the particles identified as small round cells as transitional cells, renal cells, or another small particle, a manual microscopic examination is required. In addition, studies using the UF-100 analyzer have identified an issue with false-positive results for RBCs caused by crystals, yeast, and sperm, or during analysis of urine samples transported in preservative tubes, such as BD Vacutainer Plus UA Preservative tubes (BD, Franklin Lakes, NJ), BD C&S Preservative tubes, and Greiner Stabilur Preservative tubes (Greiner Bio-One N.A., Inc., Monroe, NC).[3-5] Large quantities of amorphous precipitates in refrigerated urine specimens can also present a challenge.

Results from the UF-1000i or the UF-100 can be electronically linked to those from the urine chemistry analyzer to obtain an integrated urinalysis report. If desired, user-defined criteria can be adjusted to reduce review rate and increase productivity. When the analyzer is interfaced to an LIS, results can be compared with user-defined auto-release criteria and reported, or they can be held for review and follow-up.

Fully Automated Urinalysis Systems

Performing fully automated urinalyses requires combining a urine chemistry analyzer with a microscopy analyzer. Table 17-5 lists some fully automated urinalysis systems that are currently found in laboratories across the United States. Note that some of the system configurations listed are no longer manufactured but are still actively in use, and that other configurations are available elsewhere. Fully automated urinalysis systems

automatically identify and process each barcoded sample tube according to the tests requested in the LIS. These systems are flexible and user-friendly. Urine specimens can undergo physical and chemistry testing only, microscopy testing only, or both (i.e., complete urinalysis). After analysis, a computer system integrates the physical, chemical, and microscopic results to create a urinalysis report that can be sent to the LIS and printed.

iRICELL Urinalysis Systems. The iRICELL Automated Urinalysis Systems (iRICELL*3000*, iRICELL *2000*) (Iris Diagnostics) consists of the iChem Velocity urine chemistry analyzer companioned with the iQ200 (Figure 17-15). Before the iChem Velocity, the iQ200 was available in combination with the AUTION MAX AX-4280 chemistry analyzer. To perform a complete urinalysis, a minimum of 3 mL urine is poured into a barcode-labeled tube. Specific tubes are not required; rather a variety of tubes can be used, including commercial urinalysis tubes (e.g., KOVA, Vacuette, BD) or disposable glass test tubes (e.g., 16 × 100 mm). The tubes of urine are placed into racks (10-position) that are loaded directly onto the system and sequentially moved to the first sampling station at the iChem Velocity. The identity of each sample is determined by reading the tube's barcode label, the sample is mixed, and the urine is aspirated. After physical and chemical analyses, the rack moves across a connecting bridge to the iQ200 for microscopic analysis.

CLINITEK AUWi System. The CLINITEK AUWi System uses an ATLAS urine chemistry analyzer connected to a UF-1000i flow cytometer to perform fully automated urinalyses (Figure 17-16). For a complete urinalysis, 5 mL of uncentrifuged urine is poured into a barcode-labeled tube, which is placed into a 10-place sample rack. Tubes up to 16 mm wide can be used, but they must be "lipless" for 10 samples to fit in a rack. The sample racks are placed onto the system, and as each rack is moved to the sampling position of the ATLAS analyzer, the barcoded sample tube is automatically identified. After physical and chemical testing, the sample racks move by way of an interconnecting bridge between the instruments, from the ATLAS analyzer to the UF-1000i or the UF-100 for particle analysis.

TABLE 17-5	Fully Automated Urinalysis (UA) Systems	
Fully Automated UA System	**Chemistry Analyzer**	**Microscopy Analyzer**
iRICELL*3000*, iRICELL*2000**	iChem Velocity*	iQ200*
iQ200 Automated Urinalysis System	AUTION MAX AX-4280[†]	iQ200*
CLINITEK AUWi Work Cell System[‡]	CLINITEK Atlas[‡]	UF-1000i[§]
ADVIA Urinalysis Work Cell[‡]	CLINITEK Atlas[‡]	UF-100[§]

*Manufactured by Iris Diagnostics, Chatsworth, CA.
[†]Manufactured by ARKRAY Inc., Kyoto, Japan.
[‡]Manufactured by Siemens Healthcare Diagnostics Inc., Deerfield, IL.
[§]Manufactured by Sysmex Corporation, Mundelein, IL.

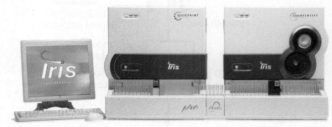

FIGURE 17-15 iRICELL*3000*, a Fully Automated Urinalysis System that combines the iChem Velocity urine chemistry analyzer and the iQ200 microscopy analyzer. *(Image courtesy Iris Diagnostics.)*

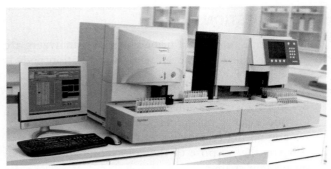

FIGURE 17-16 AUWi, a Fully Automated Urinalysis System that combines the Siemens CLINITEK Atlas chemistry analyzer and the Sysmex UF-1000i particle analyzer. *(Image courtesy Siemens Healthcare Diagnostics Inc.)*

AUTOMATION OF BODY FLUID ANALYSIS

Analysis of body fluids by manual hemacytometer methods is an ongoing challenge in clinical laboratories because these analyses are time-consuming to perform, require skilled personnel, show high interoperator variability, and are plagued by low precision (reproducibility). In contrast, automation offers better precision and turnaround times. However, body fluids with low cell counts (<30 cells/μL) present a challenge for automated systems. Despite this issue, automated analyzers could be used as a first step in triaging specimens (i.e., identifying those with low cell counts that require a manual hemacytometer count).

Note that despite the advantages of better precision, reduced interoperator variation, and shorter turnaround time, some issues with automated analyzers remain. For example, these analyzers cannot identify malignant cells. Therefore, any fluid that could potentially have malignant cells present should have a manual WBC differential performed using a stained cytospin preparation. Several analyzers that have been designed to perform body fluid cell counts are listed in Table 17-6. Note that it is the manufacturer's responsibility to have an intended use statement that clearly defines which body fluids have been approved by a regulatory agency for testing.[6] Similarly, it is the laboratory's responsibility to define the lower limits for cell counting and to clearly state when fluids must be analyzed by an alternate method (e.g., hemacytometer count).[6]

Body Fluid Cell Counts Using Hematology Analyzers

Many hematology analyzers have been used to perform body fluid cell counts; although they improve precision and turnaround time, problems have been encountered. Some of these problems occur because the matrix of body fluids differs from that of whole blood. Other problems are due to interference by large cells (mesothelial cells, macrophages, tumor cells) or noncellular

TABLE 17-6	Selected Automated Body Fluid Analyzers
Analyzer	**Body Fluids FDA Approved***
ADVIA 2120i with Body Fluids Software	Cerebrospinal fluid (CSF) Pleural Peritoneal Peritoneal dialysate Serous fluids
iQ200 using Body Fluids Module	CSF Pericardial Peritoneal Peritoneal dialysate Peritoneal lavage Pleural Serous fluids Synovial
Sysmex XE-5000 using Body Fluids mode	CSF Pleural Pericardial Peritoneal Peritoneal dialysate Serous fluids Synovial

*As of January, 2011.

particulate matter that can be present in body fluids. Last, most hematology analyzers based on impedance technology have high background counts that prevent or hinder accuracy in detecting low cell counts in body fluids (e.g., cerebrospinal fluid [CSF]). Precleaning the instrument may be required before body fluid analysis can be performed. One modification made for analyzing body fluids is that the duration of the cell count has been increased. This results in a higher number of cells counted and a concomitant increase in precision. Two hematology analyzers have been specifically modified to enhance body fluid cell counts: the ADVIA 2120i (Siemens Healthcare Diagnostics Inc., Deerfield, IL) and the Sysmex XE-5000 (Sysmex Corporation, Mundelein, IL).

Before CSF is analyzed using the ADVIA 2120i, the CSF sample must be pretreated for a minimum of 4 minutes using a special CSF reagent. This reagent fixes and converts RBCs to spheres.[7] For body fluid applications, the analyzer uses the basophil/lobularity channel, the peroxidase channel, and the RBC/platelet channel to determine the total nucleated cell count (TNC), the WBC count, and the RBC count, respectively.[8] Numeric data and scattergram results are provided. Because this analyzer is newly approved for the analysis of pleural and peritoneal fluids and peritoneal dialysates, its efficacy and statistical performance remain to be elucidated.

On the Sysmex XE-5000, a dedicated body fluids mode is used and all body fluids can be directly analyzed without dilution or pretreatment (enzyme digestion). A special software algorithm is used to count RBCs on the basis of sheath flow impedance, and because cell counting has been extended, precision is enhanced.[9] WBCs are counted using side scatter and fluorescence intensity after their nuclear DNA/RNA is stained with specific dyes. In addition to RBC and total WBC counts, a *partial* WBC differential is provided—mononuclear cells (lymphocytes and monocytes) and polymorphonuclear cells (PMNs; neutrophils, eosinophils, basophils). Macrophages and mesothelial cells are counted but are excluded from the cell counts.

Body fluid analysis using the Sysmex XE-5000 has some limitations. It is imperative that experienced users visually inspect the differential scatterplots of body fluids to (1) detect noncellular particulate matter (e.g., bacteria, cryptococcus), and (2) identify possible interference from large cells. In addition, when the WBC count is below 10×10^6 cells/L, differentiation between PMNs and mononuclear cells (MNCs) should not be done.[9]

Body Fluid Cell Counts Using iQ200

The method of cell measurement used by the iQ200 differs from that used on hematology analyzers. The iQ200, an automated microscopy analyzer primarily used to analyze cells and other particles in urine, can also be used to perform body fluid cell counts (see Table 17-6). However, its use requires the purchase of the Body Fluids software module. In contrast to hematology analyzers, body fluid analysis on the iQ200 can be performed at any time without prior cleaning or preparation of the instrument.

When the iQ200 is used, body fluids are diluted on the basis of the fluid type (e.g., CSF, serous) and its appearance (e.g., clear, bloody). Two dilutions are made in tubes: one using Iris diluent, the other using Iris RBC lysing reagent. Note that these tubes are labeled with *dilution-specific* barcodes, which enable automatic calculation of cell counts by the instrument based on the dilution prepared. The labeled tubes are placed in a sample rack and onto the instrument for analysis. The total cell count is determined using the dilution prepared with iQ diluent (unlysed), whereas the nucleated cell count is determined using the dilution prepared with the lysing agent. The difference between these two values (Total cell count − Nucleated cell count) is the RBC count.

When the iQ200 is used, the same digital flowcell imaging technology used for urine applies to body fluid analysis (see "iQ Microscopy Analyzer"). Numeric results and digital cell images are displayed for verification and manual editing, if desired.

STUDY QUESTIONS

1. When semi-automated urine chemistry analyzers are used, the color that develops on the reaction pads is measured by
   A. spectrophotometry.
   B. reflectance photometry.
   C. fluorescence photometry.
   D. comparing reaction pads with a color chart.
2. What is the purpose of the color compensation pad on reagent strips?
   A. To compensate for the effect of specific gravity on urine color
   B. To calibrate the instrument for color assessment of reaction pads
   C. To account for the contribution of urine color to the colors on the reaction pads
   D. To detect substances (e.g., phenazopyridine) that mask color development on the reaction pads
3. Select the TRUE statement regarding reflectance photometry.
   A. The amount of light that is absorbed is detected and measured.
   B. The same wavelength of light is used to evaluate all reaction pads.
   C. The intensity of light reflected from a polished surface is quantified.
   D. The relationship between reflectance and concentration is not linear.
4. Select the TRUE statement regarding semi-automated urine chemistry analyzers.
   A. Results cannot be automatically transmitted to an LIS.
   B. Specific gravity is usually determined by refractive index.
   C. Urine color and clarity are manually determined and entered into the analyzer.
   D. Well-mixed uncentrifuged urine is placed onto the intake platform for analysis.
5. The benefits of performing automated urine microscopy include all of the following EXCEPT
   A. Increases precision of microscopy results
   B. Decreases exposure to urine, a potential biohazard
   C. Increases the time required for the microscopic examination
   D. Decreases manual entry and potential transcription errors
6. Which of the following statements about the iQ200 microscopy analyzer is TRUE?
   A. Particle analysis is performed using flow cytometry.
   B. Urine particles are automatically classified into 12 categories.
   C. Concentrated urine sediments must be prepared before analysis by the analyzer.
   D. It cannot be used as a standalone instrument (i.e., it must be attached to a urine chemistry analyzer for use).

7. Which of the following statements about the UF-100 and UF-1000i urine particle analyzers is TRUE?
   A. A separate channel is used to detect bacteria.
   B. Digital images of each urine particle are available for review and archival storage.
   C. The analyzers can specifically identify pathologic casts and renal epithelial cells.
   D. Impedance technology is the primary method by which these analyzers detect and categorize particles.

8. Which of the following statements is NOT an issue for the instruments used to perform body fluid analysis?
   A. Unable to perform five-part WBC differentials
   B. Have difficulty detecting and enumerating RBCs
   C. Unable to detect and specifically identify malignant cells
   D. Unable to perform accurate and precise counting of low WBC numbers (<20 cells/µL).

REFERENCES

1. U.S. Food and Drug Administration 510(k) Premarket Notification: Sysmex UF-1000i Decision Summary k0080887, May 2, 2008: http://www.accessdata.fda.gov/scripts/cdrh/cfdocs/cfPMN/PMNSimpleSearch.cfm?db=PMN&ID=K080887. Accessed June 28, 2011.

2. Nanos NE, Delanghe JR: Evaluation of Sysmex UF-1000i for use in cerebrospinal fluid analysis. Clin Chim Acta 392:30-33, 2008.

3. Kouri T, Malminiemi O, Penders J, et al: Limits of preservation of samples for urine strip tests and particle counting. Clin Chem Lab Med 46:703-713, 2008.

4. Shayanfar N, Tobler U, von Eckardstein A, Bestmann L: Automated urinalysis: first experiences and a comparison between the iris iQ200 urine microscopy system, the Sysmex UF-100 flow cytometer and manual microscopic particle counting. Clin Chem Lab Med 45:1251-1256, 2007.

5. BD Diagnostics Technical Services Department: Tips for Urine Analysis: Q & A. Tech Talk 6(2), December 2008: http://www.bd.com/vacutainer/uap/pdfs/UAP_Tech_Talk_VS8026.pdf. Accessed June 25, 2010.

6. Clinical and Laboratory Standards Institute (CLSI): Body fluid analysis for cellular composition: approved guideline, CLSI Document H56-A, Wayne, PA, 2007, CLSI.

7. Harris N, Kunicka J, Kratz A: The ADVIA 2120 hematology system: flow cytometry-based analysis of blood and body fluids in the routine hematology laboratory. Lab Hematol 11:47-61, 2005.

8. U.S. Food and Drug Administration 510(k) Premarket Notification: ADVIA 2120/2120i Decision Summary k090346, July 28, 2010: http://www.accessdata.fda.gov/scripts/cdrh/cfdocs/cfPMN/PMNSimpleSearch.cfm?db=PMN&ID=K090346. Accessed June 28, 2011.

9. de Jonge R, Brouwer R, de Graaf MT, et al: Evaluation of the new body fluid mode on the Sysmex XE-5000 for counting leukocytes and erythrocytes in cerebrospinal fluid and other body fluids. Clin Chem Lab Med 48:665-675, 2010.

Body Fluid Analysis: Manual Hemacytometer Counts and Differential Slide Preparation

USING A HEMACYTOMETER

Manual methods using a hemacytometer are often used to perform cell counts on body fluids such as cerebrospinal fluid, synovial fluid, pleural fluid, pericardial fluid, and peritoneal fluid, as well as peritoneal dialysates, bronchoalveolar lavages, and semen. In health, the numbers of red blood cells (RBCs) and white blood cells (WBCs) in these body fluids are low, and other cells or cellular debris can be present. As discussed in Chapter 17, automated cell counting analyzers can produce erroneous results when the cell count is low. It is the responsibility of each laboratory to define its lower limit for cell counts (RBCs and WBCs) and to have a protocol for performing manual cell counts using a hemacytometer when a fluid exceeds (is below) this limit.[1]

Highly viscous body fluids (e.g., synovial fluid) and fluids that fail to appropriately liquefy (e.g., semen) require pretreatment before cell counting by manual or automated methods. Note that cell counts using a clotted body fluid are inaccurate. Because it may not be possible to obtain another body fluid specimen, every effort is made to work with the health care provider to provide valid, useful information. This may include performing a cell count and including on the report a statement such as "Specimen clotted (large clot); results may be inaccurate and must be interpreted with caution."

Manual cell counts using a hemacytometer are time-consuming, require advanced technical skills, have poor precision (reproducibility), and are subject to numerous errors owing to the multiple steps involved. Therefore it is imperative that technically proficient laboratorians perform them.

Diluents and Dilutions

The visual appearance of the body fluid aids in determining whether a dilution should be made for cell counting

TABLE 18-1	Body Fluid Dilution Guideline for Cell Counts Based on Visual Appearance	
Fluid Appearance	**WBC Count**	**RBC Count**
Clear	Undiluted	Undiluted
Hazy (slightly cloudy)	1:2* dilution	Undiluted
Blood-tinged	1:2* dilution	Undiluted
Cloudy	1:20 dilution	Undiluted
Bloody	1:2* or 1:20 dilution	1:200 dilution

RBC, Red blood cells; *WBC*, white blood cell.
*Using a diluent that lyses RBCs.

BOX 18-1	Enhancing Visualization of WBCs When Analyzing Clear Fluids

1. Rinse the inside of a disposable glass Pasteur pipette with glacial acetic acid, allow it to drain completely, and wipe off the outside and end of the pipette carefully with gauze. *CAUTION: Glacial acetic acid is caustic. Wear personal protective equipment.*
2. Place this prerinsed pipette into the well-mixed body fluid, and allow the pipette to fill by capillary action until fluid fills approximately 1 inch of its length.
3. Seal the open end of the pipette with a gloved finger, and remove the pipette from the body fluid.
4. Mix the fluid sample with the acid in the pipette by holding the pipette in a horizontal position and removing the finger from the top. Rotate the pipette carefully for 10 to 20 seconds. Be careful not to allow fluid to drip out of either end of the pipette.
5. Mount the fluid into both chambers of a hemacytometer. Allow 3 to 5 minutes for the cells to settle and the RBCs to lyse.

RBC, Red blood cell; *WBC*, white blood cell.

TABLE 18-2	Diluents for Body Fluid Blood Cell Counts*	
Diluent	**Cell Counts**	**Comments**
Isotonic saline (0.85%)	WBC count RBC count	Also known as "normal" saline
Hypotonic saline (0.30%)	WBC count	• Lyses RBCs
Dilute acetic acid (3.0%)†	WBC count	• Lyses RBCs • *Do not use* with synovial fluids; causes mucin clot and cell clumping
Turk's solution	WBC count	• Lyses RBCs • *Do not use* with synovial fluids; causes mucin clot and cell clumping
Hyaluronidase (0.1 g/L) buffer solution	WBC count RBC count	• Prevents mucin clot formation in synovial fluids • Stain enhances nucleated cell identification

RBC, Red blood cell; *WBC*, white blood cell.
*See Appendix C for diluent preparation.
†Other concentrations of acetic acid can also be used (e.g., 5%, 10%).

and what dilution should be prepared. Body fluids that are clear do not require a dilution, and the fluid can be mounted directly onto a hemacytometer. Fluids that are visibly cloudy or bloody must be diluted to obtain accurate cell counts. Table 18-1 is provided as a guide to dilution selection based on visual appearance. When diluents that do not lyse RBCs are used, a higher dilution may be necessary. Body fluids that are visibly clear indicate a low cell count, and they are evaluated undiluted. To enhance visualization of WBCs in fluid (except synovial fluid), the fluid can be "exposed" to glacial acetic acid (Box 18-1). Blood-tinged or bloody fluids can be diluted using diluents that lyse RBCs; this enhances visualization of nucleated cells.

The diluent used depends on the body fluid being evaluated. Isotonic solutions such as normal saline (0.85%) are required for RBC counts, whereas dilute acetic acid solutions are usually used for WBC counts. Acetic acid performs two functions: It lyses any RBCs present, and it enhances the nuclei of WBCs. Table 18-2 summarizes the diluents commonly used for body fluids

when WBC and RBC counts are performed. Appendix C provides details on the preparation of these diluents.

Note that synovial fluid cannot be diluted using weak acid diluents, such as acetic acid. Because of the high hyaluronic acid and protein content of synovial fluid, acetic acid will cause a mucin clot (i.e., the co-precipitation of hyaluronic acid and protein), which interferes with accurate cell counting. Instead, synovial fluid should be diluted with normal saline (0.85%), hypotonic saline (0.30%), or a hyaluronidase buffer solution. The hyaluronidase buffer solution prevents mucin clots, and when toluidine blue stain is included, it aids in the visualization and identification of cellular elements. When WBC counts are performed on synovial fluid and hypotonic saline is used as the diluent, any RBCs present are lysed but mucin formation is not initiated.

To obtain accurate cell counts, dilutions of body fluids must be made using a quantitative technique. Calibrated automatic pipettes (e.g., Pipetman, Eppendorf, Drummond) are used to prepare these dilutions manually; commercial diluting systems (e.g., Unopettes) are not available in most locations. Note that when viscous fluids, such as synovial fluid and semen, are pipetted, a positive displacement pipette must be used because an air displacement pipette cannot accurately dispense these viscous fluids. In contrast, CSF, pleural, pericardial, and peritoneal fluids and pretreated synovial fluid can be diluted using an air or a positive displacement pipette.

Pretreatment and Dilution of Synovial Fluid Specimens. Because synovial fluid is highly viscous, a positive displacement pipette must be used to accurately prepare dilutions of this fluid. Also, the viscosity of the fluid can cause an uneven distribution of cells in the hemacytometer. Some highly viscous synovial fluids may need to be *pretreated* with hyaluronidase despite the use of a hyaluronidase buffer solution as the diluent. Synovial fluid is pretreated using the enzyme hyaluronidase, which depolymerizes hyaluronic acid, thereby preventing mucin clot formation. Two pretreatment approaches using hyaluronidase are provided in Appendix C. Basically, hyaluronidase is added to an aliquot of synovial fluid, which is mixed well and incubated at 37°C.

If pretreated synovial fluid is clear, it can be evaluated undiluted for cell counts. When a dilution is needed, a diluent that does not cause a mucin clot is required, such as normal saline, hypotonic saline, or a 0.1 g/L hyaluronidase buffer solution (see Appendix C for diluent preparation).

Semen Dilution and Pretreatment of Viscous Specimens. The diluent often used to dilute semen for sperm counts is a solution of sodium bicarbonate, formalin (a fixative), and, optionally, a stain—trypan blue or gentian violet (see Appendix C for diluent preparation). Including a stain enhances visualization, which assists in differentiating between sperm, immature sperm (spermatids, spermatocytes), and WBCs—primarily neutrophils, monocytes, and macrophages.

Semen specimens that fail to liquefy adequately after 60 minutes require treatment before sperm count, sperm motility assessment, and chemical testing can be performed. One treatment approach involves diluting the seminal fluid using a physiologic medium followed by mechanical mixing—repeated aspiration and dispensing of the mixture using a pipette. Equal parts of semen and a medium such as Dulbecco's phosphate-buffered saline can be used.[2] An alternate approach consists of digestion using the proteolytic enzyme bromelain. Semen is diluted 1:2 using this enzyme solution (i.e., 1 part semen + 1 part bromelain solution). Note that any dilutions of the sample must be accounted for when the sperm concentration is calculated.

The effects that these treatments have on sperm function, morphology, or the biochemistry of the seminal plasma are not known.[2] Therefore when a semen specimen is specially treated for testing, this must be documented on the report. Note that any laboratory analyzing semen for any purpose other than postvasectomy analysis should have available the *WHO Laboratory Manual for the Examination and Processing of Human Semen.* This comprehensive and indispensible text is a vital resource for all aspects of testing when semen analysis is performed.

Hemacytometer Cell Counts

The WBC or total nucleated cell count is an important count that is requested on almost all body fluids. In contrast, little clinical value is derived from an RBC count other than to identify a traumatic puncture

---

BOX 18-2	Manual Cell Count Using a Hemacytometer

1. Using a disposable pipette, fill both sides of an "improved" Neubauer hemacytometer (Figure 18-1) with well-mixed, undiluted or appropriately diluted body fluid.
2. Allow the chamber to remain undisturbed for 3 to 5 minutes for the cells to settle (and RBCs to lyse, depending on the diluent used).
3. Examine the hemacytometer chambers for an even distribution of cells without overlap or clumping. If overlapping or clumping is present, the hemacytometer should be cleaned, the specimen mixed well or a new dilution prepared, and the chambers refilled.
4. CSF, synovial, pleural, pericardial, and peritoneal fluids:
   a. Count all the cells in the four large corner squares and the center square (the "W" squares) in both chambers of the hemacytometer. See the "W" squares in Figure 18-1.
   b. The number of cells counted in each chamber should agree within 10% to 20%. (Total area counted is 10 mm².) If not, clean the hemacytometer and repeat this procedure.
5. Semen:
   a. Spermatozoal concentration:
      i. Count all sperm present in five red blood cell squares (i.e., the four corner squares and the center square within the central large square on both sides of the hemacytometer). See the "R" squares in Figure 18-1. An alternate approach is to count two large "W" squares.
      ii. The number of sperm counted in each chamber should agree within 10% to 20%. (Total area counted is 0.20 mm².) If not, clean the hemacytometer and repeat this procedure.
   b. Round cell count:
      i. For the "round cell" (germ cells and WBCs) count, count the round cells in the four large corner squares and the center large square (the "W" squares) in both chambers of the hemacytometer (Figure 18-1).
      ii. The number of cells counted on each side should agree within 10% to 20%. (Total area counted is 10 mm².) If not, clean the hemacytometer and repeat this procedure.

---

procedure, so it may not be performed, particularly when counts are done manually. Box 18-2 summarizes a protocol for a manual cell count using a hemacytometer (Figure 18-1).

Mix body fluid specimens well for 1 to 2 minutes before filling a hemacytometer chamber with undiluted fluid or preparing a dilution of the specimen. While the body fluid is mixing, flood the hemacytometer with 70% alcohol and wipe dry. This cleans the chambers and removes dust, which can interfere with placement of the coverslip.

The number of squares counted in each chamber of the hemacytometer depends on the total number of cells present. Accuracy in cell counts is directly related to cell numbers; the higher the number of cells counted, the better the accuracy. Therefore when not needed, high dilutions should be avoided to ensure an adequate number of cells for counting. To compensate for fluids with extremely low cell counts, additional squares of the

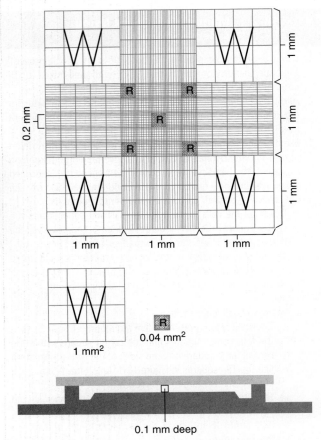

FIGURE 18-1 *Top,* View of a hemacytometer chamber with an "improved" Neubauer etched grid or rulings. *Middle,* A single "W" square that is 1 mm^2; notation derived from the use of 5 "W-sized" squares to enumerate white blood cells. A single "R" square that is 0.04 mm^2; notation derived from the used of 5 "R-sized" squares to enumerate red blood cells. *Bottom,* Side view of hemacytometer chamber demonstrating how glass coverslip rests on ridges of hemacytometer and that when properly filled, the volume of liquid in the chamber has a fixed depth of 0.1 mm.

hemacytometer grid can be counted. With fluids that have a high cell count, fewer squares can be counted. Note that regardless of the variation used, calculations must be properly adjusted for the volume of body fluid actually counted.

To ensure detection of potential errors during the preparation of body fluids for manual cell counts, dilutions should be performed and analyzed in duplicate. In other words, two separate dilutions of the body fluid are prepared and loaded into a hemacytometer—each dilution is loaded into one chamber. The cell counts obtained for each chamber are compared and must agree with the criteria established by the laboratory, usually 20% or less. If the counts between chambers are unacceptable (exceed 20%), the body fluid dilutions and counts must be repeated. Note that counting the same chamber twice or comparing two different chambers filled using the same dilution is not true replication and will not detect errors in pipetting, dilution, and mixing.

Calculations

When using a hemacytometer, regardless of the number of squares counted or the dilution used, to determine the number of cells present per microliter (or cubic millimeter) of fluid, the following general formula is used.

Equation 18-1

$$\text{Cells counted (A)} \times \text{Dilution factor (B)} \times \text{Volume factor (C)}$$
$$= \text{\# cells/}\mu\text{L (mm}^3\text{)}$$

The total number of cells counted (A) in one chamber (or side) of the hemacytometer is multiplied by the dilution factor (B), which accounts for the dilution made of the fluid, and is also multiplied by the volume factor (C), which indicates the volume of fluid actually counted in the chamber. This concentration of cells per microliter can easily be converted to the cell number per liter of fluid as follows.

Equation 18-2

$$\text{\# cells/}\mu\text{L (mm}^3\text{)} \times 10^6 \ \mu\text{L/L} = \text{\#} \times 10^6 \text{ cells/L}$$

To determine the volume factor (C), the actual volume of fluid counted in cubic millimeters (microliters) is calculated. This volume (mm^3) is determined by multiplying the area counted (mm^2) by the depth between the coverslip and the chamber, which is standardized at 0.1 mm. Note that if the chamber is overfilled or underfilled, the depth is not the assumed value of 0.1 mm. To obtain the volume factor (C) in mm^3, divide 1 by the volume of fluid counted,

Equation 18-3

$$\text{Volume factor (C)} = 1/\text{Area} \times \text{depth}$$

For example, if five large squares (5×1 mm^2) are counted, the area is 5 mm^2, the depth is 0.1 mm, and the volume of fluid counted is 0.5 mm^3. Hence the volume factor (C) is 2 (i.e., 1 divided by 0.5).

Sometimes a WBC count and a total cell count are performed on a body fluid. The RBC count is then calculated as the difference between these two counts, which is similar to the approach used by some automated cell counting analyzers (see Chapter 17).

Hemacytometer Calculation Examples

Following are some examples of hemacytometer cell counts of body fluids using undiluted and diluted fluid with appropriate calculations. Note that an additional dilution factor may be required if the fluid was "pretreated" before dilution for cell counting, which may occur with synovial fluid or semen (see Example C).

Example A: Using Undiluted Body Fluid. A well-mixed, *undiluted* cerebrospinal fluid specimen is mounted on a hemacytometer, and the WBCs in five large squares (4 "W" + Center) are counted in each chamber (i.e., 5 mm^2). The following results are obtained.

Chamber 1

A   B   C
$$15 \times 1 \times \frac{1}{(5 \times 0.1)}$$
= 30 WBCs/µL

Units Conversion

$$30 \text{ cells/µL} \times \frac{10^6 \text{ µL}}{L}$$
$$= 30 \times 10^6 \text{ WBCs/L}$$

Chamber 2

A   B   C
$$18 \times 1 \times \frac{1}{(5 \times 0.1)}$$
= 36 WBCs/µL

Units Conversion

$$36 \text{ cells/µL} \times \frac{10^6 \text{ µL}}{L}$$
$$= 36 \times 10^6 \text{ WBCs/L}$$

A, cells counted; *B*, dilution factor; *C*, volume factor.

Note that the counts from both chambers agree within 20%, which indicates that the fluid was well mixed and equivalently dispensed in both chambers. The difference in cell number between side 1 and side 2 (i.e., 18 − 15 = 3 cells) is less than 20% (or 3.6 cells = 18 × 0.20).

Example B: Using Diluted Body Fluid. A well-mixed, hazy-appearing synovial fluid specimen is diluted 1:2, *in duplicate* using hypotonic saline. Both dilutions are mounted on a hemacytometer—one dilution on each side. The WBCs in five large squares (4 "W" + Center) are counted in each chamber (i.e., 5 mm²). The following results are obtained.

Chamber 1

A   B   C
$$58 \times 2 \times \frac{1}{(5 \times 0.1)}$$
= 232 WBCs/µL

Units Conversion

$$232 \text{ cells/µL} \times \frac{10^6 \text{ µL}}{L}$$
$$= 232 \times 10^6 \text{ WBCs/L}$$

Chamber 2

A   B   C
$$44 \times 2 \times \frac{1}{(5 \times 0.1)}$$
= 176 WBCs /µL

Units Conversion

$$176 \text{ cells/µL} \times \frac{10^6 \text{ µL}}{L}$$
$$= 176 \times 10^6 \text{ WBCs/L}$$

A, cells counted; *B*, dilution factor; *C*, volume factor.

Note that the counts from both chambers *do not agree* within 20%. The difference in cell number between side 1 and side 2 (i.e., 58 − 44 = 14 cells) exceeds 20% (or 11.6 cells = 58 × 0.20), which indicates that the steps used to prepare both dilutions (mixing, pipetting, and diluting) were not equivalent. The dilutions and the cell counts should be repeated.

Example C: Sperm Count Using Diluted Semen. A semen specimen was pretreated 1:2 using a bromelain enzyme preparation to get it to liquefy. For the sperm count, the fluid is diluted 1:20, *in duplicate*. Both dilutions are mounted on a hemacytometer—one dilution on each side. The five "R" squares in the large central square (i.e., four small corner + center squares) of the hemacytometer are counted in each chamber (i.e., 0.2 mm²). The following results are obtained. Note that sperm counts are reported as the number of sperm per milliliter, which requires the use of a different units conversion factor.

Chamber 1

A   B   C   D
$$37 \times 20 \times \frac{1}{(0.2 \times 0.1)} \times 2$$
= 74,000 sperm/µL

Units Conversion to #/mL:

$$74,000 \text{ sperm/µL} \times \frac{10^3 \text{ µL}}{L}$$
$$= 74 \times 10^6 \text{ sperm/mL}$$

Chamber 2

A   B   C   D
$$42 \times 20 \times \frac{1}{(0.2 \times 0.1)} \times 2$$
= 84,000 sperm/µL

Units Conversion to #/mL:

$$84,000 \text{ cells/µL} \times \frac{10^3 \text{ µl}}{L}$$
$$= 84 \times 10^6 \text{ sperm/mL}$$

A, cells counted; *B*, dilution factor; *C*, volume factor; *D*, pretreatment dilution factor.

The dilution factor (D) accounts for the dilution made when the fluid was pretreated to get it to liquefy using the bromelain enzyme solution. In this example, the semen counts from both chambers agree within 20%. The difference in sperm number between side 1 and side 2 (i.e., 42 − 37 = 5 sperm) is less than 20% (or 8.4 sperm = 42 × 0.20), which indicates that the steps used to prepare both dilutions (mixing, pipetting, and diluting) were equivalent.

PREPARATION OF SLIDES FOR DIFFERENTIAL

Slides should be prepared as soon as possible following fluid collection. Delays will result in loss of morphologic cellular detail, as well as antigenic reactivity.[3] When preparing slides of body fluids for the WBC differential, cytocentrifugation is the preferred technique.[1] Cytocentrifugation optimizes cell recovery, concentrates the cells in a limited area on the microscope slide, and creates a monolayer that optimizes microscopic viewing. In addition, this method is fast and easy to perform. Note that wedge smears (push smears) should not be used because of their inferior ability to preserve intact cells.[1]

Several other techniques can be used to concentrate body fluids. The easiest and least expensive technique is simple centrifugation of the body fluid, but cell recovery varies, and cells can become damaged and distorted at high-speed centrifugation. Although sedimentation methods preserve cellular morphology, cell recovery is not good. Filtration techniques using commercial filters (e.g., from manufacturers Millipore Corp., Nucleopore, and Gelman Instrument Co.) also have excellent cellular recovery (≈90%). These techniques are time-consuming, and after the cells have been concentrated, a suitable smear must be prepared, which requires significant technical skill. Hence, cytocentrifugation predominates in laboratories for preparing smears from body fluids.

Before slide preparation, body fluid specimens must be gently mixed. Only fresh body fluid specimens should be used to prepare cytocentrifuge slides. If there has been a significant delay since collection (i.e., longer

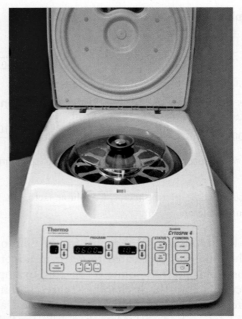

FIGURE 18-2 Thermo-Scientific Cytospin 4 cytocentrifuge *(Thermo Fisher Scientific Inc, Waltham, MA)*.

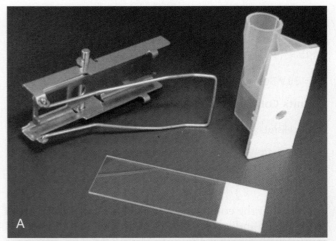

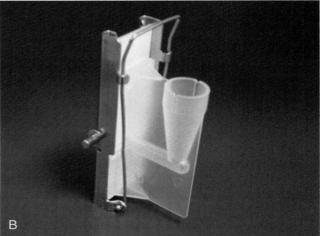

FIGURE 18-3 A, The components of an assembly for the Cytospin 4 cytocentrifuge consist of a stainless steel holder (Cytoclip), a chamber with attached filter card (Cytofunnel), and a microscope slide. Note that the opening in the filter paper is the site where sample flows from the chamber to the glass slide. **B,** Assembly ready for addition of body fluid and then placement onto the rotor of the cytocentrifuge.

than 4 hours for cerebrospinal fluid [CSF]), erroneous differential counts can occur because of cellular degeneration.[1]

Cytocentrifugation

Numerous cytocentrifuges are commercially available and require the use of specially designed assemblies for each sample (Figure 18-2). An assembly consists of a microscope slide, filter paper with a circular opening, and a chamber that holds the fluid specimen (Figure 18-3).

When the body fluid is clear, usually 5 drops (≈0.25 mL) of body fluid is added directly to the chamber. However, depending on the nucleated cell count, as few as 2 drops or as many as 10 may be used. Table 18-3 provides a guideline based on the nucleated cell count for the volume of body fluid to use when preparing a slide by cytocentrifugation. When a dilution is needed, normal saline is most often used; however, some laboratories use a diluent that lyses RBCs for bloody samples (e.g., hypotonic saline). Appropriate dilutions will reduce distortions associated with the overcrowding of cells and ensure a monolayer of cells for viewing. Note that laboratories must establish their own dilution protocols because the appropriate dilution depends on the amount of sample used, as well as the duration and speed of cytocentrifugation.

Each assembly is placed onto the rotor of the cytocentrifuge and when the instrument is activated, centrifugal force pulls the body fluid from the sample chamber to the microscope slide. The cells adhere to the

TABLE 18-3	Guideline for Body Fluid Volume When Preparing Slide by Cytocentrifugation	
Nucleated Cell Count, cells/µL	**Drops of Body Fluid**
0 to 100	10
100 to 500	5 to 6
500 to 1000	3 to 4
>1000	2

glass slide while the liquid is absorbed by the surrounding absorbent filter paper. During centrifugation the cells concentrate as a monolayer in the open circular area of the filter to form a "cell button" on the microscope slide. The centrifugal force is low (e.g., 800 × g) to minimize cell distortion; the time is long enough to ensure adequate drying of the cell button. Microscope slides specifically designed for cytocentrifugation are available, and they have a white circular ring that surrounds the cell

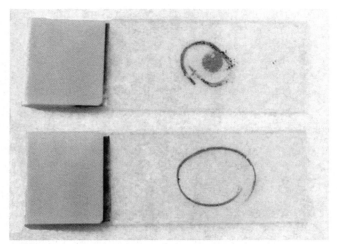

FIGURE 18-4 Cytocentrifuge prepared slides of two body fluids stained using Wright stain. The upper slide shows a visually evident cell button in the area circled by a wax pencil. In contrast, the cell button is not macroscopically evident on the lower slide. On this slide, the wax pencil circle greatly aids the microscopist in locating the proper area of the slide for viewing.

TABLE 18-4	Distortions Associated With Cytocentrifugation

- Cells at center of cell button often smaller and have denser nuclear chromatin.
- Nuclear distortions, such as clefting or lobulation or holes in nuclei
- Nuclear lobes of PMNs localized at cell periphery
- Cytoplasmic vacuoles and/or granules localized at cell periphery
- Formation of irregular cytoplasmic processes

From Kjeldsberg CR, Knight JA: Laboratory methods. In Body fluids, ed 3, Chicago, 1993, American Society of Clinical Pathologists Press.

button area. This assists the microscopist when the body fluid sample contains few cells that are not visually apparent macroscopically on the slide. Another option is to use a wax pencil to mark the backside of the glass microscope slide, indicating the region of the cell button (Figure 18-4).

During cytocentrifugation, some cells are lost to the filter paper, but this loss is not selective (i.e., all cells are equally affected); consequently, the remaining cell distribution in the cell button is accurate and representative. Several predictable cellular distortions that may be observed are listed in Table 18-4. Most are associated with high cell counts, the cytocentrifugation process (speed and time), or a time delay when an older specimen is used (i.e., not fresh).[3] To reduce these artifacts, laboratories should determine the optimal speed and time of cytocentrifugation for their instrument, use fresh specimens, and prepare appropriate dilutions of fluids with high cell counts.

For specimens that have a low protein content (e.g., CSF), adding a drop of 22% albumin to the sample chamber before adding the body fluid enhances adherence of cells to the glass slide and reduces cell distortion (smudging) or disintegration.[1,3]

Slide Preparations

Slide preparations are stained using Wright's or Wright-Giemsa stain performed manually or automatically using a slide stainer. The hand-drawn or premarked circle on the microscope slide indicates the location of the cell button (see Figure 18-4).

Adjust the microscope to low-power (100×) magnification, and thoroughly scan the entire cell button looking for cell clumps, which are characteristic of malignancies. Note that malignant cells can be present in low numbers, and even a single malignant cell is clinically significant. Also, not all cell clumps are composed of malignant cells.

The WBC differential can be performed using any area of the cell button. A systematic approach to viewing should be used (similar to that used with blood smears) to prevent erroneous repeat counting of the same cells.

STUDY QUESTIONS

1. Which of the following statements is NOT associated with the performance of cell counts using a manual hemacytometer?
   A. Procedure is time-consuming.
   B. Quantitative pipetting is required.
   C. Body fluids with low cell counts cannot be analyzed.
   D. High variability in results is obtained between laboratorians.

2. Which of the following diluents will cause synovial fluid to form a mucin clot?
   A. Hyaluronidase buffer solution
   B. Hypotonic saline
   C. Isotonic saline
   D. Turk's solution

3. Which of the following diluents should be used when an RBC count is requested?
   A. Dilute acetic acid
   B. Hypotonic saline
   C. Isotonic saline
   D. Turk's solution

4. An air displacement pipette cannot accurately dispense
   A. CSF.
   B. pleural fluid.
   C. peritoneal fluid.
   D. synovial fluid.

5. Which of the following actions will adversely affect the cell count obtained using a hemacytometer?
   A. Counting six "W" squares instead of the usual five
   B. Preparing a dilution of semen using an air displacement pipette
   C. Mixing the fluid for 3 minutes before loading it onto the hemacytometer
   D. Making three dilutions but using only two to load the hemacytometer

6. In the pretreatment of a synovial fluid with hyaluronidase, a 1:10 dilution is made, after which a WBC count is performed using a 1:20 dilution of this fluid. The WBCs in the four large corner squares ("W") and the center square are counted in each chamber (i.e., 5 mm^2). Both sides of the hemacytometer were evaluated with 37 cells and 43 cells counted in chamber 1 and chamber 2, respectively. What is the average cell count that should be reported?
   A. 160 WBCs/μL
   B. 1600 WBCs/μL
   C. 16,000 WBCs/μL
   D. 160,000 WBCs/μL

7. A WBC count is performed using a 1:2 dilution of CSF, and the four large corner squares ("W") and the center square are counted in each chamber (i.e., 5 mm^2). Both sides of the hemacytometer were evaluated with 31 cells and 23 cells counted in chamber 1 and chamber 2, respectively. What should be done next?
   A. Clean hemacytometer and repeat counts.
   B. Recount both sides of the hemacytometer.
   C. Calculate the average WBC count and report.
   D. Reload the same dilutions onto a clean hemacytometer, and repeat the counts.

8. Distortions observed on cytocentrifuge slide preparations have been associated with
   A. viscous fluids.
   B. high cell counts.
   C. use of fresh body fluid specimens.
   D. fluids that have a high protein concentration.

REFERENCES

1. Clinical and Laboratory Standards Institute (CLSI): Body fluid analysis for cellular composition: approved guideline, CLSI Document H56-A, Wayne, PA, 2007, CLSI.
2. World Health Organization: WHO laboratory manual for the examination and processing of human semen, ed 5, Geneva, Switzerland, 2010, World Health Organization.
3. Kjeldsberg CR, Knight JA: Laboratory methods. In Body fluids, ed 3, Chicago, 1993, American Society of Clinical Pathologists Press.

A

acholic stools Pale, gray, or clay-colored stools. They result when production of the normal fecal pigments—stercobilin, mesobilin, and urobilin—is partially or completely inhibited.

active transport The movement of a substance (e.g., ion or solute) across a cell membrane and against a gradient, requiring the expenditure of energy.

acute interstitial nephritis An acute inflammatory process that develops 3 to 21 days following exposure to an immunogenic drug (e.g., sulfonamides, penicillins) and results in injury to the renal tubules and interstitium. The condition is characterized by fever, skin rash, leukocyturia (particularly eosinophiluria), and acute renal failure. Discontinuation of the offending agent can result in full recovery of renal function.

acute poststreptococcal glomerulonephritis A type of glomerular inflammation occurring 1 to 2 weeks after a group A β-hemolytic streptococcal infection. Onset is sudden, and the glomerular damage is immune mediated.

acute pyelonephritis An inflammatory process involving the renal tubules, interstitium, and renal pelvis. The condition most often is caused by a bacterial infection and is characterized by sudden onset of symptoms such as flank pain, dysuria, frequency of micturition, and urinary urgency.

acute renal failure A renal disorder characterized by a sudden decrease in the glomerular filtration rate that results in azotemia and oliguria. Acute renal failure results from numerous conditions and can be categorized as prerenal (e.g., decrease in renal blood flow), renal (e.g., acute tubular necrosis), or postrenal (e.g., urinary tract obstruction). The disease course varies greatly, and survivors usually regain normal renal function.

acute tubular necrosis A group of renal diseases characterized by destruction of the renal tubular epithelium. Acute tubular necrosis is classified into two types: ischemic, caused by decreased renal perfusion that results in tissue ischemia, and toxic, resulting from the ingestion, inhalation, or injection of nephrotoxic substances.

afferent arteriole A small branch of an interlobular renal artery that becomes the capillary tuft within a glomerulus.

albuminuria The increased urinary excretion of the protein albumin.

aldosterone A steroid hormone secreted by the adrenal cortex. Aldosterone stimulates the absorption of sodium and the excretion of potassium in the distal tubules and is regulated by the renin-angiotensin-aldosterone system.

alkaptonuria A rare recessively inherited disease characterized by excretion of large amounts of homogentisic acid (i.e., alkapton bodies) caused by a deficiency of the enzyme homogentisic acid oxidase.

aminoaciduria The presence of increased quantities of amino acids in the urine.

amyloidosis A group of systemic diseases characterized by the deposition of amyloid, a proteinaceous substance, between cells in numerous tissues and organs.

antidiuretic hormone Also known as arginine vasopressin, a hormone produced in the hypothalamus and released from the posterior pituitary that regulates the reabsorption of water by the collecting tubules. Without adequate arginine vasopressin present, water is not reabsorbed.

anoxia An absence of oxygen or a deficiency in oxygen reaching tissues or organs; a severe form of hypoxia (low oxygen).

anuria (also called *anuresis*) The absence or cessation of urine excretion.

aperture diaphragm Microscope component that regulates the angle of light presented to the specimen. The diaphragm is located at the base of the condenser and changes the diameter of the opening through which the source light rays must pass to enter the condenser.

arthritis The inflammation of a joint.

arthrocentesis A percutaneous puncture procedure used to remove synovial fluid from joint cavities.

ascites The excessive accumulation of serous fluid in the peritoneal cavity.

ascorbic acid (also called *vitamin C*) A water-soluble vitamin and a strong reducing agent that readily oxidizes to its salt, dehydroascorbate.

ascorbic acid interference The inhibition of a chemical reaction by the presence of ascorbic acid. As a strong reducing agent, ascorbic acid readily reacts with diazonium salts or hydrogen peroxide, removing these chemicals from intended reaction sequences. As a result, colorless dehydroascorbate is formed, causing no or a reduced color change.

azotemia A condition characterized by increased quantities of nonprotein nitrogenous substances in the blood such as urea, creatinine, ammonia, uric acid, creatine, and amino acids. Azotemia is caused by decreased filtration and elimination of these substances by the kidneys.

B

bacterial vaginosis Noninvasive inflammation of the vagina and upper genital tract most often caused by *Gardnerella vaginalis* in association with anaerobes such as *Mobiluncus* species.

bactericidal Capable of killing bacteria.

bacteriuria The presence of bacteria in urine.

baroreceptors Sensory nerve endings found in certain blood vessels that detect changes in blood pressure within these vessels. Baroreceptors are stimulated by the stretching of the vessel wall as pressure increases.

basement membrane A trilayer structure located within the glomerulus along the base of the epithelium (podocytes) of the urinary (Bowman's) space. With the overlying slit diaphragm, the basement membrane is the size-discriminating component of the glomerular filtration barrier, limiting the passage of substances to those with an effective molecular radius less than 4 nm. Using electron microscopy, three distinct layers are evident in the basement membrane: the lamina rara interna (next to the capillary endothelium), the lamina densa (centrally located), and the lamina rara externa (next to the podocytes).

bilirubin A yellow-orange pigment resulting from heme catabolism. Bilirubin causes a characteristic discoloration of urine, plasma, and other body fluids when present in the fluid in significant amounts. When exposed to air, bilirubin oxidizes to biliverdin, a green pigment.

biological hazard A biological material or an entity contaminated with biologic material that is potentially capable of transmitting disease.

birefringent (also called *doubly refractile*) The ability of a substance to refract light in two directions.

bladder A muscular sac that serves as a reservoir for the accumulation of urine.

blood-brain barrier The physiologic interface between the vascular system and the cerebrospinal fluid. Changes in the normal regulating conditions of the blood-brain barrier result in changes in the normal chemical and cellular composition of the cerebrospinal fluid.

Bowman's capsule See *glomerulus*.

Bowman's space See *urinary space*.

brightfield microscopy Type of microscopy that produces a magnified image that appears dark against a bright or white background.

C

calculi (also called *stones*) Solid aggregates or concretions of chemicals, usually mineral salts, that form in secreting glands of the body.

casts Cylindrical bodies that form in the lumen of the renal tubules. Their core matrix is made up principally of uromodulin (formerly known as *Tamm-Horsfall glycoprotein*), although other plasma proteins can be incorporated. Because casts are formed in the tubular lumen, any chemical or formed element present—such as cells, fat, and bacteria—can also be incorporated into the matrix. Casts are enumerated and are classified by the type of inclusions present.

catabolism A degradative process that converts complex substances into simpler components.

catheterized specimen A urine specimen obtained using a sterile catheter (a flexible tube) that is inserted through the urethra and into the bladder. Urine flows directly from the bladder by gravity and collects in a plastic reservoir bag.

cerebrospinal fluid The normally clear, colorless fluid found between the arachnoid and pia mater in the brain and spinal cord. The fluid is formed primarily from plasma by selective secretions of the choroid plexus and, to a lesser extent, by intrathecal synthesis by ependymal cells of the ventricles.

Chemical Hygiene Plan An established protocol developed by each facility for the identification, handling, storage, and disposal of all hazardous chemicals. The Occupational Safety and Health Administration established the plan in January 1990 as a mandatory requirement for all facilities that deal with chemical hazards.

choroid plexus The highly vascular folds of capillaries, nerves, and ependymal cells in the pia mater. Located in the four ventricles of the brain, the choroid plexus actively synthesizes cerebrospinal fluid.

chromatic aberration The unequal refraction of light rays by a lens because the different wavelengths of light refract or bend at different angles. As a result, the image produced has undesired color fringes.

chronic glomerulonephritis A slowly progressive glomerular disease that develops years after other forms of glomerulonephritis. The condition usually leads to irreversible renal failure, requiring dialysis or kidney transplantation.

chronic pyelonephritis A renal inflammatory process involving the tubules, interstitium, renal calyces, and renal pelves, most often as a result of reflux nephropathies that cause chronic bacterial infections of the upper urinary tract. This chronic inflammation results in fibrosis and scarring of the kidney and eventually loss of renal function.

chronic renal failure A renal disorder characterized by progressive loss of renal function caused by an irreversible and intrinsic renal disease. The glomerular filtration rate decreases progressively. Chronic renal failure concludes with end-stage renal disease, characterized by isosthenuria, significant proteinuria, variable hematuria, and numerous casts of all types, particularly waxy and broad casts.

chyle A milky-appearing emulsion of lymph and chylomicrons (triglyceride) that originates from intestinal lymphatic absorption during digestion.

chylous effusion A milky-appearing effusion that persists after centrifugation; its chemical composition includes chylomicrons and an elevated triglyceride level (i.e., >110 mg/dL).

clarity (also called *turbidity*) The transparency of a urine or body fluid specimen. Clarity varies with the amount of suspended particulate matter in the specimen.

clue cells Squamous epithelial cells with large numbers of bacteria adhering to them. Clue cells appear soft and finely granular with indistinct or "shaggy" cell borders. To be considered a clue cell, the bacteria do not need to cover the entire cell, but bacterial organisms must extend beyond the cytoplasmic borders of the cell. Clue cells are characteristic of bacterial vaginosis, a synergistic infection involving *Gardnerella vaginalis* and anaerobic bacteria.

collecting duct The portion of a renal nephron following the distal convoluted tubule. Many distal tubules empty into a single collecting duct. The collecting duct traverses the renal cortex and the medulla and is the site of final urine concentration. The collecting ducts terminate at the renal papilla, conveying the urine formed into the renal calyces of the kidney.

collecting duct cells Cuboidal or polygonal cells approximately 12 to 20 mm in diameter with a large, centrally located dense nucleus. These cells form the lining of the collecting tubules and become larger and more columnar as they approach the renal calyces.

collecting tubule See *collecting duct*.

colligative property A characteristic of a solution that depends only on the number of solute particles present, regardless of their molecular size or charge. The four colligative properties are freezing point depression, vapor pressure depression, osmotic pressure elevation, and boiling point elevation. These properties form the basis of methods and instrumentation used to measure the concentrations of solutes in body fluids (e.g., serum, urine, fecal supernates). (See also *freezing point osmometer* and *vapor pressure osmometer*.)

compound microscope A microscope with two lens systems. The lens system closest to the specimen (objective forms the initial image) and the second lens system (eyepiece) further magnifies the image for viewing.

condenser Microscope component that gathers and focuses the illumination light onto the specimen for viewing. The condenser is a lens system (a single lens or combination of lenses) that is located beneath the microscope stage.

constipation Infrequent and difficult bowel movements, compared with an individual's normal bowel movement pattern. The fecal material produced is made up of hard, small, frequently spherical masses.

cortex The outer portion of the kidney, approximately 1.4 cm thick and macroscopically granular in appearance. The cortex is where the glomeruli and the convoluted tubules are located.

countercurrent exchange mechanism A passive exchange by diffusion of reabsorbed solutes and water from the medullary interstitium into the blood of its vascular blood supply (i.e., the vasa recta). A requirement of this process is that the flow of blood in the ascending and descending vessels of the U-shaped vasa recta can be in opposite directions, hence the term *countercurrent*. The countercurrent exchange mechanism simultaneously supplies nutrients to the medulla and removes solutes and water reabsorbed into the blood. As a result, the mechanism assists in maintaining the medullary hypertonicity.

countercurrent multiplier mechanism A process occurring in the loop of Henle of each nephron that establishes and maintains the osmotic gradient within the medullary interstitium. The medullary osmolality gradient ranges from being isosmotic ($\approx$300 mOsm/kg) at its border with the cortex to 1200 to 1400 mOsm/kg at the inner medulla or papilla. A requirement of this process is that the flow of the ultrafiltrate in the descending and ascending limbs must be in opposite directions, hence the name *countercurrent*. In addition, active sodium and chloride reabsorption in the ascending limb and passive water reabsorption in the descending limb are essential components of this process. The countercurrent multiplier mechanism accounts for approximately 50% of the solutes concentrated in the renal medulla.

creatinine clearance test A renal clearance test that measures the volume of plasma cleared of creatinine by the kidneys per unit of time. Reported in milliliters per minute, creatinine clearance is determined by the equation $C = U \times V/P$, in which U and P are the urine and plasma concentrations of creatinine, respectively, and V is the volume of urine excreted in a timed collection, usually 24 hours.

creatorrhea The presence of undigested meat fibers in the feces.

critical value A patient test result representing a life-threatening condition that requires immediate attention and intervention.

cryoscope See *freezing point osmometer* and *vapor pressure osmometer*.

crystals Entities formed by the solidification of urinary solutes. These urinary solutes can be made of a single element, a compound, or a mixture and are arranged in a regular, repeating pattern throughout the crystalline structure.

cystinosis An inherited recessive disorder characterized by intracellular deposition of the amino acid cystine throughout the body. Cystine deposition within renal tubular cells results in their dysfunction and the development of extensive renal disease.

cystinuria An autosomal recessive inherited disorder characterized by an inability to reabsorb the amino acids cystine, arginine, lysine, and ornithine in the renal tubules and in the intestine. This results in the presence of cystine and the other dibasic amino acids in the urine, despite normal cystine metabolism. Because cystine is insoluble at an acid pH, it readily precipitates in the renal tubules, resulting in calculus formation. The other dibasic amino acids are freely soluble and are excreted easily.

cytocentrifugation A specialized centrifuge procedure used to produce a monolayer of the cellular constituents in various body fluids on a microscope slide. The slides are fixed and stained, providing a permanent preparation for cytologic studies.

D

darkfield microscopy Type of microscopy that produces a magnified image that appears brightly illuminated against a dark background. A special condenser presents only oblique light rays to the specimen. The specimen interacts with these rays (e.g., refraction, reflection), causing visualization of the specimen. Darkfield microscopy is used on unstained specimen preparations and is the preferred technique for identification of spirochetes.

decontamination A process used to remove a potential chemical or biological hazard from an area or entity (e.g., countertop, instrument, materials) and render the area or entity "safe." Various processes to decontaminate include autoclaving, incineration, chemical neutralization, and use of disinfecting agents.

density An expression of concentration in terms of the mass of solutes present per volume of solution.

diabetes insipidus A metabolic disease characterized by polyuria and polydipsia caused by defective antidiuretic hormone production (neurogenic) or lack of renal tubular response to antidiuretic hormone (nephrogenic).

diabetes mellitus A metabolic disease characterized by the inability to metabolize glucose, resulting in hyperglycemia, glucosuria, and alterations in fat and protein metabolism. Diabetes mellitus develops because of defective (1) insulin production, (2) insulin action, or (3) both. The disease is classified as type 1 or type 2 depending on age of onset, initial presentation, insulin requirements, and other factors.

diarrhea An increase in the volume, liquidity, and frequency of bowel movements compared with an individual's normal bowel movement pattern.

diffuse Widely distributed.

disaccharidase deficiency A lack of sufficient enzymes (disaccharidases) for the metabolism of disaccharides in the small intestine. This deficiency can be hereditary or acquired (e.g., resulting from diseases or drug therapy).

distal convoluted tubular cells Oval to round cells approximately 14 to 25 mm in diameter with a small, central to slightly eccentric nucleus and a dense chromatin pattern. These cells form the lining of the distal convoluted tubules.

distal convoluted tubule A subsection of the distal tubule of a nephron. This portion of the tubule starts at the macula densa (the site of the juxtaglomerular apparatus), proceeds for two to three loops, and terminates with the collecting tubule (or duct).

distal tubule The portion of the nephron that immediately follows the loop of Henle and precedes the collecting tubule or duct. The distal tubule is subdivided into a straight portion that precedes the macula densa and a convoluted portion that begins at the macula densa and terminates with the collecting tubule.

diuresis An increase in urine excretion. Various causes of diuresis include increased fluid intake, diuretic therapy, hormonal imbalance, renal dysfunction, and drug ingestion (e.g., alcohol, caffeine).

documentation A written record. In the laboratory, documentation includes written policies and procedures, quality control, and maintenance records. Documentation may encompass the recording of any action performed or observed, including verbal correspondence, observations, and corrective actions taken.

dyspareunia Pain in the vulva, vagina, or pelvis during or after intercourse. The cause may be disease related, mechanical, or psychologic.

dysuria Pain or difficulty experienced with urination. Dysuria most often is associated with infection of the urinary tract (e.g., urethritis, cystitis). Such "internal" dysuria contrasts with "external" dysuria, which is pain experienced during urination because of the passage of urine over inflamed tissues (e.g., vulva, perineum).

E

edema The accumulation of fluid in the extracellular spaces of the tissues.

efferent arteriole The arteriole exiting a glomerulus; the efferent arteriole is formed by the rejoining of the anastomosing capillary network within the glomerulus.

effusion An accumulation of fluid in a body cavity as a result of a pathologic process.

Ehrlich's reaction The development of a red or magenta chromophore as a result of the interaction of a substance (e.g., urobilinogen, porphobilinogen) with *p*-dimethylaminobenzaldehyde (also called *Ehrlich's agent*) in an acid medium.

-emia Of or relating to the blood.

endothelium The layer of epithelial cells that line the vessels and serous cavities of the body.

epididymis A long, coiled, tubular structure attached to the upper surface of each testis and continuous with the vas deferens. The epididymis is the site of final spermatozoal maturation and the development of motility. Spermatozoa are concentrated and stored here until ejaculation.

epithelium The layer of cells that cover the internal and external surfaces of the body.

erythroblastosis fetalis A hemolytic disease of the newborn that results from a blood group incompatibility between the mother and the infant.

etiology The study of factors that cause disease, such as genetic factors, infection, toxins, or trauma.

external quality assurance The use of materials (e.g., specimens, kodachrome slides) from an external unbiased source to monitor and determine whether quality goals (i.e., test results) are being achieved. Results are compared with results from other facilities performing the same function. Proficiency surveys are one form of external quality assurance.

exudate An effusion in a body cavity caused by increased capillary permeability or decreased lymphatic absorption. An exudate is identified by a fluid-to-serum total protein ratio greater than 0.5, a fluid-to-serum lactate dehydrogenase ratio greater than 0.6, or both.

eyepiece (also called ocular) The microscope lens or system of lenses located closest to the viewer's eye. The eye-piece produces the secondary image magnification of the specimen.

F

Fanconi syndrome A complication of inherited and acquired diseases characterized by generalized proximal tubular dysfunction resulting in aminoaciduria, proteinuria, glucosuria, and phosphaturia.

fenestrated Pierced with openings.

field diaphragm Microscope component that controls the diameter of the light beams that strike the specimen and hence reduces stray light. The diaphragm is located at the light exit of the illumination source. With Köhler illumination, the field diaphragm is used to adjust and center the condenser appropriately.

field number A number assigned to an eyepiece that indicates the diameter of the field of view, in millimeters, that is observed using a 1× objective. This diameter is determined by a baffle or raised ring inside the eyepiece and sometimes is engraved on the eyepiece.

field of view The circular field observed through a microscope. The diameter of this field of view varies with the eyepiece field number and the magnifications of the objective in use plus any additional optics before the eyepiece. One can calculate the field of view (FOV) using the following formula: FOV (in millimeters) = field number/M, where M is the sum of all optics magnification, except that of the eyepiece.

first morning specimen The first urine specimen voided after rising from sleep. The night before the collection, the patient voids before going to bed. Usually the first morning specimen has been retained in the bladder for 6 to 8 hours and is ideal to test for substances that may require concentration (e.g., protein) or incubation for detection (e.g., nitrites).

fluorescence microscopy The type of microscopy modified to visualize fluorescent substances. Fluorescence microscopy uses two filters: one to select a specific wavelength of illumination light (excitation filter) that is absorbed by the specimen, and another filter (barrier filter) to transmit the different, longer-wavelength light emitted from the specimen to the eyepiece for viewing. The fluorophore (natural or added) present in the specimen determines the selection of these filters.

fluorescence polarization   An analytical technique based on the change in polarization observed in fluorescent light emitted compared with the incident polarized fluorescent light. The observed changes in the polarization of light directly result from the molecular size of the fluorophore-tagged complex. Large molecules cannot randomly orient as rapidly as small molecules. Hence fluorophores tagged to large molecular complexes emit more fluorescence in the same polarized plane as the initial incident light than fluorophores tagged to small molecular complexes.

focal   Localized or limited to a specific area.

focal proliferative glomerulonephritis   A type of glomerular inflammation characterized by cellular proliferation in a specific part of the glomeruli (segmental) and limited to a specific number of glomeruli (focal).

focal segmental glomerulosclerosis   A type of glomerular disease characterized by sclerosis of the glomeruli. Not all glomeruli are affected, hence the term *focal*, and of those that are, only certain portions become diseased, hence the term *segmental*.

free-water clearance (also called *solute-free water clearance*)   The volume of water cleared by the kidneys per minute in excess of that necessary to remove solutes. Denoted CH_2O and reported in milliliters per minute, free-water clearance is determined using the equation $CH_2O = V \times COsm$. V is the volume of urine excreted in a timed collection (milliliters per minute), and COsm is the osmolar clearance (milliliters per minute).

freezing point osmometer   An instrument that measures osmolality based on the freezing point depression of a solution compared with that of pure water. An osmometer consists of a mechanism to supercool the sample below its freezing point. Freezing of the sample subsequently is induced, and as ice crystals form, a sensitive thermistor monitors the temperature until an equilibrium is obtained between the solid and liquid phases. This equilibrium temperature is the freezing point of the sample, from which the osmolality of the sample is determined. One osmole of solutes per kilogram of solvent (1 Osm/kg) depresses the freezing point of water by 1.86° C.

fully automated urinalysis   Indicates that the entire urinalysis—physical, chemical, and microscopic examinations—is performed by analyzers with results integrated by a computer system to produce a complete urinalysis report. A urine chemistry analyzer performs the physical and chemical analyses; these are followed by urine particle.

G

galactosuria   The presence of galactose in the urine.

glomerular filtration barrier   The structure within the glomerulus that determines the composition of the plasma ultrafiltrate formed in the urinary space by regulating the passage of solutes. The glomerular filtration barrier consists of the capillary endothelium, the basement membrane, and the epithelial podocytes, each coated with a "shield of negativity." Solute selectivity by the barrier is based on the molecular size and the electrical charge of the solute.

glomerular filtration rate   The rate of plasma cleared by the glomeruli per unit of time (milliliters per minute). This rate is determined using clearance tests of substances that are known to be removed exclusively by glomerular filtration and that are not reabsorbed or secreted by the nephrons (e.g., inulin).

glomerular proteinuria   Increased amounts of protein in urine caused by a compromised or diseased glomerular filtration barrier.

glomerulonephritides (plural) or glomerulonephritis (singular)   Nephritic conditions characterized by damage and inflammation of the glomeruli. Causes are varied and include immunologic, metabolic, and hereditary disorders.

glomerulus (also called *renal corpuscle*)   A tuft or network of capillaries encircled by and intimately related to the proximal end of a renal tubule (i.e., Bowman's capsule). The glomerulus is composed of four distinct structural components: the capillary endothelial cells, the epithelial cells (podocytes), the mesangium, and the basement membrane.

glucosuria   The presence of glucose in urine.

glycosuria   See *glucosuria*.

H

hematuria   The presence of red blood cells in urine.

heme moiety   The iron-containing porphyrin ring structure that is present in hemoglobin, myoglobin, and other substances.

hemoglobinuria   The presence of hemoglobin in urine.

hemosiderin   An insoluble form of storage iron. When renal tubular cells reabsorb hemoglobin, the iron is catabolized into ferritin (a major storage form of iron). Ferritin subsequently denatures to form insoluble hemosiderin granules (micelles of ferric hydroxide) that appear in the urine 2 to 3 days after a hemolytic episode.

hyaluronate   A high-molecular-weight polymer of repeating disaccharide units secreted by synoviocytes into the synovial fluid. Hyaluronate is a salt or ester of hyaluronic acid that imparts the high viscosity to the fluid and serves as joint lubricant.

hydrometer   A weighted glass float with a long, narrow, calibrated stem used to measure the specific gravity of solutions. When placed in pure water (at a specific temperature), the hydrometer displaces a volume of water equal to its weight, and the meniscus of the water intersects the calibrated stem at the value 1.000. When placed in a solution of greater specific gravity than water, the hydrometer displaces a smaller volume of liquid, and the specific gravity is read from the calibrated stem.

hyperosmotic   See *hypertonic*.

hypersthenuric   The excretion of urine having a specific gravity greater than 1.010.

hypertonic   Term describing a solution or fluid having a higher concentration of osmotically active solutes compared with that of the blood plasma.

hypo-osmotic   See *hypotonic*.

hyposthenuric The excretion of urine having a specific gravity less than 1.010.

hypotonic Term describing a solution or fluid having a lower concentration of osmotically active solutes compared with that of the blood plasma.

I

IgA nephropathy A type of glomerular inflammation characterized by the deposition of immunoglobulin A in the glomerular mesangium. The condition often occurs 1 to 2 days after a mucosal infection of the respiratory, gastrointestinal, or urinary tract.

infectious waste disposal policy A procedure outlining the equipment, materials, and steps used in the collection, storage, removal, and decontamination of infectious material and substances.

interdigitate To interlock or interrelate.

interference contrast microscopy Type of microscopy in which the difference in optical light paths through the specimen is converted into intensity differences in the specimen image. Three-dimensional images of high contrast and resolution are obtained, without haloing. Two types available are modulation contrast (Hoffman) and differential interference contrast (Nomarski).

interstitial cells of Leydig The cells located in the interstitial space between the seminiferous tubules of the testes. These cells produce and secrete the hormone testosterone.

intrathecal Within the spinal cord or subarachnoid space.

ionic specific gravity The density of a solution based on ionic solutes only. Nonionizing substances such as urea, glucose, protein, and radiographic contrast media are not detectable using ionic specific gravity measurements (e.g., specific gravity by commercial reagent strips).

ischemia Inadequate blood supply (circulation) to an organ or area of tissue caused by constriction or obstruction of blood vessels.

isosmotic Term describing a solution or fluid with the same concentration of osmotically active solutes as the blood plasma.

isosthenuria The excretion of urine having the same specific gravity (and osmolality) as the plasma. Because the specific gravity of protein-free plasma and the original ultrafiltrate is 1.010, the inability to excrete urine with a higher or lower specific gravity indicates significantly impaired renal tubular function.

J

jaundice The yellowish pigmentation of skin, sclera, body tissues, and body fluids caused by the presence of increased amounts of bilirubin. Jaundice appears when plasma bilirubin concentrations reach approximately 2 to 3 mg/dL, that is, two to three times normal bilirubin levels.

juxtaglomerular apparatus A specialized area located at the vascular pole of a nephron. The apparatus is composed of cells from the afferent and efferent arterioles, the macula densa of the distal tubule, and the extraglomerular mesangium. The juxtaglomerular apparatus is actually an endocrine organ and is the primary producer of renin.

K

ketonuria The presence of ketones (i.e., acetoacetate, hydroxybutyrate, and acetone) in urine.

kidneys The organs of the urinary system that produce urine. Normally, each individual has two kidneys. The primary function of the kidneys is to filter the blood, removing waste products and regulating electrolytes, water, acid-base balance, and blood pressure.

KOH preparation A preparation technique used to enhance the viewing of fungal elements. Secretions obtained using a sterile swab are suspended in saline. A drop of this suspension is placed on a microscope slide, followed by a drop of 10% KOH. The slide is warmed and viewed microscopically. KOH destroys most formed elements with the exception of bacteria and fungal elements.

Köhler illumination Type of microscopic illumination in which a lamp condenser (located above the light source) focuses the image of the light source (lamp filament) onto the front focal plane of the substage condenser (where the aperture diaphragm is located). The substage condenser sharply focuses the image of the field diaphragm (located at or slightly in front of the lamp condenser) at the same plane as the focused specimen. As a result, the filament image does not appear in the field of view, and bright, even illumination is obtained. Köhler illumination requires appropriate adjustments of the condenser and the field and aperture diaphragms.

L

lamellar bodies Cytoplasmic storage granules that contain pulmonary surfactant and are secreted into the alveolar lumen from fetal type II pneumocytes lining the lungs. When electron microscopy is used, these granules have a characteristic layered or onion-like appearance, hence their name. Lamellar bodies begin to appear in the amniotic fluid at 20 to 24 weeks' gestation.

leukocyturia The presence of leukocytes, that is, white blood cells, in the urine. Compare *pyuria*.

lipiduria The presence of lipids in the urine.

liquefaction The physical conversion of seminal fluid from a coagulum to a liquid following ejaculation.

loop of Henle The tubular portion of a nephron immediately following and continuous with the proximal tubule. Located in the renal medulla, the loop of Henle is composed of a thin descending limb, a U-shaped segment (also called a *hairpin turn*), and thin and thick ascending limbs. The thick ascending limb of the loop of Henle (sometimes called *the straight portion of the distal tubule*) ends as the tubule enters the vascular pole of the glomerulus.

M

macula densa A specialized and morphologically distinct area of the distal convoluted tubule. The macula densa is located at the vascular pole and is in intimate contact with the juxtaglomerular cells of the afferent arteriole.

malabsorption The inadequate intestinal absorption of processed foodstuffs despite normal digestive ability.

maldigestion The inability to convert foodstuffs in the gastrointestinal tract into readily absorbable substances.

Maltese cross pattern A design that appears as an orb divided into four quadrants by a bright Maltese-style cross. When the microscopist uses polarizing microscopy, cholesterol droplets exhibit this characteristic pattern, which aids in their identification. Other substances, such as starch granules, can show a similar pattern.

maple syrup urine disease (MSUD) A rare autosomal recessive inherited defect or deficiency in the enzyme responsible for the oxidation of the branched-chain amino acids leucine, isoleucine, and valine. As a result, these amino acids along with their corresponding α-keto acids accumulate in the blood, cerebrospinal fluid, and urine. The name derives from the subtle maple syrup odor of the urine from these patients.

material safety data sheet (MSDS) A written document provided by the manufacturer or distributor of a chemical substance listing information about the characteristics of that chemical. An MSDS includes the identity and hazardous ingredients of the chemical, its physical and chemical properties including reactivity, any physical or health hazards, and precautions for the safe handling, storage, and disposal of the chemical.

maximal tubular capacity (T_m) See *maximal tubular reabsorptive capacity* and *maximal tubular secretory capacity*.

maximal tubular reabsorptive capacity Denoted T_m, the maximal rate of reabsorption of a solute by the tubular epithelium per minute (milligrams per minute). Reabsorptive capacity varies with each solute and depends on the glomerular filtration rate.

maximal tubular secretory capacity Also denoted T_m, the maximal rate of secretion of a solute by the tubular epithelium per minute (milligrams per minute). This rate differs for each solute.

mechanical stage Microscope component that holds the microscope slide with the specimen for viewing. The stage is adjustable, front to back and side to side, to enable viewing of the entire specimen.

meconium A dark green gelatinous or mucus-like material that represents swallowed amniotic fluid and intestinal secretions excreted by the near-term or full-term infant. The infant normally passes meconium as the first bowel movement shortly after birth.

medulla The inner portion of the kidney. Macroscopically organized into pyramids, the medulla is the location of the loops of Henle and the collecting tubules (or ducts).

melanuria The increased excretion of melanin in the urine.

melena The excretion of dark or black, pitchy-looking stools because of the presence of large amounts (50 to 100 mL/day) of blood in the feces. The coloration is due to hemoglobin oxidation by intestinal and bacterial enzymes in the gastrointestinal tract.

membranoproliferative glomerulonephritis A type of glomerular inflammation characterized by cellular proliferation of the mesangium, with leukocyte infiltration and thickening of the glomerular basement membrane. Immunologically based, the disease is slowly progressive.

membranous glomerulonephritis A type of glomerular inflammation characterized by the deposition of immunoglobulins and complement along the epithelial side (podocytes) of the basement membrane. The condition is associated with numerous immune-mediated diseases and is the major cause of nephritic syndrome in adults.

meninges The three membranes that surround the brain and spinal cord. The innermost membrane is the pia mater, the outermost membrane is the dura mater, and the centrally located membrane is the arachnoid (or arachnoidea).

meningitis Inflammation of the meninges.

mesangium The cells that form the structural core tissue of a glomerulus. The mesangium lies between the glomerular capillaries (endothelium) and the podocytes (tubular epithelium). The mesangial cells derive from smooth muscle and have contractility characteristics and the ability to phagocytize and pinocytize.

mesothelial cells Flat cells that form a single layer of epithelium, which covers the surface of serous membranes (i.e., the pleura, pericardium, and peritoneum).

micturition Urination or the passing of urine.

midstream "clean catch" specimen A urine specimen obtained after thorough cleansing of the glans penis in the male or the urethral meatus in the female. After the cleansing procedure, the patient passes the first portion of the urine into the toilet, stops and collects the midportion in the specimen container, and then passes any remaining urine into the toilet. Used for routine urinalysis and urine culture, the specimen is essentially free of contaminants from the genitalia and the distal urethra.

minimal change disease A type of glomerular inflammation characterized by loss of the podocyte foot processes. Believed to be immune mediated, the condition is the major cause of nephrotic syndrome in children.

multiple myeloma A malignant disease characterized by the infiltration of bone and bone marrow by neoplastic plasma cells. Findings include anemia, high globulin levels (e.g., immunoglobulin light chains), pathologic fractures, and renal failure.

multiple sclerosis A chronic disease of the central nervous system in which destruction of myelin and nerve axons occurs within several regions of the brain and spinal cord at different times.

myoglobinuria The presence of myoglobin in urine.

N

nephritic syndrome A group of clinical findings indicative of glomerular damage that include hematuria, proteinuria, azotemia, edema, hypertension, and oliguria. The severity and combination of features vary with the glomerular disease.

nephritis Inflammation of the kidney.

nephron The functional unit of the kidney. Each kidney contains approximately 1.3 million nephrons. A nephron is composed of five distinct areas: the glomerulus, the proximal tubule, the loop of Henle, the distal tubule, and the collecting tubule or duct. Each region of the nephron is specialized and plays a role in the formation and final composition of urine.

nephrotic syndrome A collection of clinical findings indicating adverse glomerular changes. It is characterized by proteinuria, hypoalbuminemia, hyperlipidemia, lipiduria, and generalized edema. A nonspecific disorder associated with renal as well as systemic diseases.

nocturia   Excessive or increased frequency of urination at night (i.e., the patient excretes more than 500 mL per night).

numerical aperture   A number that indicates the resolving power of a lens system. The numerical aperture (NA) is derived mathematically from the refractive index (n) of the optical medium (for air, n = 1) and the angle of light (m) made by the lens: NA = n × sin m.

O

objective   The lens or system of lenses located closest to the specimen. The objective produces the primary image magnification of the specimen.

occult blood   Small amounts of blood, not visually apparent, in the feces.

Occupational Safety and Health Administration (OSHA)   Established by Congress in 1970, OSHA is the division of the U.S. Department of Labor that is responsible for defining potential safety and health hazards in the workplace, establishing guidelines to safeguard all workers from these hazards, and monitoring compliance with these guidelines. The intent is to alert, educate, and protect all employees in every environment to potential safety and health hazards.

oligoclonal bands   Multiple discrete bands in the g region noted during electrophoresis of plasma or other body fluids (e.g., cerebrospinal fluid).

oligohydramnios   A decreased amount of amniotic fluid in the amniotic sac.

oliguria   A significant decrease in the volume of urine excreted (less than 400 mL/day).

osmolality   An expression of concentration in terms of the total number of solute particles present per kilogram of solvent, denoted osmoles per kilogram H_2O.

osmolar clearance   The volume of plasma water cleared by the kidneys each minute that contains the same amount of solutes that are present in the blood plasma (i.e., the same osmolality). Stated another way, osmolar clearance is the volume of plasma water necessary for the rate of solute elimination. Reported in milliliters per minute, osmolar clearance is determined by the equation $C = U \times V/P$, in which U and P are the urine and plasma osmolalities, respectively, and V is the volume of urine excreted in a timed collection, usually 24 hours.

osmometer   See *freezing point osmometer* and *vapor pressure osmometer.*

osmosis   The movement of water across a semipermeable membrane in an attempt to achieve an osmotic equilibrium between two compartments or solutions of differing osmolality (i.e., an osmotic gradient). This mechanism is passive, that is, it requires no energy.

oval fat bodies   Renal tubular epithelial cells or macrophages with inclusions of fat or lipids. Often these cells are engorged such that specific cellular identification is impossible.

overflow proteinuria   An increased amount of protein in urine caused by increased quantities of plasma proteins passing through a healthy glomerular filtration barrier.

P

paracellular   The transport of substances from one tissue space to another around cells via intercellular junctions.

paracentesis   A percutaneous puncture procedure used to remove fluid from a body cavity such as the pleural, pericardial, or peritoneal cavity.

parcentered   Term describing objective lenses that retain the same field of view when the user switches from one objective to another of a differing magnification.

parfocal   Term describing objective lenses that remain in focus when the user switches from one objective to another of a differing magnification.

passive transport   The movement of a substance (e.g., ion, solute) across a cell membrane along a gradient (e.g., concentration, charge). Passive transport does not require energy.

pathogenesis   The physiologic and biochemical mechanisms by which disease develops and progresses.

pericardiocentesis   A surgical puncture into the pericardial space for the aspiration of serous fluid.

pericardium   The serous membrane that surrounds the heart.

peritoneocentesis   A surgical puncture into the peritoneal space for the aspiration of serous fluid.

peritoneum   The serous membrane that lines the abdominal and pelvic walls (parietal) and the organs (visceral) that reside within.

peritubular capillaries   The network of capillaries (or plexus) that forms from the efferent arteriole and surrounds the tubules of the nephron in the renal cortex.

personal protective equipment   Items used to eliminate exposure of the body to potentially infectious agents. These barriers include protective gowns, gloves, eye and face protectors, biosafety cabinets (fume hoods), splash shields, and specimen transport containers.

phase-contrast microscopy   Type of microscopy in which variations in the specimen refractive index are converted into variations in light intensity or contrast. Areas of the specimen appear light to dark with haloes of varying intensity related to the thickness of the component. Thin, flat components produce less haloing and the best-detailed images. Phase-contrast microscopy is ideal for viewing low-refractile elements and living cells.

phenylketonuria   An autosomal recessive inherited enzyme defect or deficiency characterized by the inability to convert phenylalanine to tyrosine. As a result, phenylalanine is converted to phenylketones, which are excreted in the urine.

pleocytosis   The presence of a greater than normal number of cells in the cerebrospinal fluid.

podocytes   The epithelial cells that line the urinary (Bowman's) space of the glomerulus. These cells completely cover the glomerular capillaries with large finger-like processes that interdigitate to form a filtration slit. The term *podo*, which is Greek for "foot," relates to the footlike appearance of the podocyte when viewed in cross section. Collectively, the podocytes constitute the glomerular epithelium that forms Bowman's capsule.

polarizing microscopy   Type of microscopy that illuminates the specimen with polarized light. Polarizing microscopy is used to identify and classify birefringent substances (i.e., substances that refract light in two directions) that shine brilliantly against a dark background.

polydipsia   Intense and excessive thirst.

polyhydramnios (also called *hydramnios*) An abnormally increased amount (>1200 mL) of amniotic fluid in the amniotic sac. Polyhydramnios is often associated with malformations of the fetal central nervous system (i.e., neural tube defects) or gastrointestinal tract.

polyuria The excretion of large volumes of urine (greater than 3 L/day).

porphobilinogen An intermediate compound formed in the production of heme and a porphyrin precursor.

porphyria The increased production of porphyrin precursors or porphyrins.

porphyrinuria The presence of an increased quantity of porphyrins or porphyrin precursors in urine.

postprandial After a meal.

postrenal proteinuria An increased amount of protein in urine resulting from a disease process that adds protein to urine after its formation by the renal nephrons.

postural (orthostatic) proteinuria An increased protein excretion in urine only when an individual is in an upright (orthostatic) position.

preventive maintenance The performance of specific tasks in a timely fashion to eliminate equipment failure. These tasks vary with the instrument and include cleaning procedures, inspection of components, and component replacement when necessary.

procedure manual A written document describing in detail all aspects of each policy and procedure performed in the laboratory. For example, the manual includes supplies needed, reagent preparation procedures, specimen requirements, mislabeled and unlabeled specimen protocols, procedures for the storage and disposal of wastes, technical procedures, quality control criteria, reporting formats, and references.

prostate gland A lobular gland surrounding the male urethra immediately after it exits the bladder. The prostate is an accessory gland of the male reproductive system. The prostate is testosterone dependent and produces a mildly acidic secretion rich in citric acid, enzymes, proteins, and zinc.

protein error of indicators A phenomenon characterized by several pH indicators. These pH indicators undergo a color change in the presence of protein despite a constant pH. Described originally by Sorenson in 1909, the protein error of indicators provides the basis for protein screening tests used on reagent strips.

proteinuria The presence of an increased amount of protein in urine.

proximal convoluted tubular cells Large (approximately 20 to 60 mm in diameter) oblong or cigar-shaped cells with a small, often eccentric, nucleus (or they can be multinucleated) and a dense chromatin pattern; these cells form the lining of the proximal tubules.

proximal tubule The tubular part of a nephron immediately following the glomerulus. The proximal tubule has a convoluted portion and a straight portion, the latter becoming the loop of Henle after entering the renal medulla.

Prussian blue reaction (also called the *Rous test*) A chemical reaction used to identify the presence of iron. Iron-containing granules such as hemosiderin stain a characteristic blue color when mixed with a freshly prepared solution of potassium ferricyanide–HCl.

pseudochylous effusion An effusion that appears milky but does not contain chylomicrons and has a low (<50 mg/dL) triglyceride content.

pseudoperoxidase activity The action of heme-containing compounds (e.g., hemoglobin, myoglobin) to mimic true peroxidases by catalyzing the oxidation of some substrates in the presence of hydrogen peroxide.

pus A protein-rich product of inflammation and cellular necrosis that consists of leukocytes and cellular debris.

pyuria The presence of pus in urine. Compare *leukocyturia*.

Q

quality assurance An established protocol of policies and procedures for all laboratory actions performed to ensure the quality of services (i.e., test results) rendered.

quality control materials Materials used to assess and monitor the accuracy and precision (i.e., analytic error) of a method.

R

random urine specimen A urine specimen collected at any time, day or night, without prior patient preparation.

rapidly progressive glomerulonephritis (RPGN; also called *crescentic glomerulonephritis*) A type of glomerular inflammation characterized by cellular proliferation into Bowman's space to form "crescents." Numerous disease processes can lead to its development, including systemic lupus erythematosus, vasculitis, and infections.

reflectance The scattering or reflecting of light when it strikes a matte or unpolished surface. The intensity and wavelength of the reflected light vary depending on the color of the surface and the wavelength of the incident light used.

reflectance photometry The detection and quantification of light intensity based on reflectance.

refractive index The ratio of light refraction in two differing media (n). The refractive index is expressed mathematically using light velocity (V) or the angle of refraction (sin q) in the two media, as $n2/n1 = V1/V2$ or $n2/n1 = \sin q1/\sin q2$. The refractive index is affected by the wavelength of light used, the temperature of the solution, and the concentration of the solution.

refractometer An instrument used to measure the specific gravity of liquids based on their refractive index.

refractometry An indirect measurement of specific gravity based on the refractive index of light.

renal blood flow The volume of blood that passes through the renal vasculature per unit of time. The renal blood flow normally ranges from 1000 to 1200 mL/min.

renal clearance The volume of plasma cleared of a substance by the kidneys per unit of time. Reported in milliliters per minute, renal clearance is determined by the equation $C = U \times V/P$, in which U and P are the urine and plasma concentrations of the substance, respectively, and V is the volume of urine excreted in a timed collection, usually 24 hours. The most common renal clearance test is the creatinine clearance test.

renal pelvis The funnel-shaped structure located at the indented region of the kidney that receives the urine from the calyces and conveys it to the ureter.

renal phosphaturia A rare hereditary disease characterized by the inability of the distal tubules to reabsorb inorganic phosphorus.

renal plasma flow The volume of plasma that passes through the renal vasculature per unit of time. The renal plasma flow normally ranges from 600 to 700 mL/min.

renal proteinuria Increased amounts of protein in urine as a result of impaired renal function.

renal threshold level The plasma concentration of a solute above which the amount of solute present in the ultrafiltrate exceeds the maximal tubular reabsorptive capacity. Once the renal threshold level has been reached, increased amounts of solute are excreted (i.e., lost) in the urine.

renal tubular acidosis A renal disorder characterized by the inability of the renal tubules to secrete adequate hydrogen ions. Four types are recognized, and they can be inherited or acquired. Patients are unable to produce an acidic urine, regardless of the acid-base status of the blood plasma.

renin A proteolytic enzyme produced and stored by the cells of the juxtaglomerular apparatus of the renal nephrons. Secretion of renin results in the formation of angiotensin and the secretion of aldosterone; thus renin plays an important role in controlling blood pressure and fluid balance.

resolution Ability of a lens to distinguish two points or objects as separate. The resolving power (R) of a microscope depends on the wavelength of light used (l) and the numerical aperture of the objective lens. The greater the resolving power, the smaller the distance distinguished between two separate points.

rhabdomyolysis The breakdown or destruction of skeletal muscle cells.

S

scybala Plural of scybalum. Dry, hard masses of fecal material in the intestine.

semi-automated Indicates that some steps are performed manually and others are automated.

semi-automated urinalysis A urinalysis that is partially automated. For example, the physical and chemical examinations could be automated whereas, urine microscopic examination (if performed), is performed manually.

seminal fluid (also called *semen*) A complex body fluid that transports spermatozoa. Seminal fluid is composed of secretions from the testes, epididymis, seminal vesicles, and prostate gland.

seminal vesicles Paired glands that secrete a slightly alkaline fluid, rich in fructose, into the ejaculatory duct. Most of the fluid in the ejaculate originates in the seminal vesicles.

seminiferous tubules Numerous coiled tubules located in the testes. The seminiferous tubules are collectively the site of spermatogenesis. Immature and immotile spermatozoa are released into the seminiferous tubular lumen and are carried by its secretions to the epididymis for maturation.

serous fluid A fluid that has a composition similar to that of serum.

shield of negativity A term describing the impediment produced by negatively charged components (e.g., proteoglycans) of the glomerular filtration barrier. Present on both sides of and throughout the filtration barrier, these negatively charged components effectively limit the filtration of negatively charged substances from the blood (e.g., albumin) into the urinary space.

specific gravity A measure of the concentration of a solution based on its density. The density of the solution is compared with the density of an equal volume of water at the same temperature. Specific gravity measurements are affected by solute number and solute mass.

sperm (also called *spermatozoa*) Male reproductive cells.

spherical aberration Unequal refraction of light rays when they pass through different portions of a lens such that the light rays are not brought to the same focus. As a result, the image produced is blurred or fuzzy and cannot be brought into sharp focus.

squamous epithelial cells Large (approximately 40 to 60 mm in diameter), thin, flagstone-shaped cells with a small, condensed, centrally located nucleus (or they can be anucleated) that form the lining of the urethra in the female and the distal urethra in the male.

Standard Precautions One tier of the *Guideline for Isolation Precautions* from the Healthcare Infection Control Practices Advisory Committee (HICPAC) and the Centers for Disease Control and Prevention (CDC) that describes procedures to prevent transmission of infectious agents when obtaining, handling, storing, or disposing of all blood, body fluid, or body substances, regardless of patient identity or patient health status. All body fluids including secretions and excretions should be treated as potentially infectious.

stat An abbreviation for the Latin word *statim*, which means "immediately."

steatorrhea The excretion of greater than 6 g/day of fat in the feces.

subarachnoid space The space between the arachnid and the pia mater.

suprapubic aspiration A technique used to collect urine directly from the bladder by puncturing the abdominal wall and the distended bladder using a sterile needle and syringe. Aspiration is used primarily to obtain sterile specimens for bacterial cultures from infants and occasionally from adults.

syndrome A group of symptoms or characteristics that occur together such as the nephrotic syndrome and Fanconi's syndrome.

synovial fluid Fluid within joint cavities. Synovial fluid is formed by the ultrafiltration of plasma across the synovial membrane and by secretions from synoviocytes.

synoviocytes Cells of the synovial membrane. There are two types of synoviocytes based on their physiologic roles. The predominant type is actively phagocytic and synthesizes degradative enzymes; the second type synthesizes and secretes hyaluronate.

systemic lupus erythematosus An autoimmune disorder that affects numerous organ systems and is characterized by autoantibodies. The disease is chronic, is frequently insidious, often causes fever, and involves varied neurologic, hematologic, and immunologic abnormalities. Renal involvement, as well as pleuritis and pericarditis, is common. The clinical presentation varies greatly and is associated with a constellation of symptoms such as joint pain, skin lesions, leukopenia, hypergammaglobulinemia, antinuclear antibodies, and LE cells.

T

Tamm-Horsfall protein   See *uromodulin*.

technical competence   The ability of an individual to perform a skilled task correctly. Technical competence also includes the ability to evaluate results, such as recognizing discrepancies and absurdities.

test utilization   The frequency with which a test is performed on a single individual and how it is used to evaluate a disease process. Repeat testing of an individual is costly and may not provide additional or useful information. Sometimes a different test may provide more diagnostically useful information.

thoracentesis   A surgical puncture into the pleural space for the aspiration of serous fluid.

timed collection   A urine specimen collected throughout a specific timed interval. The patient voids at the beginning of the collection and discards this urine and then collects all subsequent urine. At the end of the timed interval, the patient voids and includes this urine in the collection. This technique is used primarily for quantitative urine assays because it allows comparison of excretion patterns from day to day; the most common are 12-hour and 24-hour collections.

titratable acids   A term representing H+ ions (acid) excreted in the urine as monobasic phosphate (e.g., NaH_2PO_4). The urinary excretion of these acids results in the elimination of H^+ ions and the reabsorption of sodium and bicarbonate. The titration of urine using a standard base (e.g., NaOH) to a pH of 7.4 (normal plasma pH) will quantitate the number of H^+ ions excreted in this form, hence the name *titratable acids*.

transcellular   The transport of substances from one tissue space to another by passing through or across cells.

transitional (urothelial) epithelial cells   Round or pear-shaped cells with an oval to round nucleus and abundant cytoplasm. These cells form the lining of the renal calyces, renal pelves, ureters, and bladder. These cells vary considerably in size, ranging from 20 to 40 mm in diameter depending on their location in the three principal layers of this epithelium, that is, the superficial layer, the intermediate layers, and the basal layer.

transudate   An effusion in a body cavity caused by increased hydrostatic pressure (i.e., blood pressure) or decreased plasma oncotic pressure. A transudate is identified by a fluid-to-serum total protein ratio of less than 0.5 and a fluid-to-serum lactate dehydrogenase ratio of less than 0.6.

tubular proteinuria   Increased amounts of protein in urine resulting from impaired or altered renal tubular function.

tubular reabsorption   The movement of substances (by active or passive transport) from the tubular ultrafiltrate into the peritubular blood or the interstitium by the renal tubular cells.

tubular secretion   The movement of substances (by active or passive transport) from the peritubular blood or the interstitium into the tubular ultrafiltrate by the renal tubular cells.

turnaround time   To the laboratorian, the time that elapses from receipt of the specimen in the laboratory to the reporting of test results on that specimen. Physicians and nursing personnel assign a broader time frame.

tyrosinuria   The presence of the amino acid tyrosine in the urine.

U

urea cycle   A passive process that occurs throughout the nephron that establishes and maintains a high concentration of urea in the renal medulla. This process accounts for approximately 50% of the solutes concentrated in the medulla. With the countercurrent exchange mechanism, the urea cycle helps establish and maintain the high medullary osmotic gradient. Because urea can passively diffuse into the interstitium and back into the lumen fluid, the selectivity of the tubular epithelium in each portion of the nephron plays an integral part in the urea cycling process.

ureter   A fibromuscular tube, approximately 25 cm long, that emerges from the renal pelvis of each kidney and extends down to connect to the base of the bladder. Peristaltic activity by smooth muscle moves the urine through the ureters down into the bladder.

urethra   A canal connecting the bladder to the exterior of the body that is approximately 4 cm long in the female and approximately 24 cm long in the male.

-uria   Of or relating to urine.

urinary space   The area in which the ultrafiltrate of plasma first forms in the nephron. This space, also known as *Bowman's space*, is located between the podocytes of the glomerulus and the specialized epithelium (Bowman's capsule) of the proximal end of the renal tubule that surrounds the glomerulus.

urinary system   The structures involved in the formation, storage, and excretion of urine. The urinary system includes the kidneys, ureters, bladder, and urethra.

urinary tract infection   The invasion and proliferation of microorganisms in the kidney or urinary tract.

urine   A fluid composed of water and metabolic waste products that is secreted by the kidneys. Urine begins as an ultrafiltrate of plasma that is modified as it passes through the renal nephrons. The composition of urine remains unchanged after passing from the renal pelvis of the kidneys into the ureters.

urine preservative   A procedure or chemical substance used to prevent composition changes in a voided urine specimen (e.g., loss or gain of chemical substances, deterioration of formed elements). The most common form of urine preservation is refrigeration.

urinometer   See *hydrometer*.

urobilin   An orange-brown pigment derived from the spontaneous oxidation of colorless urobilinogen.

urobilinogen   A colorless tetrapyrrole derived from bilirubin. Urobilinogen is produced in the intestinal tract by the action of anaerobic bacteria and is later partially reabsorbed. Most reabsorbed urobilinogen is reprocessed by the liver and re-excreted in the bile; the rest passes to the kidneys for excretion in the urine. The portion of urobilinogen that is not reabsorbed becomes oxidized to the orange-brown pigment urobilin in the large intestine, which accounts for the characteristic color of feces.

urobilins   Orange-brown pigments that impart to feces their characteristic color. Specifically, the pigments are stercobilin, mesobilin, and urobilin, which result from spontaneous intestinal oxidation of the colorless tetrapyrroles stercobilinogen, mesobilinogen, and urobilinogen.

urochrome   A lipid-soluble yellow pigment that is produced continuously during endogenous metabolism. Present in plasma and excreted in the urine, urochrome gives urine its characteristic yellow color.

uroerythrin   Pink (or red) pigment in urine that is thought to derive from melanin metabolism. Uroerythrin deposits on urate crystals to produce a precipitate described as "brick dust."

uromodulin   A glycoprotein, formerly known as *Tamm-Horsfall protein*, that is produced and secreted only by renal tubular cells, particularly those of the thick ascending limbs of the loops of Henle and the distal convoluted tubules. Studies have demonstrated that uromodulin plays a role in the following functions in the kidney: water impermeability of the tubules where it is expressed, defense against infectious agents (e.g., bacteria), and inhibition of calcium salt aggregation.

V

vaginal fornix   The arched recesses of the vaginal mucosa that surround the cervix. Of the four recesses, the posterior fornix is deeper than the anterior and lateral (right and left) fornices.

vaginal pool   The mucus and cells present in the posterior fornix of the vagina when a female is in a supine position.

vaginitis   Inflammation of the vagina.

vapor pressure osmometer   An instrument that measures osmolality based on the vapor pressure depression of a solution compared with that of pure water. The dew point of the air in a closed chamber containing a small amount of a sample is measured and compared with that obtained using pure water. A calibrated microprocessor converts the observed change in the dew point into osmolality, which is read directly from the instrument readout.

vasa recta   The vascular network of long, U-shaped capillaries that forms from the peritubular capillaries and surrounds the loops of Henle in the renal medulla.

ventricles   The four fluid-filled cavities in the brain lined with ependymal cells. The choroid plexus is located in the ventricles.

viscosity   A measure of fluid flow or its resistance to flow. Low-viscosity fluids (e.g., water) flow freely and form discrete droplets when expelled drop by drop from a pipette. In contrast, high-viscosity fluids (e.g., corn syrup) flow less freely and do not form discrete droplets; rather they momentarily form threads or strings as they are expelled from a pipette.

vulvovaginitis   Inflammation of the vulva and vagina or of the vulvovaginal glands (i.e., Bartholin's glands).

X

xanthochromia   The pink, orange, or yellowish discoloration of supernatant cerebrospinal fluid after centrifugation.

Y

yeast infection   An inflammatory condition that results from the proliferation of a fungus, most commonly *Candida* species.

ANSWER KEY

CHAPTER 1

1. D
2. D
3. D
4. B
5. A
6. A 7
   B 3
   C 5
   D 2
   E 1
   F 4
7. D
8. B
9. B
10. C
11. A
12. C
13. B
14. C
15. C
16. B
17. D
18. A
19. A
20. A 2
    B 3
    C 6
    D 5
    E 4

CHAPTER 2

1. D
2. B
3. A
4. A
5. C
6. C
7. D
8. B
9. B
10. B
11. D
12. D
13. C
14. A
15. A 3
    B 1
    C 2
    D 3
    E 3
    F 2
16. C

17. A
18. C
19. D
20. B

Case 2-1
1. E
2. C

CHAPTER 3

1. B
2. B
3. D
4. A
5. C
6. A
   B
   A
7. C
8. C
   A
   A
   A
   C
9. D
10. C
11. A
12. B
13. B

CHAPTER 4

1. A 10
   B 7
   C 6
   D 5
   E 1
   F 4
   G 3
   H 2
   I 8
   J 9
   K 11
2. C
3. A
4. C
5. A
6. A
7. D
8. A
9. A
10. D
11. D
12. A

13. A
14. C
15. C
16. A
17. C
18. A
19. C
20. D
21. B
22. D
23. C
24. A
25. B
26. C
27. C
28. D
29. A
30. B
31. A

CHAPTER 5

1. A
2. B
3. A
4. C
5. C
6. C
7. C
8. A
9. B
10. C
11. D
12. C
13. D
14. C
15. B
16. D
17. B
18. A
19. A
20. C
21. B
22. B
23. B
24. A. Yes
    B. Yes
    C. Hypo-osmotic
25. C
26. B
27. D
28. D
29. D
30. A. 42 mL/min (Note that the plasma and urine creatinine results must first be converted to the same units.)

B. 58 mL/min
C. Yes

31. A
32. B
33. B
34. A
35. C
36. C
37. A
38. D

Case 5-1

1. Surface area: 1.80
2. Normalized creatinine clearance: 55 (54.7) mL/min (using Equation 5-5)
3. 95 mg/day
4. 66 μg/min
5. 50 μg/mg creatinine

Case 5-2

1. Because of damage to the hypothalamus or the posterior pituitary, antidiuretic hormone production is partially or totally deficient. Consequently, tubular reabsorption of water does not occur and polyuria results.
2. A
3. D
4. C
5. B
6. F
7. F
8. F
9. T

CHAPTER 6

1. D
2. D
3. A
4. C
5. A 2, 3
   B 8
   C 4, 7
   D 7 (4)
   E 6 (4)
   F 3, 7
   G 1
   H 2
   I 5
6. A
7. D
8. B
9. A
10. A
11. A 1
    B 2

C 1
D 2
E 2
F 1
G 1
H 2
I 2
J 2
K 1
L 1
12. D
13. A
14. A 5
   B 3
   C 1
   D 1, 2
   E 5
   F 1, 4
15. B
16. B
17. A
18. A 1
   B 3
   C 2
   D 1
19. B
20. D
21. A
22. A
23. D
24. C
25. C
26. A
27. B
28. D

Case 6-1
1. B
2. D

Case 6-2
1. D
2. C

CHAPTER 7

1. C
2. A
3. B
4. C
5. D
6. C
7. B
8. C
9. B
10. B
11. A

12. D
13. B
14. A
15. D
16. B
17. D
18. D
19. D
20. B
21. D
22. A
23. D
24. A 3
   B 2
   C 3
   D 1
   E 4
   F 2
   G 1
   H 2
   I 3
25. A
26. A
27. C
28. B
29. D
30. D
31. B
32. D
33. B
34. D
35. C
36. C
37. D
38. B
39. D
40. C
41. B
42. D
43. C
44. D
45. D
46. A
47. B
48. A
49. D
50. D
51. C

Case 7-1
1. Abnormal findings:
   Physical examination—large amount of white foam
   Chemical examination—glucose, blood, protein
2. B
3. The changes in the glomerular filtration barrier that are now allowing increased quantities of plasma proteins to pass with the ultrafiltrate into the tubules are

also enabling red blood cells to pass. Once in the tubular lumen, red blood cells ultimately are eliminated in the urine.

4. No. To affect the protein reaction pad, large amounts of hemoglobin (>5 mg/dL) are needed, and when this amount of hemoglobin is present, the blood reaction always will read "large." However, note that it is possible to have a negative protein test with a "large" blood reaction.

5. A

6. Albumin

7. This patient has inadequate insulin resulting in a blood glucose concentration that exceeds the renal tubular reabsorptive capacity (T_m), that is, too much glucose is in the ultrafiltrate to be reabsorbed, and the excess is excreted in the urine.

Case 7-2

1. Abnormal findings:
   Physical examination—slightly cloudy
   Chemical examination—protein
   Discrepant results: Protein results by reagent strip and sulfosalicylic acid precipitation test (SSA) do not agree.

2. Protein(s) other than albumin are present.

3. B

4. C

Case 7-3

1. Abnormal findings:
   Chemical examination—Hoesch test

2. Porphobilin that has formed from the spontaneous oxidation of porphobilinogen

3. Watson-Schwartz test

4. An enzyme deficiency in the pathway of hemoglobin synthesis causes increased production of heme precursors (i.e., δ-aminolevulinic acid and porphobilinogen), which are water soluble and are excreted in the urine. Porphobilinogen becomes oxidized, causing the color change observed in this urine.

5. Acute intermittent porphyria

6. D

7. No. Neither porphobilinogen nor porphobilin is detectable by any of the commercial reagent strips available.

Case 7-4

1. Abnormal urine findings:
   Physical examination—color
   Chemical examination—blood, protein
   Abnormal blood results: creatine kinase and myoglobin

2. C

3. D

4. The trace protein result is from albumin. The amount of protein presented to the tubules for reabsorption is increased owing to myoglobin. Because this reabsorptive process is nonselective, an increased amount of albumin is not reabsorbed and is excreted in the urine.

5. During surgery while patients are under anesthesia and are placed in various positions (e.g., Simon's position), the blood supply to muscles can be inadvertently reduced, causing tissue hypoxia. The damaged muscle tissue releases myoglobin into the bloodstream, which is subsequently cleared from the plasma by the kidneys.

Case 7-5

1. Abnormal findings:
   Chemical examination—glucose, ketone
   Discrepant results: Specific gravity by reagent strip and refractometers does not agree.

2. Very high glucose concentrations cause the Clinitest reaction rapidly to turn to orange (indicates high concentration) and continue to change color. At the appropriate read time, the reaction mixture best matches the green/blue colors that represent a low glucose concentration.

3. If the entire Clinitest reaction is not observed, the pass-through effect would not be seen and a falsely low glucose result may be reported.

4. No

5. B, based on sudden onset of symptoms and age

6. Because of the inability of the body to utilize the carbohydrates (glucose) available, increased fatty acid metabolism is providing energy for bodily functions. This increases the amount of acetyl coenzyme A produced, which overwhelms the capacity of the liver to process it via the Krebs cycle and results in ketogenesis (i.e., ketonemia and ketonuria).

7. The refractometer result is detecting the glucose present, whereas the reagent strip result is not. The reagent strip specific gravity more accurately reflects the ability of the kidney to concentrate the urine (a process involving the normal and small ionic solutes usually present in urine) because it is not affected by high-molecular-weight solutes (e.g., glucose), which normally are not present in urine.

Case 7-6

1. Abnormal urine findings:
   Physical examination—color, clarity, yellow foam
   Chemical examination—protein, Ictotest

2. Bilirubin

3. The most likely reason is that the amount of bilirubin present is too low and is not detected by the reagent strip. The Ictotest has a lower detection limit than the reagent strip test.

4. Report the bilirubin as positive.

5. Once formed and conjugated by hepatocytes, bilirubin normally is conveyed to the bile ducts for excretion into the intestinal tract via the common bile duct. During inflammatory liver processes (e.g., hepatitis,

cirrhosis), conjugated bilirubin can "leak" back into the systemic circulation. In the kidneys, conjugated bilirubin readily passes the glomerular filtration barriers and appears in the urine.

6. Conjugated bilirubin, which is small enough to cross the glomerular filtration barrier. Unconjugated bilirubin in the bloodstream is bound to albumin, making it too large to pass a healthy glomerular filtration barrier.

7. The urobilinogen is normal because its formation (in the gastrointestinal tract) and processing essentially are unaffected by this patient's disorder (i.e., hepatitis). However, in severe cases of liver disease, the urine urobilinogen can be increased. This increase occurs when the liver is no longer functionally capable of removing its usual percentage (15% to 18%) of urobilinogen from the portal blood (absorbed from the intestine).

CHAPTER 8

1. D
2. D
3. C
4. B
5. A
6. C
7. D
8. D
9. B
10. C
11. D
12. B
13. A 4
    B 3
    C 1
    D 2
    E 5
14. B
15. A
16. D
17. A
18. A
19. D
20. C
21. B
22. A
23. B
24. A 3
    B 1 (2)
    C 3 (2)
    D 1, 2, 3
    E 1
    F 1 (2, 3)
    G 1
    H 1

    I 3 (2)
    J 1
    K 1
25. A 8
    B 6
    C 4
    D 5
    E 1
    F 9
    G 7
26. A
27. A
28. B
29. A
30. D
31. B
32. A
33. A
34. C
35. A

Case 8-1
1. Abnormal urine findings:
   Physical examination—cloudy
   Microscopic examination—unidentified crystals
   Discrepant results—specific gravity by refractometer and reagent strip; protein by reagent strip and SSA
2. E
3. Refractometer specific gravity of greater than 1.035 and crystalline precipitate in SSA test with no albumin present
4. Negative protein (albumin) by reagent strip. Lipiduria is always accompanied by some level of proteinuria; however, the level can vary with the patient's hydration status.
5. A

Case 8-2
1. Abnormal findings:
   Physical examination—cloudy
   Chemical examination—blood trace, protein trace
   Microscopic examination—WBCs, 10 to 25; bacteria, moderate; TE, moderate
   Note: Two to five hyaline casts is not clinically significant.
2. B
3. In a urine specimen from a woman, a large number of squamous epithelial cells often indicates that the specimen is contaminated with cells and constituents from the perineum and vagina, that is, not a clean catch. In this case, the bacteria present most likely represent normal flora from the perineum and are not from the urinary tract.
4. The nitrite test is a screening test for bacteriuria. Three reasons for a negative test despite the presence of bacteria include the following:

1. Inadequate incubation time in urine for bacterial conversion of nitrate to nitrite
2. The patient's diet does not include dietary nitrates.
3. The bacteria present are not nitrate reducers.
5. The leukocyte esterase test is a screening test for granulocytic leukocytes. Two reasons for a negative test despite the presence of white blood cells include the following:
   1. The amount of leukocyte esterase present is below the sensitivity of the test, despite increased numbers of white blood cells.
   2. The white blood cells present are lymphocytes that do not contain leukocyte esterase.
6. Increased sloughing of transitional epithelial cells at site of infection/inflammation, for example, the bladder

Case 8-3

1. Abnormal findings:
   Physical examination—large amount of foam present, slightly cloudy
   Chemical examination—glucose, blood, protein
   Microscopic examination—RBCs, fatty casts, waxy casts, oval fat bodies
2. B
3. A
4. B
5. Severe proteinuria results in hypoproteinemia. As blood protein is lost, the intravascular oncotic pressure decreases and fluid moves into the tissues.
6. Albumin. Because of its size (it is small enough to pass the glomerular filtration barrier if the shield of negativity is removed) and its high plasma concentration (compared with other plasma proteins), albumin usually is the first protein lost.
7. This patient has inadequate insulin, resulting in a blood glucose concentration that exceeds the renal tubular reabsorptive capacity (T_m), that is, too much glucose is in the ultrafiltrate to be reabsorbed, and the excess is excreted in the urine.
8. At this time, the patient has not reverted to significant lipolysis (i.e., increased fatty acid metabolism) to supply the energy needed for bodily functions.

Case 8-4

1. Abnormal findings:
   Physical examination—color, clarity
   Chemical examination— blood, protein
   Microscopic examination—RBCs, granular casts, RBC casts
2. Normally, red blood cells are too large to pass the glomerular filtration barrier. However, nephrogenic strains of streptococcus form immune complexes, which deposit in the glomerular membrane—acute poststreptococcal glomerulonephritis—causing damage to the glomerular filtration barrier and enabling the passage of red blood cells into the renal tubules.

3. B
4. A
5. Red blood cell casts

Case 8-5

1. Abnormal findings:
   Physical examination—clarity
   Chemical examination—glucose, ketone, leukocyte esterase
   Microscopic examination—WBCs, yeast, many SEs (indicates that specimen is not a clean catch)
2. Vaginal yeast infection
3. White blood cells are from vaginal fluid that is contaminating the urine.
4. Yeast and many squamous epithelial cells
5. No
6. Because of the inability of the body to utilize the carbohydrates (glucose) available, increased fatty acid metabolism is providing energy for bodily functions. This increases the amount of acetyl coenzyme A produced, which overwhelms the capacity of the liver to process it via the Krebs cycle and results in ketogenesis (i.e., ketonemia and ketonuria). This patient most likely has type 2 diabetes mellitus.

Case 8-6

1. Abnormal findings:
   Physical examination—color, clarity
   Chemical examination—blood, protein, urobilinogen
   Microscopic examination—increased number of granular casts
2. Hemosiderin is a storage form of iron that results from ferritin denaturation.
3. Free hemoglobin passes the filtration barrier and is reabsorbed primarily by the proximal renal tubule (and to a lesser degree by the distal tubules). The tubular cells catabolize the hemoglobin to ferritin and subsequently denature it to form hemosiderin. When these renal cells are sloughed, hemosiderin is found in the urine.
4. Two sources possible: the degradation (oxidation) of hemoglobin and the oxidation of urobilinogen to urobilin
5. A hemolytic episode causes the formation and excretion into the intestine of an increased amount of bilirubin. As a result, an increased amount of urobilinogen is formed and is absorbed into the enterohepatic circulation. The increased amount of urobilinogen absorbed is excreted in the urine.
6. Intravascular hemolysis results primarily in an increased amount of unconjugated bilirubin in the blood. To be soluble in plasma, unconjugated bilirubin is bound tightly to albumin, which results in a molecular complex too large to pass the glomerular filtration barrier.

Case 8-7

1. Abnormal findings:

   Chemical examination—blood, protein

   Microscopic examination—RBCs, WBCs, cellular casts

   Discrepant results: pH and crystal type do not agree; blood test and RBCs seen; color and clarity versus RBC number and microscopic elements

2. Generally, the physical and chemical examinations do not correlate with the microscopic examination. The most likely reason is a specimen handling mix-up during processing of the specimen for the microscopic examination, that is, the urine sediment is not from the same urine as the physical and chemical examinations.

CHAPTER 9

1. A
2. B
3. A
4. D
5. D
6. A
7. D
8. C
9. B
10. A
11. D
12. C
13. D
14. D
15. B
16. C
17. B
18. A
19. A
20. A
21. B
22. B
23. D
24. B
25. B
26. C
27. C
28. B
29. C
30. A
31. D
32. C
33. A
34. A
35. D
36. A
37. D
38. D
39. C
40. C
41. B
42. A

Case 9-1

1. Abnormal findings:

   Physical examination—cloudy

   Chemical examination—blood, protein/SSA, leukocyte esterase, nitrite

   Microscopic examination—25 to 50 WBCs; 2 to 5 WBC casts; moderate bacteria

2. C
3. C. Specifically, white blood cell casts, which localize the infection/inflammation to the renal tubules
4. C
5. Two different mechanisms: movement of bacteria from the lower urinary tract to the kidneys (ascending infection), or bacteria in the blood localizing in the kidneys (hematogenous infection)
6. Lysis of red blood cells has occurred; this process is enhanced in hypotonic and alkaline urine.
7. No, the reagent strip test is essentially specific for albumin. The amount of blood/hemoglobin present (trace) is insufficient to affect the protein test. If the reagent strip blood test is "large," then the possibility exists that the blood present is contributing to the protein reagent strip result.

Case 9-2

1. Abnormal findings:

   Physical examination—color, clarity

   Chemical examination—SG, protein, nitrite

   Microscopic examination—RBCs, WBCs, many calcium oxalate crystals

   Discrepant results: reagent strip blood and microscopic examination

2. Check for ascorbic acid, which can produce false-negative blood tests by reagent strip (depending on the brand of test strips used).
3. A
4. Factors that influence renal calculi formation are as follows:

   1. Increases in the concentration of chemical salts
   2. Changes in urine pH
   3. Urinary stasis
   4. The presence of a foreign body seed

Case 9-3

1. Abnormal findings:

   Physical examination—color, clarity, yellow foam

   Chemical examination—bilirubin, pH, protein

   Microscopic examination—bacteria

   Discrepant results: The glucose by reagent strip and the Clinitest do not agree.

2. Color, clarity, pH, bacteria, and crystals
3. Bilirubin
4. A reducing substance other than glucose is present.

5. Galactosemia. The presence of galactose can be confirmed by carbohydrate thin-layer chromatography. Confirm with cell culture to detect the specific enzyme deficiency.

6. No, the few bacteria present are probably a result of the length of time and the type of specimen collection. The negative or normal white blood cells, leukocyte esterase, and nitrite results support this conclusion.

Case 9-4

1. Abnormal findings:
   Physical examination—white foam noted (specific gravity and dark color indicate concentrated urine)
   Chemical examination—protein
   Microscopic examination—none
2. Protein
3. Albumin. Because of its size (it is small enough to pass the glomerular filtration barrier if the shield of negativity is removed) and its high plasma concentration (compared with other plasma proteins), albumin usually is the first protein lost.
4. Severe proteinuria results in hypoproteinemia. As blood protein is lost, the intravascular oncotic pressure decreases and fluid moves into the tissues.
5. A
6. D. The four characteristic features of nephrotic syndrome are present. Note that minimal change disease is responsible for most cases of nephrotic syndrome in children.

Case 9-5

1. Abnormal findings:
   Physical examination—slightly cloudy
   Chemical examination—blood, protein, leukocyte esterase
   Microscopic examination—RBCs, WBCs, WBC and RTE casts; moderate RTEs
2. B
3. B. Normal tubular function is altered owing to renal inflammation/allergic reaction taking place in the kidney. Because the drug is eliminated from the body by the kidneys, it becomes concentrated in the kidneys, and is the location or site of the allergic response.
4. White blood cell casts (and renal tubular epithelial casts) localize the process in the nephrons.
5. The nitrite test is a screening test for bacteriuria. Reasons for a negative nitrite test despite the presence of bacteria include the following:
   1. Inadequate incubation time in urine for bacteria to convert nitrate to nitrite
   2. The patient's diet does not include dietary nitrates.
   3. The bacteria present are not nitrate reducers.

Case 9-6

1. Abnormal findings:
   Physical examination—brown, cloudy

Chemical examination—blood, protein
Microscopic examination—RBCs, WBCs, RBC casts, increased numbers of granular casts

2. Oxidized hemoglobin, that is, methemoglobin, imparts a brown color to urine.
3. The leukocyte esterase test is a screening test for granulocytic leukocytes. Two reasons for a negative test despite the presence of white blood cells include the following:
   1. The amount of leukocyte esterase present is below the sensitivity of the test, despite the increased number of white blood cells.
   2. The white blood cells present are lymphocytes that do not contain leukocyte esterase.
4. One cannot determine conclusively using reagent strips whether blood is contributing to the protein result. The blood result is high enough to indicate that hemoglobin may or may not be contributing to the protein result. A quantitative urine protein test could determine the level of proteinuria present if deemed necessary.
5. Dysmorphic red blood cells and red blood cell casts
6. B
7. A
8. Systemic lupus erythematosus is an autoimmune disorder. Hence a possible scenario for the development of acute glomerulonephritis in this patient is that immune complexes (antibodies against glomerular tissue antigens) have formed in glomeruli, and the associated immune response/mediators are causing glomerular damage.

CHAPTER 10

1. B
2. A
3. B
4. D
5. D
6. D
7. A
8. B
9. A
10. B
11. C
12. C
13. B
14. C
15. B
16. A
17. C
18. C
19. A
20. C
21. D
22. D

23. B
24. B

Case 10-1

1. Urine abnormal findings:
Physical examination—color, clarity, yellow foam
Chemical examination—bilirubin, protein, urobilinogen
Microscopic examination—granular casts
Fecal abnormal findings: color, consistency, form, fat content
2. B
3. Steatorrhea
4. B
5. An obstruction, most likely of the common bile duct because of pancreatic cancer, is preventing bile and pancreatic enzymes from entering the intestine. Consequently, fat digestion is impaired, resulting in increased fecal fat excretion. The feces becomes pale in color (i.e., acholic) because the amount of bilirubin entering the intestine is decreased; hence the quantities of urobilins (i.e., urobilin, stercobilin, and mesobilin) that give fecal matter its normal color are decreased.
6. The sensitivity of the reagent strip urobilinogen test is limited. These tests are not able to accurately detect the absence of or decreased amounts of urobilinogen.

Case 10-2

1. Fecal abnormal findings: consistency, leukocytes, *Salmonella* spp. present
2. 326 mOsm/kg
3. C

Case 10-3

1. Abnormal findings: hemoglobin and hematocrit low; fecal occult blood positive
2. A
3. Myoglobin and cytochromes
4. D
5. D
6. C

CHAPTER 11

1. B
2. D
3. A
4. C
5. A 4
   B 7
   C 3
   D 5
   E 6
   F 8
6. B

7. D
8. C
9. D
10. C
11. B
12. D
13. C
14. D
15. B
16. D
17. A

Case 11-1

1. Abnormal seminal fluid findings: low spermatozoal concentration
Discrepant results: vitality (60%) and motility (70%) contradict each other.
2. Yes, a laboratory error is suspected because the vitality (60%) and motility (70%) determinations contradict each other.
3. Yes, low concentrations of spermatozoa are associated with infertility.
4. Fructose level in the seminal fluid; low fructose levels are associated with azospermia

Case 11-2

1. Abnormal postvasectomy seminal fluid findings: spermatozoa concentration, increased leukocytes, bacteria present
2. No, the presence of bacteria with increased leukocytes suggests an infection in the male reproductive tract.
3. Approximately 12 weeks after a successful vasectomy, the sperm concentration should be zero.

CHAPTER 12

1. C
2. C
3. D
4. C
5. A
6. B
7. A
8. D
9. B
10. A
11. B
12. D
13. D

Case 12-1

1. At 450 nm: $0.500 - 0.200 = 0.300$
2. Zone III
3. The fetus is severely affected, and the child should be delivered immediately if the lungs are mature.
4. $4.7/2.3 = 2.0$

5. 33 weeks' gestation: immature
   34 weeks' gestation: immature
   35 weeks' gestation: immature

CHAPTER 13

1. A
2. B
3. A
4. D
5. A
6. B
7. A
8. C
9. C
10. A
11. B
12. D
13. A
14. C
15. B
16. C
17. A
18. A
19. D
20. B
21. A
22. D
23. C
24. B

Case 13-1
1. Abnormal cerebrospinal fluid (CSF) findings: cloudy; leukocyte count and differential; total protein; glucose; lactate
2. CSF/glucose ratio: 0.36
3. B
4. Yes, the high lactate level (>30 mg/dL) combined with a low glucose value is associated with bacterial meningitis.
5. No, Gram stain results are not 100% sensitive because of numerous factors.
6. Increased CSF protein: Inflammatory processes involving the meninges impair the reabsorption of protein from the CSF back into the circulating bloodstream.

   Decreased CSF glucose: This occurs because of defective/ decreased transport across the blood-brain barrier and increased glycolysis within the central nervous system.

Case 13-2
1. Abnormal CSF findings: total protein, immunoglobulin G
2. CSF/serum albumin index: 6.1
3. Albumin is not produced intrathecally; therefore increased CSF albumin levels indicate changes to the blood-brain barrier, which allow increased amounts of albumin to pass.
4. CSF IgG index: 1.46
5. Multiple sclerosis
6. (1) Cerebrospinal fluid protein electrophoresis, which reveals oligoclonal banding in approximately 90% of patients with multiple sclerosis; and (2) a positive myelin basic protein test on CSF indicates an active demyelinating process consistent with multiple sclerosis.

CHAPTER 14

1. B
2. A
3. A
4. C
5. D
6. C
7. B
8. A
9. D
10. D
11. D
12. C
13. B
14. B
15. A
16. C
17. A

Case 14-1
1. Abnormal findings: blood uric acid; synovial fluid clarity; viscosity; leukocyte count and differential; crystals; glucose; total protein
2. 30 mg/dL
3. C
4. E
5. A
6. No, microscopic examination for crystals is not 100% sensitive and depends on numerous factors. For example, sometimes the synovial fluid is removed from an area of the synovium that does not contain crystals, or only a few crystals are present, which can be missed during the microscopic examination.

Case 14-2
1. Abnormal findings: synovial fluid clarity; viscosity; leukocyte count and differential; glucose; total protein; lactate; Gram stain
2. 44 mg/dL
3. D
4. D

Case 14-3
1. Abnormal findings: synovial fluid clarity, leukocyte count, crystals, glucose, total protein

2. 15 mg/dL
3. B
4. B
5. E

CHAPTER 15

1. D
2. A
3. B
4. B
5. A
6. D
7. D
8. C
9. C
10. A 1
     B 2
     C 1
     D 1
     E 1
     F 2
11. B
12. A
13. A
14. C
15. B

Case 15-1
1. Fluid-to-serum total protein ratio: 0.60
2. Fluid-to-serum lactate dehydrogenase ratio: 0.66
3. Exudates result from inflammatory processes that increase the permeability of the capillary endothelium in the parietal membrane or decrease the absorption of serous fluid by the lymphatic system.

Case 15-2
1. Fluid-to-serum total protein ratio: 0.45
2. Fluid-to-serum lactate dehydrogenase ratio: 0.42
3. Transudates result from a systemic disorder that causes an increase in hydrostatic pressure (i.e., blood pressure) or a decrease in plasma oncotic pressure in the parietal membrane capillaries.

CHAPTER 16

1. C
2. D
3. A
4. B
5. B
6. C
7. B

8. A
9. D
10. B
11. C
12. D
13. A

Case 16-1
1. Bacterial vaginosis
2. Overgrowth of anaerobic bacteria causes increased production of several metabolic by-products, including polyamines, which volatilize in an alkaline environment to produce the foul-smelling trimethylamine.
3. Seminal fluid has an alkaline pH (7.2 to 7.8). Therefore after intercourse with ejaculation, the vaginal pH becomes more alkaline and trimethylamine production is enhanced, causing the foul odor to be more pronounced.
4. For unknown and most likely complex reasons, the usually numerous *Lactobacillus* spp. of the vagina are replaced and overrun by other microbes, most often *Gardnerella vaginalis* in synergy with an anaerobe, usually *Mobiluncus* spp.
5. The presence of clue cells in the wet mount examination.
6. Bacterial vaginosis results in disruption of the normal bacterial flora of the vagina; however, the squamous epithelium is not invaded, and an inflammatory response is not initiated. Hence the disorder is termed *vaginosis* instead of *vaginitis*.

CHAPTER 17

1. B
2. C
3. D
4. C
5. C
6. B
7. A
8. B

CHAPTER 18

1. C
2. D
3. C
4. D
5. B
6. C
7. D
8. B

Reagent Strip Color Charts

The reagent strip color charts provided in this section should *not* be used to evaluate actual reagent strip results because of color variations that may have occurred in their reproduction. Note that these are only two commonly used reagent strips and that other brands are available worldwide.

The color charts in Figures A-1 and A-2 are provided as a convenient reference and show the variation in reporting parameters that exist between manufacturers. Proper orientation of the reagent strip to the color chart is critical when reading results. Figure A-3 illustrates the differences involved in properly orienting reagent strips to the manufacturer's color chart. Details regarding the chemical principles, sensitivity, and specificity for each reagent strip parameter are discussed in Chapter 7.

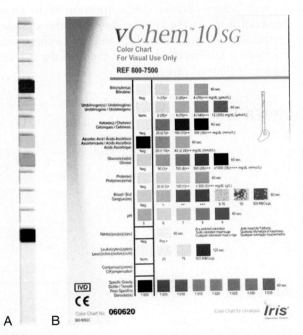

FIGURE A-1 A, vChem strip. **B,** vChem 10SG color chart. **Do not use this color chart for diagnostic testing; use chart provided with product.** *(By permission Iris Diagnostics.)*

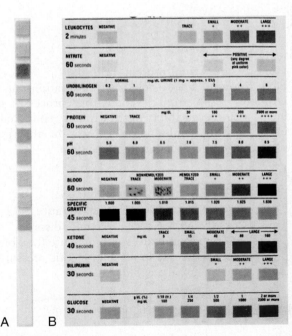

FIGURE A-2 A, Multistix strip. **B,** Multistix 10SG color chart. **Do not use this color chart for diagnostic testing; use chart provided with product.** *(By permission Siemens Healthcare Diagnostics Inc.)*

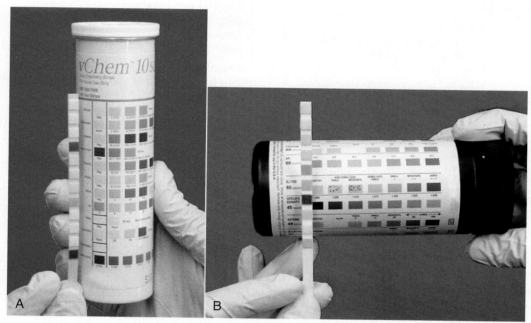

FIGURE A-3 Manufacturers vary in the proper orientation of the reagent strip to the color chart on the container when reading results. **A,** vChem 10SG Reagent Strips. **B,** Multistix 10SG Reagent Strips.

Reference Intervals

Urine (Random Specimen) Reference Intervals

Physical Examination

Component	Result
Color	Colorless to amber (varies with state of hydration, diet, health)
Clarity	Clear
Specific gravity	1.002 to 1.035 (physiologically possible 1.002 to 1.040)
Osmolality	275 to 900 mOsm/kg H_2O (physiologically possible 50 to 1400 mOsm/kg H_2O)
Volume	600 to 1800 mL/day (varies with state of hydration, diet, health)

Chemical Examination

Component	Result
Bilirubin	Negative
Glucose	Negative
Ketones	Negative
Leukocyte esterase	Negative
Nitrite	Negative
pH	4.5 to 8.0
Protein	Negative
Urobilinogen	≤1 mg/dL

Microscopic Examination*

Component	Amount	Magnification
Red blood cells	0 to 3	Per high-power field
White blood cells	0 to 8	Per high-power field
Casts	0 to 2 hyaline or finely granular[†]	Per low-power field
Epithelial cells		
Squamous	Few	Per low-power field
Transitional	Few	Per high-power field
Renal	Few	Per high-power field
Bacteria and yeast	Negative	Per high-power field

*Using the UriSystem. Note that values vary with the concentration of urine sediment, the microscope slide technique, and the optical properties of the microscope.
[†]Following physical exercise, cast numbers increase and finely granular casts are included (Haber, 1991).

Fecal Reference Intervals

Physical Examination

Color	Brown
Consistency	Firm, formed
Form	Tubular, cylindrical

Chemical Examination

Total fat, quantitative (72-hour specimen)	<6 g/day and <20% of stool
Osmolality	285 to 430 mOsm/kg H_2O
Potassium	30 to 140 mmol/L
Sodium	40 to 110 mmol/L

Microscopic Examination

Fat, Qualitative Assessment	
Neutral fat	Few globules present per high-power field
Total fat	<100 fat globules (diameter ≤4 microns) per high-power field
Leukocytes (qualitative)	None present
Meat and vegetable fibers (qualitative)	Few

Semen Characteristics Associated With Fertility

Parameter	Reference Interval*	Lower Reference Limit†
Physical Examination		
Appearance	Gray-white, opalescent, opaque	
Volume	2 to 5 mL	1.5 mL (1.4 to 1.7)
Viscosity/liquefaction	Discrete droplets (watery) within 60 minutes	
Microscopic Examination		
Motility	50% or more with moderate to rapid linear (forward) progression	40% (38% to 42%)
Concentration	20 to 250 $\times$ 10^6 sperm per mL	15 $\times$ 10^6 sperm per mL
Morphology	14% or more have normal morphology	4% normal forms
Vitality	75% or more are alive	58% (55% to 63%)
Leukocytes	Less than 1 $\times$ 10^6 per mL	
Chemical Examination		
pH	7.2 to 7.8	$\geq$7.2
Acid phosphatase (total)	$\geq$200 U per ejaculate at 37° C (*p*-nitrophenylphosphate)	
Citric acid (total)	$\geq$52 μmol per ejaculate	
Fructose (total)	$\geq$13 μmol per ejaculate	$\geq$13 μmol per ejaculate
Zinc (total)	$\geq$2.4 μmol per ejaculate	$\geq$2.4 μmol per ejaculate

*Based on the strict criteria evaluation recommended by the World Health Organization (1999) for assessing sperm morphology for fertility purposes.
†The one-sided 5th centile lower reference limit recommended by the WHO (2010) for assessing semen characteristics.

Amniotic Fluid Reference Intervals

Physical Examination	
Color	Colorless to pale yellow
Clarity	Clear to slightly turbid*
Chemical Examination	
ΔA$_{450}$ determination	
27 weeks' gestation	<0.065
30 weeks' gestation	<0.052
35 weeks' gestation	<0.035
40 weeks' gestation	<0.022
Lecithin/sphingomyelin ratio (mature)	>2.0

*Turbidity increases with gestational age.

Synovial Fluid Reference Intervals*

Physical Examination	
Total volume	0.1 to 3.5 mL
Color	Pale yellow
Clarity	Clear
Viscosity	High; forms "strings" 4 to 6 cm long
Spontaneous clot formation	No
Microscopic Examination	
Erythrocyte count	<2000 cells/mL
Leukocyte count	<200 cells/mL
Differential cell count:	
Monocytes and macrophages	≈60%
Lymphocytes	≈30%
Neutrophils	≈10%
Crystals	None present
Chemical Examination	
Glucose	Equivalent to plasma values†
Glucose: P-SF difference	<10 mg/dL†
Uric acid	Equivalent to plasma values†
Total protein	1 to 3 g/dL
Lactate	9 to 33 mg/dL‡
Hyaluronate	0.3 to 0.4 g/dL

*Values for fluid obtained from a knee joint.
†Synovial fluid values are equivalent to blood plasma values if obtained from a fasting patient.
‡Normal lactate values are assumed to be similar to those in blood and cerebrospinal fluid; actual reference intervals have yet to be established.
Data from Kjeldsberg CR, Knight JA: Synovial fluid. In Body fluids, ed 2, Chicago, 1986, American Society of Clinical Pathologists Press, pp 129-152.

Cerebrospinal Fluid Reference Intervals*

Physical Examination

Color	Colorless
Clarity	Clear

Chemical Examination

Component	Conventional Units	Conversion Factor	SI Units
Electrolytes			
Calcium	2.0 to 2.8 mEq/L	0.5	1.00 to 1.40 mmol/L
Chloride	115 to 130 mEq/L	1	115 to 130 mmol/L
Lactate	10 to 22 mg/dL	0.111	1.1 to 2.4 mmol/L
Magnesium	2.4 to 3.0 mEq/L	0.5	1.2 to 1.5 mmol/L
Potassium	2.6 to 3.0 mEq/L	1	2.6 to 3.0 mmol/L
Sodium	135 to 150 mEq/L	1	135 to 150 mmol/L
Glucose	50 to 80 mg/dL	0.5551	2.8 to 4.4 mmol/L
Total protein	15 to 45 mg/dL	10	150 to 450 mg/L
Albumin	10 to 30 mg/dL	10	100 to 300 mg/L
IgG	1 to 4 mg/dL	10	10 to 40 mg/L

Protein Electrophoresis	Percent of Total Protein
Transthyretin (prealbumin)	2% to 7%
Albumin	56% to 76%
α_1-Globulin	2% to 7%
α_2-Globulin	4% to 12%
β-Globulin	8% to 18%
γ-Globulin	3% to 12%

Microscopic Examination

Component	Conventional Units	Conversion Factor	SI Units
Neonates (<1 year old)	0 to 30 cells/µL	10^6	0 to 30×10^6 cells/L
1 to 4 years old	0 to 20 cells/µL	10^6	0 to 20×10^6 cells/L
5 to 18 years old	0 to 10 cells/µL	10^6	0 to 10×10^6 cells/L
Adults (>18 years old)	0 to 5 cells/µL	10^6	0 to 5×10^6 cells/L

Differential Cell Count	Percent of Total Count
Neonates	
Lymphocytes	5% to 35%
Monocytes	50% to 90%
Neutrophils	0% to 8%
Adults	
Lymphocytes	40% to 80%
Monocytes	15% to 45%
Neutrophils	0% to 6%

*For cerebrospinal fluid specimens obtained by lumbar puncture.

Body Fluid Diluent and Pretreatment Solutions

When the diluents and pretreatment solutions provided in this section are prepared in the laboratory, appropriate personal protective equipment should be used. Table C-1 summarizes the common uses of these diluents and the limitations associated with some body fluids (e.g., synovial fluid).

SALINE, ISOTONIC (0.85%) OR "NORMAL SALINE"

1. Into a 100 mL volumetric flask, add 0.85 g NaCl.
2. Add approximately 60 mL Clinical Laboratory Reagent Water[1] and swirl to dissolve.
3. Add water to bring the volume to the calibration mark.
4. Store at room temperature.

SALINE, HYPOTONIC (0.30%)

1. Into a 100 mL volumetric flask, add 0.30 g NaCl.
2. Add approximately 60 mL Clinical Laboratory Reagent Water[1] and swirl to dissolve.
3. Add water to bring the volume to the calibration mark.
4. Store at room temperature.

DILUTE ACETIC ACID (3.0%)

CAUTION: Acid.

1. Into a 100 mL volumetric flask, add approximately 60 mL Clinical Laboratory Reagent Water.[1]
2. Gradually add 3.0 mL glacial acetic acid to the flask. (**Note:** ALWAYS add acid to water.)
3. After acid addition, add water to bring the volume to the calibration mark.
4. Store at room temperature.

TURK'S SOLUTION[2]

This diluent lyses red blood cells (RBCs) and stains nucleated cells. As with other diluents that contain acetic acid, clumping of the body fluid will occur when a high level of protein is present. DO NOT use this solution as a diluent for synovial fluids because it will cause a mucin clot.

CAUTION: Acid.

1. To a 100 mL volumetric flask, add approximately 60 mL Clinical Laboratory Reagent Water (CLRW).[1]
2. Gradually add 3.0 mL glacial acetic acid to the flask. (**Note:** ALWAYS add acid to water.)
3. Add 1 mL of 0.5% Methylene Blue solution (provided below) *or* 1 mL of 1% Gentian Violet (aqueous solution).
4. Add water to bring volume in flask to the calibration mark.
5. Store at room temperature.

0.5% Methylene Blue Solution (Used to Prepare Turk's Solution)

CAUTION: Acid.

1. To a 100 mL volumetric flask, add 0.5 g methylene blue.

TABLE C-1	Common Uses and Limitations of Diluents	
Solution	**Use**	**Comments**
Isotonic saline (0.85%)	WBC count RBC count	Also known as "normal" saline
Hypotonic saline (0.30%)	WBC count	• Lyses RBCs
Dilute acetic acid (3.0%)*	WBC count	• Lyses RBCs • *Do not use* with synovial fluids, causes mucin clot and cell clumping
Turk's solution	WBC count	• Lyses RBCs • *Do not use* with synovial fluids, causes mucin clot and cell clumping
Hyaluronidase pretreatment solutions	Pretreatment of synovial fluid	Reduces viscosity enabling accurate cell counts
Hyaluronidase (0.1 g/L) diluent	Synovial fluid WBC count	• Prevents mucin clot formation in synovial fluids • Stain enhances nucleated cell identification
Semen pretreatment solutions	Pretreatment of semen	Reduces viscosity of semen that failed to liquefy to enable accurate sperm counts (and cell counts, when performed)
Semen diluent	Sperm count	Prepare with or without stain; stain enhances visualization of sperm

*Other concentrations of acetic acid can also be used (e.g., 5%, 10%).
Note: At all times when reagents are prepared, appropriate personal protective equipment should be used.

2. Add approximately 60 mL Clinical Laboratory Reagent Water.[1]
3. Add 0.5 mL glacial acetic acid to the flask. (**Note:** Always add acid to water.)
4. Swirl flask to mix.
5. Add water to bring volume in flask to the calibration mark.
6. Store at room temperature.

SYNOVIAL FLUID SOLUTIONS

Hyaluronidase Pretreatment for Synovial Fluid[3]

When analyzing highly viscous synovial fluids, pretreatment with hyaluronidase may be necessary to perform chemical or immunologic tests or before preparing a dilution for cell counts, even when using a diluent that contains hyaluronidase. Several approaches are available.

1. Approach A: Hyaluronidase alone
   a. Add 400 units of hyaluronidase (powder or liquid) to approximately 1 mL of fluid.
   b. Mix and incubate at 37° C for 10 minutes.[3] Note that if liquid hyaluronidase is used, the volume used must be accounted for in the cell count calculations.
2. Approach B: Buffered hyaluronidase[2]
   For each milliliter of synovial fluid, add 1 drop of 0.05% buffered hyaluronidase. Mix and incubate at room temperature for 4 minutes.[2]
   0.05% Buffered Hyaluronidase
   a. Into a 100 mL volumetric flask, add 50 mg Type 1-S hyaluronidase (EC 3.2.1.35).
   b. Add 0.912 g potassium phosphate monobasic (FW 136.09).

   c. Add approximately 60 mL Clinical Laboratory Reagent Water[1] and swirl to dissolve.
   d. Add water to bring the volume to the calibration mark.
   e. Store at 2° C to 5° C.
3. Approach C: Add 0.1 mL Type 1-S hyaluronidase (EC 3.2.1.35) to 0.9 mL synovial fluid. Mix well and incubate at 37° C for 4 hours.[2]

Hyaluronidase (0.1 g/L) Diluent for Cell Counts in Synovial Fluid[2]

Before diluting a synovial fluid, the specimen should be mixed for 5 to 10 minutes.[3] Note that for turbid specimens, the base of the tube should be flicked several times to dislodge cells before mixing. For accurate cell counts, turbid specimens must be thoroughly mixed.

To prepare 100 mL of hyaluronidase diluent:

1. Prepare 0.067 mol/L phosphate buffer as follows:
   a. Prepare 250 mL of Solution A: In a 250 mL volumetric flask, dissolve 2.279 g monobasic potassium phosphate (MW 136.09) in Clinical Laboratory Reagent Water.[1] Store at 2° C to 5° C. Stable for 3 months.
   b. Prepare 500 mL of Solution B: In a 500 mL volumetric flask, dissolve 4.756 g dibasic sodium phosphate (MW 141.96) in Clinical Laboratory Reagent Water.[1] Store at 2° C to 5° C. Stable for 3 months.
   c. Combine 13 mL solution A, 87 mL solution B, and 13 mL absolute methanol. Store at 2° C to 5° C. Stable for 3 months.
2. In a 100 mL volumetric flask, add the following chemicals:
   a. 10.0 mg hyaluronidase, Type 1-S (EC 3.2.1.35)
   b. 40.0 mg dextrose
   c. 8.0 mg toluidine blue O (CAS 92-31-9)

3. Fill flask to approximately half-full using 0.067 mol/L phosphate buffer. Swirl flask to dissolve chemicals. Bring volume to calibration mark using buffer.

4. Store at 2° C to 5° C. Stable for 3 months. Filter before use, if necessary.

SEMEN SOLUTIONS

Semen Pretreatment Solutions

Two treatment solutions are provided that can be used to reduce the viscosity of mucoid semen specimens that fail to liquefy adequately after 60 minutes. The effects of these treatments on sperm motility, sperm morphology, and biochemical tests of seminal plasma are not known. Document use of these solutions, and account for the volume used when performing sperm concentration calculations.

A. Dilution With Physiologic Solution. Prepare a 1 to 2 dilution of the semen (one part semen + one part diluent) using Dulbecco's Phosphate-Buffered Saline (pH 7.4). After the dilution is prepared, liquefaction can be enhanced by repeatedly pipetting the mixture.

Dulbecco's Phosphate-Buffered Saline (pH 7.4)[4]

1. Into a 1 L volumetric flask, add the following substances:

    Approximately 750 mL Clinical Laboratory Reagent Water (CLRW)[1]
    8.00 g sodium chloride (NaCl)
    1.00 g D-glucose
    0.20 g potassium chloride (KCl)
    0.20 g potassium dihydrogen phosphate (KH_2PO_4)
    2.16 g disodium hydrogen phosphate heptahydrate ($Na_2HPO_4 \bullet 7H_2O$)
    0.10 g magnesium chloride hexahydrate ($MgCl_2 \bullet 6H_2O$)

2. In a 10 mL volumetric flask, dissolve 0.132 g of calcium chloride dihydrate ($CaCl_2 \bullet 2H_2O$).

3. *To prevent precipitation,* add the calcium chloride dihydrate solution (10 mL) to the 1 L flask *slowly and with stirring.*

4. Bring to within ≈3 mL of calibration mark using CLRW and mix.

5. Adjust to pH 7.4 using 1 mol/L sodium hydroxide (NaOH).

6. After pH adjustment, bring volume to 1 L calibration mark using CLRW.

B. Digestion With Bromelain. The proteolytic enzyme bromelain can be used to enzymatically digest and liquefy the semen specimen. Prepare a 1 to 2 dilution of the semen (i.e., one part semen + one part bromelain solution) using Bromelain Solution (see below), and mix well. After the dilution is prepared, incubate at 37° C for 10 minutes. Mix well before analysis.

Bromelain Solution (10 IU/mL)[4]

1. Into a 100 mL volumetric flask, add 1000 IU of Bromelain (EC 3.4.22.32).

2. Add approximately 60 mL Dulbecco's phosphate-buffered saline (for preparation, see above).

3. Swirl flask to dissolve, then bring volume to calibration mark using buffered saline.

Semen Diluent for Sperm Counts

1. Into a 100 mL volumetric flask, add the following substances:

    ≈60 mL Clinical Laboratory Reagent Water[1]
    5 g sodium bicarbonate
    1 mL 35% (v/v) formalin
    Optional (to enhance visualization of sperm heads):
    25 mg Trypan Blue or 5 mL saturated Gentian Violet (>4 mg/mL)[4]

2. Swirl to dissolve.

3. Bring volume to 100 mL calibration mark using Clinical Laboratory Reagent Water.[1]

4. Store at 4° C. If crystals form, filter before use.

REFERENCES

1. Clinical and Laboratory Standards Institute (CLSI): Preparation and testing of reagent water in the clinical laboratory: approved guideline, CLSI Document C03-A4, Wayne, PA, 2006, CLSI.
2. Kjeldsberg CR, Knight JA: Laboratory methods. In Body fluids, ed 3, Chicago, 1993, American Society of Clinical Pathologists Press.
3. Clinical and Laboratory Standards Institute (CLSI): Body fluid analysis for cellular composition: approved guideline, CLSI Document H56-A, Wayne, PA, 2007, CLSI.
4. World Health Organization: WHO laboratory manual for the examination and processing of human semen, ed 5, Geneva, Switzerland, 2010, World Health Organization.

INDEX

Page numbers followed by "f" indicate figures, "t" indicate tables, and "b" indicate boxes.